Becoming a Health Care Professional

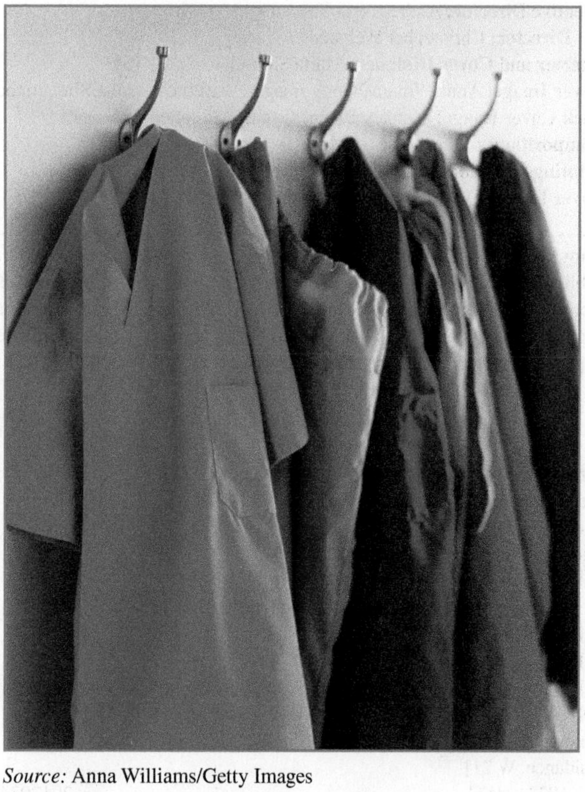

Source: Anna Williams/Getty Images

Sherry Makely, PhD, R.T. (R)
Shirley A. Badasch, M.Ed, RN
Doreen S. Chesebro, B.Ed, LVN

PEARSON

Boston Columbus Indianapolis New York San Francisco Upper Saddle River Amsterdam
Cape Town Dubai London Madrid Milan Munich Paris Montréal Toronto Delhi
Mexico City São Paulo Sydney Hong Kong Seoul Singapore Taipei Tokyo

Publisher: Julie Levin Alexander
Publisher's Assistant: Regina Bruno
Editor-in-Chief: Marlene McHugh Pratt
Executive Editor: Joan Gill
Project Management: Emergent Learning, LLC
Copy Editor: Jill Rembetski
Associate Editor: Melissa Kerian
Editorial Assistant: Stephanie Kiel
Director of Marketing: David Gesell
Marketing Manager: Katrin Beacom
Senior Marketing Coordinator: Alicia Wozniak
Managing Production Editor: Patrick Walsh
Production Liaison: Julie Boddorf
Production Editor: Peggy Kellar
Senior Media Producer: Amy Peltier
Media Project Manager: Lorena Cerisano
Manufacturing Manager: Lisa McDowell
Creative Director: Andrea Nix
Art Director: Christopher Weigand
Interior and Cover Designer: Marta Samsel
Cover Image: Anna Willams/Getty Images, wavebreakmedia/Shutterstock
Back Cover Image: Monkey Business Images/Shutterstock
Composition: Aptara®, Inc.
Printing and Binding: LSC Communications
Cover Printer: LSC Communications

Library of Congress Cataloging-in-Publication Data
Makely, Sherry.
Becoming a health care professional/Sherry Makely, Shirley A. Badasch, Doreen S. Chesebro.—1st ed.
p.; cm.
Includes bibliographical references and index.
ISBN-13: 978-0-13-284323-2
ISBN-10: 0-13-284323-4
I. Badasch, Shirley A., (date) II. Chesebro, Doreen S., (date) III. Title.
[DNLM: 1. Health Occupations. 2. Career Choice. 3. Health Personnel—ethics. 4. Professional-Patient Relations. 5. Vocational Guidance. W 21]
362.1023—dc23 2012034890

6 17

PEARSON

ISBN-10: 0-13-284323-4
ISBN-13: 978-0-13-284323-2

Contents

Preface

Becoming a Health Care Professional is designed for students who are interested in exploring, planning, and preparing for a career in health care. The information provided in the textbook and its supplemental resources applies to all health occupations and health care settings, including hospitals, outpatient clinics, physician offices, dental practices, nursing homes, rehabilitation facilities, biotechnology research and development labs, and so forth.

The text presents the essential information that students need in order to prepare for success as health care workers. The content is comprehensive, informative, inspiring, and timely. Real-world insights emphasize the challenges and rewards that students can expect as they prepare for and begin a career in the rapidly changing health care industry.

While technical competence remains a high priority, good character, a strong work ethic, and personal and professional traits and behaviors are becoming more important in the health care workplace than ever before. Statistics indicate a growing concern on the part of employers with theft, fraud, and behavioral problems. Poor attendance, interpersonal conflicts, disregard for quality, and disrespect for authority all too often lead to employees being fired from their jobs. With a growing emphasis on customer service, patient satisfaction, cultural competence, quality improvement, patient safety, and corporate compliance, health care employers are increasingly seeking workers with strong *soft skills* and *people skills*—people who communicate appropriately, work well on teams, respect and value differences, use limited resources efficiently, and interact effectively with coworkers, patients, and guests.

To be successful, students must understand the importance of professionalism and the need to perform in a professional, ethical, legal, and competent manner. Developing and strengthening professional traits and behaviors has become a major challenge for students, teachers, and employers. *Becoming a Health Care Professional* helps meet that challenge. This text presents the professional standards that apply to all health care workers and the information that students need to choose, plan, and prepare for the health occupation that best matches their individual interests, skills, and abilities.

Textbook Features

The chapters in the textbook include several features to stimulate, clarify, and reinforce learning. These features include:

- ***Chapter Quote.*** Each chapter begins with a quote to generate discussion among the students and their teachers.
- ***Getting Started.*** The Getting Started activity at the beginning of each chapter serves as a *bell-ringer* to engage students in the subject at hand.
- ***Background.*** The Background description *sets the stage* for the material to be covered in each section.
- ***Objectives.*** Each list of Objectives identifies the major concepts to be learned in that section of the text.
- ***Key Terms.*** As each Key Term is presented for the first time in the text, it appears in bold font, and a margin glossary provides the term's pronunciation and definition.
- ***Apply It.*** Apply It recommends activities to help students apply the information they are learning in the section.
- ***Consider This.*** The Consider This feature helps stimulate thinking about topics presented in the chapter.
- ***Recent Developments.*** The Recent Developments feature highlights a current trend or issue related to chapter content.
- ***Build Your Skills.*** The Build Your Skills feature provides additional information to help students develop skills related to the material presented.
- ***The More You Know.*** The More You Know feature includes details to expand learning about chapter topics.
- ***Language Arts, Math, and Science Links.*** Language Arts, Math, and Science Links enable students to apply health care information and concepts to their core curriculum courses.
- ***Community Service.*** The Community Service feature recommends opportunities for students to expand their learning by interacting with local community organizations.
- ***Reality Check.*** Reality Check provides a direct, *get-real* message at the end of each section to reinforce how important concepts apply to the students.
- ***Key Points.*** The Key Points listed at the end of each section presents a quick review of the important topics covered.
- ***Section and Chapter Review Questions.*** Section and Chapter Review Questions enable the students to self-assess their learning as related to the material presented.
- ***Chapter Review Activities.*** Chapter Review Activities present additional activities to supplement learning.
- ***What If? Scenarios.*** Each chapter concludes with a list of What If? Scenarios to stimulate the students' critical thinking, decision-making, and problem-solving skills as related to real-life workplace situations.

- ***Learn by Doing/Student Activity Guide Worksheet Assignments.*** Each section in the text has a Learn by Doing list of worksheets that students should complete in their *Student Activity Guide* to review, reinforce, expand, and apply their learning.
- ***Media Connection.*** Media Connection is a reminder for students to take advantage of the supplemental learning resources posted on the companion website for the textbook.
- ***Portfolio Connection.*** Guidelines in the Portfolio Connection feature of each chapter encourage students to create a career portfolio and expand its contents both during the course and after the course has ended.
- ***Glossary.*** The Glossary for this text lists more than 625 key terms with definitions.
- ***Index.*** The Index provides a quick reference to locate specific information within the textbook.

Supplemental Resources

In addition to the comprehensive information provided in the textbook, several supplemental resources are available for students and teachers.

Resources for Students

Supplemental learning resources for students include the following:

- ***Student DVD.*** The Student DVD provides an Audio Glossary of Key Terms, a variety of informative videos, and several additional learning resources.
- ***Student Activity Guide.*** Closely aligned with the sections in the text, the *Student Activity Guide* presents more than one hundred different learning activities to develop and strengthen critical thinking skills and to assist students in reviewing and applying what they have learned.
- ***Companion Website*** (www.myhealthprofessionskit.com). The Companion Website aligns with chapters in the text and provides an array of supplemental learning resources, many of which are interactive and provide immediate feedback. These resources include Self-Assessments with Next Step Improvement Plans, Chapter Quizzes, Videos, Video Scenario Analysis Quizzes, an Audio Glossary of Key Terms, the Golden Personality Type Profiler, and the Think Watson Critical Thinking Assessment.

Resources for Teachers

Resources for teachers include the following:

- ***Teacher's Resource Manual.*** The printed *Teacher's Resource Manual* provides information and additional content to help teachers develop and present course material. Content includes Section Topics, Objectives, Key Terms, Lesson Plans, Discussion Topics, and Experiential Learning activities for each section in the textbook.
- ***Teacher's Resource DVD.*** The *Teacher's Resource DVD* provides a test bank, PowerPoint Slides, *Teacher's Resource Manual* files, and answers to the questions in the *Student Activity Guide*.

Acknowledgments

Sincere appreciation is extended to the many people who helped develop and produce this book.

REVIEWERS

Beverly Campbell
President, *BECGroup* Consulting
Cameron Park, CA

Shari Cloud, RN, BSN, NBCT
Medical Science Instructor
South Mecklenburg High School
Charlotte, NC

Gail A. Eckerle, RN
Health Occupations Instructor/School Nurse
Jasper High School
Jasper, IN

Rebecca Walters, MEd, ATC
Assistant Athletic Trainer,
Health Science Instructor
Pelion High School
Pelion, SC

SPECIAL THANKS

A special thank you is extended to:

- Jennifer Olson for Chapter Five content.
- Vanessa Austin for Chapter Eight content.
- Jasmine Laseter and George Sullivan for research assistance.
- Carmen Martin for photographic services.
- The health care students and faculty members who appeared in photographs.
- Jen Frew for the Bonus Section on Life Cycles and for her encouragement, support, and personal commitment to quality.
- Jill Rembetski for her copy-editing and attention to detail.
- Peggy Kellar for her dedication throughout the project.

Notice: The term *patients* used throughout this textbook includes people who might typically be referred to as *clients*, nursing home *residents*, and others who seek, and benefit from, medical and health care services. The term *health care organizations* refers to public, private, for profit, not-for-profit, and government health care facilities and providers.

About the Authors

Sherry Makely, PhD, RT(R), is a Radiologic Technologist with a Master's degree in Education from Indiana University and a Ph.D. in Human Resources from the Union Institute. Dr. Makely managed allied health and professional development programs, state and federal grant projects, and workforce training and employment programs for more than 40 years as manager of Employee Education and Development for Clarian Health Partners/Indiana University Health in Indianapolis, Indiana. She has authored books on health careers, cross-training, and professionalism including Pearson Education's textbook *Professionalism in Health Care: A Primer for Career Success*, currently in its fourth edition. Dr. Makely chaired the Advisory Board of the Metropolitan Indianapolis/Central Indiana AHEC (Area Health Education Center) and served as a CAAHEP Commissioner (Commission on Accreditation of Allied Health Education Programs) and member of the National Health Care Skill Standards Review Committee. Dr. Makely was honored as the 1991 Baxter Fellow for Innovation in Health Management by the American Hospital Association's Research and Educational Trust and the Baxter Foundation.

Shirley A. Badasch, MEd, RN, is a graduate of California State University at Long Beach. Her career includes acute care nursing, office nursing, industrial nursing, Director of Nursing for a developmentally disabled nursing facility, and Assistant Administrator in Long Term Care. Ms. Badasch's teaching experience includes co-developing the Medical Occupations Program, teaching for nine years in a Regional Occupation Program, and part-time instructor in the Educational Psychology department, California State University at Long Beach. She also taught in the teacher certification program at Cal Poly Pomona and California State University at Sacramento. During her career she worked as a contract consultant to the California State Department of Education, presenting seminars, writing materials, developing programs, and consulting on program development. Ms. Badasch completed her career as the Director of Education for Bristol Park Medical Group. She continues to research and participate in health occupations as a volunteer in her community and as a member of the California Association of Health Career Educators.

Doreen S. Chesebro, BEd, LVN, is a graduate of California State University at Long Beach. Her nursing career includes ambulatory care, long-term care, and acute care nursing primarily in intensive care and coronary care units. Ms. Chesebro's teaching experience includes co-developing and teaching the Medical Occupations Program in a Regional Occupation Program. This program includes long-term care nurse assistant, advanced nurse assistant, home health aide, front and back office medical assistant, and hospital health occupations. She also served as a Program Specialist for the Long Beach Unified School District and has experience as a part-time instructor for teacher certification at California State University at Sacramento and Cal Poly Pomona. As Director of Education in the ambulatory care setting, she was responsible for development, implementation, and oversight of disease prevention and management classes through patient education and for staff development programs ranging from new employee orientation to management/leadership preparation and mentorship. Ms. Chesebro is currently the Director of Mission Services for the ambulatory care setting of the St. Joseph Health System in California's Central Orange County Region.

Navigating Your Textbook and Supplemental Resources

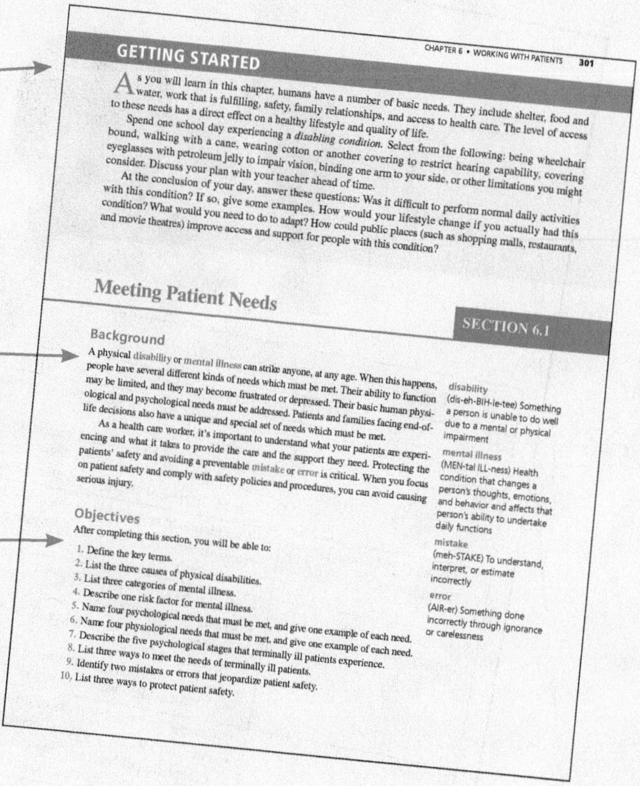

CHAPTER 6 • WORKING WITH PATIENTS 301

GETTING STARTED

As you will learn in this chapter, humans have a number of basic needs. They include shelter, food and water, work that is fulfilling, safety, family relationships, and access to health care. The level of access to these needs has a direct effect on a healthy lifestyle and quality of life.

Spend one school day experiencing a *disabling condition*. Select from the following: being wheelchair bound, walking with a cane, wearing cotton or another covering to restrict hearing capability, covering eyeglasses with petroleum jelly to impair vision, binding one arm to your side, or other limitations you might consider. Discuss your plan with your teacher ahead of time.

At the conclusion of your day, answer these questions: Was it difficult to perform normal daily activities with this condition? If so, give some examples. How would your lifestyle change if you actually had this condition? What would you need to do to adapt? How could public places (such as shopping malls, restaurants, and movie theatres) improve access and support for people with this condition?

Meeting Patient Needs

SECTION 6.1

Background

A physical disability or mental illness can strike anyone, at any age. When this happens, people have several different kinds of needs which must be met. Their ability to function may be limited, and they may become frustrated or depressed. Their basic human physiological and psychological needs must be addressed. Patients and families facing end-of-life decisions also have a unique and special set of needs which must be met.

As a health care worker, it's important to understand what your patients are experiencing and what it takes to provide the care and the support they need. Protecting the patients' safety and avoiding a preventable mistake or error is critical. When you focus on patient safety and comply with safety policies and procedures, you can avoid causing serious injury.

disability
(dis-eh-BIH-le-tee) Something a person is unable to do well due to a mental or physical impairment

mental illness
(MEN-tal ILL-ness) Health condition that changes a person's thoughts, emotions, and behavior and affects that person's ability to undertake daily functions

mistake
(meh-STAKE) To understand, interpret, or estimate incorrectly

error
(AIR-er) Something done incorrectly through ignorance or carelessness

Objectives

After completing this section, you will be able to:

1. Define the key terms.
2. List the three causes of physical disabilities.
3. List three categories of mental illness.
4. Describe one risk factor for mental illness.
5. Name four psychological needs that must be met, and give one example of each need.
6. Name four physiological needs that must be met, and give one example of each need.
7. Describe the five psychological stages that terminally ill patients experience.
8. List three ways to meet the needs of terminally ill patients.
9. Identify two mistakes or errors that jeopardize patient safety.
10. List three ways to protect patient safety.

GETTING STARTED

Each chapter opens with a Getting Started bell-ringer activity to help you engage in the subject at hand.

BACKGROUND

Background information introduces the chapter topics and sets the stage for your learning.

OBJECTIVES

Section Objectives help you focus on the essential concepts presented in each chapter. The Objectives state what you should know and be able to do after reading the section and completing its activities.

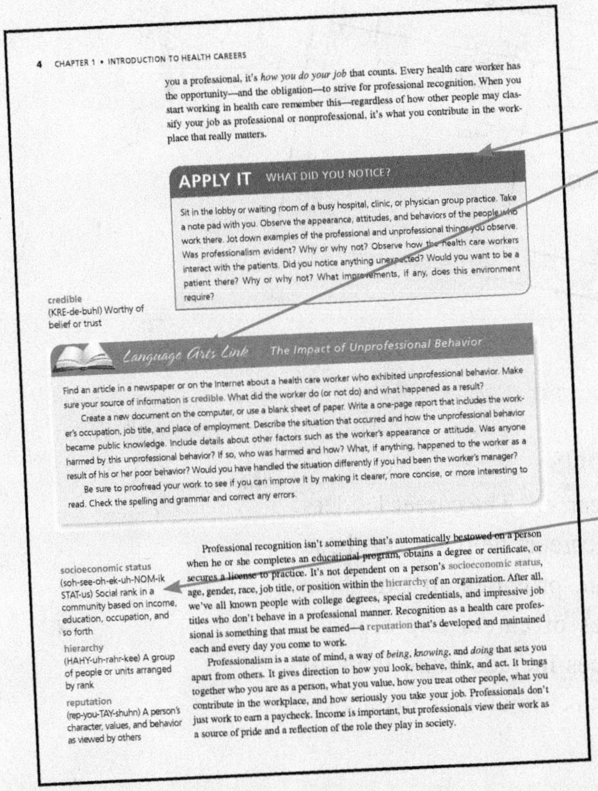

4 CHAPTER 1 • INTRODUCTION TO HEALTH CAREERS

you a professional, it's *how you do your job* that counts. Every health care worker has the opportunity—and the obligation—to strive for professional recognition. When you start working in health care remember this—regardless of how other people may classify your job as professional or nonprofessional, it's what you contribute in the workplace that really matters.

APPLY IT WHAT DID YOU NOTICE?

Sit in the lobby or waiting room of a busy hospital, clinic, or physician group practice. Take a note pad with you. Observe the appearance, attitudes, and behaviors of the people who work there. Jot down examples of the professional and unprofessional things you observe. Was professionalism evident? Why or why not? Observe how the health care workers interact with the patients. Did you notice anything unexpected? Would you want to be a patient there? Why or why not? What improvements, if any, does this environment require?

credible
(KRE-de-buhl) Worthy of belief or trust

Language Arts Link The Impact of Unprofessional Behavior

Find an article in a newspaper or on the Internet about a health care worker who exhibited unprofessional behavior. Make sure your source of information is credible. What did the worker do (or not do) and what happened as a result?

Create a new document on the computer, or use a blank sheet of paper. Write a one-page report that includes the worker's occupation, job title, and place of employment. Describe the situation that occurred and how the unprofessional behavior became public knowledge. Include details about other factors such as the worker's appearance or attitude. Was anyone harmed by this unprofessional behavior? If so, who was harmed and how? What, if anything, happened to the worker as a result of his or her poor behavior? Would you have handled the situation differently if you had been the worker's manager?

Be sure to proofread your work to see if you can improve it by making it clearer, more concise, or more interesting to read. Check the spelling and grammar and correct any errors.

Professional recognition isn't something that's automatically bestowed on a person when he or she completes an educational program, obtains a degree or certificate, or secures a license to practice. It's not dependent on a person's socioeconomic status, age, gender, race, job title, or position within the hierarchy of an organization. After all, we've all known people with college degrees, special credentials, and impressive job titles who don't behave in a professional manner. Recognition as a health care professional is something that must be earned—a reputation that's developed and maintained each and every day you come to work.

Professionalism is a state of mind, a way of *being*, *knowing*, and *doing* that sets you apart from others. It gives direction to how you look, behave, think, and act. It brings together who you are as a person, what you value, how you treat other people, what you contribute in the workplace, and how seriously you take your job. Professionals don't just work to earn a paycheck. Income is important, but professionals view their work as a source of pride and a reflection of the role they play in society.

socioeconomic status
(soh-see-oh-ek-uh-NOM-ik STAT-us) Social rank in a community based on income, education, occupation, and so forth

hierarchy
(HAHY-uh-rahr-kee) A group of people or units arranged by rank

reputation
(rep-you-TAY-shuhn) A person's character, values, and behavior as viewed by others

ACTIVE LEARNING

Each chapter in your textbook includes special features to help you understand and apply the concepts you are learning. These include Apply It, The More You Know, Consider This, Recent Developments, Build Your Skills, and Community Service. Language Arts, Math, and Science Links help you apply health care information and concepts to your core curriculum courses.

MARGIN GLOSSARY

For your convenience, the definition and pronunciation for each of the more than 625 Key Terms appear in the margin when each term is first introduced in the text. A complete Glossary is provided at the end of your book.

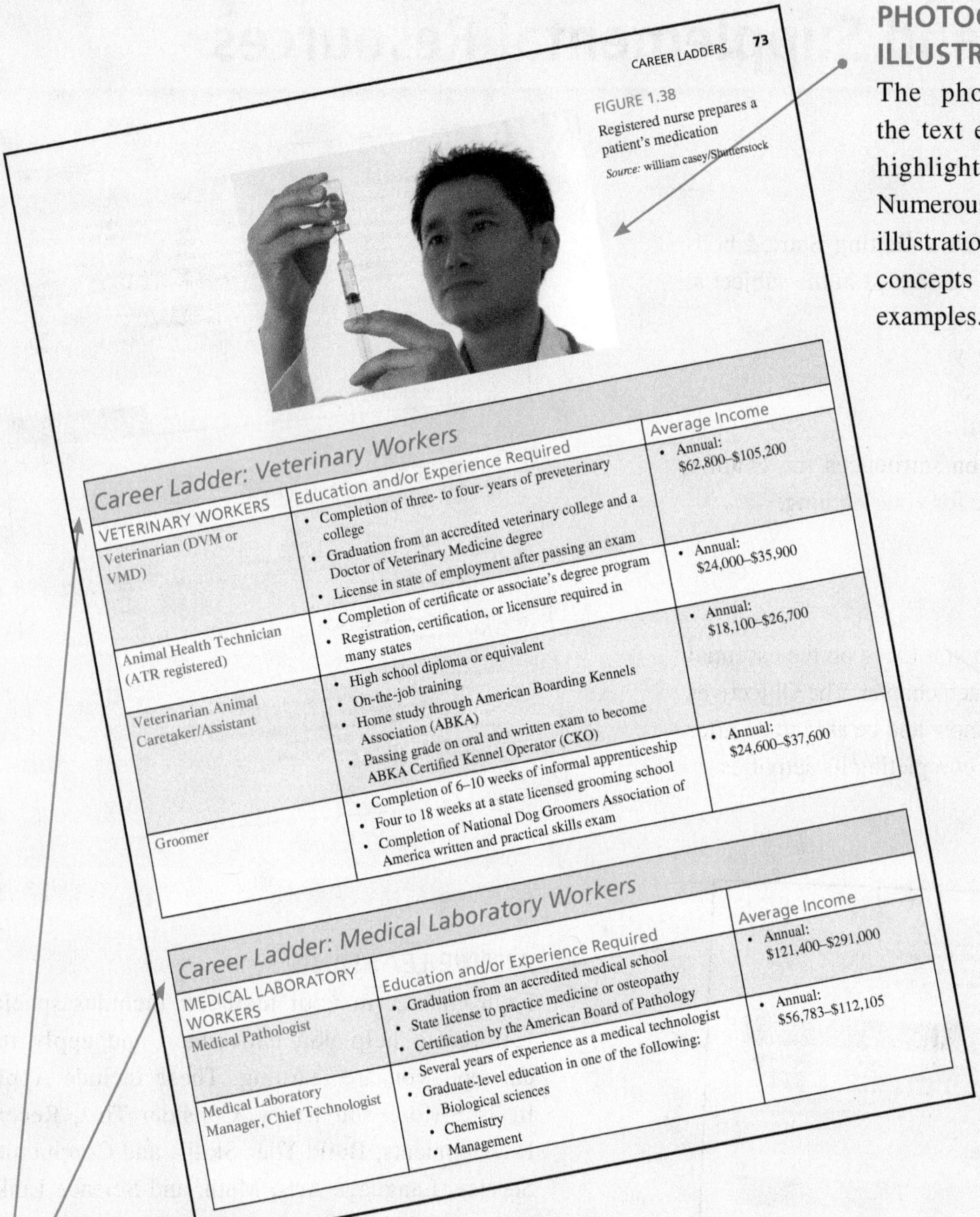

FIGURE 1.38
Registered nurse prepares a patient's medication
Source: william casey/Shutterstock

Career Ladder: Veterinary Workers

VETERINARY WORKERS	Education and/or Experience Required	Average Income
Veterinarian (DVM or VMD)	• Completion of three- to four- years of preveterinary college • Graduation from an accredited veterinary college and a Doctor of Veterinary Medicine degree • License in state of employment after passing an exam	• Annual: $62,800–$105,200
Animal Health Technician (ATR registered)	• Completion of certificate or associate's degree program • Registration, certification, or licensure required in many states	• Annual: $24,000–$35,900
Veterinarian Animal Caretaker/Assistant	• High school diploma or equivalent • On-the-job training • Home study through American Boarding Kennels Association (ABKA) • Passing grade on oral and written exam to become ABKA Certified Kennel Operator (CKO)	• Annual: $18,100–$26,700
Groomer	• Completion of 6–10 weeks of informal apprenticeship • Four to 18 weeks at a state licensed grooming school • Completion of National Dog Groomers Association of America written and practical skills exam	• Annual: $24,600–$37,600

Career Ladder: Medical Laboratory Workers

MEDICAL LABORATORY WORKERS	Education and/or Experience Required	Average Income
Medical Pathologist	• Graduation from an accredited medical school • State license to practice medicine or osteopathy • Certification by the American Board of Pathology	• Annual: $121,400–$291,000

Medical Laboratory Manager, Chief Technologist	• Several years of experience as a medical technologist
	• Graduate-level education in one of the following:
	  • Biological sciences
	  • Chemistry
	  • Management
		• Annual: $56,783–$112,105

PHOTOGRAPHS AND ILLUSTRATIONS

The photo-rich design of the text engages readers and highlights important topics. Numerous tables, figures, and illustrations add clarity to the concepts and provide helpful examples.

CAREER LADDERS AND OCCUPATIONAL DESCRIPTIONS

What does it take to choose, prepare for, and qualify for a health career? The career ladders and occupational descriptions for more than 100 different health careers help answer these questions. Chapter Five, *Finding the Right Occupation for You*, provides an extensive discussion to guide you through self-discovery and the stages of career exploration, planning, and preparation. In addition, your companion resources include more than 40 Career Focus Videos describing a wide variety of health occupations from which to choose.

REALITY CHECK

Reading concepts in a textbook is helpful, but the most important thing is to think about how the information actually applies to you. The Reality Check feature at the end of each section brings home the information in a direct, get real message to help you understand the concepts and recognize what will be expected of you as a health care professional.

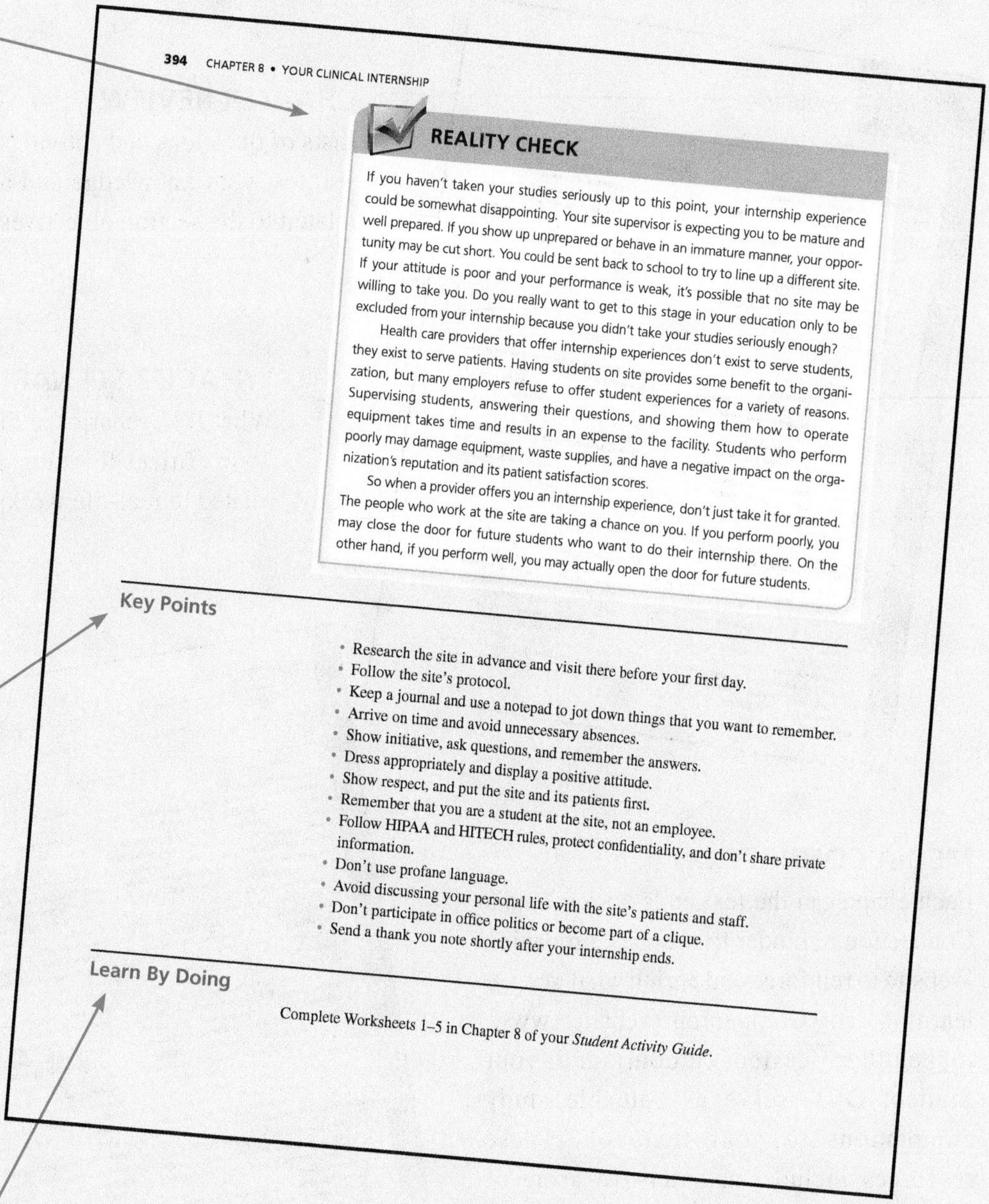

394 CHAPTER 8 • YOUR CLINICAL INTERNSHIP

REALITY CHECK

If you haven't taken your studies seriously up to this point, your internship experience could be somewhat disappointing. Your site supervisor is expecting you to be mature and well prepared. If you show up unprepared or behave in an immature manner, your opportunity may be cut short. You could be sent back to school to try to line up a different site. If your attitude is poor and your performance is weak, it's possible that no site may be willing to take you. Do you really want to get to this stage in your education only to be excluded from your internship because you didn't take your studies seriously enough?

Health care providers that offer internship experiences don't exist to serve students, they exist to serve patients. Having students on site provides some benefit to the organization, but many employers refuse to offer student experiences for a variety of reasons. Supervising students, answering their questions, and showing them how to operate equipment takes time and results in an expense to the facility. Students who perform poorly may damage equipment, waste supplies, and have a negative impact on the organization's reputation and its patient satisfaction scores.

So when a provider offers you an internship experience, don't just take it for granted. The people who work at the site are taking a chance on you. If you perform poorly, you may close the door for future students who want to do their internship there. On the other hand, if you perform well, you may actually open the door for future students.

Key Points

- Research the site in advance and visit there before your first day.
- Follow the site's protocol.
- Keep a journal and use a notepad to jot down things that you want to remember.
- Arrive on time and avoid unnecessary absences.
- Show initiative, ask questions, and remember the answers.
- Dress appropriately and display a positive attitude.
- Show respect, and put the site and its patients first.
- Remember that you are a student at the site, not an employee.
- Follow HIPAA and HITECH rules, protect confidentiality, and don't share private information.
- Don't use profane language.
- Avoid discussing your personal life with the site's patients and staff.
- Don't participate in office politics or become part of a clique.
- Send a thank you note shortly after your internship ends.

Learn By Doing

Complete Worksheets 1–5 in Chapter 8 of your *Student Activity Guide*.

KEY POINTS

The Key Points listed at the end of each section provides a quick summary and review of the major concepts presented in the section.

LEARN BY DOING

Each section ends with a Learn By Doing reminder to complete the worksheets in your Student Activity Guide. The Student Activity Guide presents more than 100 activities designed to strengthen your knowledge and skills and help you apply what you are learning.

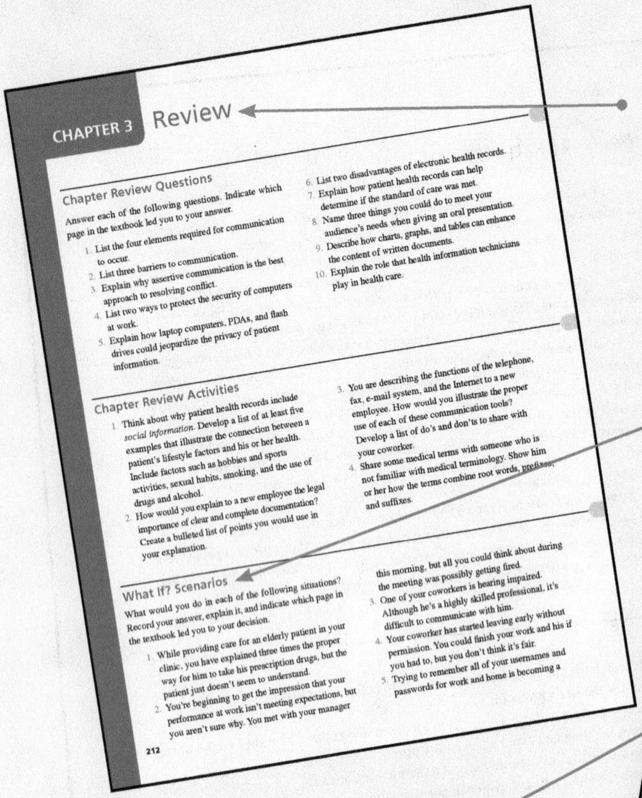

CHAPTER 3 Review

Chapter Review Questions

Answer each of the following questions. Indicate which page in the textbook led you to your answer.

1. List the four elements required for communication to occur.
2. List three barriers to communication.
3. Explain why assertive communication is the best approach to resolving conflict.
4. List two ways to protect the security of computers at work.
5. Explain how laptop computers, PDAs, and flash drives could jeopardize the privacy of patient information.
6. List two disadvantages of electronic health records.
7. Explain how patient health records can help determine if the standard of care was met.
8. Name three things you could do to meet your audience's needs when giving an oral presentation.
9. Describe how charts, graphs, and tables can enhance the content of written documents.
10. Explain the role that health information technicians play in health care.

Chapter Review Activities

1. Think about why patient health records include *social information*. Develop a list of at least five examples that illustrate the connection between a patient's lifestyle factors and his or her health. Include factors such as hobbies and sports activities, sexual habits, smoking, and the use of drugs and alcohol.
2. How would you explain to a new employee the legal importance of clear and complete documentation? Create a bulleted list of points you would use in your explanation.
3. You are describing the functions of the telephone, fax, e-mail system, and the Internet to a new employee. How would you illustrate the proper use of each of these communication tools? Develop a list of do's and don'ts to share with your coworker.
4. Share some medical terms with someone who is not familiar with medical terminology. Show him or her how the terms combine root words, prefixes, and suffixes.

What If? Scenarios

What would you do in each of the following situations? Record your answer, explain it, and indicate which page in the textbook led you to your decision.

1. While providing care for an elderly patient in your clinic, you have explained three times the proper way for him to take his prescription drugs, but the patient just doesn't seem to understand.
2. You're beginning to get the impression that your performance at work isn't meeting expectations, but you aren't sure why. You met with your manager this morning, but all you could think about during the meeting was possibly getting fired.
3. One of your coworkers is hearing impaired. Although he's a highly skilled professional, it's difficult to communicate with him.
4. Your coworker has started leaving early without permission. You could finish your work and his if you had to, but you don't think it's fair.
5. Trying to remember all of your usernames and passwords for work and home is becoming a

212

CHAPTER REVIEW

Lists of questions and activities at the end of each chapter help you test your knowledge and apply what you have learned as related to the section objectives.

WHAT IF? SCENARIOS

What If? Scenarios at the end of each chapter stimulate your critical thinking and decision-making skills as related to real-life workplace situations.

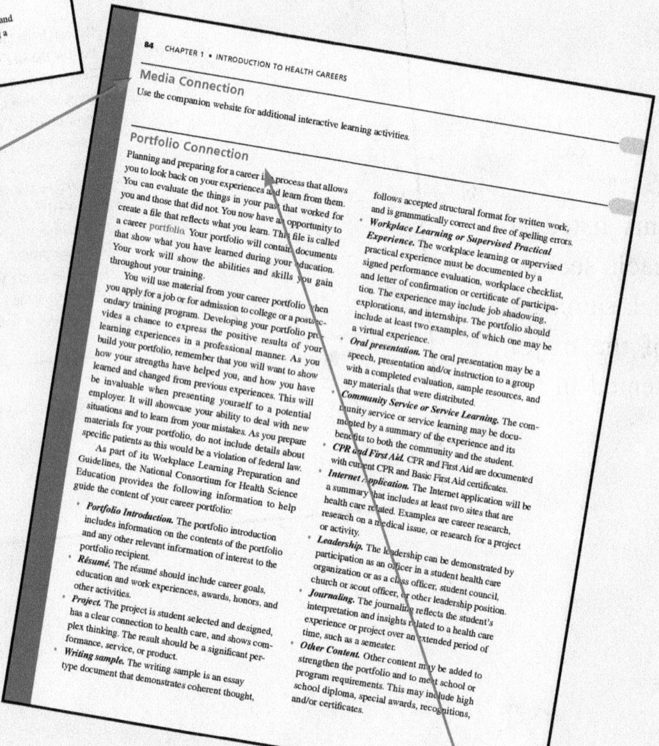

84 CHAPTER 1 • INTRODUCTION TO HEALTH CAREERS

Media Connection

Use the companion website for additional interactive learning activities.

Portfolio Connection

Planning and preparing for a career is a process that allows you to look back on your experiences and learn from them. You can evaluate the things in your past that worked for you and those that did not. You now have an opportunity to create a file that reflects what you learn. This file is called a career portfolio. Your portfolio will contain documents that show what you have learned during your education. Your work will show the abilities and skills you gain throughout your training.

You will use material from your career portfolio when you apply for a job or for admission to college or a postsecondary training program. Developing your portfolio provides a chance to express the positive results of your learning experiences in a professional manner. As you build your portfolio, remember that you will want to show how your strengths have helped you, and how you have learned and changed from previous experiences. This will be invaluable when presenting yourself to a potential employer. It will showcase your ability to deal with new situations and to learn from your mistakes. As you prepare materials for your portfolio, do not include details about specific patients as this would be a violation of federal law.

As part of its Workplace Learning Preparation and Guidelines, the National Consortium for Health Science Education provides the following information to help guide the content of your career portfolio:

- ***Portfolio Introduction.*** The portfolio introduction includes information on the contents of the portfolio and any other relevant information of interest to the portfolio recipient.
- ***Résumé.*** The résumé should include career goals, education and work experiences, awards, honors, and other activities.
- ***Project.*** The project is student selected and designed, has a clear connection to health care, and shows complex thinking. The result should be a significant performance, service, or product.
- ***Writing sample.*** The writing sample is an essay type document that demonstrates coherent thought, follows accepted structural format for written work, and is grammatically correct and free of spelling errors.
- ***Workplace Learning or Supervised Practical Experience.*** The workplace learning or supervised practical experience must be documented by a signed performance evaluation, workplace checklist, and letter of confirmation or certificate of participation. The experience may include job shadowing, explorations, and internships. The portfolio should include at least two examples, of which one may be a virtual experience.
- ***Oral presentation.*** The oral presentation may be a speech, presentation and/or instruction to a group with a completed evaluation, sample resources, and any materials that were distributed.
- ***Community Service or Service Learning.*** The community service or service learning may be documented by a summary of the experience and its benefits to both the community and the student.
- ***CPR and First Aid.*** CPR and First Aid are documented with current CPR and Basic First Aid certificates.
- ***Internet Application.*** The Internet application will be a summary that includes at least two sites that are health care related. Examples are career research, research on a medical issue, or research for a project or activity.
- ***Leadership.*** The leadership can be demonstrated by participation as an officer in a student health care organization or as a class officer, student council, church or scout officer, or other leadership position.
- ***Journaling.*** The journaling reflects the student's interpretation and insights related to a health care experience or project over an extended period of time, such as a semester.
- ***Other Content.*** Other content may be added to strengthen the portfolio and to meet school or program requirements. This may include high school diploma, special awards, recognitions, and/or certificates.

MEDIA CONNECTION

Each chapter in the text ends with a Media Connection reminder to use the Companion Website to reinforce and enrich what you are learning. The Companion Website (www.myhealthprofessionskit.com) and your Student DVD serve as valuable study companions to your textbook. These resources include an extensive array of videos plus chapter-related self assessments, next step improvement plans, quizzes, audio glossaries, and flash cards to support interactive learning. Helpful tools include the Golden Personality Type Profiler, and the Think Watson Critical Thinking Assessment. Additional Student Activities are presented along with an informative Bonus Section on Life Cycles, describing the human progression of life stages from infancy through old age, or senescence.

PORTFOLIO CONNECTION

The Portfolio Connection at the end of each chapter guides you through the process of developing a career portfolio. Your portfolio demonstrates your learning and your personal and professional growth during the course and after the course has ended. Your portfolio will be of special value when you apply for a health care educational program and for employment after graduation.

Chapter 1

Introduction to Health Careers

Source: Stephen Coburn/Fotolia

SECTIONS

"Opportunity is missed by most because it is dressed in overalls and looks like work."

THOMAS ALVA EDISON, INVENTOR, 1847–1931

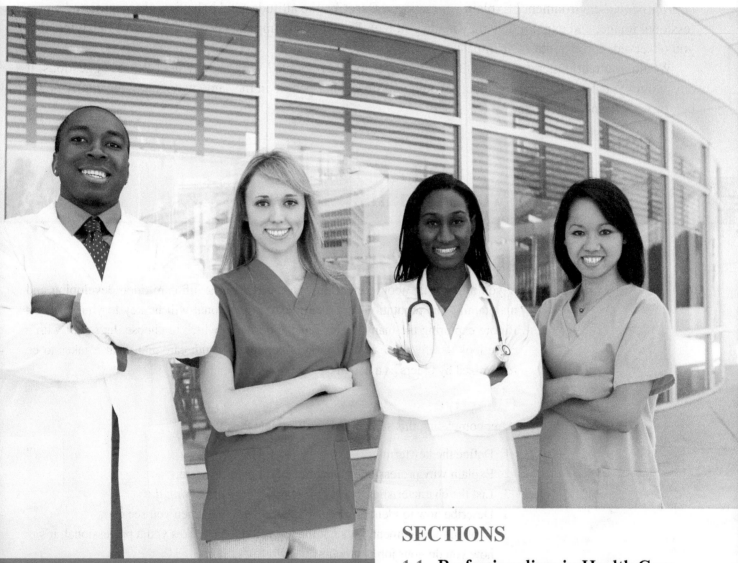

GETTING STARTED

Think about when you were a patient yourself, or when you were with a family member or friend who was a patient. This could be at a doctor's office, clinic, hospital, emergency room, dental practice, eye doctor, nursing home, and so forth. Make a list of things that you noticed about the people who worked in that environment. How did they treat you or your family member or friend? How did they dress? What did they say? How did they behave? How did they interact with their coworkers? Include any details you can remember.

Given what you observed and experienced, would you consider this a *professional* environment or an *unprofessional* environment? Explain your answer. Describe the attitudes and behaviors that supported a professional image, and explain how they made you feel. Describe any unprofessional attitudes or behaviors that you observed, and explain their impact.

Would you recommend this health care provider to other people? Why or why not? What suggestions, if any, would you offer for improvement? Would you treat other people in the same way you, your family member, or your friend was treated?

SECTION 1.1 Professionalism in Health Care

Background

If you're thinking about embarking on a career in health care, then developing and maintaining the reputation of a health care professional will be key to your success. Before exploring the many health occupations from which to choose, let's start with a close look at why professionalism is important in health care and what it takes to be recognized by others as a health care professional yourself.

Objectives

After completing this section, you will be able to:

1. Define the key terms.
2. Explain why professionalism is important in health care.
3. List the characteristics that define a *health care professional.*
4. Describe how to identify a health care professional when you see one.
5. Explain the statement, "It's not the job you do that makes you a professional, it's how you do your job that counts."
6. Discuss the impact that a successful health career can have on your self-esteem and self-worth.
7. Explain why health care workers need an attitude that supports service to others.
8. List five steps you can take now to begin developing your professional reputation.

RECOGNITION AS A HEALTH CARE PROFESSIONAL

There's no doubt about it. When you're sick or injured or when a family member or friend needs health care, you want to be certain that you and your loved ones are cared for by **professionals**. Think about a time when you were a patient in a doctor's office, clinic, or

professionals (pruh-FESH-uh-nls) People with experience and skills who are engaged in a specific occupation for pay or as a means of livelihood

hospital; you probably encountered several different types of health care workers. Although most of them performed their duties in a professional manner, it is likely a few did not. We would like to think that everyone who works in health care functions as a professional, but experience proves that this is not always the case.

What is a professional? Why is professionalism important? How can you recognize a professional when you see one? What does *taking a professional approach* to one's work mean? What should you learn as a student to prepare for your future recognition as a health care professional?

According to *Webster's New World Dictionary of the American Language, College Edition*, a *professional* is a person "with much experience and great skill in a specified role" who is "engaged in a specific occupation for pay or as a means of livelihood." (*Webster's New World Dictionary of the American Language, College Edition.* Reproduced with permission of John Wiley & Sons.) As we look around us, we see many examples of professionals in different walks of life. In sports, for example, professional status is awarded to gifted athletes who have surpassed amateur events and moved into high-paying, major league competitions. In medicine, law, and science, doctors, lawyers, and engineers are considered professionals because of their expertise, advanced education, and special **credentials** such as **licenses** and **certifications**. However, truck drivers, hair stylists, and photographers also consider themselves professionals, as do bankers, insurance underwriters, and investment counselors. Exactly what is a professional and who is qualified to be one?

Occupations are sometimes divided into "professional" and "nonprofessional" categories based on criteria such as the following:

- Carving out a unique and exclusive **scope of practice**
- Setting minimum standards for education and training
- Establishing **accreditation** of educational programs
- Enforcing minimum standards for entry into practice
- Requiring credentials such as licenses or certifications
- Sponsoring **professional associations** with codes of **ethics** and standards of **competence**

When we apply these criteria to the health care workforce, then doctors, registered nurses, pharmacists, physical therapists, surgical technologists, dental hygienists, radiographers, and the like are all classified as professionals. However these criteria may leave other types of health care workers, such as nurse aides, insurance processors, secretaries, food service workers, and housekeepers, in the nonprofessional category. Exclusion from the list of professionals may be demeaning to people who work hard and make their jobs a top priority in their lives.

In health care it's important to acknowledge another set of criteria that gives all health care workers the opportunity to be viewed as professionals whether they provide direct patient care or function in a support role

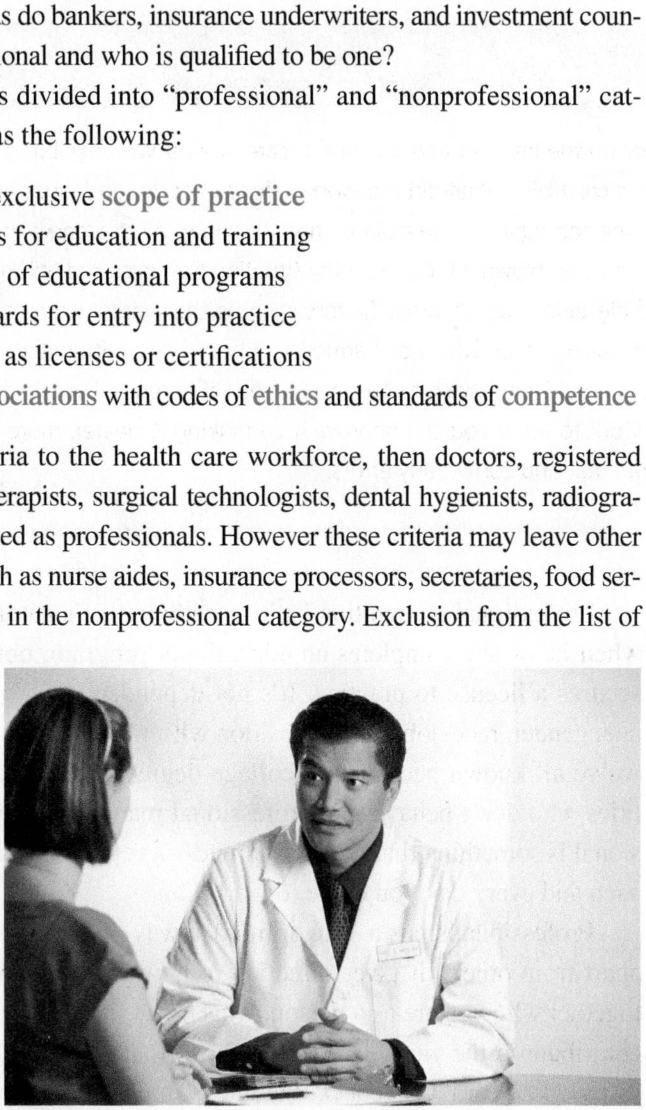

FIGURE 1.1

Physician assures a patient that she is being cared for by professionals

Source: iofoto/Shutterstock

credentials
(kri-DEN-shuhls) Letters or certificates given to a person to show that he or she has the right to exercise a certain authority

licenses
(LIE-suhns-ez) Credentials from a state agency awarding legal permission to practice; must meet pre-established qualifications

certifications
(sur-teh-fi-KAY-shuhns) Credentials from a state agency or a professional association awarding permission to use a special professional title; must meet pre-established competency standards

scope of practice
(skohp ov PRAK-tis) Boundaries that determine what a worker may and may not do as part of his or her job

accreditation
(uh-KRED-it-day-shun) Certified as having met set standards

professional associations
(pruh-FESH-uh-nl uh-soh-see-AY-shuhns) Organizations composed of people from the same occupation

ethics
(ETH-iks) Standards of conduct and moral judgment

competence
(KOM-peh-tens) Possessing necessary knowledge and skills

behind the scenes: it's not *the job you do* that makes you a professional, it's *how you do your job* that counts. Every health care worker has the opportunity—and the obligation—to strive for professional recognition. When you start working in health care remember this—regardless of how other people may classify your job as professional or nonprofessional, it's what you contribute in the workplace that really matters.

APPLY IT WHAT DID YOU NOTICE?

Sit in the lobby or waiting room of a busy hospital, clinic, or physician group practice. Take a note pad with you. Observe the appearance, attitudes, and behaviors of the people who work there. Jot down examples of the professional and unprofessional things you observe. Was professionalism evident? Why or why not? Observe how the health care workers interact with the patients. Did you notice anything unexpected? Would you want to be a patient there? Why or why not? What improvements, if any, does this environment require?

credible
(KRE-de-buhl) Worthy of belief or trust

Language Arts Link The Impact of Unprofessional Behavior

Find an article in a newspaper or on the Internet about a health care worker who exhibited unprofessional behavior. Make sure your source of information is **credible**. What did the worker do (or not do) and what happened as a result?

Create a new document on the computer, or use a blank sheet of paper. Write a one-page report that includes the worker's occupation, job title, and place of employment. Describe the situation that occurred and how the unprofessional behavior became public knowledge. Include details about other factors such as the worker's appearance or attitude. Was anyone harmed by this unprofessional behavior? If so, who was harmed and how? What, if anything, happened to the worker as a result of his or her poor behavior? Would you have handled the situation differently if you had been the worker's manager?

Be sure to proofread your work to see if you can improve it by making it clearer, more concise, or more interesting to read. Check the spelling and grammar and correct any errors.

socioeconomic status
(soh-see-oh-ek-uh-NOM-ik STAT-us) Social rank in a community based on income, education, occupation, and so forth

hierarchy
(HAHY-uh-rahr-kee) A group of people or units arranged by rank

reputation
(rep-you-TAY-shuhn) A person's character, values, and behavior as viewed by others

Professional recognition isn't something that's automatically bestowed on a person when he or she completes an educational program, obtains a degree or certificate, or secures a license to practice. It's not dependent on a person's **socioeconomic status**, age, gender, race, job title, or position within the **hierarchy** of an organization. After all, we've all known people with college degrees, special credentials, and impressive job titles who don't behave in a professional manner. Recognition as a health care professional is something that must be earned—a **reputation** that's developed and maintained each and every day you come to work.

Professionalism is a state of mind, a way of *being*, *knowing*, and *doing* that sets you apart from others. It gives direction to how you look, behave, think, and act. It brings together who you are as a person, what you value, how you treat other people, what you contribute in the workplace, and how seriously you take your job. Professionals don't just work to earn a paycheck. Income is important, but professionals view their work as a source of pride and a reflection of the role they play in society.

Professionalism is something that every organization seeks in its employees. How can you spot a health care professional when you see one? It's easy. Health care professionals are good at what they do, and they like doing it. They enjoy helping others and knowing they've made a difference. Professionals *have their act together*, and it shows. They set high standards for their performance and achieve them. They see *the big picture* in health care and know where they fit in. Professionals care about quality and how to improve it. They treat everyone they meet with dignity and respect. Professionals continually strive to grow and to learn.

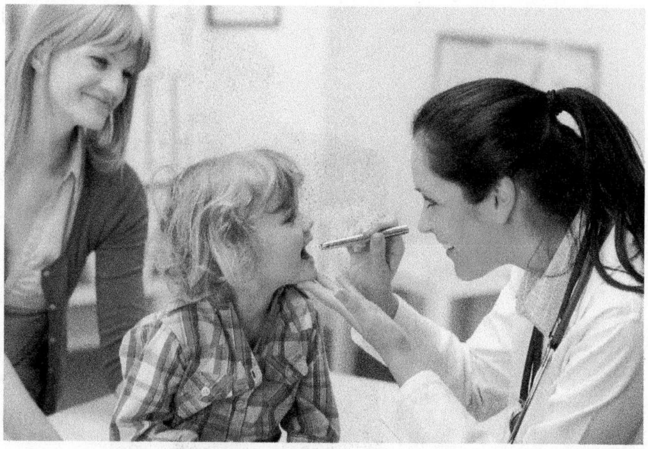

FIGURE 1.2

Health care professional examining a young patient.

Source: CandyBox Images/Fotolia LLC

dignity
(DIG-ni-tee) The degree of worth, merit, honor

respect
(ri-SPEKT) Feeling or showing honor or esteem

APPLY IT YOUR STRONGEST TRAITS

When you think about the need for professionalism among health care workers, make a list of what you consider to be your five strongest **traits**. Then ask someone who knows you well—a family member, friend, teacher, or clergyman—to create the same list. Compare the two lists. What have you learned about yourself that can be useful information when considering a future career in health care?

traits
(TREYTS) Characteristics or qualities related to one's personality

Spotting a health care professional may be easy, but becoming one yourself is another matter. It's something you have to concentrate on every day, but it's worth the effort. To *be* a professional, you must *feel like* a professional. In today's society, the amount of education that a person has and what he or she does for a living have become important contributors to an individual's self-esteem and sense of self-worth. *What we do* has become *who we are*. When you graduate from school, complete a training program, earn a degree, or obtain a license or certification, you experience the exhilaration of knowing you've accomplished something worthwhile. Being recognized by others as a professional brings value and meaning to your efforts. It reminds you that what you do really counts. This is true whether you care for patients, process specimens, prepare meals, clean public areas, interact with vendors or work in any one of hundreds of different health care jobs. It's also true whether you work in a hospital, physicians' office, dental practice, clinic, rehabilitation facility, or another type of health care organization. No matter what your role involves, how you view your work and how you approach it can have a tremendous impact on your life as well as on the lives of those you serve.

self-esteem
(celf ih-STEEM) Belief in oneself, self-respect

self-worth
(CELF-wurth) Importance and value in oneself

vendors
(VEN-ders) People who work for companies with which your company does business

WHY HEALTH CARE NEEDS PROFESSIONALS

When you're sick or injured, health care can become a basic need for survival. Each year, millions of Americans receive health services in doctors' offices, hospitals, clinics, mental health facilities, and at home. Patients rely on health care professionals to

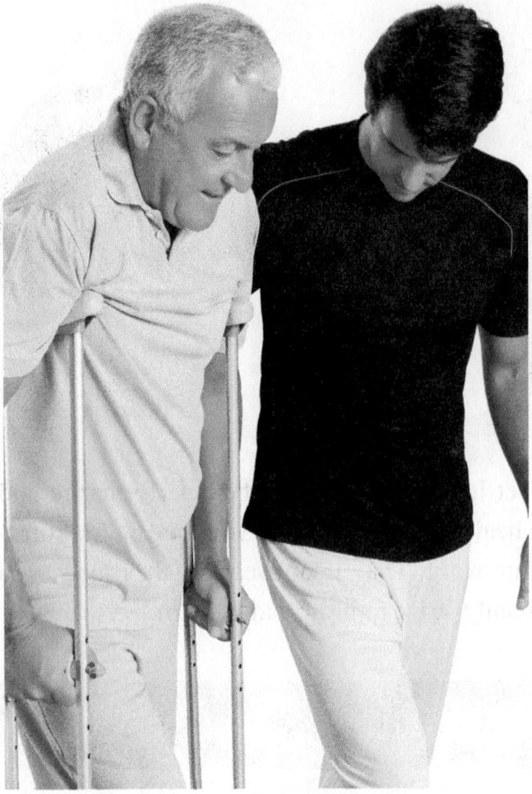

FIGURE 1.3

Physical therapist assistant helps a patient learn to use crutches

Source: Tyler Olson/Shutterstock

provide affordable, state-of-the-art **diagnostic** and **therapeutic** procedures to help them overcome illnesses, injuries, and other challenges that affect their health and quality of life.

It's important to remember that health care is also a business. Finding ways to provide health care for more patients, using fewer resources, while achieving better outcomes, has become a major challenge for health care **providers** and **payers**. Meeting these challenges requires a crew of health care workers who are committed to providing quality care, customer service, and cost effective operations. People who fail to take a professional approach to their work are often late, absent, unreliable, and sloppy. Their actions may endanger patient care, customer service, safety, and the efficient use of limited resources.

diagnostic
(dahy-uhg-NOS-tik) Deciding the nature of a disease or condition

therapeutic
(thair-uh-PYOO-tik) Treating or curing a disease or condition

providers
(pruh-VIE-ders) Doctors, health care workers, and health care organizations that offer health care services

payers
(PAY-ers) Someone that covers the expense for goods received or services rendered

APPLY IT UNEXPECTED SURGERY

Imagine yourself as a 25-year-old man or woman who has just broken your leg after slipping on ice during a winter storm. You arrive by ambulance at a nearby hospital and are told you'll need surgery to repair your fracture, followed by several weeks in a cast. You're a single parent who works full-time at a fast-food restaurant to support two young children ages three and five. You've never been in the hospital before, let alone undergone surgery.

Describe how you would feel when finding yourself in this situation. Make a list of the concerns that you might have and the decisions you would need to make. Given your situation, list the attitudes, behaviors, and other characteristics that you would like to see in the health care workers who will care for you. What role would *professionalism* play?

attitude
(A-teh-tood) A manner of acting, feeling, or thinking that shows one's disposition or opinion

trust
(TRUHST) To place confidence in the honesty, integrity, and reliability of another person

caregivers
(KAIR-giv-ers) Health care workers who provide direct, hands-on patient care

Working in health care requires special skills and an **attitude** that supports service to others. Patients seek health care services during some of the most vulnerable times in their lives, when they're sick, injured, and *at their worst*. Each patient-worker interaction must build confidence and **trust**. The decisions and actions of those who care for patients or those who work behind the scenes to support the efforts of **caregivers** can have an immediate and lasting impact.

REALITY CHECK

If you're seriously considering a career in health care, it's time to get real about what it's going to take to achieve your **goals**. The first step is completing your education. Few positions exist in health care organizations for people without a high school diploma or the equivalent, and those jobs offer only limited opportunities for advancement. You'll also need a high school diploma, or **GED**, to qualify for admission into college and/or a **postsecondary** training program. Grades, exam scores, and attendance in high school all matter, so it's never too soon to start laying the groundwork for your future. The information in this textbook can serve as your roadmap. Regardless of which health occupation you choose, rest assured that you will play a vital role in caring for patients because *every* job and *every* worker is important.

Start pulling together the knowledge, skills, attitudes, and commitment you'll need to become the very best health care professional you can be. If your education includes an **internship**, before long you'll be interacting with health care workers, physicians, and patients to gain some *real-life experience* even before you graduate. Here are some things you can do now to begin developing good habits and to lay the foundation for a professional career:

- Take your studies seriously. Almost everything that you hear, observe, read, learn, and experience in school will be important at some point in your health career.
- Earn high grades and score well on exams. Admission into college and postsecondary training programs is competitive. Final grades and exam scores matter.
- Show up for school every day, arrive on time, and apply yourself. Good attendance, punctuality, and the ability to concentrate are vital in school and at work.
- Encourage and support your fellow classmates, and strengthen your interpersonal relationships with family members and friends.
- Participate in extracurricular activities and join volunteer organizations to develop your leadership and teamwork skills.
- Enhance your communication skills. Pay attention to *what you say* and *how you say it*, and consider the impact that your comments make on other people.
- Interact with people from other **cultures** and explore your differences and similarities.
- Improve your time management, organizational, and study skills. Find healthy ways to relieve your stress and balance the **priorities** in your life.
- Increase your self-dependence and make careful, thoughtful decisions.

goals
(GOHLS) Aim, objects, or ends that one strives to attain

GED
(gee-ee-dee) General Educational Development test; a high school equivalency credential

postsecondary
(pohst SEK-uhn-der-ee) After high school

internship
(in-TURN-ship) A real-life learning experience obtained through working on-site in a health care facility while enrolled as a student

cultures
(kKUHL-chers) Groups of people who share the same values, norms, and behaviors

priorities
(prahy-OR-eh-tees) Having precedence in time, order, and importance

Key Points

- Developing a professional reputation is the key to success for all health care workers.
- Health care is a basic need for survival. People want to know that they and their loved ones are being cared for by professionals.
- All health care workers have the opportunity—and the obligation—to strive for professional recognition regardless of their job title, education, credentials, or years of work experience.

- Regardless of whether your job is classified as *professional* or *nonprofessional*, it's what you contribute in the workplace that really matters.
- It's not *the job you do* that makes you a professional; it's *how you do your job* that counts.
- Graduating from a training program or earning a college degree doesn't automatically make you a professional. You must earn and maintain a professional reputation each and every day you come to work.
- Professionalism is a state of mind, a way of *being*, *knowing*, and *doing* that sets you apart from others. It gives direction to how you look, behave, think, and act.
- Working in health care requires special skills and an attitude that supports service to others in order to build confidence and trust.
- Start developing your professional skills and habits now, while you're still in school. Use this textbook as your roadmap to success.

Section Review Questions

Answer each of the following questions. Indicate which page in the textbook led you to your answer.

1. List two things that might happen if a patient witnesses unprofessional behavior by a health care worker.
2. Give one example to illustrate the statement, "It's not the job you do that makes you a professional, it's how you do your job that counts."
3. Describe why health care workers need an attitude that supports *service to others*.
4. List three behaviors or traits that help you identify a health care professional when you see one.
5. Discuss the meaning of the statement, "To *be* a professional, you must *feel like* a professional."

Learn By Doing

Complete Worksheets 1–4 in Section 1.1 of your *Student Activity Guide*.

SECTION 1.2 Overview of Health Careers

Background

Hundreds of different kinds of jobs are available in health care. This section describes occupations that represent some of the career choices available. Health occupations with similar characteristics are grouped together in *clusters* and *pathways*, supported by the National Health Care Skills Standards and designed to help you achieve success as a health care worker. After learning about the wide variety of careers, you can identify and research the occupations that sound like a good match for you.

Objectives

After completing this section, you will be able to:

1. Define the key terms.
2. Describe the purpose of the National Career Clusters™ Framework.
3. List three of the sixteen Career Clusters in addition to Health Science.
4. List the five Health Science pathways.
5. Describe the purpose of the National Consortium for Health Science Education.
6. Name three of the eleven foundation standards topics covered by the National Health Care Skills Standards.
7. Describe the role that each of the following services plays in health care: Therapeutic, Diagnostic, Health Informatics, Support, and Biotechnology Research and Development.
8. Name one health occupation for each of the five Health Science service areas.
9. Name two health occupations aligned with systems of the human body.
10. Name two careers in alternative health services.
11. Name two careers in medicine.

CAREER CLUSTERS AND HEALTH SCIENCE

Health care, like other fields, requires more knowledge, skills, and abilities than ever before.

Millions of students are currently enrolled in Career Technical Education (CTE) programs offered in high schools and community colleges throughout the United States. These individuals must meet standards to prove they have learned what they need to know in order to achieve success on the job.

standards
(STAN-derds) Accepted basis of comparison in measuring quality or value

APPLY IT WHO WORKS IN HEALTH CARE?

Make a list of all of the different health occupations or jobs with which you are familiar. Start with doctors, nurses, pharmacists, and dentists and keep adding to the list. Include people who work in the various types of health care settings, such as doctors' offices, hospitals, clinics, nursing homes, and so forth. How many occupations can you name? Compare your list with those of your classmates. Which occupations did they mention that you didn't, and vice versa? Combine all the health occupations into one master list and add up the total. How many health occupations did you and your classmates identify? How many more health occupations do you think may exist?

In an effort to help students explore different career options and prepare for the occupation of their choice, the National Career Clusters™ Framework focuses on sixteen Career Clusters™ and related Career Pathways. Career clusters link what students learn in school with the knowledge, skills, and abilities they will need for success in future careers or educational pursuits. Career clusters and pathways also help schools and communities develop their courses and educational programs. Partnerships that involve states, schools, educators, and industries are creating guidelines, technical standards, and assessments for these career clusters.

Health Science is one of the sixteen career clusters. (Reprinted with permission by the NASDCTEc/NCTEF 2012, www.careertech.org.) Some of the other clusters include:

- Agriculture, Food, and Natural Resources
- Business Management and Administration
- Education and Training
- Finance
- Hospitality and Tourism
- Manufacturing
- Transportation, Distribution, and Logistics

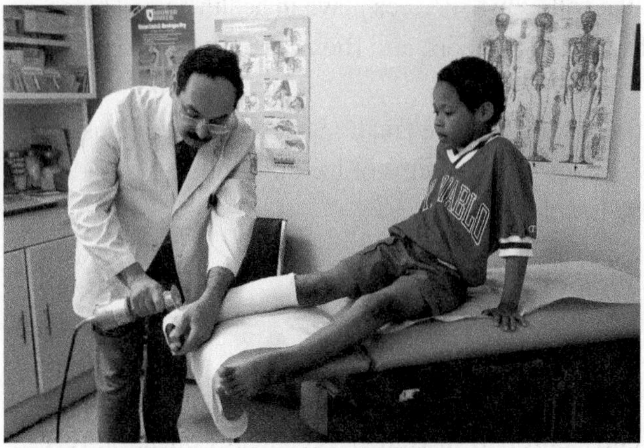

FIGURE 1.4

Working on a plaster cast to repair a broken leg

Source: Michal Heron/Pearson Education

For more information, visit the National Association of State Directors of Career Technical Education Consortium (NASDCTEc) website at www.careertech.org.

Health care is one of the largest and fastest growing industries in the United States. The Health Science Career Cluster is defined as "planning, managing, and providing therapeutic services, diagnostic services, health informatics, support services, and biotechnology research and development." The following information describes the types of services and careers included within the Health Science cluster pathways:

- ***Therapeutic Services*** focus on the changing health status of the patient over time. Professionals work directly with the patient; they provide care, treatment, counseling, and education. Some examples include physical therapists, respiratory therapists, athletic trainers, and dental hygienists.
- ***Diagnostic Services*** address the tests and evaluations that help to detect, diagnose, and treat disease, injuries, and other physical conditions. Some examples include medical laboratory technicians, pathologists, radiographers, and electroneurodiagnostic (END) technologists.
- ***Health Informatics Services*** include managing patient data and information, handling financial information, using computer applications to perform processes and procedures, and developing programs to improve quality of care and health care delivery. Some examples are admitting clerks, medical coders, financial analysts, medical librarians, and medical transcriptionists.
- ***Support Services*** include occupations that help provide a safe, supportive environment for the delivery of health care. These positions can start as **entry-level** with housekeepers (environmental services workers) or food service workers, for example, and may lead to management, technical, and professional careers. Some examples include dietitians, equipment repair technicians, hospital maintenance engineers, and telecommunications operators.

entry-level
(en-TREE LEV-uhl) A starting position for someone with little or no experience

- ***Biotechnology Research and Development Services*** address bioscience applications to human health. These individuals may conduct research to find new treatments for diseases, improve diagnostic testing, or create new medical devices to advance medical care. Some of the occupations in this field include biomedical engineers, biochemists, microbiologists, clinical trials coordinators, and research assistants.

APPLY IT MASTER LIST OF HEALTH OCCUPATIONS

Review the master list of health occupations that you and your classmates developed. Consider each occupation and decide if it belongs in Therapeutic Services, Diagnostic Services, Health Informatics Services, Support Services, or Biotechnology Research and Development Services. Into which category did most of the occupations fall? Why do you think that you and your classmates were most familiar with these types of occupations? Which category had the fewest occupations identified, and why do you think this is the case?

Another organization that's geared to strengthening the knowledge, skills, and abilities of health care students is the National Consortium for Health Science Education (NCHSE). This collaborative effort among educators, health care leaders, policy makers, and professional organizations has produced National Health Care Skills Standards, including *pathway standards,* for each of the five health care pathways. Pathway standards answer the question, "What does a worker need to know and be able to contribute to the delivery of safe and effective health care?" Foundational standards outline the *core expectations* required for occupational success for most health care workers. They provide *accountability criteria* to help measure student achievement, and a common language and shared goals for educators, employers, and consumers. Foundation standards cover the following topics:

- Academic foundation
- Communications
- Systems
- Employability skills
- Legal responsibilities
- Ethics
- Safety practices
- Teamwork
- Health maintenance practices
- Technical skills
- Information Technology/Applications

To learn more about the National Consortium for Health Science Education and to view the National Healthcare Foundation Standards and Accountability Criteria, visit www.healthscienceconsortium.org.

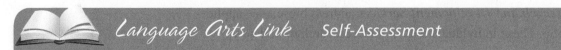

Language Arts Link Self-Assessment

Determining your likes, dislikes, and priorities is an important part of deciding your career path. Do you prefer working alone or as part of a team? Would you be willing to work the night shift at your local hospital or would the day or evening shift be better for you? Do you want to work in a small setting or in a large organization? Only you can answer these questions. Create a new document on the computer, or use a blank sheet of paper. Create a letter to your teacher describing your work-related priorities and needs. Include a thesis statement (a sentence stating your main ideas) in the opening paragraph. Be sure to incorporate information on the major factors that would influence what career path you take. Explain the importance of identifying your personal likes, dislikes, and priorities when choosing a career path. Be sure to proofread your work to see if you can improve it by making it clearer, more concise, or more interesting to read. Check the spelling and grammar and correct any errors.

EDUCATION AND CAREER PLANNING

With such a variety of occupations to consider, and so many educational standards to meet, you've probably realized that making the best career decisions for you might be a challenge. You don't have to make major decisions about your future right now. The first step is to learn more about the health care industry and what will be expected of you as a health care professional.

This chapter presents a broad overview of the health occupations that employ the largest numbers of workers. Before examining these occupations, let's take a look at some of the choices you'll need to make about where you would like to work and how you will need to prepare to launch your health career successfully.

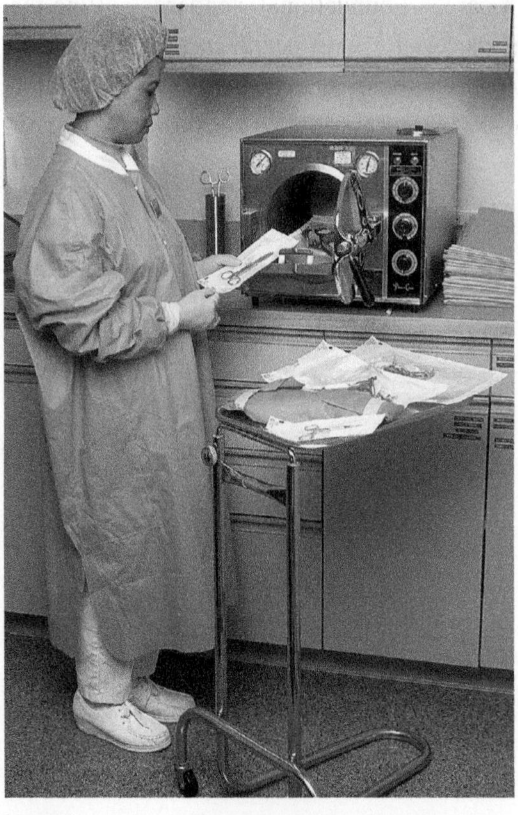

FIGURE 1.5

Operating an autoclave to sterilize surgical instruments

Source: Craig X. Sotres/Pearson Education

One of the benefits of pursuing a health career is having a variety of environments in which to work. In the mid-twentieth century, most health care was delivered at a doctor's office or in a hospital. Now the focus is moving from hospitals to the **outpatient** environment where patients can be cared for more quickly and at less expense. Job opportunities are growing in clinics, urgent care centers, satellite imaging and surgery centers, occupational health centers, step-down and short-term stay units, rehabilitation facilities, extended care facilities, and so forth.

outpatient
(OUT-pey-shuhnt) A place to receive medical care without being admitted to a hospital, or a person who receives medical care someplace other than a hospital

You also have several options for education, training, and entry points into health care employment. These include:

- *On-the-job Training:* You can apply for an entry-level job and receive on-the-job training after you've been hired. This is a good way to *get your foot in the door*, start earning an income, and explore career options while working in that particular setting. Most of these jobs require a high school diploma or GED. If you want to work toward advancement and increase your income, you'll need additional training and possibly a college degree and/or a license or professional certification depending on the occupation you choose. Some health care employers provide tuition assistance, tutoring, or on-site training programs to help entry-level employees advance within the organization.
- *Postsecondary Training Programs:* You can apply for admission into a health care training program after completing your high school education. These programs typically award a Certificate of Completion once you've met the necessary requirements to graduate. In addition to completing a *certificate program*, you may also need to obtain a license or a professional certification to be eligible for employment. Typically, students don't earn college credits when enrolling in certificate programs. However some colleges and universities will award college credits later once you have earned a license or certification and gained work experience in the field.
- *College Degree Programs:* Several health occupations require a college degree to be eligible for employment. Students can earn an associate's degree, bachelor's degree, master's degree, or doctorate degree depending on the career chosen. In addition, you may also need to obtain a license or professional certification. Some occupations require a specific amount of continuing education each year and even periodic retesting in order to maintain the *active status* of a license or certification. Once you've earned your first degree and gained some work experience, you may need to return to school at some point in your career to earn an advanced degree in order to advance in your field.

It's helpful to remember that in health care you'll need to *learn more to earn more.* Taking the on-the-job training route may sound good since you can begin a job right after high school and start earning a paycheck. However, unless you acquire additional education and training fairly soon, you may find yourself working in an entry-level job with little hope for advancement. Compare the information provided in "The Connection between Education and Income" on the following page with the different levels of education required for various health careers and the average salary for each.

Most health care disciplines offer **career ladders** that identify *next steps* and opportunities for advancement within the field. Career ladders help you move upward within your discipline. For example, radiographers might earn a Computerized Tomography (CT), Magnetic Resonance Imaging (MRI), or Mammography certification to increase their career options and income. **Career lattices** allow you to use your **transferable skills** to move from one discipline to another. For example, medical assistants might add an Electrocardiography (EKG) certification to expand their career options, or continue their education to become registered nurses or cardiovascular technologists. Because there are so many different health careers to consider, both career ladders and lattices provide many choices.

career ladder
(kuh-REER LAD-er) A vertical sequence of job positions to increase rank and pay

career lattice
(kuh-REER LAT-is) Related job positions offering vertical and lateral movement

transferable skills
(trans-FURABL SKILLS) Skills acquired in one job that are applicable in another job

THE MORE YOU KNOW

The Connection between Education and Income

According to the report "Education Pays 2010: The Benefits of Higher Education for Individuals and Society" by the College Board Advocacy and Policy Center, continuing your education after high school can really pay off. What follows are some interesting findings from the College Board's research (note: *high school graduate* statistics include people with a GED):

- People with bachelor's degrees working **full-time** earned almost $22,000/year more than those with a high school education. Anyone who completed some college, but not a degree, still earned 17% more per year than high school graduates.
- In 2008, women age 25 to 34 with a bachelor's degree or higher earned 79% more than women with a high school education; men with a bachelor's degree or higher earned 74% more. The income gap is widening. In 1998, the difference in earnings was 60% for women and 54% for men.
- People with bachelor's degrees will earn about 66% more over the course of their working lives than people with a high school education.
- People with higher education are more likely to work full-time, year-round. The unemployment rate at the end of 2009 for young adults age 20 to 24 was 2.6 times higher for high school graduates than for college graduates. The unemployment rate for people with at least a bachelor's degree is about half of the unemployment rate for those with just a high school education.

To learn more, go to http://trends.collegeboard.org/downloads/Education_Pays_2010.pdf to access the College Board report.

full-time
(FUL-time) Working approximately 40 hours per week

multiskilled
(MUHL-tee skild) Cross-trained to perform more than one function, often in more than one discipline

clerical
(KLER-i-kuhl) Of or pertaining to keeping records, filing, typing, or other general office tasks

You may also become **multiskilled** at some point in your career, cross-trained to perform more than one function and often in more than one discipline. For example, a general practice dental assistant might be cross-trained to also function as an orthodontic or pedodontic assistant. You might decide to make a *lateral move*, switching to another job or a different discipline at the same pay level as your current job. Lateral moves often don't lead to immediate pay increases but may create more opportunities for future job advancements. For example, a department secretary might become an accounts payable clerk in order to start working her way up the career ladder to become a financial analyst. Some health care workers are already multiskilled when they enter the workforce. Medical assisting is a good example. MAs acquire both clinical and **clerical** skills, working in the *back office* to assist physicians in providing patient care and also in the *front office* to schedule patients, handle financial transactions, and coordinate paperwork and medical records.

As you learn about the different health careers and start thinking about which occupation might be best for you, also consider the educational requirements for each level of worker. Remember, you can *start at the bottom* and work your way up if you want to. Nursing is a good example. You can begin your nursing career in an entry-level job right

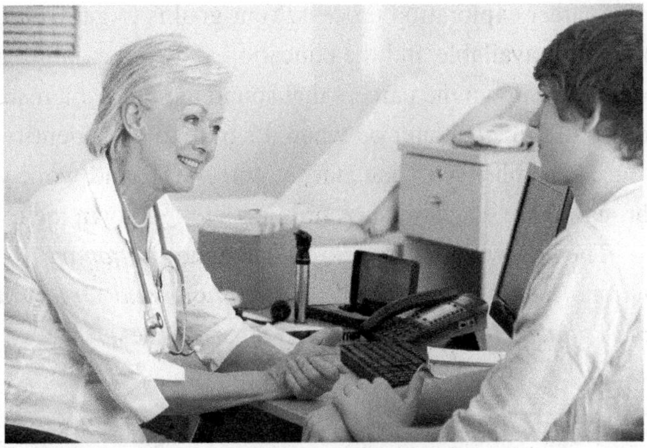

FIGURE 1.6

A multiskilled medical assistant reports test results for a patient

Source: Monkey Business Images/ Shutterstock

out of high school, or you can enroll in college and start your nursing career at a higher level. An entry-level position in this field would be the nursing assistant.

Nursing assistants complete a short-term training program that includes both classroom and clinical time, and they must pass an examination to become Certified Nursing Assistants (CNAs). The Licensed Practical Nurse (LPN) or Licensed Vocational Nurse (LVN) role requires completing one year of formal education and passing a board examination. The Registered Nurse (RN) requires the minimum of a two-year associate's degree or up to a four-year bachelor's degree plus passing a board exam. Registered nurses with graduate degrees, such as a master's degree in nursing, can practice at a higher level as a Nurse Practitioner (NP), diagnosing, treating, and supporting patients with simple medical problems or promoting higher standards of care for a specific population of patients, such as **geriatric** patients. Registered nurses may pursue advanced degrees to function as Physician Assistants (PAs). Registered nurses who complete a doctoral degree in nursing, and earn the credential DNS, are prepared to participate in research and a more advanced scientific role in nursing.

geriatric
(jer-ee-A-trik) Specializing in health care for elderly patients

Admission into an associate's or bachelor's degree program in nursing is often very competitive. Applicants who are certified nursing assistants typically have an advantage over those who are not.

Often times, life situations can dictate the factors you use to make decisions about your education and career goals. Here are some questions people typically ask themselves:

- How much time can I devote to my education right after high school?
- Do I have the support I need from my family and friends to continue my education?
- Do I have sufficient financial resources to enroll in college or a postsecondary training program?
- If I must borrow money for school, will I eventually make enough money to repay my school loans?
- Should I start at a lower level now and make plans to seek more education and training later?

Taking the time to investigate thoroughly the job duties and education, training, and credentialing requirements for the occupations that sound appealing to you will help you make the best decisions for you and your family.

As mentioned previously, occupations within the Health Science Cluster are divided into pathways. Start reading about Therapeutic Services and work your way through all five pathways. You'll also find some additional lists of health occupations toward the end of this chapter, organized in several different ways. Before you start reading, be aware. What follows is a lengthy list of occupations and job titles, many of which may sound unfamiliar and confusing to you. Try not to become overwhelmed at this stage of your career exploration process. Your goal is to gain a *big picture view* of the vast array of careers available and the education and credentialing requirements involved. As you read, write down the careers that sound the most interesting and most practical for you. You'll use this list later on when it's time to start identifying the best career choices for you. Remember, you can start at entry-level and work your way up the career ladder through more education and training later on down the road.

The following information is from the *Dictionary of Occupational Titles*, the *Occupational Outlook Handbook, Descriptions and Organizational Analysis for Hospitals and Related Health Services,* and other sources.

BUILD YOUR SKILLS *Researching References*

An important aspect of learning is the ability to conduct research and find credible information when you need it. The Internet provides large databases of information that can be especially helpful when researching the different health careers. The O*NET Resource Center is a good example. This website serves as an occupational information network (sponsored by the U.S. Department of Labor, Employment and Training Administration) that provides occupational information on hundreds of different jobs to help people explore career options. Resources include occupational descriptions and the necessary training, credentialing, and work experience requirements. It also lists the knowledge, skills, and abilities that people need to be successful in each specific field. Interactive tools and assessments help people identify careers that best match their individual needs and interests. The website also provides information on wages and labor trends. Go to www.onetcenter.org to explore this rich and robust reference, and begin sharpening your research skills.

CAREERS IN THERAPEUTIC SERVICES

Therapeutic service workers observe the patient, instrumentation, and environment. They report results and assist the treatment team by performing procedures accurately. They also assist in reaching treatment goals.

Respiratory Therapy/Respiratory Care Workers

Every breath is the breath of life, and helping patients with their breathing is an important part of health care. Patients may live without water for a few days. They may live without food for a few weeks. But without air, they will suffer brain damage within a few minutes and may die after nine minutes.

Respiratory therapy workers and respiratory care practitioners evaluate, treat, and care for patients of all ages who have breathing problems. Therapists test lung capacity and check blood for oxygen and carbon dioxide content. They give treatments and teach self-care to patients with **chronic** respiratory problems. They also provide emergency care following drowning, stroke, shock, heart failure, and other emergencies. Other duties may include keeping records and making minor repairs to equipment.

chronic
(KRON-ik) Occurs frequently over a long period of time

Respiratory care workers have many career options and work in acute care hospitals, cardiopulmonary laboratories, ambulatory care units, health maintenance organizations, home health agencies, and nursing homes. They work indoors and may be exposed to flammable gases and body fluids. Their jobs may require shift work and weekend work. They stand for long periods of time and carry or push equipment throughout the facility.

acute
(uh-KYOOT) Severe but over a short period of time

Thoracic Surgeons

A thoracic surgeon is a surgeon who specializes in treating conditions affecting organs in the chest. General thoracic surgeons specialize in the lungs and esophagus. Cardiothoracic surgeons also care for the heart and major blood vessels. Using minimally invasive procedures, thoracic surgeons perform heart bypass operations and heart and lung transplants. They also remove cancerous tumors. Thoracic surgeons treat patients during and after surgery, as well as while they are in critical care. Thoracic surgeons attend medical school and then complete five years in a general surgery residency and at least two years in a residency focusing on thoracic surgery.

invasive
(in-VEY-siv) Entering the body

Pulmonologists

Pulmonologists are physicians who are specially trained to treat diseases and conditions of the chest. These conditions, which affect the lungs and bronchial tubes, include such things as pneumonia, asthma, tuberculosis, and emphysema. Pulmonologists do not perform major surgical procedures, but they do often obtain samples from the lining of a lung or the chest wall for diagnostic testing. Pulmonology is a subspecialty of internal medicine. This means that in order to become a pulmonologist, you must first become certified in internal medicine. It takes at least seven years to accomplish this. Once this is completed, you must continue your studies for two or three more years focusing on conditions specifically related to the respiratory system.

specialists
(SPESH-uh-lists) People devoted to a particular occupation or branch of study

Respiratory Therapists

Respiratory therapists work with patients who have breathing or other cardiopulmonary disorders. Working under the direction of a physician, these specialists evaluate, treat, and care for patients and are primarily responsible for all respiratory care therapeutic treatments and diagnostic procedures. They also supervise respiratory care technicians, who perform many of these same functions. Respiratory therapists work with a variety of patients. For example, they may work with premature babies whose lungs are not fully developed. They may also work with elderly patients

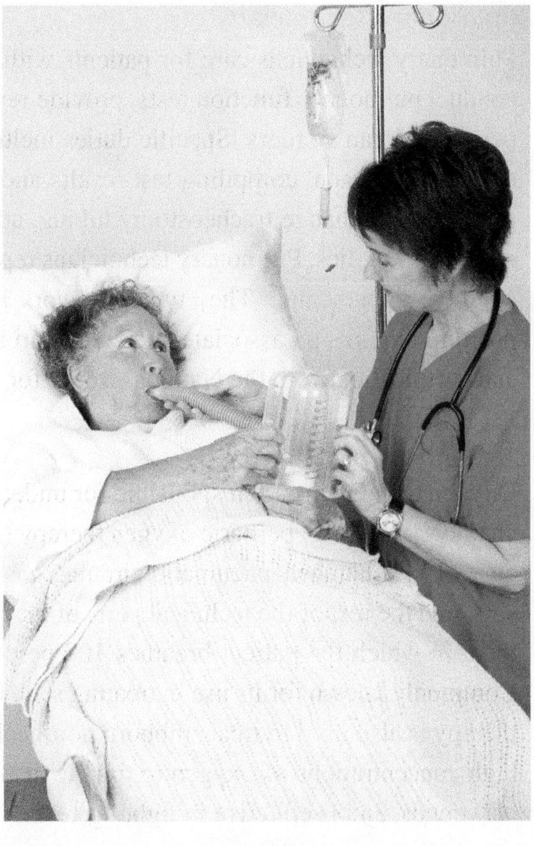

FIGURE 1.7

Undergoing a respiratory therapy procedure

Source: Lisa F. Young/Shutterstock

whose lungs are diseased. Many respiratory therapists work in hospitals. Some work for home health care agencies and travel to patients' homes. Many programs at colleges, universities, medical schools, and vocational/technical schools offer programs in respiratory therapy. Some programs offer an associate's degree, which would prepare you for an entry-level position. Others offer bachelor's degrees, which would prepare you for an advanced position in this field. Graduates must then pass a test to become either a Registered Respiratory Therapist (RRT) or a Certified Respiratory Therapist (CRT).

Tasks—Respiratory Therapy Aides

- Spend most time taking care of equipment
- Follow tasks under the direction of a respiratory therapist
- Scrub and wash equipment, such as respirators, intermittent positive pressure breathing machines, pulmonary function machines, and oxygen administration sets
- Inspect equipment for damage, and report problems to supervisor
- Start and test gauges, and notify supervisor of malfunctioning equipment
- Deliver oxygen tanks and other equipment where needed
- Assist in administration of gas or aerosol therapy as directed
- Record amount of oxygen used by patient, and prepare billing forms

For more information, write or go online:

American Association for Respiratory Care
9425 N. MacArthur Blvd. Suite 100
Irving, TX 75063-4706
www.aarc.org

Pulmonary Technicians

Pulmonary technicians care for patients with lung-related problems. These technicians conduct pulmonary function tests, provide respiratory-related care, and treat patients as per a physician's orders. Specific duties include educating patients on medications and the use of oxygen, compiling test results and reviewing them with physicians, helping physicians to change tracheostomy tubing, and maintaining pulmonary function equipment and supplies. Pulmonary technicians report to a nurse manager, physician, or other appropriate personnel. They typically work in a clinic, hospital, or other facility. This position requires an associate's degree from an accredited respiratory therapy program and certification from the National Board for Respiratory Care.

Oxygen Technicians

Oxygen technicians are responsible for understanding the use of the hyperbaric oxygen chamber, used in hyperbaric oxygen therapy (HBOT) programs. They have to check and control the chamber, pneumatic circuits, gas or compressed air reserves, air-compressors, and the rest of the technical parts of the facility. This is a specialized medical treatment in which the patient breathes 100 percent oxygen inside a pressurized chamber. Commonly known for its use in treating scuba diving complications, modern hyperbaric therapy is also used to treat stubborn non-healing wounds. The therapy quickly delivers high concentrations of oxygen to the bloodstream, which assists in the healing process of wounds, and is effective in fighting certain types of infections. These technicians are high-level specialists, needing a degree with a specialty in Pneumatic Systems, Hyperbaric Technology, or the like.

Pharmacy Workers

Pharmacy workers prepare and dispense medications prescribed by physicians, podiatrists, dentists, and other health care professionals. They provide information to health care professionals and to the public about medicines. Another important task is to review the medicines that patients are taking. This reduces the chance that the patient will have a drug interaction that can cause illness or an allergic reaction. They also help in the strict control of the distribution and use of government-controlled products, such as narcotics and barbiturates. Because vaccines and other drugs deteriorate over time, pharmacy workers are responsible for careful inventory control.

dispense
(dih-SPENS) To distribute or pass out

Pharmacy workers have many career options and work in acute hospitals, community pharmacies, health maintenance organizations, home health agencies, and clinics. A pharmacist may also work for state and local health departments, as well as for pharmaceutical manufacturers. Pharmacy workers work indoors and may be required to work in a restricted environment, such as areas where sterile solutions are prepared. In large hospitals or community pharmacies, they may work in shifts. Their work requires lifting, carrying, pushing items, and climbing ladders in storage areas. They need good vision for close-up work. They stand for long periods of time and must take proper safety precautions when working with products that can be dangerous.

Tasks—Pharmacy Assistants and Technicians

- Type labels for medications
- Maintain records and transactions in the pharmacy log
- Attach typed labels to medication requests and deliver to the pharmacist
- Assign prescription numbers
- Copy physician's instructions for use of medication
- Calculate charges, type billing slips for prescriptions, and enter charges on medication forms
- Compile periodic reports from log book
- Label pharmaceutical preparations by using a typewriter, printer, or computer, and maintain records and files
- Rotate stock to keep dated items current and order supplies
- Run errands and deliver orders
- Clean equipment and work areas according to department procedures
- Destroy damaged drugs according to department standards
- Use aseptic techniques, follow procedure for working under purification hood, and wear appropriate clothing and disposable caps

aseptic
(uh-SEP-tik) Free from the living germs of disease

For more information, write or go online:

American Association of Colleges of Pharmacy
1727 King Street
Alexandria, VA 22314
www.aacp.org

Occupational Therapy Workers

Occupational therapy workers treat people who are mentally, physically, developmentally, or emotionally disabled. They evaluate the self-care, work, and leisure skills of their patients. They plan and develop programs that help restore, develop, and maintain patients' abilities to manage the activities of daily living. The goal is to optimize the patient's functional independence by helping them compensate for their limitations.

Occupational therapy workers have many career options and work in general hospitals, schools, nursing homes, outpatient clinics, rehabilitation centers, day care centers, mental health agencies, special workshops, health maintenance organizations, and psychiatric hospitals. They work a 40-hour week and may have to work evenings or weekends occasionally. The work environment depends on the type of facility. In a large rehabilitation center, therapists may work in a spacious room equipped with machines, hand tools, and other devices. In a psychiatric hospital, they may work on the ward. They carry and lift equipment and transfer patients from wheelchairs. Their work requires both standing and sitting. Occupational therapists need to be creative; they have to design equipment and tools for their patient's individual needs.

Tasks—Occupational Therapy Aides

- Transport patients, assemble equipment, and prepare and maintain work areas
- Perform clerical tasks, restock and order supplies, answer the phone, and schedule appointments

Tasks—Occupational Therapy Assistants

- Teach work-related skills such as the use of power tools
- Help patients with rehabilitative activities and exercises
- Teach proper method of moving from a wheelchair to bed
- Observe patient activities for progress and make reports to aid in evaluation of patient progress
- Assist in adaptation of equipment, splints, and other self-help devices
- Transport patients
- Store equipment, clean work areas, and help maintain tools and equipment
- Perform other clerical duties such as filing

FIGURE 1.8

Undergoing physical therapy to regain stability

Source: Tyler Olson/Fotolia LLC

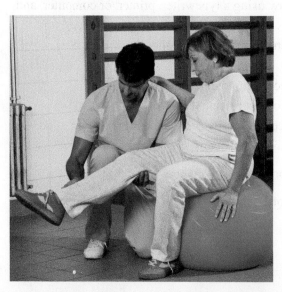

For more information, write or go online:

American Occupational Therapy Association, Inc.
Division of Credentialing
4720 Montgomery
PO Box 31220
Bethesda, MD 20824-1220
www.aota.org

Physical Therapy and Sports Medicine Workers

Physical therapy workers help people with injuries or diseases of the muscles, nerves, joints, and bones to overcome their disabilities. The patient may be disabled from an accident, a stroke, or a disease. Some of the conditions that require treatment are multiple sclerosis, cerebral palsy, nerve injuries, amputations, fractures, arthritis, and heart disease. Patients vary in age from newborn to elderly. Physical therapy workers help the patient regain as close to normal activity as possible. A subset of this category includes sports medicine, or sports therapy workers, who specialize in treating disabilities caused by sports-related injuries.

Physical therapy workers have many career options and work in acute care and long-term care facilities, ambulatory care units, health maintenance organizations, rehabilitation centers, schools, public health agencies, home health care agencies, and sports medicine centers. Some physical therapists are in private practice. They contract to work for health care agencies or may have an office where they provide care. They work in specially equipped physical therapy departments, in clinics, and in private homes. Their work requires lifting and carrying up to 50 pounds, stooping, pushing, and pulling patients and equipment. They stand and walk during their shifts.

Physical Therapists

Physical therapists (PTs) work with accident victims and people who suffer from disabling conditions such as lower back pain, fractures, heart disease, and cerebral palsy. PTs help these patients restore function, improve mobility, relieve pain, and prevent or limit permanent physical disabilities. PTs test and measure everything from a patient's strength and range of motion to their balance and coordination. They develop individualized treatment plans that may include things such as electrical stimulation, hot packs and cold compresses, ultrasound, traction, or deep-tissue massage. Physical therapists typically work a 40-hour week. Most PTs work in hospitals, clinics, and private offices. To become a physical therapist, you must graduate from an accredited physical therapy program with either a master's or a clinical doctorate degree and pass a state-administered national exam. With additional training and clinical experience, physical therapists may specialize in sports medicine. Sports physical therapists help athletes prevent and treat injuries and improve their performance.

Physical Therapist Assistants

Physical therapist assistants (PTAs) work under the direct supervision of a licensed physical therapist. They assist in implementing patient treatment plans, teach patients how to use crutches and walkers, and help people learn how to exercise properly to build strength and coordination. To become a physical therapist assistant, you must graduate from an accredited physical therapist assistant educational program and meet state licensure or certification requirements.

Physical Therapist Aides

Physical therapist aides provide support for therapists and assistants. Some are trained on-the-job and others complete a short-term vocational program.

Tasks—Physical Therapist Aides

- Prepare equipment such as hydrotherapy pools, paraffin baths, and hot packs
- Assist patients:
  - With walking and gait training
  - To dress and undress
  - To position themselves
  - To remove and replace braces, splints, and slings
- Change linens on beds and tables
- Fold linens
- Clean equipment and work area
- May inventory materials and supplies

Sports Medicine Professionals

Sports medicine is one of the fastest growing fields in medicine. It includes working with professional sports teams, high school and college athletes, and individuals with sports-related injuries. Sports medicine professionals include sports medicine assistants and aides, exercise physiologists, athletic trainers, personal trainers, health fitness specialists, and exercise instructors.

Sports Medicine Assistants

Under the direct supervision of a physician, a sports medicine assistant works specifically with athletes. Duties include helping diagnose, treat, and prevent injuries, as well as assisting athletes with their nutrition, training, and conditioning. Specifically, a sports medicine assistant might recommend protective gear, supervise trainers, or develop training or rehabilitation programs.

Sports medicine assistants can be found in school athletic departments, community recreation programs, health and fitness clubs, sports centers, resorts, clinics specializing in sports medicine, or even in a private practice. To become a sports medicine assistant, you need a four-year degree. This is a growing profession, and the qualifications required are rapidly evolving.

Sports Medicine Aides

One subspecialty of working as a physical therapy aide is working as a sports medicine aide. Sports medicine aides perform the duties of physical therapy aides but deal with the practical aspects of sports injury prevention, recognition, and treatment of sports-related injuries.

Tasks—Sports Medicine Aides

- Perform all the duties of a physical therapy aide
- Prepare equipment such as massage tables
- Assist in injury treatments, evaluations, and rehabilitation of athletes

- Assist or perform taping, wrapping, protective bracing, and equipment fitting
- Assist in pre-practice preparations and post-practice follow-up
- Assist in event coverage

Athletic Trainers

Athletic trainers prevent, diagnose, and treat injuries and illnesses of the muscles and bones. They work under the direct supervision of a physician or another health care professional, and may meet with sports team physicians and athletic directors on a regular basis. To become an athletic trainer, you need a bachelor's or master's degree from an accredited program. Most states require certification or licensure.

Tasks—Athletic Trainers

- Apply tape, bandages, and braces
- Recognize and evaluate injuries
- Provide emergency care and first aid
- Treat injured athletes via rehabilitation techniques
- Design programs to prevent athletic injuries and illnesses
- Maintain records and write reports

For more information, write or go online:

American Physical Therapy Association
1111 North Fairfax Street
Alexandria, VA 22314-1488
www.apta.org

American College of Sports Medicine
401 West Michigan Street
Indianapolis, IN 46202-3233
www.acsm.org

National Athletic Trainers' Association
2952 Stemmons Freeway #200
Dallas, TX 75247
www.nata.org

FIGURE 1.9

Applying a therapeutic technique in sports medicine

Source: Guy Cali/Corbis Images

Radiation Therapy Workers

Radiation therapy workers assist physicians (radiation oncologists) in using ionizing radiation to treat patients with cancer. They expose specific areas of the patient's body to radiation using high-energy linear accelerators, particle generators, and radioactive isotopes. Radiation therapy technologists or therapists work in hospitals and cancer treatment centers. They spend most of their time standing and lifting patients and equipment. Unlike many other types of health care workers, radiation therapists typically work only on weekdays and during the day shift, except when called in after hours for emergencies. Therapists must be ever mindful of radiation safety procedures, and they may experience stress in working with cancer patients. Most states require certification and licensure for radiation therapy workers.

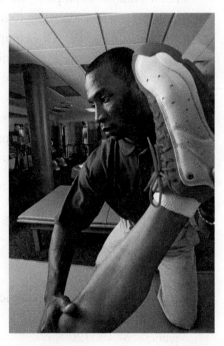

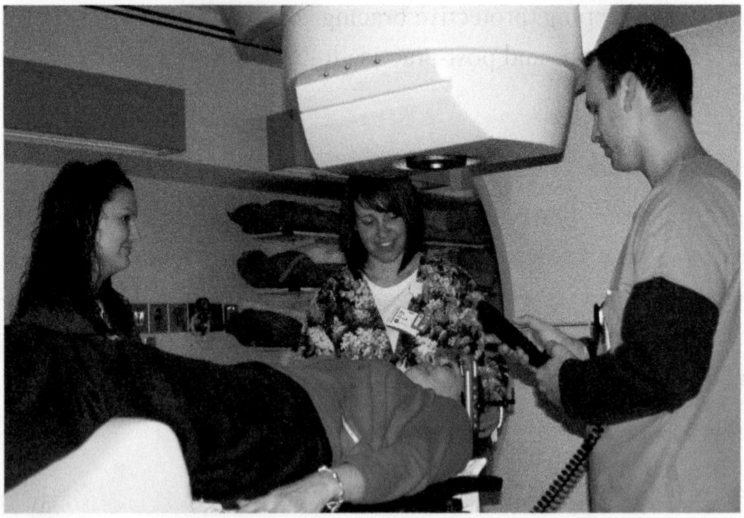

FIGURE 1.10
Positioning a patient for a radiation therapy treatment

Source: Carmen Martin/Pearson Education

Tasks—Radiation Therapy Technologists/Therapists

- Produce images to pinpoint the location of the patient's tumor
- Apply procedures according to the patient's treatment plan
- Position the patient and the equipment for the treatment
- Explain the procedure to the patient
- Operate the equipment according to established protocols
- Monitor the patient's physical condition during the treatment
- Report complications and adverse patient reactions
- Maintain strict radiation safety procedures
- Document treatments and maintain medical records

For more information, write or go online:

American Society of Radiologic Technologists
15000 Central Ave. SE
Albuquerque, NM 87123-3909
www.asrt.org

American Registry of Radiologic Technologists
1255 Northland Drive
Mendota, MN 55120
www.arrt.org

Science Link *Ionizing Radiation*

Radiation therapists and diagnostic imaging workers use ionizing radiation to diagnose and treat medical conditions. Go online to learn more about ionizing radiation, how it is produced, how it is controlled, and how it creates both benefits and risks for patients and workers. Identify places where ionizing radiation is used outside of the health care industry. (Clue—check manufacturing.) What science courses do radiation therapy and diagnostic imaging students need to master in order to use ionizing radiation safely and appropriately in the medical setting?

Surgery Workers

A variety of people work on teams to perform surgical procedures. These include general and specialized surgeons, surgical assistants, surgical nurses, and surgical technologists.

Surgeons

Surgeons are physicians who operate on patients to cure or prevent a disease, repair an injury, or solve other health problems. They review the patient's medical history and examine the patient to decide if surgery is necessary. They consult with the patient and the patients' other doctors to assess the surgical risks and determine the appropriateness of a surgical procedure. General surgeons perform a variety of operations. Specialized surgeons perform complex operations on certain parts of the body, such as the heart or brain. Other areas of specialization include orthopedics, pediatrics, neurosurgery, plastic surgery, and thoracic surgery. Most surgeons work in hospitals or in ambulatory (outpatient) surgery centers. They spend long hours standing on their feet, often working in cramped spaces, and frequently perform emergency operations. Eligibility to practice as a surgeon requires about five years of medical residency and internship experience after medical school, plus passing licensure and board exams.

For more information, write or go online:

American College of Surgeons
633 N Saint Clair Street
Chicago IL 60611-3211
www.facs.org

Surgical Assistants

Working under the direct supervision of a surgeon, surgical assistants help the surgeon perform safe operations on patients. They assist with pre- and post-surgery patient care. During surgical procedures, surgical assistants position the patient, handle surgical supplies and instruments, maintain a sterile field, clamp and cut tissue, close wounds, and insert drainage tubes. They assist in general surgeries and in specialized procedures such as obstetrical surgery, trauma surgery, and cardiac surgery. Graduates of surgical assisting educational programs may become a Certified First Assistant (CSFA) through the National Board of Surgical Technology and Surgical Assisting (NBSTSA).

For more information, write or go online:

National Surgical Assistant Association
2615 Amesbury Road
Winston Salem, NC 27103
www.nsaa.net

Association of Surgical Assistants
6 West Dry Creek Circle, Suite 210
Littleton, CO 80120
www.surgicalassistant.org

Surgical Nurses

A registered nurse with a bachelor's degree in nursing may elect to specialize in surgical procedures and become a surgical nurse (also called **perioperative** nurse, circulating nurse, or operating room nurse). With an acute awareness of the patient's physical,

perioperative
(per-ee-AWE-per-a-tiv) Three phases of surgery, from the time a decision is made to have surgery, through the operation itself, and until the patient has recovered

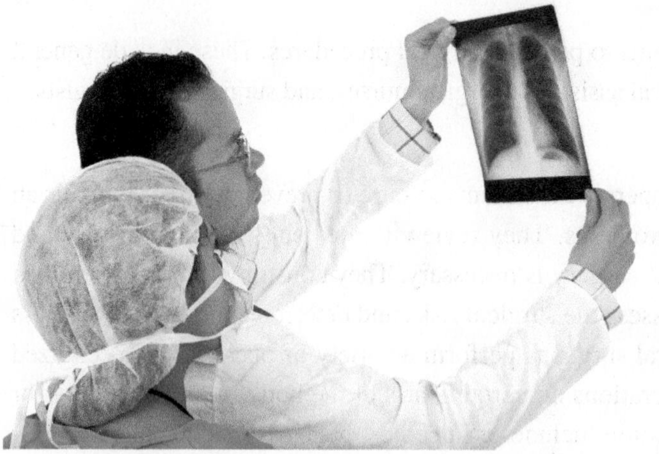

FIGURE 1.11
Reviewing medical records to prepare for surgery
Source: Andresr/Shutterstock

emotional, and psychological condition, the surgical nurse coordinates the patient's care before, during, and after the operation. The nurse assesses the patient's readiness for surgery, develops the patient's perioperative nursing care plan, and explains the procedure to the patient. Working in tandem with surgical technologists and other team members, the nurse helps maintain the sterile field and provides support to obtain optimal patient outcomes. After about two years of work experience in surgery, RNs may become certified as perioperative nurses.

For more information, write or go online:

Association of peri Operative Registered Nurses (AORN)
2170 South Parker Road, Suite 400
Denver, CO 80231
www.aorn.org

Surgical Technologists

Surgical technologists, also known as operating room technicians or scrub techs, are members of the surgical team who work under the supervision of surgeons and surgical nurses. Surgical technologists function as the sterile member of the surgical team. They "scrub" their hands and forearms, wear sterile gowns and gloves, and pass sterile instruments, sponges and sutures to the surgeon during operations. Surgical technologists work primarily in hospitals and ambulatory surgery centers. They spend long hours on their feet, taking few breaks, and often function in small spaces where sterile fields must be maintained. After completing a one- or two-year educational program, surgical technologists may become certified through the National Board of Surgical Technology and Surgical Assisting (NBSTSA). With additional education and work experience, technologists may become Surgical First Assistants.

Tasks—Surgical Technologists

- Prepare the operating room
- Set up equipment
- Organize supplies and instruments
- Arrange sterile drapes
- Wash and shave the patient
- Cover the incision site with sterile drapes
- Monitor the patient's vital signs
- Hold retractors
- Suction the incision site

For more information, write or go online:

Association of Surgical Technologists
6 West Dry Creek Circle, Suite 200
Littleton, CO 80120-8031
www.ast.org

Emergency Medical Service Workers

First responders are often the first trained people to treat patients. They provide emergency medical care before emergency medical technicians (EMTs) reach the scene. They may be law enforcement officers, members of the fire service, company employees, or private citizens.

Emergency medical technicians are providers of pre-hospital medical care in an emergency. A heart attack, unscheduled birth, automobile accident, or near drowning all require immediate attention. The EMT administers basic life support and transports sick and injured people to medical facilities. Paramedics, on the other hand, work within many emergency room settings in a similar role as a registered nurse. They can make independent medical emergency decisions, unlike an EMT. The difference between an EMT and a paramedic is the difference between basic and advanced life support training.

Emergency medical service workers have many career opportunities and may work in rescue, police, and fire departments, hospital emergency departments, private ambulance services, and ski patrols. They usually work shifts and weekends and work inside and outside in all weather conditions. They may be exposed to body fluids. Emergency medical service workers must be in good physical condition. For example, they must have good eyesight, hearing, and speech. They must also be able to lift heavy loads, reach, stoop, and climb as the job requires. Emergency medical service workers must be prepared to assess a situation quickly and to take steps for basic life saving actions.

Tasks—First Responders

- Gain access to patient, assess patient, provide appropriate care, and report assessment and care given
- Lift or move patient to a safe place if necessary

Tasks—Emergency Medical Technicians/A (Basic)

- Drive an ambulance
- Determine the nature of the victim's illness or injury
- Provide the following appropriate care:
  - Open and maintain the airway
  - Restore breathing
  - Control bleeding
  - Treat for shock
  - Immobilize fractures
  - Bandage wounds
  - Assist with childbirth

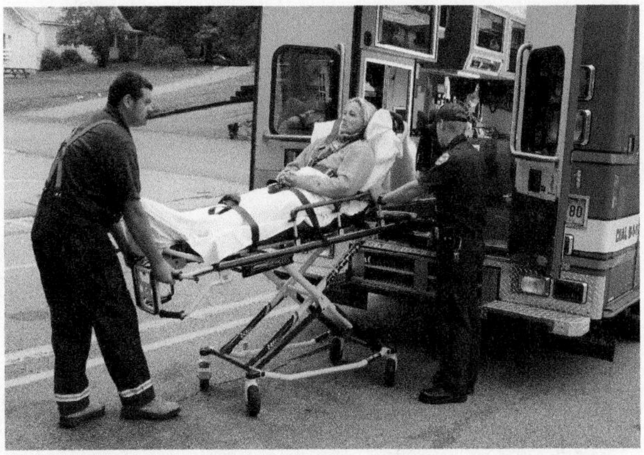

FIGURE 1.12
EMS professionals transporting a patient by ambulance

Source: Michal Heron/Pearson Education

  - Give initial care to poison and burn victims
  - Use automated external defibrillators
  - Use correct equipment and techniques to remove trapped victims safely
- Transport patients to hospital:
  - Place patient on stretcher
  - Constantly watch patient while in transport
  - Notify hospital of arrival
- Report to the emergency staff observations of and care given to the victim
- Maintain clean, well-equipped ambulance
- Ensure ambulance is in good running order:
  - Check gas, oil, tire pressure, siren, communication equipment

For more information, write or go online:

National Association of Emergency Medical Technicians
PO Box 1400
Clinton, MS 39060-1400
www.naemt.org

National Registry of Emergency Medical Technicians
PO Box 29233
Columbus, OH 43229
www.nremt.org

Medical Assistants

Medical assistants are responsible for the efficient operation of a physician's office. They also work in clinics, health maintenance organizations, and ambulatory care units. Medical assistants have varied duties. Some specialize in back office (clinical) procedures, while others choose to work in the front office. They work indoors in a clean environment, 40 hours a week, and some weekends.

MAs have varied job opportunities, and their work requires standing most of the day (back office), lifting, reaching, and helping patients. They may be exposed to body fluids. The front office worker sits at a desk for long periods at a time. The current trend toward large medical groups has relocated administrative/front office responsibilities. Billing, insurance verification, medical records, appointment scheduling, and payroll have been relocated to departments that specialize in handling work for the increased number of patients. See "Administrative Support Service Workers" later in this section for more information.

Tasks—Administrative/Front Office Medical Assistants

- Greet patients
- Answer phones
- Handle mail
- Make appointments
- Arrange hospital admissions
- Arrange for laboratory services
- Prepare insurance forms such as Medicare, medical insurance, workers' compensation
- Type medical reports

- Maintain patient files
- May handle billing and receipts
- Prepare payroll for office staff

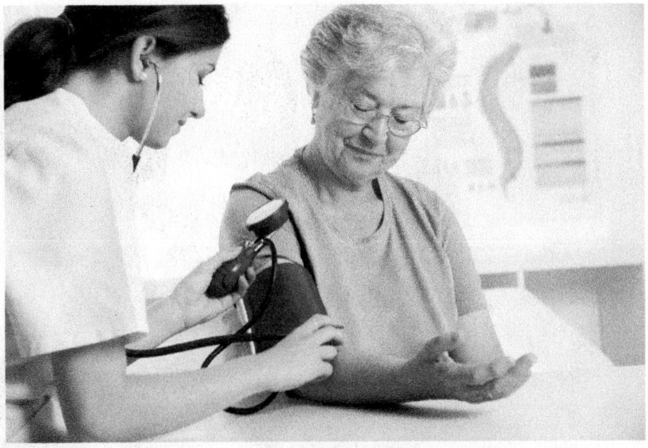

FIGURE 1.13

Medical assistant taking a patient's blood pressure

Source: Alexander Raths/Fotolia LLC

Tasks—Clinical/Back Office Medical Assistants (tasks vary according to state law)

- Sterilize instruments using an autoclave
- Prepare patients for examination
- Assist physician during examination
- Give injections
- Take and record temperature, pulse, respiration, and blood pressure
- Measure height and weight
- Perform routine urinalysis
- Collect blood samples
- Perform simple blood tests
- Record electrocardiograms
- Assist with minor surgery
- Direct patients in preparation for x-rays and tests
- Instruct patients about medication and special diets

For more information, write or go online:

American Association of Medical Assistants
20 North Wacker Drive, Suite 1575
Chicago, IL 60606-2903
www.aama-ntl.org

American Medical Technologists
10700 W. Higgins, Suite 150
Rosemont, IL 60018
www.americanmedtech.org

Dental Workers

Dental workers are responsible for maintaining oral health and repairing dental abnormalities. They emphasize treatment and prevention of problems associated with the hard and soft tissues of the mouth. According to their level of education, dental workers have many different opportunities. They work in private practices, dental schools, hospital dental departments, private clinics, health maintenance organizations, and state and local public health departments. Dental laboratory technicians work in a dental laboratory. Dental workers work indoors in a clean environment. They are subject to respiratory infections due to close contact with patients and may be exposed to body fluid. Their work requires standing most of the day, reaching, and handling dental instruments, equipment, and supplies.

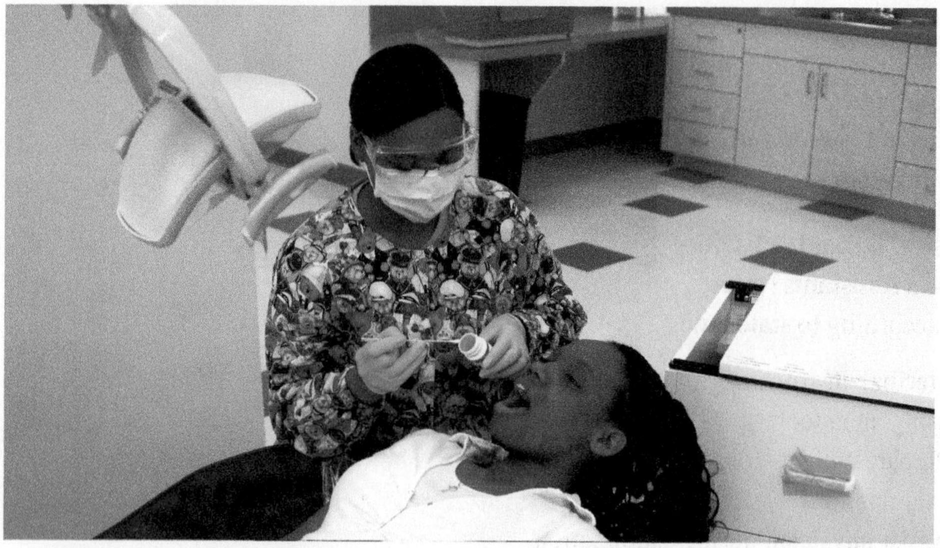

FIGURE 1.14
Patient receiving dental care
Source: Carmen Martin/Pearson Education

Tasks—Dental Assistants

- Work directly with the dentist in the treatment room
- Prepare and clean dental treatment rooms following infection control guidelines
- Prepare necessary equipment and instrumentation for dental procedures
- Process and mount dental x-rays
- Care for and maintain dental equipment
- Teach patients oral hygiene methods
- Take and pour study models (may be an expanded role in your state)
- Possibly perform front office duties
- Expose radiographs (x-rays); requires completion of a state-approved radiography course or examination

For more information, write or go online:

American Dental Association
211 East Chicago Avenue, Suite 1814
Chicago, IL 60611
www.ada.org

American Dental Assistants Association
35 East Wacker Drive, Suite 1730
Chicago, IL 60601-2211
www.dentalassistant.org

Nursing Service Workers

Nursing service workers provide many varied and essential services. They care for patients who are physically ill or disabled and provide preventive care such as immunizations. They work in industry, community health nursing, general hospitals, long-term care facilities, government agencies, schools, educational institutions, visiting nurse associations, clinics, physicians' offices, ambulatory care units, homes, and health maintenance organizations. Nurses work indoors. They may have rotating shifts and work on weekends. Their work requires standing, walking, lifting, and pushing patients, carts, and wheelchairs. They are exposed to unpleasant odors and body fluids.

preventive
(pri-VEN-tiv) Actions taken to avoid a medical condition

Registered Nurses

Registered nurses (RNs) care for patients in hospitals, clinics, doctor's offices, nursing homes, and patients' homes. Registered nurses take care of sick and injured people and work directly with patients and their families. They monitor and track vital signs and are the primary point of contact. Some RNs work with the public rather than with individual patients. They educate the public on warning signs and symptoms of various conditions and tell them where to get help. Some RNs run immunization clinics and blood drives. Some are trained in grief counseling. RNs account for the largest occupation in health care. Although they may work in a variety of settings, roughly three out of every five RNs work in a hospital.

With additional training and work experience, nurses may specialize in many different areas. Some examples include midwifery, obstetrics, pediatrics, labor and delivery, behavioral care, surgery, anesthesiology, cardiovascular care, orthopedics, interventional radiography, gerontology, home health care, hospice, and medical research.

Tasks—Registered Nurses

- Conduct physical assessments
- Collaborate with physicians and other health care team members to develop a treatment plan for the patient
- Direct the health care team
- Coordinate delivery of care and evaluate outcome of care
- Administer treatment and medications
- Educate patients about their medical conditions
- Provide advice and emotional support to patients and their families
- Record medical histories and symptoms
- Help perform diagnostic tests and analyze results
- Operate medical equipment
- Administer treatment and medications

Nurse Practitioners

A nurse practitioner (NP) is a registered nurse who has received additional education and clinical training in the diagnosis and treatment of illnesses. Most NPs have completed a two- or three-year master's degree program. Some have a doctorate degree in their specialty area, such as acute care, adult or family health, gerontology health, neonatal health, oncology, pediatric/child health, psychiatric/mental health, and women's health. NPs may further specialize in everything from allergy and immunology to urology. Nurse practitioners work in a variety of settings. They can be found everywhere, from clinics, hospitals, and private practices to nursing homes, schools, and public health departments. On the job, they order, perform, and interpret diagnostic tests, diagnose and treat common acute illnesses and injuries, prescribe medications and therapies, perform procedures, and educate patients and their families on living a healthy lifestyle.

Licensed Practical and Licensed Vocational Nurses

A licensed practical nurse (LPN), or licensed vocational nurse (LVN) as they are called in some states, provides basic care for patients. Their responsibilities are limited because all of their duties are conducted under the direct supervision of a physician or a registered

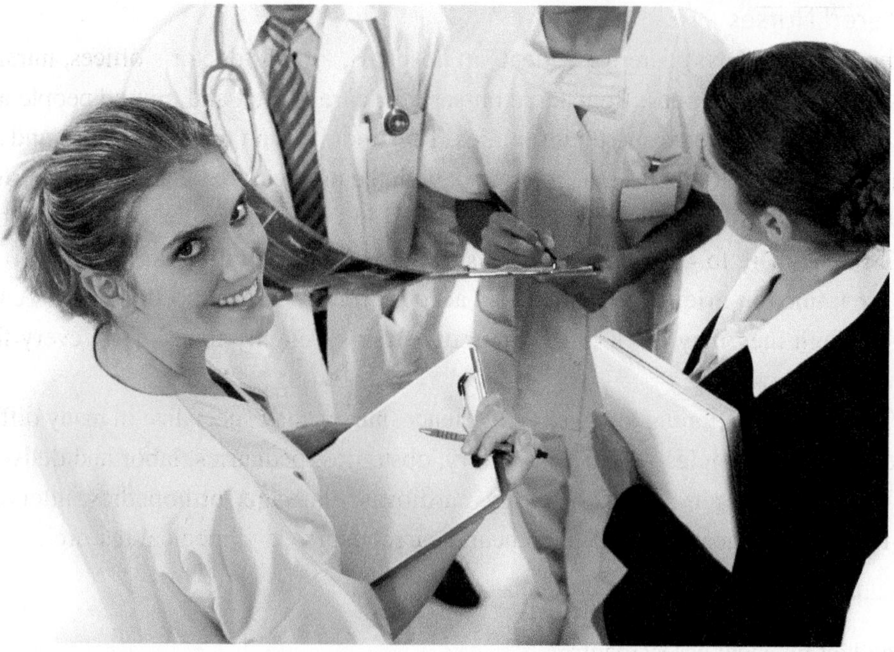

FIGURE 1.15

Nurses comparing notes and medical records to create a patient's treatment plan

Source: auremar/Fotolia LLC

nurse. A common task for an LPN/LVN is to take a patient's vital signs, which includes temperature, blood pressure, pulse, and respiration. LPN/LVNs also give injections and enemas, monitor catheters, collect samples, and conduct routine laboratory tests. They also apply dressings, treat bedsores, and give alcohol rubs and massages. They observe patients and report any adverse reactions to medications or treatments. They also help patients with personal hygiene and ensure the patients' comfort. Those wishing to become an LPN/LVN can attend a one-year program at a vocational or technical school and then pass a licensing examination. Many LPN/LVNs work in hospitals and nursing-care facilities. Others work in physicians' offices, outpatient-care facilities, or for pubic health care agencies.

Tasks—Licensed Practical/Vocational Nurses

- Provide technical care for the sick, injured, convalescent, and disabled under the direction of the registered nurse and physician
- Measure and record vital signs
- Prepare and give injections
- Dress wounds
- Assist with bathing, dressing, and personal hygiene
- Collect samples for testing
- Record food and fluid intake/output
- Clean and monitor medical equipment
- Monitor patients
- Teach family how to care for patients

For more information, go to www.nurse.org to find a state organization for nurses.

Nursing Assistants

Nursing assistants (NAs) work under the direct supervision of a nurse (RN). They have extensive daily contact with patients and are the caregivers who help patients perform day-to-day tasks, such as bathing, feeding, and dressing. They help patients walk and go to the bathroom. They transport patients, take vital signs, make beds, and set up equipment. Nursing assistants aid patients with activities of daily living and work as part of a collaborative team in the delivery of health care. Because of the physical requirements of the job, good physical conditioning is a plus. Nursing assistants work in hospitals, physicians' offices, home health agencies, nursing homes, private homes, and mental health institutions. To become a nursing assistant, you need at least a high school diploma followed by 120 hours of training. Some employers offer onsite training. Courses are also offered through high school health science programs, as well as at community and state colleges. Once training is complete, the nursing assistant may have the opportunity to be certified as a nursing assistant (CNA).

Tasks—Nursing Assistants

- Collaborate with the licensed nurse in charge of the patient's care to establish a plan of care and goals for care
- Answer patient call lights
- Bathe patients
- Dress and undress patients
- Assist with personal hygiene such as shaving, hair care, oral care, and dental care
- Serve and collect food trays and feed patients who need help
- Provide between-meal nourishment and fresh drinking water
- Transport patients in wheelchair or stretcher or help patients walk
- Take and record temperature, pulse, respiration, and blood pressure
- Record food and liquid intake and output
- Apply ice bags or heat packs as needed
- Give back rubs, if appropriate
- Observe and report any unusual conditions
- Tidy patients' rooms, change bed linens, and collect soiled linens
- Document in patients' charts

Home Health Aides

Home health aides care for patients in their homes instead of in a health facility. They care for patients of all ages who need more care than their families can give. Their job requires them to go to different homes. Similar to nurse assistants, home health aides stand, walk, and lift patients and may push wheelchairs. They may be exposed to body fluids.

Tasks—Home Health Aides

- Transfer patients from place to place and assist with bathing, walking, and prescribed exercises
- Assist with medication routines
- Help with braces or artificial limbs
- Check and record temperature, pulse, respiration, and blood pressure
- Change nonsterile dressings
- Provide emotional support

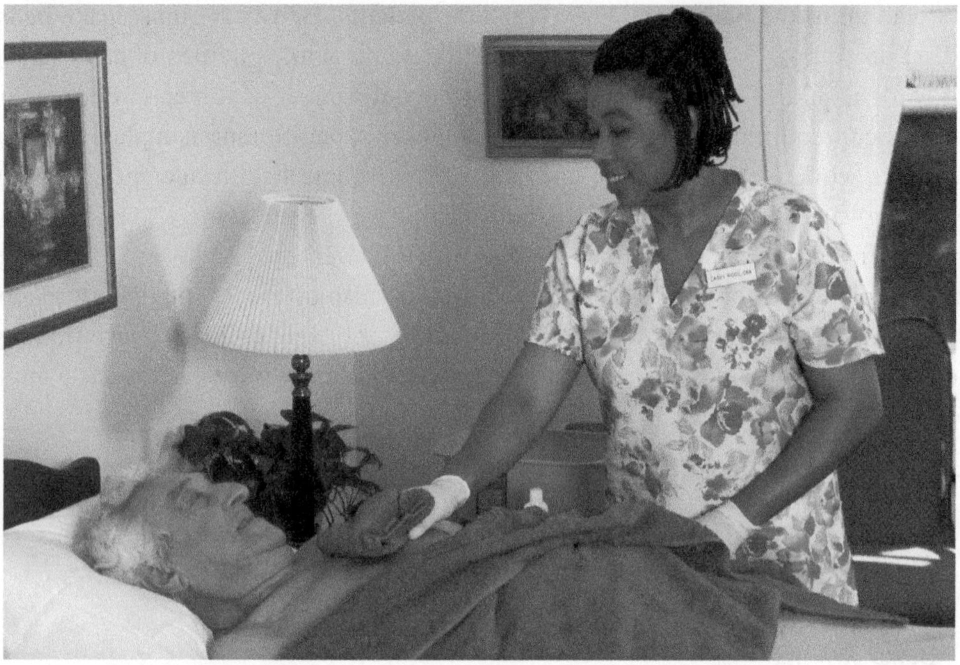

FIGURE 1.16
Home health aide cares for a patient in his home
Source: Michal Heron/Pearson Education

- Change bed linens, clean laundry, and clean patients' living quarters
- Shop for patients' food and prepare meals
- Report findings and observations to supervisors
- Act as a companion on shopping trips, doctor visits, and outdoor activities

For more information, write or go online:

National Association for Home Care & Hospice
228 Seventh Street SE
Washington, DC 20003
www.nahc.org

Veterinary Workers

Veterinary assistant animal caregivers usually care for small animals such as dogs and cats. They provide basic care such as feeding, grooming, cleaning cages, exercising animals, providing companionship, and observing animals for behavioral changes that can indicate an illness or injury. Other positions in animal care include working with horses, zoo animals, and laboratory animals used for research.

Animal care workers have many career opportunities. They may work in kennels, animal shelters, veterinary hospitals and clinics, stables, laboratories, aquariums, and zoological parks. Job titles and duties vary by employment setting. In some positions shift work may be required because the animals need 24-hour care. The work environment depends on the type of facility. Some kennels have outdoor animal runs; veterinary offices have exam and treatment rooms. Concern for and interest in animals may cause workers emotional upset due to witnessing the results of abuse or having to **euthanize** the animal. The work can be physically demanding as it may require lifting large bags of food, kneeling, bending, crawling, and restraining animals. A chance of injury caused by bites and scratches exists. Odors can be unpleasant.

euthanize
(YOO-thuh-nahyz) To painlessly end the life, or permit the death, of a hopelessly sick or injured animal or individual for reasons of mercy

Tasks—Animal Caretaker/Assistant

- Keep constant eye on condition of animals in their charge
- Monitor animals recovering from surgery
- Check dressings on wounds
- Observe animals' overall attitude
- Notify doctor of anything out of the ordinary
- Maintain sanitary conditions

Tasks—Kennel Staff

- Clean cages and dog runs
- Fill food and water dishes
- Exercise animals

Tasks—Experienced Attendants

- Provide basic animal health care
- Bathe animals
- Trim nails
- Attend to other grooming needs
- Sell pet food and supplies
- Assist in obedience training
- Help with breeding

Tasks—Groomers

- Perform initial brush-out
- Clip hair with electric clippers, cobs, and grooming shears
- Cut nails
- Clean ears
- Bathe animal
- Blow-dry animal
- Perform final clipping and styling

Tasks—Groomer/Owners

- Operate own grooming business
- Answer telephones
- Schedule appointments
- Discuss pets' grooming needs
- Collect information on pets' disposition
- Collect information on pets' veterinarian
- Inspect and report medical problems such as skin or ear infection

For more information, write or go online:

The Humane Society of the United States
2100 Street NW
Washington, DC 20037-1598
www.hsus.org

RECENT DEVELOPMENTS

Questioning Credibility

You're probably familiar with the saying, "Don't believe everything you hear." With so much information now available on the Internet, this warning should include, "Don't believe everything you read online." Let's face it—anyone can post just about anything they want on the web.

When information is credible, it can be trusted and believed. You must first ask several questions when judging the credibility of online information. According to a tutorial presented by the University of California Berkeley's Teaching Library (a *credible source*, at http://www.lib.berkeley.edu/TeachingLib/Guides/Internet/Evaluate.html), you can start by looking at the URL. Who is responsible for the web page? Can you identify the author? How much does the author really know about the subject? Does the author provide details about his or her sources of information? What can you discover by examining the author's links to other websites? Do other websites link to the author's site? How old is the webpage? Is the information up-to-date? Why was the information put on the web?

Visit UC Berkeley's website tutorial yourself. Review the questions to ask and the implications of each. Then use these questioning techniques yourself to assess the credibility of *your* sources.

CAREERS IN DIAGNOSTIC SERVICES

Diagnostic service workers help with the diagnosis of illnesses and diseases. Some diagnostic service workers have direct contact with the patient, whereas others do not. They plan services and prepare and perform tests accurately. They also understand quality control and report results in a timely manner.

Medical Laboratory Workers

Medical laboratory workers perform many varied tests. Some of these tests are highly technical, while others are less technical. In many cases, tests are performed on computerized equipment. Medical laboratory workers determine changes that have occurred in the blood, urine, lymph, and body tissues. They identify increases or decreases in white or red blood cells, cross-match blood for transfusions, identify microscopic changes in cells, and determine the presence of parasites, viruses, or bacteria in the blood, tissue, or urine. These tests help the physician make an accurate diagnosis and correctly treat the patient.

Medical laboratory workers have many career opportunities. They work for acute care hospitals, private laboratories, physicians' offices, clinics, ambulatory care units, health maintenance organizations, public health agencies, pharmaceutical firms, and research institutions. Their work requires a lot of walking, standing, reaching, stooping, lifting, and carrying of equipment. In addition, they need good eyesight for close work. They work indoors and may be exposed to unpleasant odors and body fluids and have frequent contact with water and cleaning solutions. Their jobs often require them to work shifts and weekends.

Pathologists

A pathologist is a medical doctor who examines tissue specimens, cells, and body fluids through laboratory tests and then interprets the results to gain an accurate diagnosis. An accurate diagnosis is necessary if the patient is to receive proper treatment. Currently, more than 2,000 different tests can be performed on blood and body fluids. Many times, a pathologist helps a patient's team of doctors select the most appropriate test to gain a complete diagnosis. A pathologist is a critical member of a patient's core medical team. To become a pathologist, one must complete medical school and an approved residency in pathology. Medical school generally takes four years. Residency training for pathologists takes from three to six years depending upon the specialty. Pathologists work in hospitals, clinics and independent laboratories.

Microbiologists

A microbiologist is a scientist who studies microbes, or living organisms and infectious agents that are too small to be seen with the naked eye. Because many different species of microbes exist, microbiologists usually select one type of microbe to study, focusing their research and building their careers in that area. A small sampling of specialties includes: bacteriologists, who study bacteria; virologists, who study viruses; and immunologists, who study the human body and how it defends itself against disease. Microbiologists work in almost every industry, and careers in this field are quite varied. At the lowest level are laboratory assistants, who generally have a two-year technical training degree. Those with a four-year degree in biology or microbiology work as research assistants and medical technologists. A master's degree is required for supervisory, technical support, and teaching positions. Microbiologists who perform independent research, teach at the university level, or hold executive-level positions have doctoral degrees.

Laboratory Technologists and Technicians

Laboratory workers include medical laboratory technologists (also known as clinical laboratory scientists), medical laboratory technicians, medical laboratory assistants and aides, and medical phlebotomists. Medical laboratory workers may specialize in blood banking, microbiology, clinical chemistry, immunology, toxicology, and other areas.

For more information, write or go online:

American Society for Clinical Laboratory Science
6701 Democracy Boulevard, Suite 300
Bethesda, MD 20817
www.ascls.org

Board of Certified Laboratory Assistants
9500 South California Avenue
Evergreen Park, IL 60642

Diagnostic Imaging Workers

Diagnostic imaging workers, sometimes referred to as radiologic technologists or x-ray techs, operate x-ray equipment and other types of medical technology to take pictures of the internal parts of the body. The images they produce, called radiographs or scans,

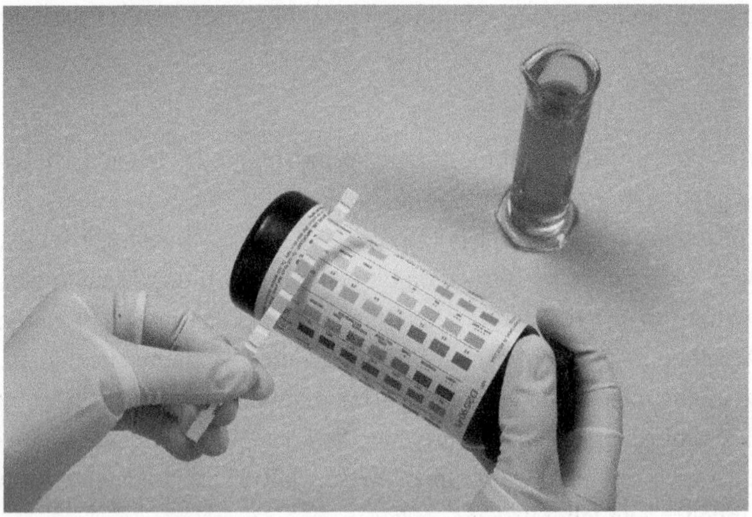

FIGURE 1.17

Medical laboratory worker reads reagent strips

Source: Michal Heron/Pearson Education

provide valuable information for the diagnosis and treatment of patients. For example, radiographs of the chest help detect lung diseases, such as lung cancer and tuberculosis. Some of the diseases or injuries that x-rays help a physician diagnose and treat include ulcers, blood clots, cancer, and fractures.

The term *diagnostic imaging* refers to general radiography as well as an array of imaging techniques, including computerized tomography (CT), diagnostic medical sonography, mammography, nuclear medicine technology, positron emission tomography (PET), and magnetic resonance imaging (MRI). Diagnostic imaging workers may start their careers as general radiographers and then specialize in an imaging modality to become mammographers or CT technologists. Workers may also begin their careers by training in a modality, such as nuclear medicine technology or diagnostic medical sonography. Each imaging area requires special training, and some areas require professional certifications and licenses to practice. Some states permit the use of *limited radiographers* who are trained to assist registered radiographers and/or perform certain procedures of the chest, extremities, skull/sinuses, and spine or podiatric radiography.

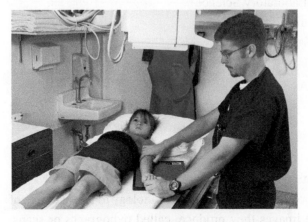

Diagnostic imaging workers have a variety of job opportunities and may work in hospitals, physician practices, satellite imaging and surgery centers, trauma centers, chiropractic offices, clinics, occupational health centers, and ambulatory care facilities. They work indoors and may be in confined areas. They wear protective gloves, aprons, and film badges when the hazards of radiation are present. Shift work and evening work may be part of their schedule. Their work requires the lifting and positioning of patients, standing during most of the shift, and pushing mobile equipment. They may be exposed to body fluids.

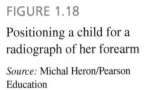

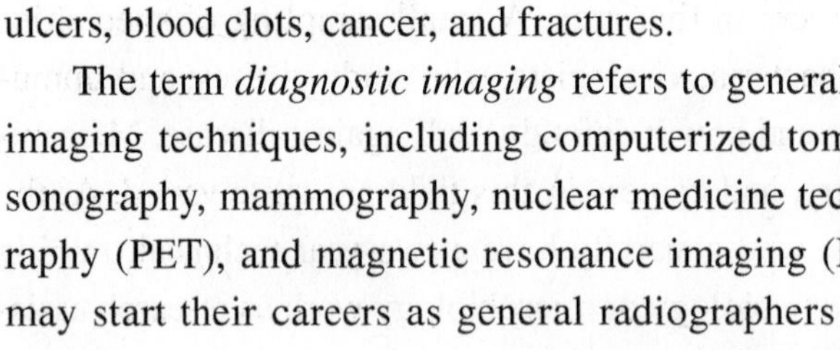

FIGURE 1.18

Positioning a child for a radiograph of her forearm

Source: Michal Heron/Pearson Education

Tasks—Radiographers/Diagnostic Imaging Technologists

- Prepare the patient and explain the procedure
- Set up and operate imaging equipment safely and correctly
- Conduct procedures to produce radiographs, scans, or other images
- Take radiographs or scans in surgery and at the patients' bedside
- Assess the quality of images to ensure diagnostic value
- Assist physicians (radiologists) with sophisticated procedures
- Maintain equipment and report malfunctions

For more information, write or go online:

American Society of Radiologic Technologists
15000 Central Ave. SE
Albuquerque, NM 87123-3909
www.asrt.org

Diagnostic Medical Sonographers

As part of the diagnostic imaging team, medical sonographers (also called ultrasound technologists) use diagnostic ultrasound to transmit sound waves at high frequencies into the patient's body. Images are viewed on a screen and automatically recorded on a printout strip or video. The use of ultrasound is important in prenatal care and for cardiology patients. Sonographers work in hospitals and clinics or in group practices with obstetrics specialists. Unlike most other types of health care workers, many sonographers typically work only on weekdays.

prenatal (pree-NEYT-l) Occurring before birth

For more information, write or go online:

American Society of Radiologic Technologists
15000 Central Avenue SE
Albuquerque, NM 87123-3917
www.asrt.org

American Registry of Radiologic Technologists
1255 Northland Drive
Mendota, MN 55120
www.arrt.org

Society of Diagnostic Medical Sonographers
12770 Coit Road, Suite 708
Dallas, TX 75251
www.sdms.org

Cardiovascular Workers

A variety of professionals focus on the cardiovascular system. These include cardiologists, cardiovascular technologists, cardiopulmonary technicians (also known as perfusionists), echocardiographers, and electrocardiographic technicians.

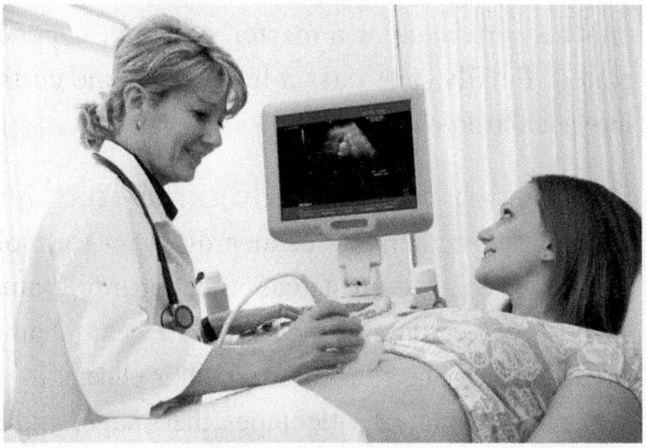

FIGURE 1.19

Patient undergoing a sonography (ultrasound) procedure

Source: Alexander Raths/Shutterstock

Cardiologists

Cardiologists are medical doctors who diagnose, treat, and try to prevent problems in the cardiovascular system. The cardiovascular system includes the heart and blood vessels. Patients are usually referred to a cardiologist by their **primary care** physician. If a problem is suspected, the cardiologist checks the medical records, discusses signs and symptoms, conducts tests, and recommends a course of treatment. This may involve medication, lifestyle changes, or surgery. In the case of surgery, patients are sent to a cardiovascular surgeon. Cardiologists typically work in clinics and hospitals. Some choose to specialize in their practice, such as pediatric or adult cardiology. To become a cardiologist, you must graduate from college and then medical school. You must complete a residency and become certified in internal medicine. Finally, you must complete another residency and become certified in cardiology. Further specialization requires another residency and certification.

primary care
(PRI-mer-ee KAIR) Basic medical care that a patient receives upon first contact with the health care system, before being referred to specialists

Cardiovascular Technologists

Cardiovascular technologists perform diagnostic and therapeutic procedures involving the heart and blood vessels. They work in invasive and noninvasive cardiology, noninvasive peripheral vascular ultrasound, or cardiac electrophysiology. Cardiovascular technologists review and record clinical data and participate in procedures, including echocardiography, exercise stress testing, cardiac catheterization, balloon angioplasty, stent insertion, and pacemaker and/or implantable defibrillator insertion. They work in hospitals and in invasive and noninvasive laboratories. Requirements to work in this profession include one to four years of training and professional certification.

Cardiopulmonary Technicians or Perfusionists

A cardiopulmonary technician, also called a perfusionist, is a professional who operates a heart-and-lung machine. This life-supporting equipment replaces the function of the heart and lungs when they must be temporarily stopped, such as during cardiac surgery. Cardiopulmonary technicians must pay close attention to detail and notice even the slightest change in heart or lung function during surgery as any change could indicate a problem. Cardiopulmonary technicians may work for hospitals, surgeons, or in group practices. Some are independent contractors who work for one or more different employers. There are several different routes to work in this profession. In general, though, you need a four-year college degree with an emphasis on medical technology, respiratory therapy, or nursing. You must then complete a training program that can take from one to four years. This will result in either a certificate or a master's degree, depending upon the type of program completed. Finally, you pass a test to become certified by the American Board of Cardiovascular Perfusion.

Echocardiographers or Echocardiogram Technologists

Echocardiographers, or echocardiogram technologists, use ultrasound equipment to perform specialized tests called echocardiograms. During these tests, high-frequency sounds waves are transmitted into the heart chambers, valves, and blood vessels to create an image. The echocardiographer checks the images on screen for any abnormalities, photographs or videotapes the image, and sends the images and a report to the patient's physician for evaluation. Nearly three-fourths of all echocardiographers work in cardiology departments in hospitals. Others are employed in physicians' offices or diagnostic laboratories. Although some are trained on the job, most have completed a two- or four-year program in this specialty. Professional certification is available.

Electrocardiographic (EKG/ECG) Technicians

Electrocardiographic technicians operate an EKG (or ECG) machine to record the electrical changes that occur during a heartbeat. These recordings help physicians diagnose any irregularities or changes in the patient's heartbeat. These tests are done routinely on patients after they reach a certain age, before surgery, and as a diagnostic tool. EKG technicians also apply Holter monitors. EKG technicians have many job opportunities and work in acute care hospitals, clinics, private physicians' offices, health maintenance organizations, and ambulatory care facilities. They work indoors and may work shifts, evenings, and weekends. They spend a lot of their time standing and walking.

Tasks—Electrocardiographic Technicians

- Escort patient to treatment room
- Take portable equipment to patient's room
- Explain the test procedure
- Paste or attach electrodes to correct areas on patient's chest, arms, legs; connect leads from EKG machine to electrodes; and operate selector switch on EKG machine

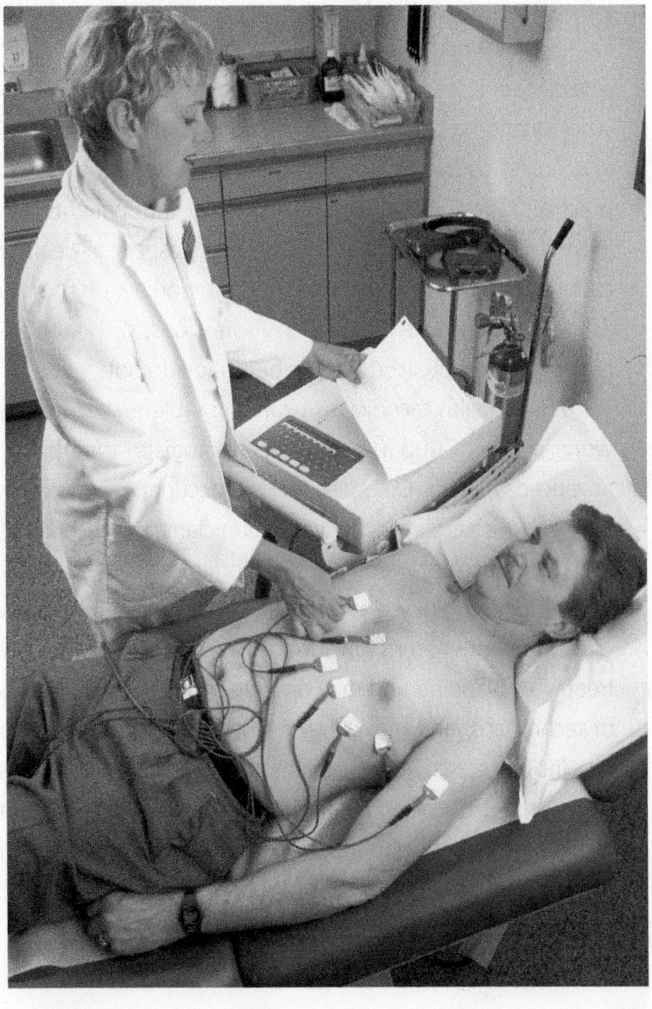

FIGURE 1.20

EKG technician performing an electrocardiogram

Source: Craig X. Sotres/Pearson Education

deviation
(dee-vee-EY-shuhn)
Departure from a standard or norm

- Reposition chest electrodes to record various positions
- Check recording for accuracy (leads placed incorrectly give an incorrect reading)
- Recognize significant **deviations** from normal heartbeat and report immediately
- Edit and mount final results
- Send copy of graph to the physician
- Maintain EKG records
- Type physician's diagnosis
- Care for equipment by cleaning electrodes and maintain inventory of supplies
- Conduct vectorcardiograms (multidimensional traces), stress testing (exercise tests), and pulse recordings
- Perform Holter monitoring (12- to 24-hour recording of an EKG)

For more information, write:

National Society for Cardiovascular Technology
120 Falcon Drive, Suite 3
Fredericksburg, VA 22408

Consider This *Allied Health Defined*

What is *allied health*? Almost everyone knows that doctors and nurses are part of the health care workforce. But the 5 million people who work within the *allied health professions* are less widely known. These are the technicians, technologists, and therapists who function in approximately 80 different career fields. They work alongside doctors and nurses as part of the health care team, and some may also operate independent practices. They work directly or indirectly with patients, function in a variety of different job titles, and are found in virtually every aspect of health care. Colleges that offer educational programs to train allied health workers often group their programs together in Schools of Allied Health, Health Professions, or Health Science. Some colleges include nursing as part of allied health, but many do not.

Allied health technicians usually complete about two years of training or less. Their work is directly supervised by technologists, therapists, or other professionals with advanced training. Examples include occupational therapy assistants, pharmacy technicians, and emergency medical technicians. Allied health technologists and therapists must undergo more extensive training and often earn college degrees at the bachelor's level or higher. They play key roles in diagnosing and treating patients, and may also work behind the scenes in supportive roles. Technologists and therapists are involved in treatment planning and may operate sophisticated technology. They supervise the work of technicians, and may advance into leadership, education, and research roles. Examples include cardiovascular technologists, radiation therapists, and perfusionists.

Many of the allied health disciplines have their own professional associations composed of members who are highly involved in the education, credentialing, and practice of future workers. For more information, visit the Association of Schools of Allied Health Professions (ASAHP) at http://www.asahp.org/.

CAREERS IN HEALTH INFORMATICS SERVICES

Information service workers provide important support to all other medical services. These workers analyze, extract, and document information using automated systems. They understand the sources, routes, and flow of information within the health care environment. They may also have special skills and advanced training in computer programming and assist in the development of software that ensures delivery of high quality and cost effective care.

extract
(ik-STRAKT) Identify and take out or emphasize

Administrative Support Service Workers

Administrative support service workers (medical clerical workers) handle customer complaints, interpret and explain policies or regulations, prepare payrolls, resolve billing disputes, and collect delinquent accounts. They are responsible for the everyday situations that medical organizations must deal with smoothly and efficiently to maintain business operations and good customer service. The following list of occupations is included in administrative support services:

- Patient registration clerk
- Claims representative
- Insurance processor or enrollment clerk
- Billing and account collector
- Clerical worker
- Computer or data processor
- Receptionist
- Appointment scheduler
- Material/supply and distribution clerk or purchasing clerk
- Payroll and timekeeping clerk
- Personnel clerk
- Secretary or word processor
- Telephone operator

Admitting Department Workers

Admitting department workers are responsible for admitting and discharging patients in a hospital. They interview patients for information necessary for accurate record keeping and are usually the first hospital employees whom the patient sees. Employees in this department help the patient feel confident about the hospital and the care they will receive. Admitting workers have a variety of job opportunities and work in an acute care hospital and in the short stay hospital setting. They may assist with lifting patients and carrying their belongings. They may also push wheelchairs or stretchers. Their work is in an office environment and requires sitting and reaching. They may work shifts and evenings.

discharging
(dis-CHAHRJ-ing) The act of releasing or allowing to leave

Tasks—Admitting Clerks

- Interview incoming patients and record information required for admission
- Assign rooms
- Prepare identification band
- Explain hospital rules and policies
- Store patients' valuables in hospital safe and arrange escort to room
- Send admitting forms to appropriate departments

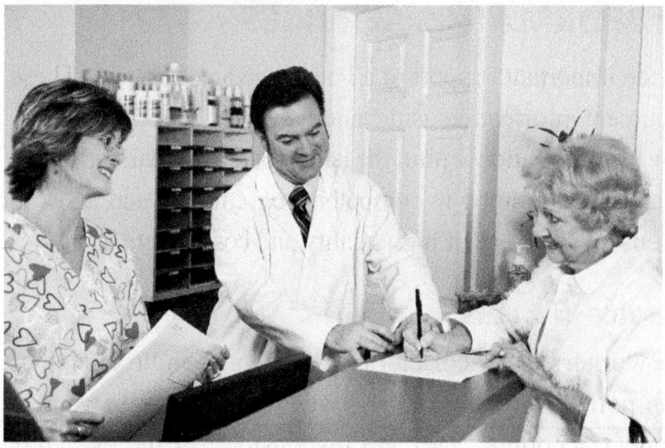

FIGURE 1.21
Completing paperwork for admission to the hospital
Source: Lisa F. Young/Fotolia LLC

- Prepare daily census and preadmission forms and arrange transfers
- Perform cashier and receptionist duties as needed (depending on the size of the facility)
- Use a computer for records

For more information, write or go online:

American Hospital Association
One North Franklin
Chicago, IL 60606-3421
www.aha.org

Medical Records/Health Information Management Workers

Medical records/health information management workers keep permanent records that describe the patient's condition and the treatment that he or she receives. Physicians and allied health personnel use medical records to provide care for the patients. Medical records are also legal documents that can be used in a court of law. Insurance companies use the records to determine what they will pay for the patient's care. Records are used in medical research, as well. Medical records must be accurate and carefully filed or logged into a computer. Medical records/health information management workers have many job opportunities and are employed by acute care hospitals, long term care facilities, public health departments, manufacturers of medical record systems, and insurance companies. Medical records/health information management specialists may have a private practice as a consultant. Their work requires frequent reaching and stretching for files, long periods of time at a desk, and some lifting of records.

Tasks—Medical Records/Health Information Management Clerks

- File and access paper and electronic medical records
- Maintain a sign-out system for paper medical records
- Update medical records and check for prior records of newly admitted patients
- Apply established procedures for maintaining and sharing medical records
- Answer routine staff requests for information about patients
- Gather statistics for state health department
- Transcribe reports of operations, x-rays, and laboratory examinations

For more information, write or go online:

American Health Information Management Association
233 N. Michigan Avenue, 21st Floor
Chicago, IL 60601-5800
www.ahima.org

Unit Secretaries and Health Unit Coordinators

Unit secretaries and health unit coordinators are responsible for clerical, reception and communication duties in nursing units. They facilitate the organized and efficient operation of the unit and communication among patients, visitors, physicians, nurses, and other staff. The unit secretary serves as a resource for the patient care team, freeing up nurses to devote more time to patient care. Health unit coordinators have various career options and may be employed in acute care hospitals, long-term care facilities, and clinics. Their work is indoors and may require shifts and weekends. Their work requires sitting at a desk for long periods of time, operating a computer, and making frequent phone calls. To function in this job, a person requires strong communication and organizational skills, and the ability to use computer programs to access, enter, and retrieve patient information.

Tasks—Health Unit Coordinators

- Greet patients and families, answer questions, and provide directions as necessary
- Prepare and compile records, including patient's name, address, and names of attending physicians
- Copy information into charts and/or enter information into computer programs
- Submit requisitions for procedures such as laboratory and radiology tests
- Maintain inventory of supplies and ensure proper storage
- Answer patients' call lights and send appropriate person for request
- File reports in paper or electronic charts

For more information, write or go online:

National Association of Health Unit Coordinators, Inc.
1947 Madron Road
Rockford, Illinois 61107-1716
www.nahuc.org

Medical Coders

The health care that a patient receives must be documented before a doctor or a hospital can file a claim to be paid for the services rendered. Before medical billers can submit a *clean* claim that is likely to be paid rather than denied, a medical coder must review the patient's medical records, verify that services were provided, and assign the appropriate codes. Reference books and online resources help guide the medical coder in determining which codes to assign based on the level of health services provided. Medical coding and medical billing may be performed by the same worker or by different people depending on where they work.

Medical coders must be detail-oriented, with a comprehensive knowledge of human anatomy and physiology and medical terminology, in order to assign accurate codes. They must be familiar with the different types of health insurance plans, current procedures for billing and reimbursement, and how to comply with regulations. Because health insurance and coding procedures change frequently, workers must keep up with the latest information. Medical coders have several options for professional certifications, and it's not unusual for a coder to be certified in more than one area. Coders may also specialize in auditing and compliance responsibilities.

Tasks—Medical Coders

- Perform a comprehensive review of the patient's medical documentation
- Determine if the final diagnosis and procedures are valid, complete, and accurately reflect the services provided
- Assess the records for compliance with insurance policies and procedures
- Assign proper codes using classification manuals
- Use computer programs and clinical databases

For more information, write or go online:

American Association of Procedural Coders (AAPC)
2480 South 3850 West, Suite B
Salt Lake City, UT 84120
www.aapc.com

American Health Information Management Association (AHIMA)
233 N. Michigan Avenue, 21st Floor
Chicago, IL 60601-5809
www.ahima.org

CAREERS IN SUPPORT SERVICES

Many health care workers function in support roles, often in areas *behind the scenes*. They help provide a clean and safe environment for the delivery of care. They repair and maintain medical and general equipment, and follow aseptic procedures.

Central Processing/Supply Workers

Central processing/supply workers supply various departments with equipment and materials. The equipment must be in good working condition since malfunctioning equipment is life- threatening. The workers keep an inventory of supplies and equipment. Supplies and equipment are properly packaged, cleaned, and sterilized. The workers in this department are key members of the health care team. Other health care workers cannot provide necessary patient care without the proper tools. Central processing/supply workers work in acute care hospitals and large outpatient clinics. The department is often in a basement or at the rear of the building. Lifting and moving articles and equipment are required. The workers stand on their feet for long periods of time and may be exposed to body fluids.

Tasks—Central Processing/Supply Technicians

- Use solutions to scrub and wash surgical instruments, containers, syringes, and equipment

- Sterilize articles such as instruments, equipment, and linens using the steam autoclave, gas autoclave, or antiseptic solution
- Prepare packs of supplies, instruments, dressings, and treatment trays; carefully wrap, label, and seal each pack
- Store and inventory prepared articles, supplies, and equipment
- Fill requisitions (gathering supplies and equipment as requested) and post charges
- Check expiration dates on sterilized materials

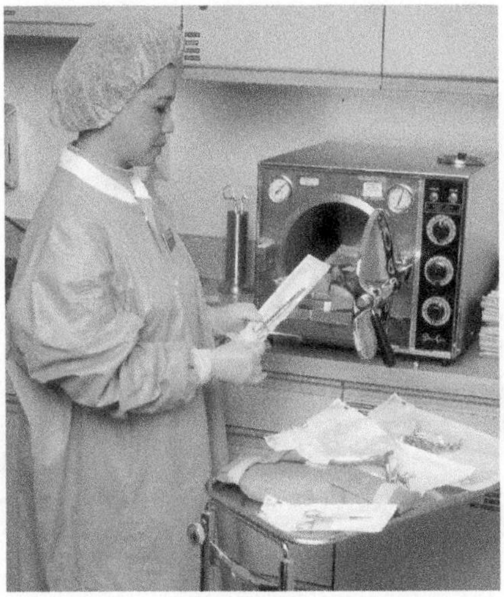

FIGURE 1.22

Central supply technician loading instruments for sterilization

Source: George Dodson/Pearson

For more information, write or go online:

American Hospital Association
One North Franklin
Chicago, IL 60606-3421
www.aha.org

International Association of Healthcare Central Service Materiel Management (IAHCSMM)
213 West Institute Place, Suite 307
Chicago, IL 60610
www.ashcsp.org

Hospital Housekeepers/Environmental Services Technicians

Housekeepers, also called environmental services technicians, are responsible for the cleanliness of the health care environment. Cleanliness helps prevent the spread of infection and creates a more pleasant environment for patients, staff, and visitors. Environmental services workers have many job opportunities and work in long-term care facilities, acute hospitals, and clinics. They have frequent contact with water and cleaning solutions. They walk, stand, and stoop during their shift. They also push and pull equipment, climb on ladders when necessary, and may be exposed to body fluids. Their hours may include shift work and weekend work.

Tasks—Hospital Housekeepers

- Load service cart
- Clean assigned areas such as rooms, offices, laboratories
- Dust, vacuum, and clean blinds, floors, furniture, and equipment
- Polish floors using a buffing machine
- Wash walls, ceilings, windows
- Empty trash
- Scour sinks, tubs, and mirrors
- Disinfect bedsprings and unit equipment
- Replenish soap and towels
- Replace cubicle curtains and soiled draperies

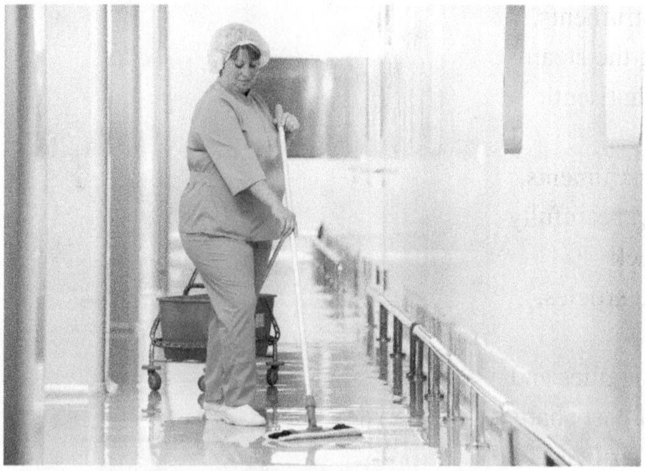

FIGURE 1.23

Housekeeping attendant cleaning a public area

Source: Dmitry Kalinovsky/Shutterstock

- Report malfunctioning equipment
- Move furniture, equipment, and supplies and turn mattresses

For more information, write or go online:

Institute of Sanitation Management
1710 Drew Street
Clearwater, FL 33515

International Executive Housekeepers Association
1001 Eastwind Drive, Suite 301
Westerville, OH 43081-3361
www.ieha.org

Food Service Workers and Dietary Aides

Food service workers are responsible for providing nutritional care to patients. They plan special and balanced diets. They also distribute menus, prepare food trays, and deliver food to the patients throughout the facility. Food service workers have many career options and may work in acute care hospitals and long-term care facilities.

Dietary aides prepare and deliver food trays to patients in hospitals or facilities such as nursing homes. Duties may include: reading menu cards to determine which items to place on a tray, placing items on trays, helping the cook prepare food items, preparing foods for soft or liquid diets, pushing a food cart, serving meals to patients, collecting dirty dishes, washing dishes, and recording the amount and type of special foods served to patients.

Food service workers and dietary aides generally work 40 hours a week and may work in shifts. Their work areas might be very warm, with much activity in a relatively small area. Some lifting, reaching, equipment moving, and occasional bending are required. They walk and stand most of the shift. To become a food service worker or dietary aide, a high school diploma is recommended and sometimes required.

Tasks—Food Service Workers and Dietary Aides

- Prepare and deliver food trays to patients
- Read color-coded menu cards to determine appropriate items to place on trays

- Measure food servings according to diet list; prepare individual servings of salad, desserts, sandwiches
- Prepare foods for soft or liquid diets using a blender
- Check trays for accuracy and completeness, push food tray carts to patient floors, and serve trays to patients (according to hospital policy)
- Stock the nutrition kitchen in patient care areas
- Return food tray carts to kitchen
- Clean work area, wrap silverware, and restock condiments for tray line

For more information, write or go online:

American Dietetic Association
120 South Riverside Plaza, Suite 2000
Chicago, IL 60606-6995
www.eatright.org

American Home Economics Association
2010 Massachusetts Avenue NW
Washington, DC 20036

CAREERS IN BIOTECHNOLOGY RESEARCH AND DEVELOPMENT SERVICES

The field of Biotechnology Research and Development is especially exciting. As scientists and other researchers discover, invent, and develop new kinds of drugs, medical equipment and devices, diagnostic tests, and therapeutic treatments, new occupations and jobs are sure to follow. Let's take a look at some of the biotech jobs that currently exist.

Biomedical Engineers

Biomedical engineers combine the study of engineering with the life sciences, and speak the language of both engineering and medicine. They work in hospitals and research labs, and in industry and sales with a variety of people, including laboratory scientists, physicians, nurses, and other engineers. Biomedical engineers who work in hospitals are known as clinical engineers. They design and evaluate medical devices such as prosthetics, cardiac pacemakers, and laser systems used for corrective eye surgery.

Bioengineering is a relatively new occupation, and the number of universities that offer degrees in this field is growing. Students examine the connections between living systems and non-living materials and systems through coursework in biomaterials, biomechanics, and bioelectricity. They study electromagnetics, fluid dynamics, and heat transfer along with molecular biology, pharmacology, and anatomy and physiology. Students can earn a bachelor's degree in Biomedical Engineering by completing an integrated curriculum that combines traditional engineering with biomedical applications. Or, they can complete a traditional bachelor's degree in Engineering (electrical, chemical, or mechanical) followed by a master's degree in Biomedical Engineering. Opportunities for specialization are based on specific diseases, body systems, and technologies. Most Biomedical engineers with B.S. degrees continue their education by earning master's or doctorate degrees, and some pursue careers in medicine, dentistry, and law.

FIGURE 1.24

Scientist conducting a controlled experiment

Source: Brady/Pearson Education

Cell Biologists

Using microscopes and assay instruments, cell biologists conduct experiments to study how cells act alone and with other cells in molecules and tissues to discover new drugs, vaccines, and the causes of disease. Cell biologists work in research laboratories, using hazardous chemicals and operating complex pieces of equipment. They harvest and grow cells, study DNA, and use cloning techniques to produce identical organisms.

Some research assistant jobs are available for people with an associate's degree, but most biologists enter the field with a bachelor's degree in chemistry, physics, biology, or microbiology. Cell biologists continue their education with additional studies in mathematics for statistical analyses and computing for modeling and simulating biological processes. Most cell biologists have a master's or doctorate degree, and may specialize in studying human cells, animal cells, or plant cells. The study of human cells includes genetics, genomics, biochemistry, and immunology.

CAREERS ALIGNED WITH SYSTEMS OF THE HUMAN BODY

Some health care workers perform both therapeutic and diagnostic procedures, or their job duties may cross over into health informatics, support services, or biotechnology research and technology roles. In addition to categorizing health careers via the five different service areas (therapeutic, diagnostic, and so on), occupations may also be organized according to the systems of the human body in which workers specialize. For example, cardiology workers focus on the circulatory system, orthopedic workers focus on the musculoskeletal system, and neurology workers focus on the nervous system. What follows in the next section are some more occupational descriptions based on anatomic systems.

Skeletal and Muscular Systems

Several health care professionals focus on the skeletal and muscular systems. These include orthopedists, orthopedic technicians, prosthetists, and myologists.

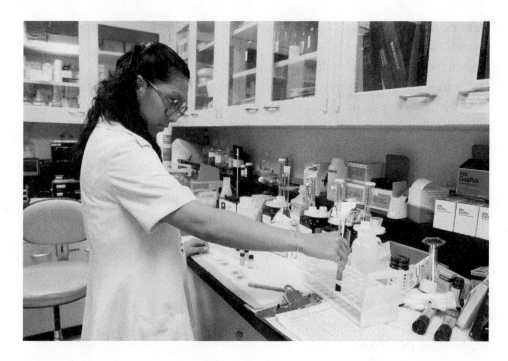

Orthopedists

An orthopedist, also called an orthopedic surgeon, is a physician who specializes in treating disorders of the musculoskeletal system. The musculoskeletal system is comprised of bones, joints, muscles, tendons, ligaments, nerves, skin, and any of the structures related to these body parts. Orthopedists use casts to repair broken bones; they prescribe exercise and medication for the treatment of musculoskeletal injuries or diseases, and they perform surgeries, such as implanting artificial joints or reconstructing damaged limbs. Although historically orthopedists primarily worked with children, modern orthopedists have patients of all ages. Some orthopedists specialize in one area, such as sports injuries, but most treat a wide variety of conditions.

Orthopedic Technicians

An orthopedic technician, also known as an orthopedic technologist or cast technician, helps physicians and orthopedic surgeons care for and treat patients with orthopedic needs. This work is generally done in a hospital, clinic, or private practice. The duties of an orthopedic technician are three-fold. First, they perform work directly related to patient care by assisting with such tasks as the application, adjustment, and removal of casts, splints, and braces. They also help set up, adjust, and maintain traction devices. Another aspect of the job is organizational. Orthopedic technicians are responsible for maintaining the cast room as well as orthopedic equipment and devices. The third prong is clerical. Orthopedic technicians manage insurance, medical billing, and coding for orthopedic procedures.

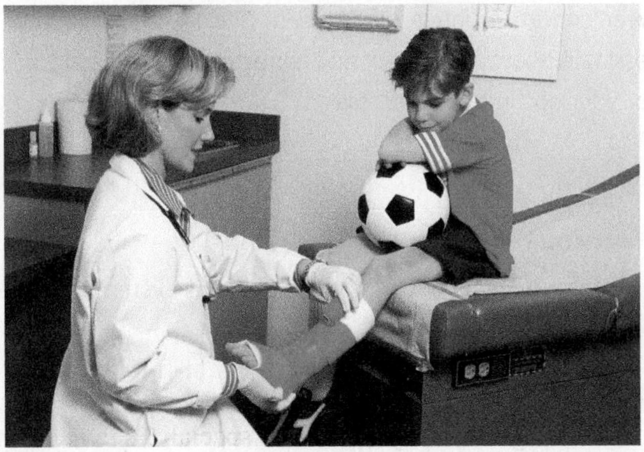

FIGURE 1.25

Orthopedic technician checks a child's leg cast

Source: Michal Heron/Pearson Education

Three different career levels exist for orthopedic technicians. Level I, or entry-level positions, require a high school diploma and at least one year of full-time, on-the-job experience working with orthopedic patients. Level II requires certification from the National Board of Certification for Orthopaedic Technologists (NBCOT), plus either two years of experience, completion of an orthopedic technology training program, or completion of a related program and one year of full-time experience. Level III requires certification, completion of a training program, and up to eight years of experience.

Prosthetists

A prosthetist is a medical professional who evaluates, designs, and creates artificial limbs, or prostheses, for patients who have lost all or part of a limb due to disease or injury. A prosthetist works with a team comprised of physicians, nurses, and physical and occupational therapists. Once the prosthesis is created, the prosthetist periodically evaluates the device and makes adjustments as needed. To become a prosthetist, you must earn a B.S. degree and then complete a certificate program in prosthetics. It typically takes four years to earn a B.S. degree. Certificate programs in prosthetics, which include both coursework and clinical experience, take between six months to one year to complete.

Myologists

An orofacial myologist diagnoses and treats abnormal patterns of the mouth and face caused by things such as thumb sucking, tongue thrusting, nail biting, and jaw clenching. Left untreated, these habits lead to problems with teeth alignment, speech, chewing, swallowing, and breathing. The myologist works in conjunction with physicians and dentists to help patients develop new habits that lead to the proper usage and placement of the tongue, lips, and jaw. Myologists include professionals such as speech pathologists, physicians, dentists, and dental hygienists who have sought further training in this specialty. To become certified by the International Association of Orofacial Myology, candidates who are already practicing professionals in another area must complete an approved 28-hour introductory course or internship, be a member in good standing for one year, and pass a take-home proficiency exam and an on-site evaluation.

Language Arts Link Career Study

Many health care workers focus on one specific body system, such as the reproductive system, the respiratory system, or the skeletal system. Select an occupation that aligns with a system of the human body and learn more about the job opportunities for that career. In paragraph form, describe the position, including its job requirements and skills, and earning potential for health care workers in that field. If possible, interview professionals in your selected field to find out how they became interested in this specialty area and what a typical day is like on the job. Be sure to proofread your work to see if you can improve it by making it more clear, concise, or interesting to read. Check the spelling and grammar and correct any errors. Exchange your report with a classmate. Provide feedback and corrections as necessary, and then exchange back. Read your classmate's comments and revise your document as necessary.

Nervous System

Professionals who focus on the nervous system include neurologists and electroneurodiagnostic technologists.

Neurologists

A neurologist is a physician who specializes in nervous system disorders. This includes diseases of the brain, spinal cord, nerves, muscles, and the blood vessels that relate to these structures. Neurologists examine the nerves of the head or neck and test muscle strength and movement. They see how well a patient moves and balances. They also test reflexes and examine a patient's sense of sensation, memory, speech, language, and other cognitive abilities. They do many tests to complete these assessments, including CT scans, MRIs, and spinal taps. To become a neurologist, you must complete medical school followed by a one-year internship. At least eight months of that internship must be spent in internal medicine. Then, you must complete a three-year residency in neurology and pass an exam to become a certified neurologist. If you choose to pursue a specialty area, such as child neurology, clinical neurophysiology, or pain medicine, you must complete one to three years of additional training.

Electroneurodiagnostic Technologists

Electroneurodiagnostic (END) technologists use computers to record electrical impulses transmitted by the brain and the nervous system. They perform several different neurological tests including electroencephalograms (EEGs), evoked potentials (EPs), nerve conduction studies (NCSs), polysomnographs (PSG/sleep studies), and surgical monitoring. EEGs assist in the diagnosis of various brain disorders such as seizures, stroke, head trauma, and brain tumors. EPs are performed on patients with possible multiple sclerosis, brainstem tumors, and spinal cord problems. NCSs evaluate peripheral nervous system problems such as carpal tunnel syndrome. Sleep studies are performed on patients to diagnose sleep disorders such as sleep apnea and narcolepsy. The brain, nerves, and/or muscles can be monitored by END technologists during various brain and spinal cord surgeries.

After completing an accredited two-year associate's degree program in END Technology and gaining work experience, technologists may seek registration in one or more of the five specialty areas by the American Board of Electroencephalographic and Evoked Potential Technologists. END technologists have many job opportunities. They work in hospitals, neurologists' and neurosurgeons' offices, sleep centers, and psychiatric facilities. Some positions may require on-call duty, and sleep disorder technologists usually work evenings and nights.

Tasks—Electroneurodiagnostic Technologists

- Take medical histories
- Apply electrodes for the procedure being performed
- Record and monitor the patient's waveforms on a computer
- Interact with patients to reduce anxiety during tests
- Interact with neurologists and other health care staff
- Write technical reports (possibly)
- Keep records
- Schedule appointments
- Order supplies
- Maintain equipment

For more information, write or go online:
The Neurodiagnostic Society
402 East Bannister Road, Suite A
Kansas City, MO 64131-3019
www.aset.org

Lymphatic System

Immunologists and immunology technologists focus their work on the lymphatic system.

Immunologists

An immunologist is someone who studies and/or treats the immune system. An immunologist may be a research scientist who works in a laboratory. The scientist investigates the components needed for a healthy immune system or the diseases that disrupt the immune system. An immunologist can also be a doctor who treats people with immune system disorders, including allergies or autoimmune diseases. Some immunologists perform both duties and combine research with patient care. Immunologists who conduct independent research usually have an advanced degree such as a PhD or MD, although some jobs only require a master's degree. Training must include a combination of coursework, laboratory research, and a thesis or dissertation, followed by two to four years in a postdoctoral training fellowship. Physicians who work as immunologists typically go to medical school, complete a residency in internal medicine, pediatrics, or a medicine-pediatrics program, and then spend two more years specializing in allergies/immunology.

Immunology Technologists

Immunology technologists study the human immune system and how it responds to foreign invaders. They strive to diagnose, treat, and prevent infections by studying the organisms that cause disease and how they attack the immune system. This work is done under the supervision of an immunologist or a physician. Because of the nature of their work, they often work with other scientists, including chemists, pathologists, geologists, and civil engineers. Immunology technologists work in a variety of academic and health-related centers. Some work for hospitals; others are employed by research facilities or diagnostic laboratories. People can enter this profession with a BS degree in immunology or by completing an immunology technology program at a college or technical institute. Some states require immunology technologists to be licensed.

Digestive System

Professionals who focus on the digestive system include gastroenterologists, hepatologists, dietitians, and dietary aides.

Gastroenterologists

A gastroenterologist is a physician who specializes in the digestive system. A gastroenterologist treats diseases of the gastrointestinal tract, which includes the esophagus, stomach, small intestine, colon and rectum, pancreas, gallbladder, bile ducts, and liver. A gastroenterologist treats conditions including colon polyps, cancer, hepatitis, gastroesophageal reflux (heartburn), and irritable bowel syndrome. Gastroenterologists are trained in endoscopy, which is the use of narrow, lighted tubes with built-in cameras. By utilizing these instruments, they can see the inside of the intestinal tract. To become a gastroenterologist, you must complete medical school followed by a three-year residency in internal medicine. Finally, you must complete additional specialized training in gastroenterology, which lasts two to three years.

Hepatologists

A hepatologist is a physician who specializes in treatment of the liver. As a hepatologist, you might deal with hepatitis, cirrhosis, genetic or metabolic liver diseases, liver cancer, liver transplants, or metabolic or immunologic issues related to the liver. To become a hepatologist, you must first be trained as a gastroenterologist, and then complete another one-year fellowship in which you will receive both clinical and research training specific to hepatology. Once this training is complete, you must pass an exam to become certified in this field.

Dietitians

Dietitians plan food and nutrition programs that help treat or prevent disease. They are often part of a medical team in a hospital, private practice, or other health care facility. Dietitians promote healthy eating habits, evaluate patients' diets, and suggest modifications. Some dietitians specialize in the management of overweight or critically ill patients. Because they help identify and treat health ailments, they require a detailed

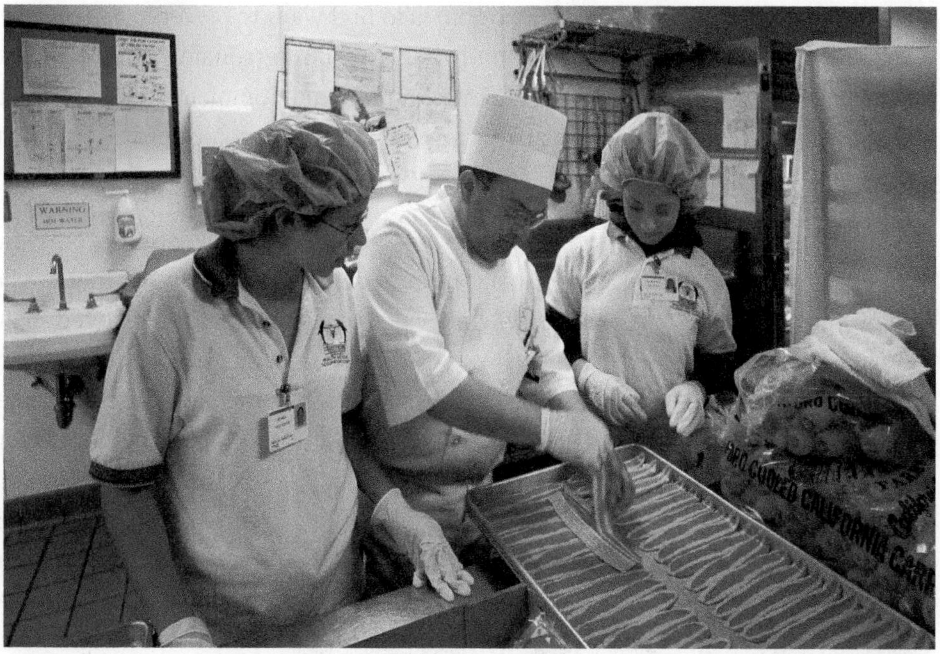

FIGURE 1.26
Food service workers preparing meals
Source: Spencer Grant/PhotoEdit

knowledge of growth and development, metabolism, and biochemistry of nutrients and food components. To become a registered dietitian, you must have at least a bachelor's degree in nutrition or dietetics and complete a 6- to 12-month internship at a health care facility, food service company, or nonprofit agency. You must also pass an exam given by the Commission on Dietetic Registration.

Urinary System

Professionals who focus on the urinary system include urologists, nephrologists, and dialysis technicians.

Urologists

Urologists specialize in issues related to the male and female urinary tracts and the male reproductive organs. People see urologists for issues ranging from discomfort while urinating to male infertility. Urologists examine a patient's urine for signs of infection, blood, or excess sugars or protein, which could indicate diabetes or other kidney problems. Because urologists encounter such a wide variety of issues, they must have a broad knowledge of internal medicine, pediatrics, gynecology, and other specialties. Urologists must graduate from medical school and then complete an accredited urology residency program. This program can last up to five years and involves a combination of surgical and clinical training. Urologists can specialize in a variety of areas, including urologic oncology, male infertility, female urology, or pediatric urology. To practice as a pediatric urologist, one more year of training is required. All urologists must also pass an exam to become certified in this field.

Nephrologists

A nephrologist, also called a renal physician, is a medical doctor who specializes in the treatment of patients with kidney diseases. This includes patients with diabetes, polycystic kidney disease, and chronic kidney failure. Many patients must receive dialysis therapy and some will require kidney transplants. Nephrologists are trained in internal medicine. They do not perform surgery. However, they may perform a kidney biopsy to obtain a sample of kidney tissue. Their goal is to find ways to preserve patients' remaining kidney function. To become a nephrologist, you must graduate from medical school, complete an internal medicine residency program, and complete a two- to three-year fellowship in nephrology. You must also take an exam to become certified in this field.

Dialysis Technicians

A dialysis technician is the primary caregiver for patients who are undergoing dialysis, which is a process through which waste products are filtered from the blood when the kidneys are not functioning properly. Under the supervision of a registered nurse, the dialysis technician performs the actual dialysis treatment, while the nurse is responsible for overall patient care. Job duties include assembling supplies, preparing the machine for use, obtaining patient vital signs, administering local anesthetics and drugs under supervision, and closely monitoring the patient before, during, and after dialysis treatment. Dialysis technicians work in hospitals, out-patient facilities, and home dialysis programs. To become a dialysis technician, you must have a high school diploma. A dialysis technician may be trained on the job, through an employer-sponsored training program, or at a vocational school or community college.

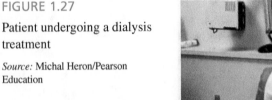

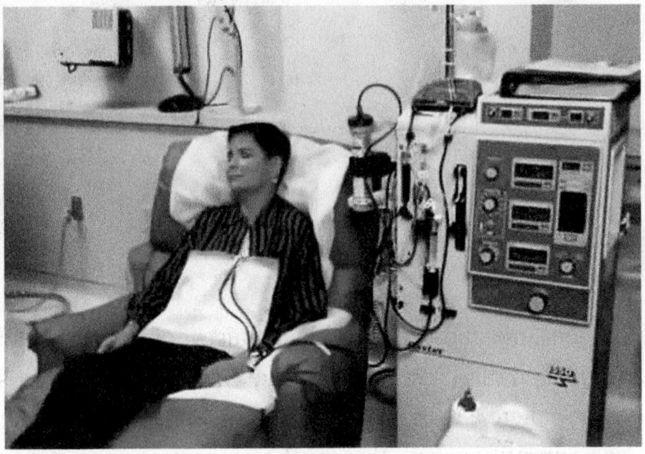

FIGURE 1.27

Patient undergoing a dialysis treatment

Source: Michal Heron/Pearson Education

Reproductive System

Embryologists, gynecologists, obstetricians, and midwives focus their work on the reproductive system.

Embryologists

Embryologists study the early growth and formation of life. Clinical embryologists work with human embryos. They study the stages of pregnancy and watch how embryos grow and change day by day. Many embryologists work in infertility clinics to help infertile couples have children. To do this, they collect eggs and sperm from patients for examination and check fertility levels. Sometimes, they prepare egg and sperm samples for in vitro fertilization. Other times, an embryologist will combine the egg and sperm so that it grows into an embryo, which can be preserved and implanted at a later date. Embryologists may also study abnormalities in embryos. Their goal is to discover why abnormalities occur and how they may be prevented. Embryologists are highly trained in advanced laboratory techniques. They may work in hospitals, clinics, laboratories, or for a government agency, pharmaceutical company or biotechnology firm.

The minimum requirement for this position is a four-year bachelor's degree in embryology, microbiology, or biochemistry. You must also have a background in genetics. This will qualify you to be a laboratory assistant or technician. To become a senior researcher, you must have a master's degree or a PhD.

Gynecologists

Gynecologists are physicians who specialize in the female organs and reproductive system. They manage hormonal disorders, treat infections, perform Pap smears, diagnose cancers of the reproductive system, and perform operations such as hysterectomies. Much of a gynecologist's work is to perform routine check-ups to prevent the development of serious problems. Some gynecologists specialize in a specific area, such as gynecologic oncology, or reproductive endocrinology. To become a gynecologist, you must graduate from college and medical school. You must then complete a four-year gynecology residency and two years of clinical practice. One to three additional years of training are required if you decide to pursue a specialty area. All gynecologists must pass an exam to become certified before practicing in this field.

Obstetricians

An obstetrician is a physician who cares for women throughout pregnancy and childbirth. Some of their patients are women who are having complications during pregnancy. Obstetricians closely monitor the mother's health and diagnose any abnormalities or health issues in the developing fetus. If an issue does arise, the obstetrician may refer the mother to a specialist for treatment. Many doctors who become obstetricians also train as gynecologists. To become an obstetrician, you must complete college and medical school. You must also complete a four-year residency specializing in obstetrics and gynecology and two more years of clinical practice. One to three more years of training are required for those who pursue an area of specialization. All obstetricians must also pass a national examination to become certified to practice in this field.

Midwives

Midwives are trained medical professionals who care for and support women throughout normal pregnancies. This care extends from the onset of pregnancy to just after delivery. Midwives stress the importance of communication with the mother and provide individualized health care information, emotional and social support, and continuous hands-on assistance during labor and delivery. If any problems arise, the midwife does not deliver the baby, but calls for an obstetrician. Two types of midwives exist in the United States: direct-entry midwives and nurse-midwives. Direct-entry midwives are not nurses. However, they have at least a bachelor's degree, have completed specific health science courses, graduated from an accredited midwifery education program, and passed a national exam to become certified. Nurse-midwives are registered nurses who have completed an accredited midwifery program and passed an exam to become certified.

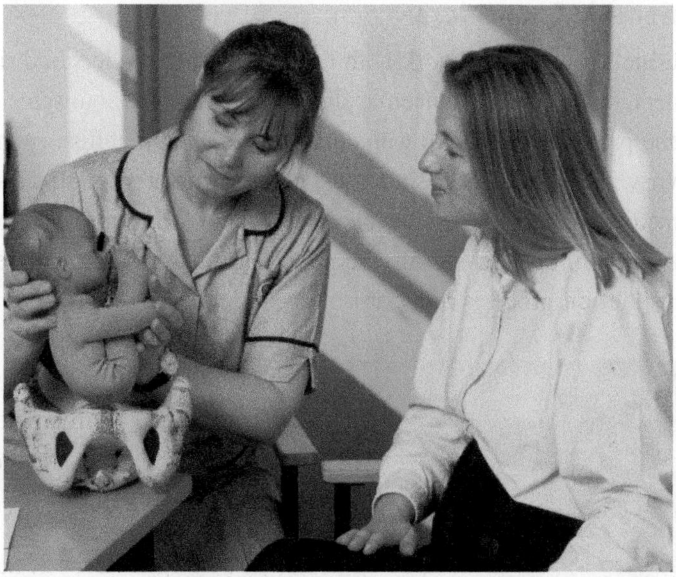

FIGURE 1.28

Midwife demonstrates the breech position to a pregnant woman

Source: Ruth Jenkinson/MIDIRS/Photo Researchers, Inc.

CAREERS IN GENETICS

Career opportunities in the field of medical genetics are opening up as a result of advances in genetic technology and The Human Genome Project. Job tasks in genetics include isolation, identification, and analysis of genes, which assists with research into gene function, as well as the causes of inherited diseases. Three main areas of jobs in genetics exist; these include:

genes
(JEENS) A portion of DNA that contains instructions for a trait

- *Cytogenetics* professionals study chromosomes and how they are connected to disease and human body development.
- *Bioinformatic* professionals focus on managing genetics data, providing databases and computing tools for gathering, sorting, analyzing, and merging data. Computations and statistical analysis are required for sequencing projects.
- ***Genetics Laboratory Research Assistants*** perform genetics testing and research for a variety of purposes, including law enforcement, pharmaceutical research, and clinical medical diagnoses and treatments.

Geneticists

A geneticist is a scientist who is certified to work in medical and scientific areas related to genes. This work may involve experiments that explore and determine laws and environmental factors that affect the origin, transmission, and development of inherited traits. Geneticists may devise methods to alter traits or produce new traits. A geneticist may specialize in developing resistance methods to diseases and disorders, understanding the relationship between heredity and fertility, or evaluating the genetic makeup that has caused a disorder or disability in order to help a patient manage a condition. To become a geneticist, a doctoral degree and approximately two years of training in an accredited laboratory for certification are required.

Genetic Counselors

Genetic counselors work with families to fully understand risks of certain genetic disorders, such as neuromuscular diseases. A genetic counselor evaluates a family's history and provides information and insight into what that history means from a genetic point of view. The genetic counselor must patiently and thoroughly record details of each patient's medical history and then evaluate that data. This part of the job requires a scientific-based approach, but the job also requires caring support of patients as they go through the evaluation process and learn of risks and difficulties associated with their genetics. A genetic counselor must have a master's degree, preferably in the field of human genetics and/or counseling. Certification is recommended.

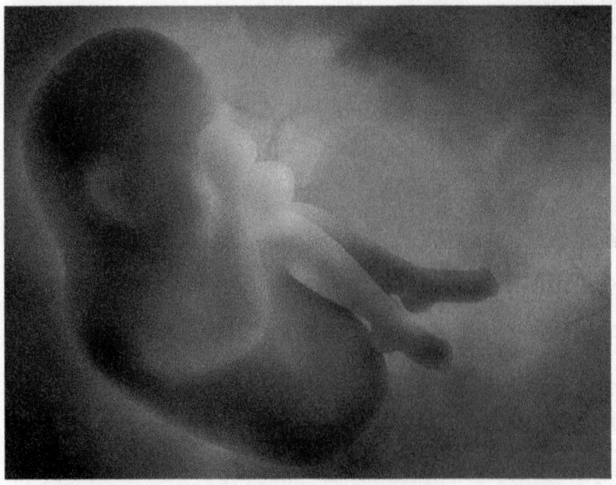

FIGURE 1.29
Genetic testing helps explain the relationship between heredity and fertility
Source: zven0/Fotolia LLC

Genetic Nurses

Genetic nurses specifically care for the genetic health of patients who have genetic issues, such as Huntington disease, hereditary breast cancer, and cystic fibrosis. Care includes screening, early detection, risk identification, treatment, and testing. A genetic nurse usually has long-term relationships with patients and their families. Because the outcomes for patients with genetic problems are often negative, a genetic nurse must be able to deal with this emotionally and help families deal with this eventuality as well. Genetic nurses need additional training, education, and certification to work in this field.

CAREERS IN ALTERNATIVE HEALTH SERVICES

A wide variety of careers also exist outside of the mainstream medical world. These careers fall under the category of **alternative medicine**. In addition to less familiar job roles, physicians and nurses also specialize in alternative medicine, such as homeopathy and naturopathic medicine. A career in alternative health care areas will require entrepreneurship to establish a practice. Some occupations are well known; others less so. The following are some examples of alternative health care and related occupations.

alternative medicine
(awl-TUR-*n*uh-tiv MED-uh-sin)
Using healing arts which are not part of traditional medical practice in the United States

- ***Homeopathy:*** Developed in Germany in the eighteenth century, homeopathic remedies are created from plant, animal, or mineral products greatly diluted in water or alcohol.
- ***Massage therapy:*** A wide variety of physical manipulative techniques promote relaxation and treats conditions caused by tension, such as headaches or insomnia.
- ***Naturopathic medicine:*** Although similar to traditional medicine, naturopathic medicine avoids drugs, major surgery, and cutting-edge technologies and relies instead on treatments designed to strengthen the body's own healing capabilities. For example, preparations such as vitamins, nutritional supplements, and herbs might be used to treat and prevent disease.
- ***Prayer and spirituality:*** Often considered "alternative" by conventional medical standards, prayer and spirituality help patients maintain a sense of purpose, meaning, and hope in the face of pain, suffering, and uncertainty.
- ***Chinese traditional medicine:*** Utilizing methods such as herbal remedies, acupuncture, diet, meditation, and exercises such as qigong and tai chi, this therapy seeks to achieve overall balance of health in preventing as well as treating illnesses. Qigong is an aspect of traditional Chinese medicine which involves the coordination of different breathing patterns with various physical postures and motions of the body. Tai chi is a gentle exercise program derived from martial arts, but composed of slow, deliberate movements, meditation, and deep breathing, which enhance physical health and emotional well-being.
- ***Biofeedback specialists:*** These specialists are trained to use a form of alternative medicine that involves measuring a patient's bodily processes such as blood pressure, heart rate, skin temperature, galvanic skin response (sweating), and muscle tension. They convey such information to the patient in real time in order to raise his or her awareness and conscious control of the related physiological activities. Specialists must pass a certification exam.
- ***Parish nurse specialists:*** These registered nurses commit to the healing missions of a church. They work to help fellow parishioners find support in crisis or with day-to-day struggles. They also work directly with parish staff to educate on wellness and improving life quality. Parish nurses must be registered and meet the standard nursing educational requirements.

- ***Acupressurists:*** These specialists use a form of traditional Chinese medicine in which the health care provider stimulates certain pressure points of the body to encourage the flow of vital energy (Qi) along the specific pathways called meridians. This is often used to control chronic pain such as migraine headaches or backaches. Acupressure is generally classified as massage, and training may be offered through massage schools or independent seminars.
- ***Acupuncturists:*** Acupuncturists use a form of traditional Chinese medicine that treats specific health disorders with the insertion of fine needles into the body at specific points where the flow of energy is thought to be blocked. To be certified, they must attend an accredited school of acupuncture and pass a licensing exam.
- ***Palliative care specialists:*** Palliative care is the active, total care of patients whose disease does not respond to curative treatment. It includes controlling a patient's pain and other symptoms, and addressing psychological, social, and spiritual problems. The goal is to provide the best possible quality of life for patients and their families. Palliative care specialists typically work in teams and usually are needed when the disease is advanced, life expectancy is short, and problems become complex and more urgent. Palliative care specialists are board certified physicians and must meet all of the standard requirements.
- ***Ayurvedic practitioners:*** These practitioners use a traditional system of Indian medicine in which the basic texts analyze the human body in terms of earth, water, fire, air, and ether, as well as the three bodily humors (wind, bile, and phlegm). To prevent illness, these practitioners emphasize hygiene, exercise, herbal preparations, and yoga. To cure ailments, they rely on herbal medicines, physiotherapy, and diet. Specialists must take specific courses and pass a certification exam.
- ***Chiropractors:*** Chiropractors treat patients whose health problems are associated with the body's muscular, nervous, and skeletal systems, especially the spine. Chiropractors use manipulation and specific adjustment of body structures, such as the spinal column, to rebalance the nervous system and the body. They must be licensed, which requires two to four years of undergraduate education and passing national and state exams.

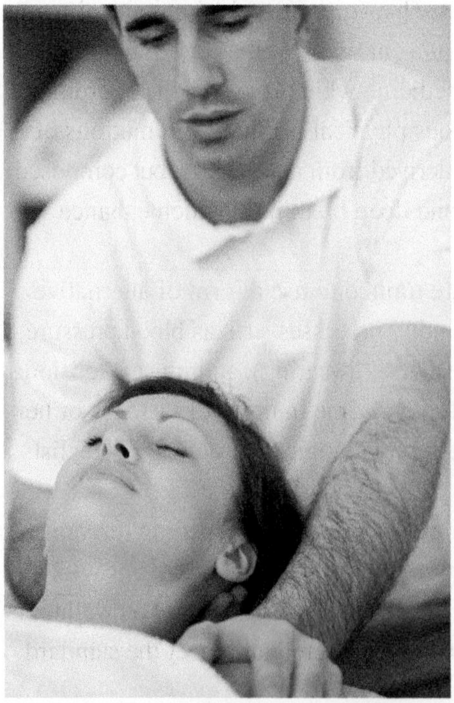

FIGURE 1.30

Chiropractor holds a patient's head to perform an alignment

Source: wavebreakmedia/ Shutterstock

- ***Aromatherapists:*** Aromatherapists use essential oils extracted from plants as therapy to promote health and well-being. These can be inhaled by patients, introduced internally, or applied topically. They must pass a training course and receive a certificate.
- ***Hypnotists:*** Hypnotists are trained in inducing trance states and therapeutic suggestions to improve a wide range of medical and psychological issues, such as fears, phobias, anxiety, sleep disorders, etc. Hypnotists must take a course (about one month long) and pass a test to be certified.

Community Service Organizations Involved in Health Care

Make a list of community organizations that are involved in health care. Identify the purpose of each organization. Select three of the organizations and describe what might happen if these organizations did not exist.

CAREERS IN MEDICINE

If you are considering becoming a doctor, medicine offers a wide variety of career options from which to choose. Physicians have doctorate degrees in Medicine (MD) or in specialty areas such as optometry (Doctor of Optometry or OD), osteopathy (Doctor of Osteopathic Medicine or DO), veterinary medicine (DVM or VMD), and so forth.

Medical Doctors (MD)

A medical doctor is a licensed physician who is responsible for comprehensive patient care. An MD promotes and maintains health, and treats both injuries and disease. Duties include, but are not limited to, examining patients; obtaining medical histories; ordering, performing, and interpreting diagnostic tests; counseling patients on health-related issues; and prescribing medicines. It is not uncommon for an MD to work 60 or more hours a week, and most work in small, private offices or clinics. Some practice in large health care organizations, which may allow for a less demanding work schedule. The education and training for an MD are among the most strenuous of any profession. In general, MDs complete four years of undergraduate school, four years of medical school, and three to eight years of internship and residency, depending upon the specialty pursued. All candidates must also pass a licensing exam, and they must continue to study throughout their careers to keep up with advances in medical science and technology.

Many physicians with an MD go on to specialize in other areas. For example, cardiologists study and treat the structure and function of the heart; pediatricians study and treat the care and health of babies and children, and dermatologists study and treat the makeup and pathology of skin. Other specialists include anesthesiologists, gerontologists, psychiatrists, orthopedists, neurologists, gynecologists, oncologists, pathologists, urologists, ophthalmologists, radiologists, surgeons, and orthodontists. Osteopaths are doctors who provide holistic care, considering both the physical and mental needs of patients. Physicians who specialize in the care of animals are called veterinarians.

What follows are more examples of physician specialties.

Family Medicine Physicians

Formerly known as "general practice," the field of Family Medicine became a distinct medical specialization in 1969 when it was decided that a one-year internship after medical school was no longer sufficient to prepare doctors for the full range of medical services required. A three-year residency program was implemented, physicians became eligible for board certification, and "family practice" became "family medicine." Family medicine physicians diagnose and treat illnesses and injuries for patients of all ages. They help patients manage chronic ailments and provide preventive care, including

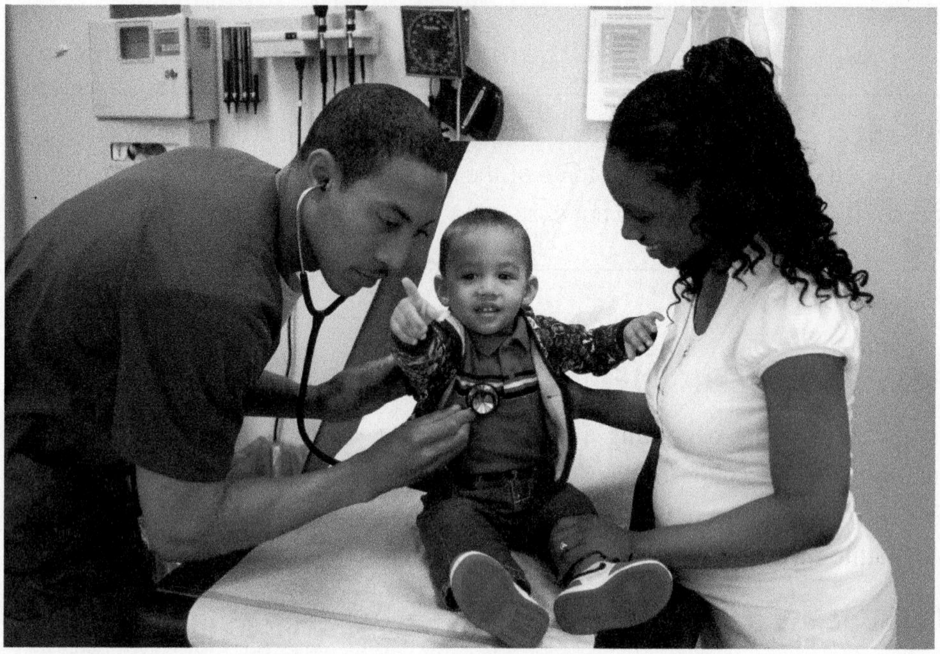

FIGURE 1.31

Family medicine physician examines a pediatric patient

Source: Carmen Martin/Pearson Education

screening tests, routine physical exams, and immunizations. They conduct health-risk assessments and counsel patients on how to lead healthier lives. Many family medicine physicians also provide prenatal care and deliver babies. About one out of every four visits to a doctor's office involves a family medicine doctor.

Internists (Internal Medicine Physicians)

An internist is a physician who may provide either primary or long-term comprehensive care. They also may specialize in fields such as cardiology, critical care, infectious disease, or pulmonology. Internists, as the name implies, focus on the health of internal organs. They generally treat illnesses such as high blood pressure or diabetes, which do not require surgery. The majority of an internist's patients are adults. Internists must complete medical school followed by a three-year residency in which they receive training focused on internal medicine. In order to specialize in a particular area, internists must complete another one to three years of training. Between 20 and 25 percent of all physicians are internists.

Dermatologists

A dermatologist is a physician trained to treat conditions and diseases of the skin, hair, and nails. This may involve skin allergies, cancer, melanomas, moles, acne, or even some sexually transmitted diseases. Dermatologists must be able to perform various types of dermatologic surgery and be able to analyze and interpret cultures. They must also have a broad base of knowledge that includes things such as allergies and immunology, environmental and industrial medicine, radiology, microbiology and surgery. To become a dermatologist, you must complete college and medical school. Following medical school, all dermatologists must complete one year of clinical training. Next, they spend three to four years as a resident specializing in dermatology. Those who choose to specialize must train for one more year in that area.

Epidemiologists

Epidemiologists study the occurrence and frequency of disease in large populations and determine the sources and causes of infectious disease epidemics. For example, epidemiologists might study childhood obesity, avian influenza, or AIDS. Epidemiologists have a master's degree in public health or a doctorate degree. Most are physicians who work in the community, universities, hospitals, or government agencies, such as the Centers for Disease Control and Prevention (CDC).

Podiatrists

Podiatrists diagnose and treat diseases and injuries of the foot, including corns, calluses, bunions, skin and nail infections, and deformities. After earning a bachelor's degree, students attend a four-year college of podiatry followed by a four-year residency at a hospital or medical clinic. They must pass a written and oral exam to become licensed by the state in which they plan to practice.

Optometrists

Optometrists are physicians who diagnose and treat vision problems. They examine the eyes for diseases such as glaucoma, nearsightedness and farsightedness, and depth and color perception. Optometrists prescribe eyeglasses and contact lenses. After earning a bachelor's degree, students must complete a four-year Doctor of Optometry degree program and become licensed to practice.

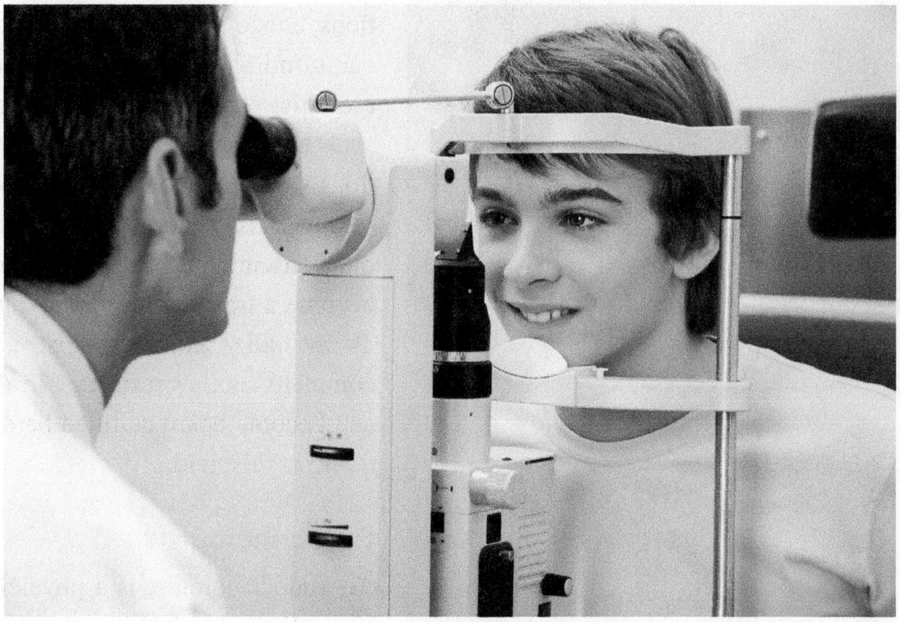

FIGURE 1.32

Patient undergoing an eye examination

Source: Tyler Olson/Fotolia LLC

Ophthalmologists

An ophthalmologist is a medical doctor who specializes in the eye and the visual system. Their job is to diagnose and treat eye diseases. They also treat eye injuries. This may entail routine eye exams, diagnosis and treatment of eye disorders or diseases, prescribing eyeglasses or contact lenses, surgery, or managing problems caused by systemic illness. To become an ophthalmologist, you must complete college and medical school, and then a one-year clinical internship and at least three years as a hospital resident in ophthalmology. To specialize in a specific area, such as a disease, an eye part, or pediatrics, you must complete one or two years of additional training. Once training is complete, ophthalmologists must pass an exam to become certified in this profession.

Otorhinolaryngologists

An otorhinolaryngologist, commonly known as an ENT, is a physician/surgeon who specializes in problems associated with the ear, nose, throat, and neck. Common ailments addressed include: head and neck cancer; tumors; sinus and allergic disease; thyroid and parathyroid problems; snoring and sleep apnea; and pediatric ear, nose and throat issues. An otorhinolaryngologist might perform surgery on the salivary or thyroid glands or reconstructive surgery of the head or neck. Other procedures include microsurgery of the middle ear, sinus surgery, or surgery at the base of the skull. To become an otorhinolaryngologist, students must complete medical school, one year of general surgery residency, and four years of otorhinolaryngology training.

Otologists

An otologist, also known as a neurotologist, is a physician who specializes in conditions affecting the ears. These conditions include problems with balance and dizziness, all types of hearing loss, noises in the ear, facial nerve disorders, persistent infections, congenital ear malformations, and ear tumors. Trained as a surgeon, an otologist performs surgical procedures, such as the repair of eardrum perforations, hearing reconstruction, and tumor removal. To become an otologist, you must attend medical school and then become a trained otorhinolaryngologist. To specialize as an otologist, you must complete another residency in that area and become board certified before practicing in this field.

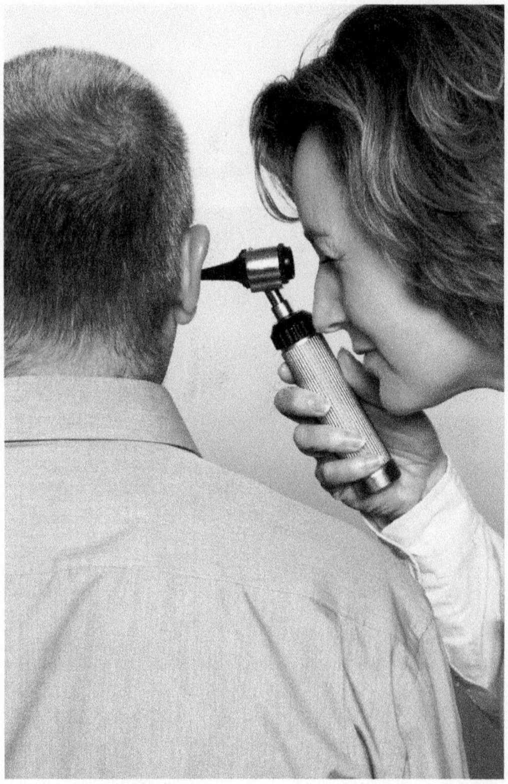

FIGURE 1.33

Patient having his ear checked with an otoscope

Source: RTimages/Fotolia LLC

Endocrinologists

An endocrinologist is a physician who specializes in the endocrine system. These doctors treat conditions that affect your glands. This may include diabetes, thyroid diseases, metabolic disorders, osteoporosis, hypertension, lack of growth, infertility, or cancer. Endocrinologists treat these hormone problems and try to restore a normal balance of hormones in their patients. Endocrinologists also do research to learn how glands work and find the best treatments for patients with glandular problems. As in many other specialties, to become an endocrinologist you must first complete medical school and then complete a two- to three-year residency to become certified in internal medicine. Following that, you must then spend two or three more years studying the endocrine system. It takes more than ten years to become trained as an endocrinologist.

ADDITIONAL HEALTH CAREERS

Health care offers many other job opportunities. Here are some more examples.

Health Educators

Health educators encourage a healthy lifestyle and focus on wellness by educating individuals and communities about health issues such as the importance of exercise and nutrition. These educators conduct lectures and classes, provide health screenings, and distribute videos and brochures. Health educators should be good communicators since they work with the public, have strong public speaking skills, and be sensitive of cultural differences.

Environmental Health Specialists

Environmental health specialists enforce regulations that protect food and water, safeguard hazardous materials, and dispose of infectious wastes. They collect and analyze samples, consult with physicians about environmental health hazards, prepare reports, and make suggestions on how to correct problems. Environmental health specialists work in hospitals, health departments, and wildlife parks.

Biomedical Equipment Technicians

Biomedical equipment technicians ensure that medical equipment is serviceable, safe, and properly configured. Their responsibilities include installation, inspection, repair, calibration, maintenance of, and education about biomedical equipment. Biomedical equipment technicians are employed by hospitals, clinics, and the military.

Research Scientists

Research specialists plan, develop, conduct, and evaluate scientific research in the lab, field, or teaching environment.

Social Workers

Social workers help individuals and families cope with problems or situations that occur in everyday life such as relationship issues, individuals with disabilities or illnesses, unemployment, or substance abuse. Social workers must be objective and sensitive to people, their cultures, and their problems.

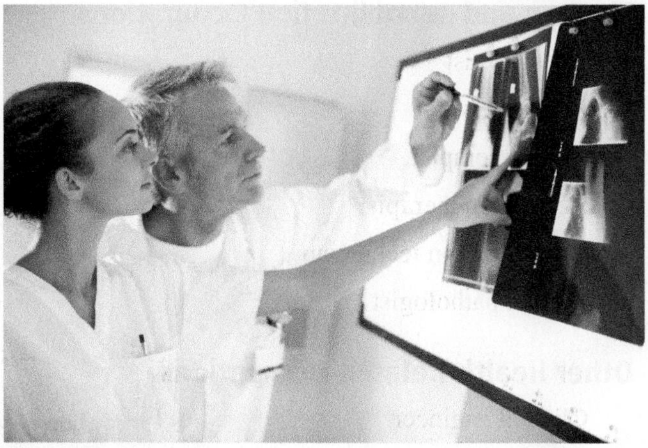

FIGURE 1.34
Physician and physician assistant discussing a patient's surgical procedure

Source: Yuri Arcurs/Fotolia LLC

Physician Assistants

Physician assistants, also referred to as PAs, practice medicine under the supervision of a physician or surgeon. They are trained to provide diagnostic, therapeutic, and preventive services. Physicians assistants take medical histories, examine patients, order and interpret tests, and make diagnoses. Most physician's assistants work in primary care facilities.

Psychologists

Psychologists study human behavior and the human mind. There are many different fields of psychology including clinical, educational, and research.

MORE HEALTH CAREERS

Health care offers many other occupational options, including the following:

Dental Occupations

Dental ceramist

Dental radiographer

Vision Services

Contact lens technician

Ophthalmic technician

Optician/dispensing optician

Technologists, Technicians, Assistants, and Aides

Audiometrist

Electroencephalographic (EEG) technologist

Medication aide

Patient transporter

Mental/Social Services Occupations

Mental health counselor

Mental retardation assistant

Psychiatric aide

Therapy and Rehabilitation Occupations

Art therapist

Audiologist

Music therapist

Recreation therapist

Rehabilitation technician

Speech pathologist

Other Health-Related Occupations

Clinical engineer

Funeral director/mortician

Grounds maintenance/landscaper

Health service administrator/health care administrator

Insurance clerk

Medical illustrator

Medical writer

Morgue attendant/embalmist

Nursing home administrator

A large percentage of health care workers have jobs that also occur in other kinds of organizations and industries. These include cooks, lawyers, business analysts, personnel workers, telephone operators, instructors, audio-visual technicians, beauticians and barbers, marketing specialists, computer techs, secretaries, payroll clerks, and so forth. When you stop to think about it, many large and urban hospitals employ such a diverse workforce they begin to resemble small towns.

CAREER LADDERS

One of the best advantages of working in health care is having career ladders to climb. Here are several examples. Be sure to check with the state where you plan to work to identify state-specific requirements for education, training, and certification.

Career Ladder: Respiratory Therapy Workers		
RESPIRATORY THERAPY WORKERS	Education and/or Experience Required	Average Income
Respiratory Therapist (RRT)	• High school diploma or equivalent • Completion of AMA-approved respiratory therapist training program in a community college or a four-year bachelor's degree program • Two years of experience in the field following training • Passing grade on a written examination given by the National Board of Respiratory Therapy	• Annual: $45,300–$62,570
Respiratory Therapy Technician (CRTT)	• High school diploma or equivalent • Completion of AMA-approved respiratory therapy technician training program • One year of work experience in the field following training • Passing grade on a written examination given by the National Board of Respiratory Therapy	• Annual: $35,900–$54,900
Respiratory Therapy Aide	• High school diploma or equivalent (preferred) • Completion of a vocational training program in respiratory therapy	• Annual: $24,300–$31,200

Career Ladder: Pharmacy Workers

PHARMACY WORKERS	Education and/or Experience Required	Average Income
Pharmacist	• Completion of a Doctor of Pharmacy degree (Pharm.D.) from an accredited school • One year of pharmacy internship • Passing grade on two exams to be licensed by the state • One year of pharmacy internship • License in state of employment after passing an exam	• Annual: $95,800–$123,300
Pharmacy Technician	• Two to twelve months of on-the-job training, completion of a high school pharmacy technician course, or completion of a one- to-two-year program in a community college • Some states offer a pharmacy technician certification upon successful completion of an examination • A national certification, offered by the Pharmacy Technician Certification Board, is required for employment by some hospitals and retail pharmacies	• Annual: $23,000–$33,800
Pharmacy Clerk/Pharmacy Helper	• High school diploma or equivalent • Good typing skills • Two to three months of on-the-job training or completion of a pharmacy vocational program	• Annual: $18,000–$25,000

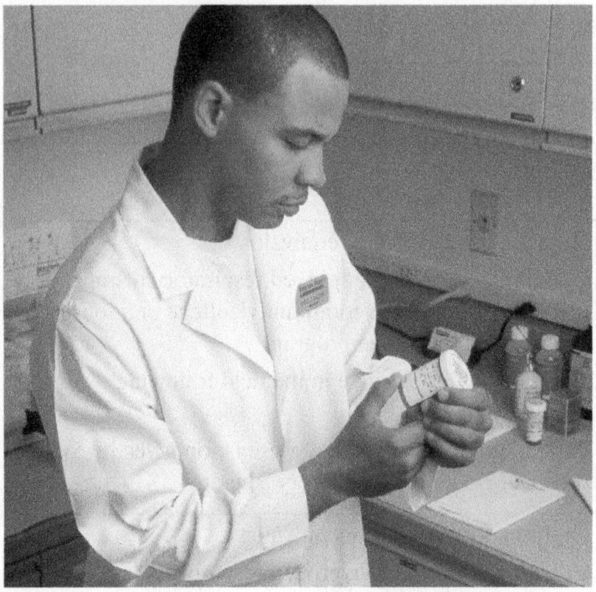

FIGURE 1.35

Pharmacist prepares a patient's medication

Source: George Dodson/Pearson

Career Ladder: Occupational Therapy Workers

OCCUPATIONAL THERAPY WORKERS	Education and/or Experience Required	Average Income
Physiatrist	• Graduation from an accredited medical school • License to practice medicine or osteopathy in state of employment • Residency in physical medicine and rehabilitation	• Annual: $124,800–$220,900

Occupational Therapist (OT) (OTR registered)	• Bachelor's degree in occupational therapy (four-year course in an approved program) • Certification by the Board of Registry of the American Occupational Therapy Association • Up to six months of on-the-job training	• Annual: $57,200–$84,200
Certified Occupational Therapy Assistant (COTA)	• High school diploma or equivalent • Completion of a two-year program in a community college • Completion of a certified vocational or technical program • Supervised fieldwork • Completion of a two-year program approved by the American Occupational Therapy Association (AOTA)	• Annual: $41,200–$59,900
Occupational Therapy Aide	• High school diploma or equivalent • On-the-job training • Completion of a vocational education program as an occupational therapy aide	• Annual: $19,500–$33,200

Career Ladder: Physical Therapy Workers

PHYSICAL THERAPY WORKERS	Education and/or Experience Required	Average Income
Physical Therapist (PT)	• Masters or doctorate degree in physical therapy • Supervised clinical internship • Passing grade on a state licensure examination	• Annual: $62,300–$87,900
Physical Therapist Assistant (PTA)	• Graduation from an accredited physical therapist assistant program • May be required to pass a state licensure or certification examination	• Annual: $39,100–$57,800
Physical Therapist Aide	• High school diploma or equivalent (preferred) • On-the-job training • Completion of a vocational education program as a physical therapy aide	• Annual: $20,100–$28,900

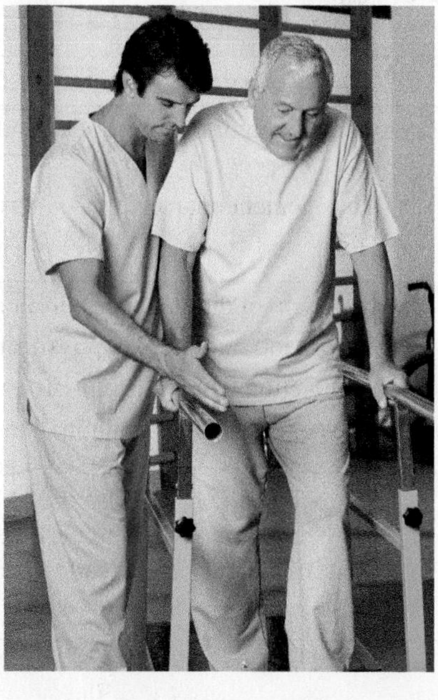

FIGURE 1.36

Physical therapist helps a patient walk

Source: Tyler Olson/Shutterstock

Career Ladder: Emergency Medical Workers

EMERGENCY MEDICAL WORKERS	Education and/or Experience Required	Average Income

Registered EMT-Paramedic	• Completion of EMT-paramedic training in an approved program offered by one of the following:
	  • Vocational school
	  • State educational facility
	  • Community college
	  • Hospital
	  • Medical school
	  • University
	• Six months of field experience as an EMT-paramedic
	• Passing grade on a written and practical examination given by the National Registry of Emergency Medical Technicians or the state emergency medical systems board
		• Annual: $31,000–$46,200

Registered EMT-Ambulance/I (Intermediate)	• Graduation from an approved EMT Basic program and 35–55 hours of additional instruction • Passing grade on a written and practical examination given by the National Registry of Emergency Medical Technicians or the state emergency medical systems board	• Annual: $23,700–$34,200
Basic EMT-Ambulance/A (Basic)	• At least 18 years of age • High school diploma or equivalent • Valid driver's license • Completion of a minimum 110-hour program offered in vocational programs and community colleges • Passing grade on a written and practical exam given by the National Registry of Emergency Medical Technicians or the state emergency medical systems board	• Annual: $21,300–$31,800

Career Ladder: Medical Assistants

MEDICAL ASSISTANTS	Education and/or Experience Required	Average Income
Office Manager	• Completion of administrative and clinical medical assistant program • Management courses, workshops, seminars • Home study courses	• Annual: $30,900–$47,100
Clinical/Back Office Medical Assistant (MA)	• High school diploma or equivalent • On-the-job training in a physician's office • Completion of a medical assistant training program • Passing grade on an examination by American Association of Medical Assistants to become a certified medical assistant (CMA), or by American Medical Technologists to become a registered medical assistant (RMA); certification is optional but preferred or required by many employers	• Annual: $27,300–$32,600

Administrative/Front Office Medical Assistant (MA)	• High school diploma or equivalent • On-the-job training in a physician's office • Completion of a medical assistant training program • Passing grade on an examination by American Association of Medical Assistants to become a certified medical assistant (CMA), or by American Medical Technologists to become a registered medical assistant (RMA); certification is optional but preferred or required by many employers	• Annual: $28,500–$37,000

Career Ladder: Dental Workers

DENTAL WORKERS	Education and/or Experience Required	Average Income
Dentist	• Graduation from a dental school approved by the American Dental Association • Passing grade on written and practical examinations • State licensure by passing written examinations given by the National Board of Examiners	• Annual: $119,700–$155,800
Dental Hygienist (DH)	• Graduation from an accredited dental hygienist program in a two-year community college, a four-year bachelor's degree program, or a five-year master's degree program • Passing grade on a written and clinical examination • License in the state of employment (given by the National Board of Dental Examiners)	• Annual: $55,600–$80,000
Dental Laboratory Technician	• High school diploma or equivalent • Two-year vocational program • On-the-job training (three to four years) • May become certified by passing a written and practical examination given by the National Board for Certification	• Annual: $27,000–$45,100
Dental Assistant	• High school diploma or equivalent • On-the-job training • Completion of a one- or two- year community college or vocational training program • Completion of an examination by the Certifying Board of the Dental Assisting National Board (CDA) (optional) • Some states offer a state certificate and also require a dental x-ray certification	• Annual: $27,500–$39,800

FIGURE 1.37

Dentist and dental assistant work as a team to provide dental care

Source: Monkey Business/Fotolia LLC

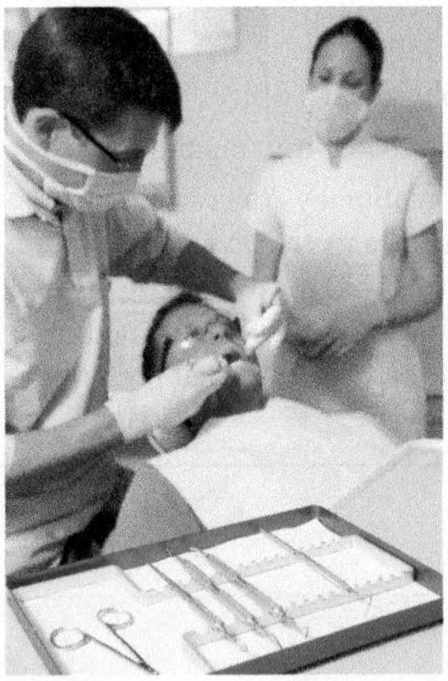

Career Ladder: Nursing Service Workers

NURSING SERVICE WORKERS	Education and/or Experience Required	Average Income
Nurse Practitioner (NP)	• All requirements for becoming a registered nurse • Completion of an accredited course in nurse practitioner training • License for the state of employment after passing an exam	• Annual: $69,900–$94,600
Registered Nurse (RN)	• High school diploma or equivalent • Graduation from a two-year community college • Graduation from a four-year college or university • Graduation from an accredited school of nursing • Graduation from a diploma school (three-year hospital schools are being phased out) • License for the state of employment after passing an exam	• Annual: $52,500–$78,000 • $58,300–$103,500 with advanced education
Licensed Practical Nurse (LPN)/Licensed Vocational Nurse (LVN)	• High school diploma or equivalent • Graduation from a recognized 1-year to 18-month program • License for the state of employment after passing an exam	• Annual: $33,900–$47,200
Unlicensed Assistive Personnel (Nursing Aide or Attendant, Orderly, Patient Care Assistant)	• Completion of on-the-job training or short-term training in a high school or vocational program • May require passing grade on a state competency exam as a nurse assistant • May require certification as a nurse assistant	• Annual: $20,200–$31,200
Home Health Aide (HHA)	• High school diploma or equivalent (preferred) • Completion of a vocational education program as a home health aide • State certification may be required	• Annual: $17,700–$24,300
Nurse Assistant/Geriatric Aide	• High school diploma or equivalent (preferred) and/or participation in a high school nursing assistant program • Hospital-conducted on-the-job training • Completion of an OBRA approved 1987 Omnibus Budget Reconciliation Act nurse assistant program • License for the state of employment after passing an exam	• Annual: $20,500–$29,000

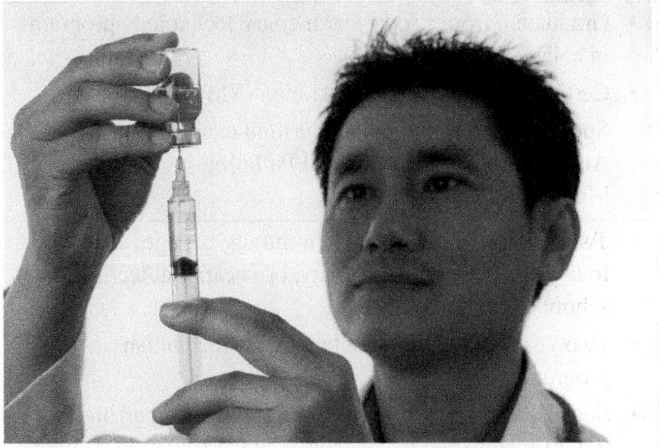

FIGURE 1.38
Registered nurse prepares a patient's medication
Source: william casey/Shutterstock

Career Ladder: Veterinary Workers

VETERINARY WORKERS	Education and/or Experience Required	Average Income
Veterinarian (DVM or VMD)	• Completion of three- to four- years of preveterinary college • Graduation from an accredited veterinary college and a Doctor of Veterinary Medicine degree • License in state of employment after passing an exam	• Annual: $62,800–$105,200
Animal Health Technician (ATR registered)	• Completion of certificate or associate's degree program • Registration, certification, or licensure required in many states	• Annual: $24,000–$35,900
Veterinarian Animal Caretaker/Assistant	• High school diploma or equivalent • On-the-job training • Home study through American Boarding Kennels Association (ABKA) • Passing grade on oral and written exam to become ABKA Certified Kennel Operator (CKO)	• Annual: $18,100–$26,700
Groomer	• Completion of 6–10 weeks of informal apprenticeship • Four to 18 weeks at a state licensed grooming school • Completion of National Dog Groomers Association of America written and practical skills exam	• Annual: $24,600–$37,600

Career Ladder: Medical Laboratory Workers

MEDICAL LABORATORY WORKERS	Education and/or Experience Required	Average Income
Medical Pathologist	• Graduation from an accredited medical school • State license to practice medicine or osteopathy • Certification by the American Board of Pathology	• Annual: $121,400–$291,000

Medical Laboratory Manager, Chief Technologist	• Several years of experience as a medical technologist
	• Graduate-level education in one of the following:
	  • Biological sciences
	  • Chemistry
	  • Management
		• Annual: $56,783–$112,105

Medical Laboratory Technologist (Clinical Laboratory Scientist) (MT)	• Graduation from a four-year medical technology program in college or university • Certification (CMT) or registration (RMT) • Successful completion of a written examination by American Society of Clinical Pathologists or American Medical Technologists	• Annual: $45,800–$65,100
Medical Laboratory Technician (MLT)	• Two years of training in a community college, four-year college or university, or vocational/technical school • Two years of training in a laboratory technician program • Successful completion of requirements for certification (CLT) established by the National Certification Agency for Medical Laboratory Personnel	• Annual: $28,800–$45,400
Medical Laboratory Assistant Blood and Plasma	• High school diploma or equivalent • Completion of an approved 12-month medical laboratory technician certificate program in a community college, vocational school, or private program	• Annual: $20,800–$41,600
Medical Phlebotomist	• High school graduate or equivalent • Ten to 20-hour certification program in a hospital, physician's office, or laboratory • Completion of a vocational education program as a phlebotomist • Some states require certification to practice	• Annual: $26,000–$32,300
Medical Laboratory Aide	• High school diploma or equivalent • On-the-job training for at least two months • Completion of a vocational education program as a laboratory aide	• Annual: $24,000–$31,500

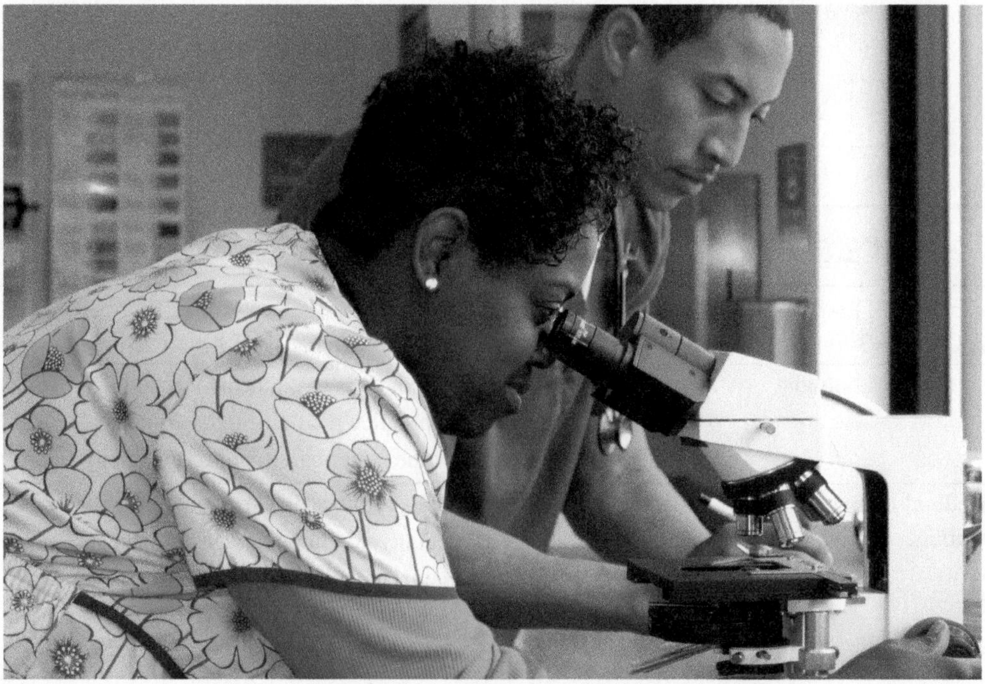

FIGURE 1.39

Examining a microscopic slide to ensure an accurate diagnosis

Source: Carmen Martin/Pearson Education

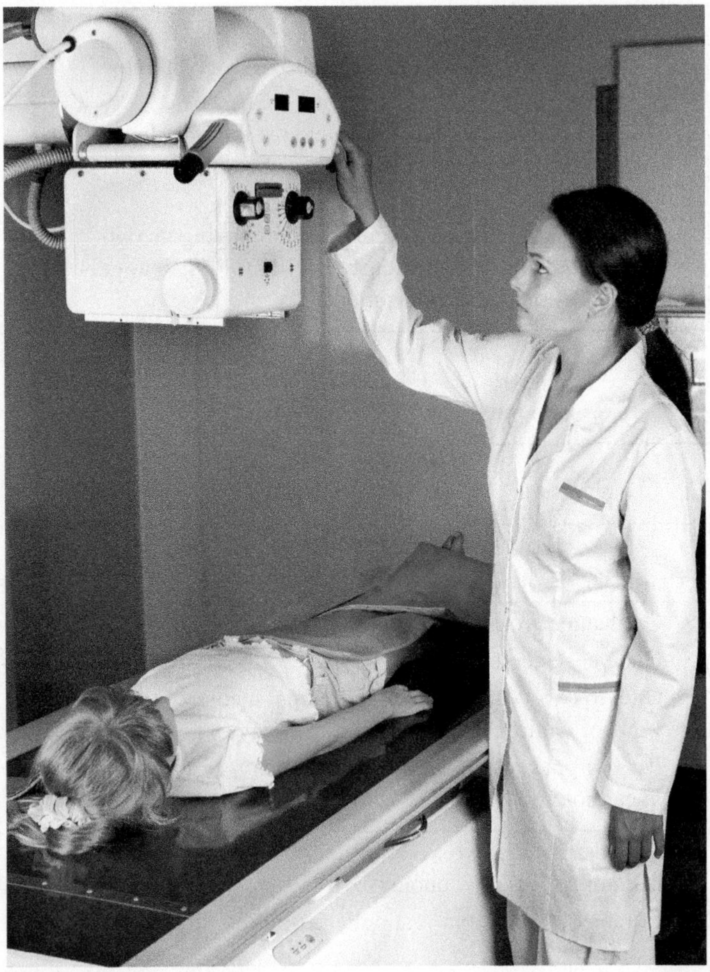

FIGURE 1.40

Patient undergoing a radiographic procedure

Source: Gennadiy Poznyakov/Fotolia

Career Ladder: Diagnostic Imaging Workers

DIAGNOSTIC IMAGING WORKERS	Education and/or Experience Required	Average Income
Radiologist	• Graduation from an accredited medical school • License to practice medicine in the state of employment • Three year residency program in radiology • Passing grade on examinations for board certification in radiology	• Annual: \$93,500–\$329,600
Chief Technologist	• Graduation from an accredited radiologic technology program • Registered as a radiologic technologist through the American Registry of Radiologic Technologists (ARRT) • Bachelor's degree in radiologic technology or equivalent • Training and experience in two or more imaging modalities, such as nuclear medicine, CT, MRI, PET, or sonography	• Annual: \$43,500–\$74,400

Radiographer, Diagnostic Imaging Technologist, Diagnostic Medical Sonographer	• High school diploma or equivalent • Graduation from an accredited radiologic technology program • Registered as a radiologic technologist through the American Registry of Radiologic Technologists (ARRT) • Additional training and experience in imaging modalities, such as nuclear medicine, CT, MRI, PET, sonography, fluoroscopy, and mammography	• Annual: $53,300–$63,600

Career Ladder: Cardiovascular Workers

CARDIOVASCULAR WORKERS	Education and/or Experience Required	Average Income
Cardiologist	• Graduation from an accredited school of medicine • One-year internship • One- to two-year residency in internal medicine to two years of clinical fellowship in cardiology • Passing grades on examinations for board certification in cardiology	• Annual: $101,300–$378,400
Cardiovascular Technologist	• Completion of a two-year community college program in cardiovascular technology • Completion of a four-year college or university program	• Annual: $33,700–$63,000
EKG Technician	• High school diploma or equivalent • One to six months of on-the-job training • Completion of a vocational education program as an EKG technician • One to two years of study at a community college	• Annual: $27,200–$35,500

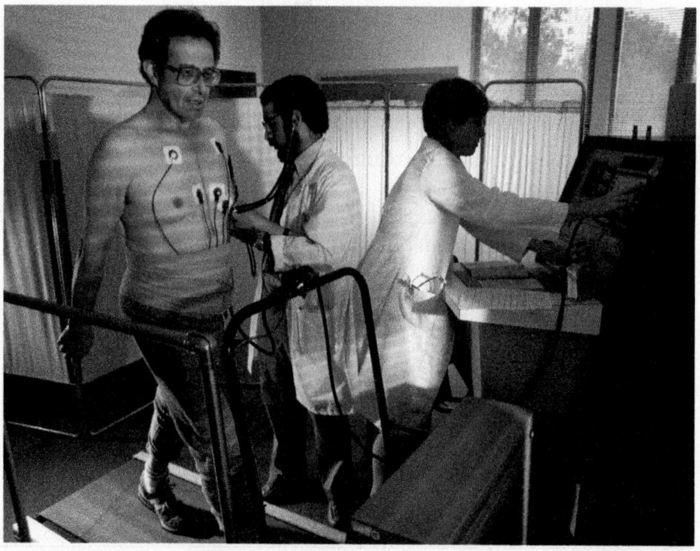

FIGURE 1.41

Patient undergoing an exercise treadmill stress test to detect a cardiovascular condition

Source: Nathan Benn/Alamy

Career Ladder: Admitting Department Workers

ADMITTING DEPARTMENT WORKERS	Education and/or Experience Required	Average Income
Admitting Officer	• High school diploma or equivalent • Bachelor's degree • Two to three months of on-the-job training • One to two years of experience working in a health care facility (may be required)	• Annual: $41,400–$55,400
Admitting Clerk	• High school diploma or equivalent • Computer skills • One to two months of on-the-job training	• Annual: $25,300–$31,800

Career Ladder: Medical Records/Health Information Management Workers

MEDICAL RECORDS/ HEALTH INFORMATION MANAGEMENT WORKERS	Education and/or Experience Required	Average Income
Registered Medical Records Administrator (RRA)	• Bachelor's degree from an accredited college program • Passing grade on the certification examination given by the American Health Information Management Association (AHIMA)	• Annual: $54,500–$78,000
Medical Coder	• High school diploma or equivalent • Completion of a 12- to 18-month training program or associate's degree program • Passing grade on certification exam(s) by AHIMA and the American Academy of Professional Coders (AAPC)	• Annual: $32,899–$56,520
Medical Records Technician	• Graduation from a program accredited by AHIMA or the AHIMA Independent Study Program • Passing grade on the AHIMA certification exam	• Annual: $34,300–$42,200
Medical Transcriptionist	• High school diploma or equivalent • On-the-job training • Completion of a vocational education program in the area of medical transcriptionist • Completion of a correspondence course	• Annual: $27,200–$39,000
Medical Records/Health Information Management Clerk	• High school diploma or equivalent • Typing and filing skills • Knowledge of office methods and medical terminology • Three to six months of on-the-job training • Completion of a vocational education program in the area of medical records clerk	• Annual: $24,000–$28,900

FIGURE 1.42

Health information technician pulls medical records for review

Source: Craig X. Sotres/Pearson Education

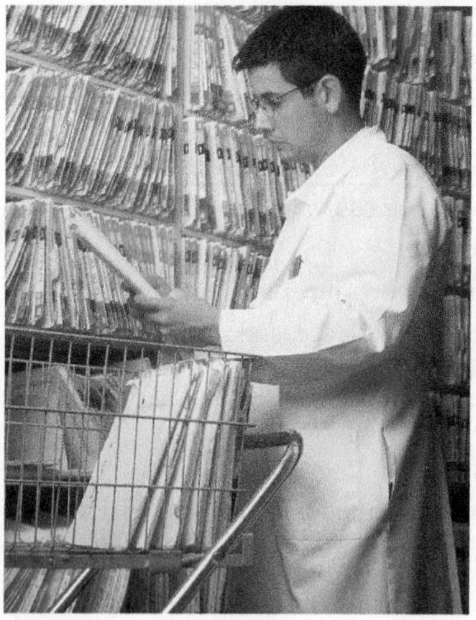

Career Ladder: Health Unit Coordinators

HEALTH UNIT COORDINATORS	Education and/or Experience Required	Average Income
Manager of Health Unit Coordinators	• High school diploma or equivalent • Associate's degree from a community college in unit management as a health unit coordinator	• Annual: $32,500–$48,700
Unit Secretary/Health Unit Coordinator	• High school diploma or equivalent • Completion of a hospital-based, vocational, or community college training program	• Annual: $24,900–$32,000

Career Ladder: Central Processing/Supply Workers

CENTRAL PROCESSING/ SUPPLY WORKERS	Education and/or Experience Required	Average Income
Central Processing Manager	• CRCST certification by the International Association of Healthcare Central Service Materiel Management (IAHCSMM) • Bachelor's degree or online, self-study, management courses and workshops • Passing grade on IAHCSMM exam • Certification in Healthcare Leadership (CHL) (optional)	• Annual: $53,605–$88,551
Technician/Certified Registered Central Service Technician (CRCST)	• High school diploma or equivalent • On-the-job training (six months), online or self-study course • Completion of a vocational education program as a central supply technician • Passing grade on IAHCSMM certification exam (optional)	• Annual: $21,300–$35,300

Career Ladder: Housekeeping/Environmental Services Workers

HOUSEKEEPING/ ENVIRONMENTAL SERVICES WORKERS	Education and/or Experience Required	Average Income
Director of Housekeeping Services/Environmental Services	• College degree in management and/or completion of courses in environmental services management • Supervisory experience	• Annual: $52,959–$98,323
Housekeeping/ Environmental Services Crew Leader/Supervisor	• High school diploma or equivalent • Completion of courses in hospital housekeeping and environmental services • One to four months of on-the-job training in supervision • Up to two years of experience as a housekeeper/ environmental services technician	• Annual: $22,900–$34,000
Housekeeper/Environmental Services Technician	• One to six months on-the-job training • Completion of a vocational education program	• Annual: $17,200–$26,700

Career Ladder: Food Service Workers

FOOD SERVICE WORKERS	Education and/or Experience Required	Average Income
Administrative Dietitian	• Must be a registered dietitian • Graduate study credits in institutional or business administration	• Annual: $41,700–$67,400
Registered Dietitian	• Bachelor's degree with a major in foods and nutrition or institutional management • Six to twelve month internship in a dietary department	• Annual: $42,400–$63,500
Dietetic Intern	• Bachelor's degree with a major in foods and nutrition or institutional management	• Annual: $28,900–$38,800
Dietetic Technician	• Completion of a dietetic technician program in a community college	• Annual: $21,100–$34,700
Food Service Worker/ Dietetic Assistant	• On-the-job training • Completion of a vocational education program as a food service worker	• Annual: $16,400–$23,500

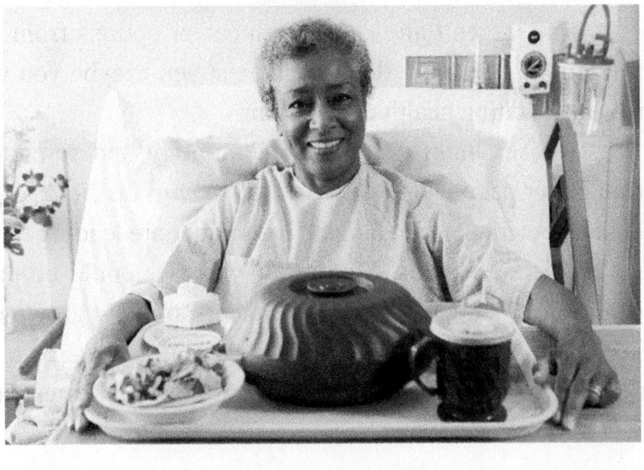

FIGURE 1.43

Hospital patient benefits from a healthy meal planned and prepared by food service workers

Source: Monkey Business Images/ Shutterstock

RECENT DEVELOPMENTS

Job Growth in the Health Care Industry

The rapidly growing elderly population in the United States is increasing the demand for health care services and health care workers. Health care provided about 14.3 million jobs in 2008. Approximately 40% of employees worked in hospitals, 21% in nursing homes and other residential care locations, and about 16% worked in physician practices. When the economic downturn occurred, the U.S. economy lost about 7.5 million jobs overall, but employment in health care increased. In fact, 22% of the job growth that did occur in the U.S. since 2008 was in health care, representing twice as much growth as in manufacturing. Ten of the twenty occupations growing most rapidly in the U.S. are in health care or health care related fields.

This represents just the beginning of a major, multi-year growth spurt in health care employment. By the year 2050, one out of every four Americans will be age 65 or older, increasing the demand for health care services even more. According to the Bureau of Labor Statistics, by the year 2020 health care and social assistance jobs will add about 5.6 million additional workers, becoming the industry with the largest number of job gains.

According to the Bureau of Labor Statistics, employment in the following jobs will grow substantially between 2008 and 2018:

- *Biomedical engineers:* 72% increase; average salary $82,421
- *Computer software engineers:* high demand for those with bachelor's degrees; average salary $97,581
- *Customer service representatives:* fast growth due to high turnover; great opportunities for bilingual workers; average salary $29,314
- *Home health aides:* jobs are growing as the elderly population increases; average salary $28,173
- *Medical assistants:* projected to grow by 33.9%; average salary $37,571
- *Registered nurses:* the largest segment of the health care workforce will grow by 22.2%; average salary $71,692.

HEALTH CAREERS AND THE FUTURE

As if there weren't already enough career options from which to choose, many health care jobs of the future don't even exist yet. Maybe you will play a role in one of these new and exciting health occupations.

Advancements in medical technology and science have caused an increasing demand for people who are qualified to work in biology, genetics, and the life sciences. Stem cell therapies and cloning techniques are leading the way as the study of regenerative medicine evolves. Many fatal diseases could be prevented with tissue or organ replacement, so doctors and researchers are now growing organs from a patient's own cells. For example, a patient's bladder cells can be grown in a petri dish and layered into a bladder. Within a few weeks, a 3-D mold will create a new bladder. Once it has grown and is functioning properly, the new bladder can be implanted into the patient. State of the art labs are now growing a wide array of tissues and organs including muscle, blood vessels, kidneys, hearts, and livers.

APPLY IT RESEARCHING FUTURE DEMAND

Choose one of the health occupations described in this chapter. Do some online research to learn more about the occupation and its future. What is the future demand for these workers? What new types of jobs might emerge within the next few years?

REALITY CHECK

By now you've probably realized that there are far more occupations in health care than you ever imagined. If you're feeling overwhelmed by the long list of choices and confused by some of the unusual job titles (*electroneurodiagnostic technologist*, *prosthetist,* or *otorhinolaryngologist*, for example), don't be concerned. You are not alone. Most people are familiar with the roles that doctors, nurses, pharmacists, and dentists play in health care. But the majority of people, including those who have worked in health care for many years, aren't familiar with *all* of the different occupations available.

If you pursue a career in health care, help may soon be on the way. Once you start learning medical terminology, these job titles won't sound so foreign anymore. For example, when you break down *otorhinolaryngologist* into its parts (oto = ear; rhin = nose; laryng = larynx or throat) you'll quickly realize that an otorhinolaryngologist is an ear-nose-and-throat doctor, also known as an ENT doctor.

Other health care workers may have job titles that lend few clues to their actual job duties. Examples include *Clinical Associate*, *Care Team Specialist*, *Patient Care Technician*, *Unit Support Tech*, and *Multiskilled Technician*. Some workers who perform the same job, even within the same organization, may have different job titles. Don't hesitate to pursue a health career because the options are too overwhelming to figure out. By the time you finish reading this book and completing your assignments, you'll have narrowed down the list of choices and identified a few of the occupations that sound good to you. Wading through this information and figuring out where *you* fit in will be well worth your time and energy.

According to the U.S. Bureau of Labor and Statistics, health care generates more jobs than any other industry in the country. The aging population and expected advancements in medical technology and gene therapy ensure that the demand for health care workers will continue into the future. By choosing a career in health care, you'll be well on your way to enjoying a productive and rewarding career. Because you'll need to meet several standards along the way, your next step is to take a closer look at what it's like to work in health care and what will be expected of you as a health care professional.

portfolio
(port-FOE-lee-oh) Collection of materials that demonstrate knowledge, skills, and abilities

Key Points

- The National Career Clusters™ Framework links what students learn in school with the knowledge, skills, and abilities they will need for career success.
- As one of the sixteen Career Clusters, the Health Science cluster includes a wide variety of health occupations in Therapeutic Services, Diagnostic Services, Health Informatics Services, Support Services, and Biotechnology Research and Development Services.
- The National Consortium for Health Science Education (NCHSE) provides *pathway standards* for the five health care pathways, detailing *core expectations* and *accountability criteria* that must be met to deliver safe and effective health care services.
- The health occupations offer a variety of work environments from which to choose.
- Options for education, training, and entry points into health care include on-the-job training and completion of a post-secondary program or college degree.
- In health care, you must *learn more to earn more*.
- Most health occupations offer career ladders and career lattices to support growth and advancement. You can often *start at the bottom* and work your way up over time.
- Health occupations are divided into five pathways, with each area offering an extensive array of options from which to choose.
- Some health occupations align with body systems, such as the circulatory or digestive system.
- The study and practice of genetics, medicine, and alternative health care services provide additional health career options.
- Employment opportunities in health care will continue to grow, with new occupations that have yet to emerge.

Section Review Questions

Answer each of the following questions. Indicate which page in the textbook led you to your answer.

1. List two questions you should answer when using online references to make sure the information on the site is credible.
2. Give one example of how ionizing radiation is used in health care.
3. Name the website sponsored by the U.S. Department of Labor, Employment and Training Administration that provides comprehensive occupational information on hundreds of different jobs.
4. Compare the income/financial benefits of earning a bachelor's degree versus a high school diploma or GED.
5. Break *otorhinolaryngologist* into its separate word parts and define the term.
6. Discuss labor projections for the health care industry.
7. Explain the difference between allied health technicians and technologists.

Learn by Doing

Complete Worksheets 1–4 in Section 1.2 of your *Student Activity Guide*.

CHAPTER 1 Review

Chapter Review Questions

Answer each of the following questions. Indicate which page in the textbook led you to your answer.

1. List three reasons why professionalism is important in health care.
2. Explain how having a successful health career can positively impact your self-esteem and self-worth.
3. Explain the purpose of the National Career Clusters™ Framework.
4. Describe the purpose of the National Consortium for Health Science Education.
5. Identify one health occupation for each of the five Health Science pathways.
6. Name two health occupations aligned with systems of the human body.
7. List two careers in alternative health services and two careers in medicine.

Chapter Review Activities

1. Select one health occupation that's described in this chapter that sounds interesting to you, and then list the reasons why. Next, choose an occupation that doesn't sound appealing to you, and list the reasons why. Do you notice any patterns or similarities in your reasoning?
2. Go online to find the National Health Care Skills Standards at http://www.healthscienceconsortium.org. Prepare a poster that summarizes the standards. Select a foundation standard and prepare a brief oral presentation describing the knowledge and skills required for it.
3. Go online to find information about the States' Career Clusters Initiative (SCCI) at http://www.careertech.org/. Identify and list the sixteen major occupational categories. Discuss how the clusters can be helpful to both students and teachers.

What If? Scenarios

What would you do in each of the following situations? Record your answer, explain it, and indicate which page in the textbook led you to your decision.

1. While visiting your aunt in a nursing home, you overhear one of the nursing assistants using obscene language while speaking with one of the other residents.
2. Your department is sponsoring an upcoming workshop entitled "Customer Service Concepts for Health Care Professionals". Invitations are being sent to the doctors, nurses, and allied health personnel, but the housekeeping and dietary workers aren't included.
3. A coworker was just laid off because of a corporate downsizing. She's depressed and beginning to wonder if she's worthy of finding another job.
4. You're due to graduate from high school in less than one year, but a relative calls to say he has a full-time job waiting for you if you'll quit school and move across town.
5. You've heard that it doesn't take long to become a pharmacy technician, but you don't know anything about the profession or the requirements for entry into practice.
6. After a visit to your eye doctor to have an eye exam and to order new glasses, you think you might be interested in pursuing a career that involves diagnosing and treating vision problems, but you don't know where to go to find more information.

Media Connection

Use the companion website for additional interactive learning activities.

Portfolio Connection

Planning and preparing for a career is a process that allows you to look back on your experiences and learn from them. You can evaluate the things in your past that worked for you and those that did not. You now have an opportunity to create a file that reflects what you learn. This file is called a career **portfolio**. Your portfolio will contain documents that show what you have learned during your education. Your work will show the abilities and skills you gain throughout your training.

You will use material from your career portfolio when you apply for a job or for admission to college or a postsecondary training program. Developing your portfolio provides a chance to express the positive results of your learning experiences in a professional manner. As you build your portfolio, remember that you will want to show how your strengths have helped you, and how you have learned and changed from previous experiences. This will be invaluable when presenting yourself to a potential employer. It will showcase your ability to deal with new situations and to learn from your mistakes. As you prepare materials for your portfolio, do not include details about specific patients as this would be a violation of federal law.

As part of its Workplace Learning Preparation and Guidelines, the National Consortium for Health Science Education provides the following information to help guide the content of your career portfolio:

- ***Portfolio Introduction.*** The portfolio introduction includes information on the contents of the portfolio and any other relevant information of interest to the portfolio recipient.
- ***Résumé.*** The résumé should include career goals, education and work experiences, awards, honors, and other activities.
- ***Project.*** The project is student selected and designed, has a clear connection to health care, and shows complex thinking. The result should be a significant performance, service, or product.
- ***Writing sample.*** The writing sample is an essay type document that demonstrates coherent thought, follows accepted structural format for written work, and is grammatically correct and free of spelling errors.
- ***Workplace Learning or Supervised Practical Experience.*** The workplace learning or supervised practical experience must be documented by a signed performance evaluation, workplace checklist, and letter of confirmation or certificate of participation. The experience may include job shadowing, explorations, and internships. The portfolio should include at least two examples, of which one may be a virtual experience.
- ***Oral presentation.*** The oral presentation may be a speech, presentation and/or instruction to a group with a completed evaluation, sample resources, and any materials that were distributed.
- ***Community Service or Service Learning.*** The community service or service learning may be documented by a summary of the experience and its benefits to both the community and the student.
- ***CPR and First Aid.*** CPR and First Aid are documented with current CPR and Basic First Aid certificates.
- ***Internet Application.*** The Internet application will be a summary that includes at least two sites that are health care related. Examples are career research, research on a medical issue, or research for a project or activity.
- ***Leadership.*** The leadership can be demonstrated by participation as an officer in a student health care organization or as a class officer, student council, church or scout officer, or other leadership position.
- ***Journaling.*** The journaling reflects the student's interpretation and insights related to a health care experience or project over an extended period of time, such as a semester.
- ***Other Content.*** Other content may be added to strengthen the portfolio and to meet school or program requirements. This may include high school diploma, special awards, recognitions, and/or certificates.

You can develop many of your career portfolio components by completing the activities outlined in this textbook and by participating in student leadership events and activities. So let's get started.

Think about a time when you surprised yourself by accomplishing something that you were not sure you could do. What caused you to try it when you were unsure about it? What went well in that experience? What would you do differently? Explain your answers in a short paper. Your explanation must clearly identify your self-evaluation and show how you would approach uncertain experiences in the future. This assignment helps you review and evaluate your past experience. Some of the future assignments for your portfolio will require a similar process, with a focus on your career training.

CHAPTER 2

Working in Health Care

Source: Monkey Business Images/Shutterstock

SECTIONS

"Character is like a tree and reputation like its shadow. The shadow is what we think of it; the tree is the real thing."

Abraham Lincoln, 16th U.S. President, 1809–1865

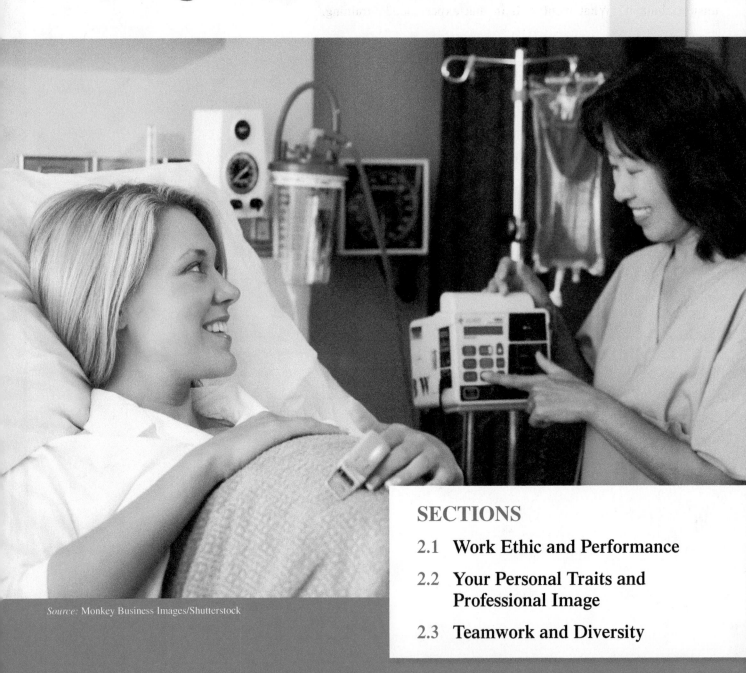

GETTING STARTED

Imagine that you own a health care organization that employs about two hundred people. Because of the economic downturn, you receive at least thirty applications for every job vacancy that you post. Think about the kind of people whom you would want working for your organization. List the top ten characteristics that you would seek when selecting the best candidates. What qualifications, attitudes, and behaviors would be important to you? What would you expect from your employees once they've been hired? How would you evaluate job performance and award pay raises? What factors would you consider when promoting people into higher paying jobs? What policies and procedures would you expect your employees to follow in order to create a safe and professional work environment? List five behaviors that would cause you to dismiss an employee from his or her job.

Work Ethic and Performance

SECTION 2.1

Background

Achieving success as a health care worker requires knowing what is expected of you and then meeting (or better yet, exceeding) those expectations. To develop and maintain a professional reputation, you must commit to your job each and every day and demonstrate a strong work ethic. Your attendance, reliability, and attitude all play a role, as well as your use of effective problem solving and critical thinking skills. Working within your scope of practice, protecting patient confidentiality, and complying with all laws, regulations, and policies related to your job are extremely important. Let's start by taking a look at how health care workers must depend on one another to get the work done, and done well.

work ethic
(WERK EH-thik) Attitudes and behaviors that support good work performance

Objectives

After completing this section, you will be able to:

1. Define the key terms.
2. Explain the difference between *soft skills* and *hard skills* and discuss why health care workers need both types of skills.
3. Define *interdependence* and *systems perspective* and explain their importance in health care.
4. Explain why it's important to be "present in the moment" at work.
5. Define *critical thinking* and list three things that critical thinkers do to make good decisions.
6. List five factors that demonstrate a strong work ethic.
7. Describe the attitudinal differences between optimists and pessimists.
8. Discuss the importance of confidentiality, HIPAA, and the HITECH Act.
9. Identify how competence and scope of practice impact quality of care.
10. List two things you should do when representing your employer.
11. Explain the purpose of performance evaluations.
12. Differentiate between objective and subjective evaluation criteria.

MAKING A COMMITMENT TO YOUR JOB

Health care employs about 10% of all American workers. One of the best benefits of working in health care is the opportunity to improve the quality of people's lives. Premature babies struggle to survive, injured athletes strive to regain strength, people with ailments attempt to lead normal lives, and terminally ill patients face end-of-life decisions. Health care workers are at their patients' sides from cradle to grave, providing crucial diagnostic and therapeutic procedures, compassionate care, and helpful encouragement and support. It's a privilege to work in health care and touch the lives of those you serve.

As a service industry, health care requires not only technical competence but also **people skills** that enhance your ability to interact effectively with other people. Also called **soft skills** or **interpersonal skills**, these characteristics relate more to *who you are* than *what you know*. Once you've completed training, employers will assume you are competent to perform the hands-on, technical, **hard skills** duties of your job. While hard skills can be learned and improved over time, soft skills are part of your **personality** and much more difficult to acquire and change. Employers are increasingly screening, hiring, paying, and promoting for soft skills to ensure that their employees work harmoniously with other people.

When you work in health care, you must commit to your job and take a professional approach to your work. Failure to do so can result in some bad outcomes for both you and the patients you serve. What could go wrong if someone fails to take his or her job seriously? Consider the following scenarios:

- What if a phlebotomist confuses blood samples and labels them incorrectly?
- What if a clerical worker misspells a medical term on a patient's health record?
- What if a technician doesn't sterilize surgical instruments properly?
- What if a radiographer fails to position a patient correctly for a diagnostic imaging exam?

Interdependence

The ability to view *the big picture* in health care and know where you fit in starts with examining your job and seeing how it connects with the roles of other workers. This means developing a **systems perspective**—standing back, viewing the entire process of how a patient moves through your organization, and understanding how your role fits into that process. No one in health care works alone—everyone's work is interconnected. This reliance on one another is called **interdependence**, and without it, the work flow breaks down.

Think about your role and responsibilities.

- How do your responsibilities connect with those of other workers?
- What other workers do you rely on to get your work done?
- What other workers must depend on you to get their work done?
- Where do the patients fit into this picture?

Many employers have an **organizational chart**—an illustration showing the components of the company and how they fit together. Typical organizational charts include the hierarchy of the organization—in other words, *who* reports *to whom*. Large organizations have detailed illustrations showing the flow of work processes within and

people skills
(PEE-puhl skils) Personality characteristics that enhance your ability to interact effectively with other people; also known as soft skills

soft skills
(SAWFT skils) Personality characteristics that enhance your ability to interact effectively with other people; also known as people skills

interpersonal skills
(in-ter-PUR-suh-nl skils) The ability to interact with other people

hard skills
(HAHRD skils) The ability to perform the technical, hands-on duties of a job

personality
(pur-suh-NAL-i-tee) Distinctive individual qualities of a person, relating to patterns of behavior and attitudes

systems perspective
(SIS-tuhm per-SPEK-tiv) Stepping back to view an entire process to see how each component connects with the others

interdependence
(in-ter-di-PEN-duhns) The need to rely on one another

organizational chart
(awr-guh-nuh-ZEY-shuhnal CHART) Illustration showing the components of a company and how they fit together

across departments. Regardless of an organization's size and structure, one common thread always exists: all departments and employees must work together and depend on one another to get the work done and done well.

From a systems perspective, ask yourself what would happen if you:

- Don't show up for work on time and fail to notify someone?
- Get sloppy and make an error?
- Appear for work **impaired** by alcohol or by an illegal or prescription drug?

impaired
(im-PAIRD) A reduced ability to function properly

How would these behaviors affect other workers who are counting on you? If you fail to commit to your job, you won't be an employee there for long. You may be able to hide incompetence, sloppiness, and indifference for a little while, but eventually poor performance will catch up with you. What's worse, someone could be harmed by your lack of commitment and professionalism in the meantime.

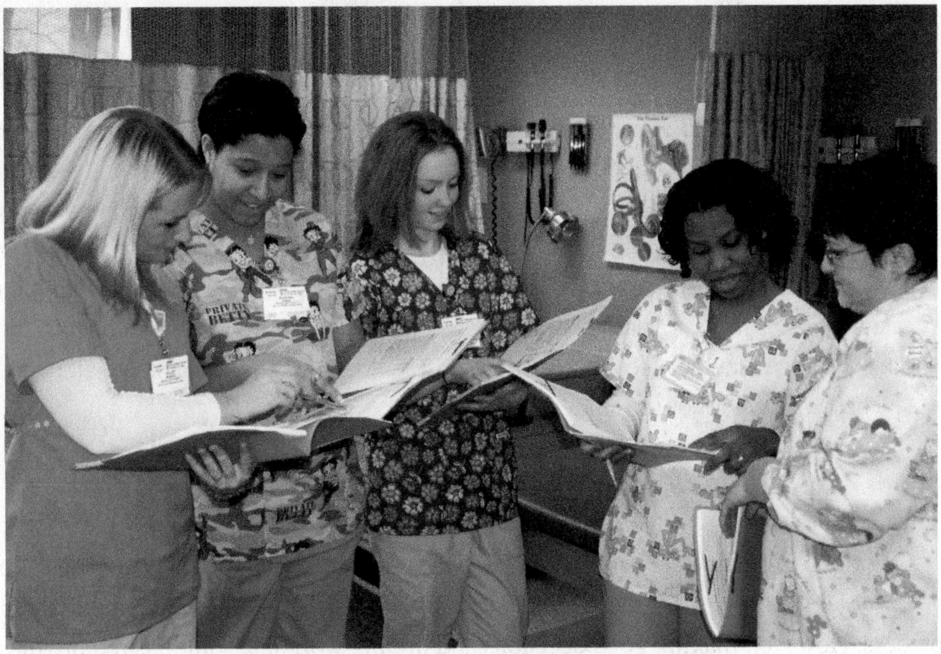

FIGURE 2.1

Medical assistants collaborating to organize the day's activities

Source: Carmen Martin/Pearson Education

Self-Awareness

One of the challenges of working in a busy environment is the ability to avoid distractions and pay attention to what's going on around you. This requires a certain degree of **self-awareness**, or understanding where you are, what you're doing, and why you're doing it at any point in time. This concept is also called *being present in the moment*. When you are *present in the moment*, you can filter out distractions and concentrate on what's in front of you at any given time. This ability to focus is absolutely critical in avoiding mistakes and errors. It's important to stop and think before you act. Everything you say and do should be **intentional**. This means thinking things through and doing and saying things on purpose rather than just quickly reacting to whatever situation occurs.

self-awareness
(CELF uh-WAIR-nis) Understanding where you are, what you're doing, and why you're doing it

intentional
In-TEN-shuh-nl) Something done on purpose

When you're at work you need to filter out distractions from your personal life, which is easier said than done. Family conflicts, an argument with a friend, bill collectors tracking you down at work, children left unsupervised, legal issues and court dates, and your own medical concerns are just a few examples of how your personal life can cause distractions at work. Let's face it—you're just one person, and it's not easy to keep everything in balance. Concentrating on the task at hand when there's so much else going on around you can be challenging, but it's something you must work hard to achieve.

One of the best ways to reduce distractions at work is to avoid becoming a distraction yourself. Remember, you aren't there to sell things, convince coworkers to adopt your political or religious beliefs, plan social gatherings, spread gossip, text friends, visit social networking sites, shop online, wager bets, or collect donations for your favorite charity. You're there to work, not to advance your personal agenda. Once at work, you must save such distracting activities for your personal time after work hours.

social networking sites (SOH-shuhl NET-wur-king SITES) Internet places for people to publish and share personal information

BUILD YOUR SKILLS *Study Skills*

It's important to build your study skills as early in your education as possible. Avoiding distractions by finding a good place to study, learning how to concentrate, developing productive study habits, and taking advantage of study groups will go a long way toward enhancing your learning and improving your grades. The study skills you acquire now will also pay off in the future as you undergo your initial training and then work toward future career advancement. To learn about the "Ten Study Habits of Successful Students" and other helpful study tips recommended by Dr. Charles T. Mangrum II and Dr. Stephen S. Strichart, visit www.how-to-study.com.

Working in health care is stressful. Each day you'll face a variety of decisions to make and problems to solve. The facts and data that you learn in school will certainly help this process. However, making good decisions and finding workable solutions require the ability to fully understand, explore, question, and apply the information you've learned in the past. When it comes to patient care, finding one right way to do things isn't always possible. You must instead think through each situation, decide on a strategy, test it, observe the results, and adjust accordingly. This is where critical thinking and problem solving skills become valuable.

critical thinking (KRIT-i-kuhl THING-king) Using reasoning and evidence to make decisions about what to do or believe without being biased by emotions

problem solving (PROB-luhm solv-ing) Using a systematic process to solve problems

Critical Thinking and Problem Solving Skills

By using critical thinking skills and a step-by-step, systematic approach to decision making, you can reduce your stress and find an effective solution to almost any problem. What is critical thinking? Critical thinking is using reasoning and evidence to make the best decisions about what to do, or what to believe, without being influenced by emotions. When you think critically, you:

- Look at things from a rational and practical perspective
- Ask essential questions to get to the heart of the matter
- Identify and analyze relevant information and evidence

systematic (sis-tuh-MAT-ik) A methodical procedure or plan

reasoning (REE-zuh-ning) Forming conclusions based on coherent and logical thinking

rational (RASH-uh-nl) Based on reason, logical

- Differentiate between facts, opinions, and personal feelings
- Think with an open mind and question assumptions
- Exercise caution in drawing conclusions
- Test conclusions against relevant standards

When faced with a problem, you can use critical thinking skills to help you:

- Avoid jumping to conclusions
- Identify and clarify the problem
- Gather as much information as you can
- Examine the evidence you've found
- Identify options to solve the problem
- Decide which option would work best
- Implement your solution
- Evaluate the results

A good solution almost always exists for every problem, but it may require an investment of your time and energy to find it.

Effective problem solving and critical thinking skills are mandatory to achieve a well-orchestrated personal and professional life. Interpreting the *small print* on credit card agreements, creating a budget for your family, comparing options for car insurance, and figuring out how to resolve an argument with a friend are just a few examples of where critical thinking skills can help you personally. Selecting the appropriate equipment settings, revising a patient's treatment plan, interpreting blood test results, and deciding whether to apply for a promotion are just a few examples of how critical thinking skills can help guide you in the right direction professionally. Developing critical thinking and problem solving skills takes time, but it is well worth the investment. The more you use your skills, the sharper they will become.

Language Arts Link — Organizational Skills

The ability to follow-through on assignments may require the development of strong organizational skills. Learning how to become and stay organized will help you both in school and at work. Organizational skills can help you manage your time, meet your deadlines, and avoid issues and problems caused by disorganization.

Go online and identify three credible sources of information on improving your organizational skills. After reviewing the information, write a list of steps that you could take to become better organized. In paragraph form, describe the benefits of organizational skills and the actions you will take to develop or enhance your skills. Also explain how you will measure your improvements. For example, were you able to reduce your study time by thirty minutes as a result of improved organizational skills? Or, did you turn in an assignment before the deadline because the research phase of your project was better organized? If you have the opportunity to interview someone who is known to have strong organizational skills, you may use that interview as one of your three sources of information.

Be sure to proofread your work to see if you can improve it by making it more clear, concise, or interesting to read. Check the spelling and grammar and correct any errors. Exchange your report with a classmate and compare your strategies to become better organized.

DEVELOPING A STRONG WORK ETHIC

When employers are asked to identify which characteristics make the best employees, most include "having a strong work ethic" on their list. Having a strong work ethic means positioning your job as a high priority in your life, and making sound decisions about how you approach your work. Employees with a strong work ethic:

- Stay focused and leave their personal problems at home.
- Apply themselves to the task at hand.
- Get their work done right the first time.
- Exercise self-discipline and self-control.
- Know what management expects of them, and they measure up.
- Act instead of waiting to be told what to do.
- Demonstrate a positive attitude and enthusiasm for their work.

Let's examine some additional factors that define a strong work ethic.

Attendance and Punctuality

punctual
(PUHNGK-choo-uhl) Arriving on time

It's nearly impossible to demonstrate a commitment to your job without being there. Performing your job duties requires showing up for work every day and being punctual.

Poor attendance usually results in other people having to cover for you when you aren't there yourself. How would you feel if your coworkers called in sick frequently, leaving you to do your work plus their work? How would your coworkers feel if your attendance falls below expectations? Many health care organizations are already lean on staffing and can't afford to have people absent on a regular basis. When people are counting on you, it's important to be there and to arrive on time.

When you arrive late for work:

- The patient's diagnosis, treatment, surgery, or discharge from the hospital might be delayed.
- Necessary supplies might not get delivered on time.
- Paperwork might get filed too late to meet a deadline.
- Other people might have to work late to catch up.

Remember how the roles of health care workers are interconnected? You may think arriving late won't cause a problem for your work group, but what complications might you be causing other people?

corrective action
(kuh-REK-tiv ACK-shuhn) Steps taken to overcome a job performance problem

dismissal
(dis-MIS-uhl) I Involuntary termination from a job

contingency plans
(kuhn-TIN-jen-see plans) Backup plans in case the original plans don't work

Almost everyone must miss work or arrive late on occasion. But when poor attendance or punctuality becomes a habit, it may result in a performance issue leading to corrective action or dismissal.

What steps can you take to ensure good attendance and punctuality?

- Make a commitment to show up for work every day and arrive on time.
- When your shift starts, make sure you are in the area and ready to go.
- Have contingency plans to cover situations when your children or spouse gets sick or when your transportation becomes unreliable.
- Protect your health and safety to keep from getting sick or injured.
- Eat well, get plenty of sleep, and get an annual flu shot.

Allow some extra time at the end of your shift in case you get held over. Never leave a patient or coworker *hanging* by rushing out the door the minute your shift ends. Ensure a smooth transition between shifts and don't leave your work for other people to complete. Remember interdependence? Other people are counting on you to arrive on time and get your part of the work done.

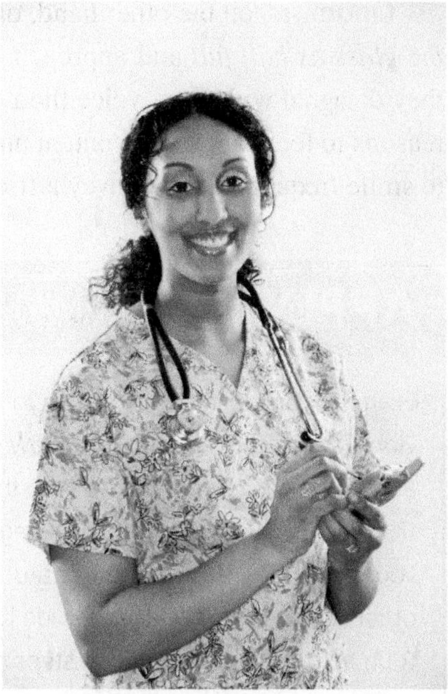

FIGURE 2.2
A health care professional arrives on time and is ready to work

Source: Don Mason/Corbis Images

Reliability and Accountability

Reliability and accountability are key factors in a strong work ethic. **Reliable** people can be counted on to keep their word. If they've agreed to do something, their coworkers know they will follow through. Following through on commitments is a big part of team effort. If you are there for other people when you say you will be, it's more likely they will be there for you when you need them.

reliable
(ri-LIE-uh-buhl) Can be counted on; trustworthy

People who are accountable accept **responsibility** for the consequences of their actions. They *own up* to what they've done and don't blame other people. If you make a mistake, admit it and accept full responsibility. Apologize to those who have been inconvenienced. Remember, while it's important to apologize for a mistake, your apology doesn't erase the fact that a mistake was made. Learn from the experience and avoid making the same mistake twice. Your supervisor and coworkers will appreciate your *the buck stops here* attitude.

responsibility
(ri-spon-suh-BIL-i-tee) A sense of duty binding someone to a course of action

Show **initiative**—don't wait to be told what to do. Follow through on all work assignments that you are qualified and prepared to perform. If you're given a work assignment that you are not qualified or prepared to perform, discuss the situation with your supervisor immediately. Refusal to complete a task as assigned may be construed as **insubordination** and grounds for dismissal.

initiative
(ih-NISH-ee-uh-tiv) Taking the first step or move

insubordination
(in-suh-BAWR-din-ay-shun) Refusal to complete an assigned task

When serving the needs of patients, it's important to avoid passing judgment or projecting your own personal beliefs on others. If you object to an assignment because it conflicts with your religious beliefs or values, you must discuss these concerns with your supervisor. It's best to resolve such issues when you first consider a job offer. If you do not wish to participate in abortions, sex change operations, end-of-life procedures, or other such activities, many employers will allow you to opt out. But this must be discussed ahead of time so that patient care isn't delayed or jeopardized.

Attitude and Enthusiasm

How often have you witnessed another person's behavior and thought to yourself, "What a bad attitude"? For some people, negativity is a way of life. As **pessimists**, they see *the glass as half empty*. From this perspective, a situation is always bad and getting worse. Pessimists complain about everything and seem satisfied by nothing. They rarely smile, appear happy, or convey enthusiasm about their work. They spread negativity to everyone around them and undermine morale, teamwork, and a spirit of **cooperation**.

pessimists
(PESS-uh-mists) People who look on the dark side of things

cooperation
(koh-op-uh-rey-shuhn) Acting or working together for a common purpose

optimists (OPP-tuh-mists) People who look on the bright side of things

Optimists, on the other hand, display a positive attitude most of the time. They see *the glass as half full* and approach life with enthusiasm. When they experience things they disagree with, they voice their complaints in a constructive manner. They look for reasons to feel happy and content and appreciate the small things in life. Optimists tend to smile frequently and convey a friendly, cooperative attitude.

APPLY IT OPTIMIST OR PESSIMIST?

Examine your point of view. Do you consider yourself to be an optimist or a pessimist? How would other people who know you well answer that question? (If you aren't sure, ask a few of them.) Write a paragraph that answers the following questions. Do you focus on the positives of a situation or the negatives? What impact does your point of view have on your attitude? How does your attitude affect your school work and your relationships with other people? Is a positive attitude helping you move forward in life, or is a negative attitude holding you back? What steps can you take to develop a more positive outlook?

Working in health care can really challenge your attitude. People who have worked in health care for several years may feel as if things are getting worse. They may be critical, resentful, and angry about some of the changes they've seen occur. Perhaps cutting staff to reduce expenses has resulted in longer work hours, additional duties, and more holiday shifts to cover. Some of the benefits they enjoyed in the past may have been reduced or eliminated to save money. Their job titles and job duties might have been altered as part of a reorganization or merger of companies.

As mentioned earlier, health care is constantly changing. When workers feel like something of value has been taken away, their attitudes can suffer. It's important to look for the advantages that come with change and avoid focusing on the negatives.

People who are relatively new in their health careers may also face attitudinal challenges. Young workers may become impatient when job promotions and pay raises don't occur quickly enough. They might question long-standing policies and procedures that no longer seem relevant. Wearing a uniform or following dress code requirements that bar visible tattoos, facial piercings, and non-traditional hair colors and styles may cause discontent.

The bottom line is this—no job or place of employment will ever be perfect. Although organizations may work hard to enhance employees' job satisfaction and become an **employer of choice**, people will still find things to complain about. That's just human nature. The key to maintaining a positive attitude is to always look for what's good in any situation and remain optimistic that things will improve.

employers of choice (im-PLOI-ers of chois) Companies where people like to work

Displaying enthusiasm and a positive attitude is an important part of a professional's work ethic. If you want to excel and advance in your career, a positive attitude is a must.

- If you are an optimist, make sure your positive attitude is evident at work.
- If you are a pessimist, put some effort into changing your outlook.
- Look for the bright side in any situation and focus on the positives.
- Seize opportunities to feel happy and appreciate the small things in life.
- When you must complain, express your concerns to the appropriate person and in a constructive manner.

If you feel *stressed out* get some help right away. Health care workers who don't alleviate their stress run the risk of damaging their health and spreading their stress among coworkers. Smile every chance you get, even when speaking on the telephone. By adopting a positive attitude, you will experience more joy and greater satisfaction in life, and your optimism and enthusiasm will spread to those around you.

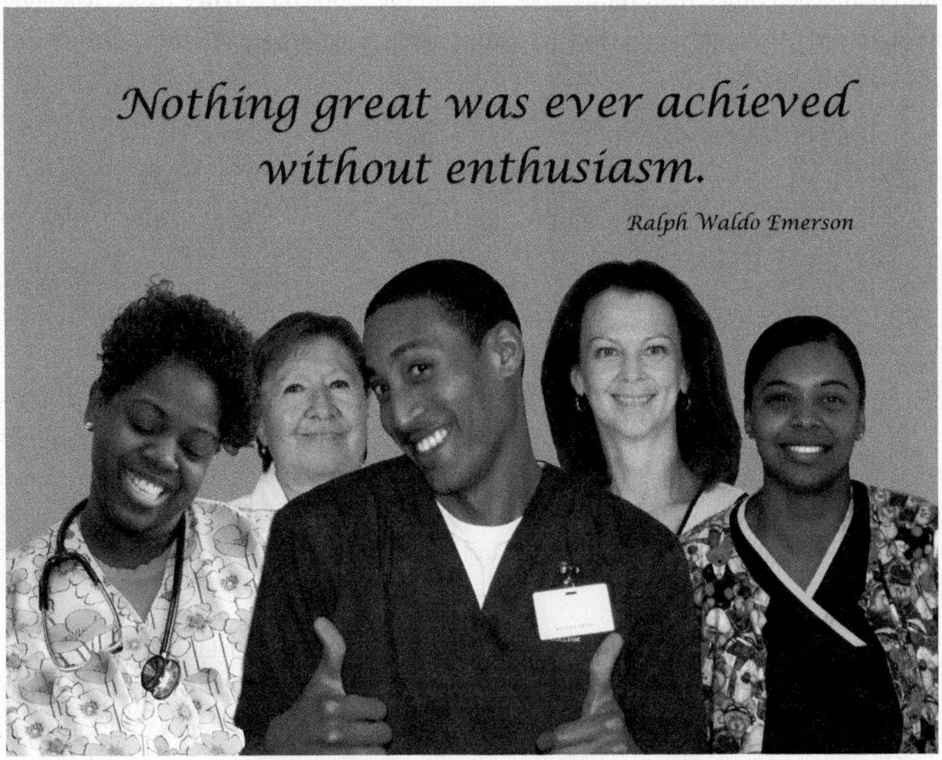

FIGURE 2.3

Enthusiastic workers creating a positive work environment

Source: Carmen Martin/Pearson Education

Competence and Quality of Work

Regardless of where your job falls within the organization, the quality of your work is extremely important. What does quality mean to you? What does it mean to your employer and your patients? How can you support quality improvement? Let's start with the importance of competency. Consider the following:

- Make sure you're well trained and competent to perform every function of your job.
- Never take a chance and just *wing it.*
- Keep your knowledge up-to-date and your skills sharp.
- Learn about the latest procedures, techniques, and new equipment.
- Attend in-service sessions, register for continuing education workshops, and read professional publications in your field.
- Don't hesitate to ask questions or request help.

Keep in mind that your education won't end when you graduate from school. Nothing stays **stagnant** in health care. As a professional, it's your responsibility to continue learning, strengthening your skills, and improving the quality of your work.

stagnant (STAG-nuhnt) Without motion; dull, sluggish

Perhaps you've heard the saying "quality is in the details." This means paying attention to even the smallest things, because making a small mistake or overlooking a minor detail can have a big impact on quality. Stocking items on the wrong shelf, misfiling a patient's record, losing a phone number, miscalculating a bill, or missing an important meeting can all negatively impact quality. Each day brings many opportunities to overlook details. Being **diligent** about quality and careful in your work will help prevent such problems.

diligent
(DIL-i-juhnt) Careful in one's work

Contributing to quality improvement efforts organization-wide is an important aspect of your work ethic. No one has a better handle on how to improve work processes and quality outcomes than the people who do the work on a daily basis. Management can't improve the organization's quality without the help of their **subordinates**. Consider the following:

subordinates
(suh-BAWR-din-eyts) People at a lower rank

- When you have a suggestion for quality improvement, submit it to your supervisor.
- When you spot a potential problem, report it.
- If your work unit receives periodic quality-related data, pay attention to the reports and do your best to support improvements.

Sometimes you may be asked to do things that don't fall within your job duties. Responding to one of these requests by saying, "That's not my job!" isn't acceptable. Doing what's asked of you might not fall within your job duties, but one of two things needs to happen. Either you should perform the task because you are capable and willing to do it, or you should refer the matter to the appropriate person and make sure he or she follows through with it.

No task is too menial when working in health care. For example, consider the following:

- If a patient or visitor becomes ill in the parking lot, offer assistance or send for help.
- If someone looks lost, provide directions; if possible, guide them to their destination.
- If you notice a spill in a public area, don't wait for a housekeeper to discover it. Clean it up yourself (using safety precautions), or report it to the appropriate person and stay in the area until it's cleaned up to prevent possible injuries.
- If you observe that a piece of equipment is not working properly or spot a situation that could pose a health or safety hazard, take action. Don't just ignore things and go on about your business.

A commitment to quality requires paying attention to what's going on around you and addressing concerns before they escalate into serious problems.

COMPLIANCE

Health care workers have limited authority and responsibility. This means a worker is only allowed to do certain things as part of his or her job. Job duties are typically stated in a written **job description** for each position in the organization. You should be familiar with your job description and the authority and responsibilities you are expected to fulfill.

job description
(JAWB dih-SKRIP-shuhn) A document that describes a worker's job duties

Compliance is extremely important in health care. Ignoring a rule, violating a policy, or breaking the law can compromise quality of care, harm a patient or coworker, and result in your termination. Consider what might happen if employees:

compliance
(kuhm-PLY-uhns) Acting in accordance with laws and with a company's rules, policies, and procedures

- Didn't wear their identification badges at work?
- Shared private business matters or confidential patient information?

- Made threats against other employees?
- Exceeded their authority?
- Didn't fulfill the responsibilities in their job descriptions?
- Attempted to perform duties beyond their scope of practice?

Scope of Practice

Health care workers must always function within their scope of practice. Performing duties beyond what you're legally permitted to do is highly risky and illegal. Some jobs require a special license to practice. State agencies grant licenses only to people who have met pre-established qualifications, and only licensed workers may legally perform the job. Other jobs may require a special certification. State agencies and professional associations certify people who have met certain competency standards. Although non-certified people may legally perform the job, employers may prefer to hire only those workers who possess certification and who are eligible to use the professional title associated with that certification. When a license, certification, or some other special credential is required for your job, make sure you meet those requirements and maintain *active status*. In some professions this means completing annual continuing education requirements or periodic competency retesting.

APPLY IT PROFESSIONAL CREDENTIALS

Form groups of four students. Each group member should choose a health occupation. Research and list the licenses, certifications, or registrations necessary for your chosen profession. Find out if additional educational or training requirements are needed to move ahead in your chosen field.

Rules and policies are established for good reasons, and everyone has the responsibility to comply with them. Health care organizations usually have written policies and procedures plus employee handbooks to communicate their expectations. Know where to find these documents and, if you don't understand something, ask for clarification.

Complying with laws and policies has always been important in health care. However, compliance is currently gaining even more attention because the government is stepping up its efforts to identify violators and prosecute them. Some organizations have hotlines to help employees report compliance concerns anonymously with no fear of backlash.

Violating a law, regulation, or policy can get you and your employer in serious trouble. You could be terminated, prosecuted, fined, or incarcerated. Your employer could face stiff fines and exclusion from vital government programs like Medicare or Medicaid. Complying with laws, regulations, and policies because you have to is important, but there's more to it than that. Professionals comply because *it's the right thing to do.*

- Make sure you're aware of and understand all of the laws, regulations, and policies pertaining to your job.
- Become familiar with medical/legal issues specific to your profession.
- Learn about fire safety procedures and how to protect the security of your patients, coworkers, and organization.

- Know what your employer expects of you in terms of sound business practices.
- Know what laws, regulations, and policies apply to you and your job. If you are accused of an illegal activity, claiming that you weren't aware of the law isn't an acceptable legal defense.
- Ask for clarification if you're uncertain about compliance responsibilities.

APPLY IT POLICIES AND PROCEDURES

Research the organizational policies and procedures at a health care facility in your community. Write a description of the issues and situations that the policies and procedures address. In your description, interpret at least three of the policies and explain why you think the facility provides those policies and procedures for its employees. Discuss your interpretations with a classmate.

HIPAA
(HIPAA) Health Insurance Portability and Accountability Act of 1996; national standards to protect the privacy of a patient's personal health information

HITECH Act
(HITECH Act) Health Information Technology for Economic and Clinical Health Act of 2009; national standards to protect the confidentiality of electronically transmitted patient health information

reimbursement
(ree-im-BURS-ment) To pay back or compensate for money spent

conflict of interest
(KON-flikt of IN-ter-ist) An inappropriate relationship between personal interests and official responsibilities

unethical
(uhn-ETH-i-kuhl) A violation of standards of conduct and moral judgment

fraud
(FRAWD) I Intentional deceit through false information or misrepresentation

sexual harassment
(SEK-shoo-uhl HAR-uhs-muhnt) Unwelcome, sexually-oriented advances or comments

hostile workplace
(HOS-tl WURK-pleys) An uncomfortable or unsafe work environment

A major part of compliance in health care is protecting the confidentiality of patient medical records. The Health Insurance Portability and Accountability Act of 1996 (**HIPAA**) enacted national standards for this purpose. Protecting confidentiality has become even more critical with the advent of electronic medical records. The Health Information Technology for Economic and Clinical Health (**HITECH**) Act was signed into law in February of 2009 as part of the American Recovery and Reinvestment Act of 2009 (ARRA). Portions of the HITECH Act address the confidentiality of health information transmitted electronically and strengthen the enforcement and penalties associated with HIPAA rules.

Become familiar with what you need to do to comply with HIPAA and the HITECH Act to prevent the inappropriate disclosure of confidential information and avoid potential fines against you and your employer. Also make sure you maintain the confidentiality of financial information and other materials your employer deems private. If you work for more than one health care organization at the same time, or move from employer to employer, it's important to not share private information among employers.

Other areas of risk that can result in compliance concerns include safety and environmental precautions, labor laws, records retention, Medicare billing and **reimbursement**, licenses and credentials, and **conflict of interest**.

Examples of illegal or **unethical** behaviors include:

- **Fraud**, such as charging for a test or treatment that wasn't performed
- Improperly changing or destroying medical, financial, or other types of records
- **Sexual harassment**
- Creating a **hostile workplace**
- Stealing property

Issues related to sexual harassment can cause major problems at work. Avoid any suggestion of unwelcome sexually-oriented advances or comments that could lead to sexual harassment charges being filed against you. Examples include verbal communication, visual and written materials, unwanted touching, sexually explicit texting or postings on social networking sites, or any other actions that have the potential to make another person uncomfortable. Even if you think your actions are harmless, the other person, or someone else present at the time, might see things differently.

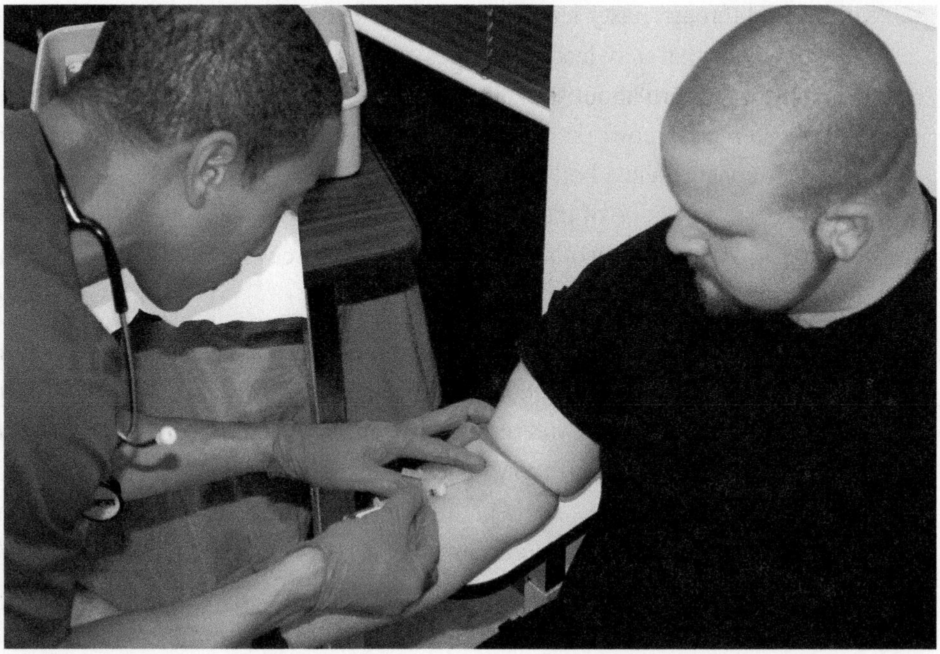

FIGURE 2.4

Professional working within his scope of practice to obtain a blood sample

Source: Carmen Martin/Pearson Education

If you are the victim of sexual harassment or intimidation, report the incident to your supervisor or another superior immediately. Keep written notes on what you've observed or experienced, including details such as the date, time, place, who was present, what exactly happened, and what you did to follow up. Information such as this will be very important should an investigation take place.

Far too many examples of compliance issues exist to list them all. Here are some important things related to compliance to keep in mind:

- Don't modify or destroy patient or financial records without proper authority.
- If your job involves preparing bills for patient procedures, make sure the codes you use to identify specific diagnoses or procedures are accurate; never **up-code** a procedure to increase reimbursement.
- Always work within your scope of practice.
- Don't accept pay for hours that you did not work.
- Avoid any suggestion of a conflict of interest.
- Avoid inappropriate relationships between your personal interests and your official responsibilities.
- If your job involves awarding contracts to outside companies, don't accept gifts or free meals in exchange from these vendors.
- Don't ask a vendor that your organization has contracted to give you a special discount on a personal purchase.
- Don't refer patients to one of your relatives who works in the health care business.

up-code
(UHP-code) Modifying the classification of a procedure to increase financial reimbursement

Inappropriate Behavior

Inappropriate behavior can result in serious compliance issues. As a professional, you would never knowingly engage in an illegal or unethical act yourself, but you might observe someone else doing something suspicious. Or you might feel that you are a victim of sexual harassment or a hostile work environment. Consider the following:

- You should never bring a weapon to work or create an environment where someone else could feel intimidated or unsafe.

- Avoid verbal threats, nasty letters or e-mail or text messages, or other forms of hostile behavior that may lead to charges of intimidation.
- If you have a concern about something you see occurring at work that might place you, your employer, coworkers, or patients at risk, let your supervisor know or report your concern via a hotline if one is available.
- If your supervisor is one of the people involved in the suspicious activity, report the matter to your supervisor's boss, a human resources representative, or someone in legal services.

Stay alert! If you see something, say something. If you find yourself in a situation where you aren't sure how to proceed, ask yourself some questions. Is what's going on legal and ethical? Is it in the best interests of my employer and patients? How would this look to others outside my organization? Then take action.

whistle blower (WISS-uhl BLOH-er) A person who exposes the illegal or unethical practices of another person or of a company

You've probably heard the term **whistle blower**—a person who notifies authorities when another person or an organization is involved in wrongdoing. *Blowing the whistle* can be a scary proposition for employees, but the law protects whistle blowers from retribution. In fact, whistle blowers might receive a portion of the fine the government collects when a health care provider is found guilty of Medicare fraud, for example. Consider the following:

- If you suspect someone of illegal or unethical behavior, it's your responsibility to report it.
- Try to resolve your concerns within your organization first. Avoid going to the government or the media unless repeated internal attempts have failed.
- If you've tried your best to report and stop illegal or unethical practices without success, you might need to think about finding a job at another organization.

Consider This *The Fastest and Largest Growing Occupations*

According to the U.S. Department of Labor, the occupations expected to grow the fastest between 2006 and 2016 fall within health care and social and mental health services. These occupations include home care aides, medical assistants, substance abuse and mental health counselors, social and human service assistants, pharmacy technicians, physical therapists and physical therapist assistants, dental hygienists and dental assistants, and physician assistants. The aging population and advances in medical technology are driving this rapid growth. Most of these jobs require postsecondary training and an associate's or bachelor's degree for entry into practice.

Registered nurses are on the list of the nation's largest growing occupations, along with several of the jobs listed above. Also included are general occupations which can be found in health care organizations, such as housekeepers, food service workers, receptionists and information clerks, accountants and auditors, executive secretaries and administrative assistants, computer systems analysts, customer service representatives, and accounting clerks. Most of these jobs require short-term or on-the-job training, or an associate's degree for entry-level positions.

Visit http://www.dol.gov/wb/factsheets/Qf-HotJobs3.htm for more information.

REPRESENTING YOUR EMPLOYER

When you accept a job offer, show up for work, and receive a paycheck, you become a representative of the organization. To patients, visitors, guests, and vendors, *you are the organization that you work for*. Everything you do and say can have an impact on the organization's reputation. By accepting employment, you not only agree to follow your employer's rules and policies, but you also agree to support its mission and values.

Review your organization's **corporate mission** and **corporate values** and think about what you could do to support your employer. Although you don't own the organization, you should take an active interest in it and get involved. Here are some more steps you can take to support your employer:

corporate mission
(kawr-per-it mish-uhn)
Special duties, functions, or purposes of a company

corporate values
(KAWR-per-it VAL-yoos)
Beliefs held in high esteem by a company

- Learn about the history and structure of your organization in order to discuss it intelligently with other people.
- Read your employer's newsletters and keep up with the latest news and events.
- Participate in your organization's social activities and sports teams.
- Volunteer to serve on committees and help plan special events.
- Represent your employer in community service projects.
- Substitute words such as *we* and *us* for *they* and *them*. For example, instead of saying, "They told us they are going to open a new clinic next year," it would be better to say, "We are opening our new clinic next year."

Take pride and ownership in the organization for which you work. It's part of being a professional.

Community Service Health and Wellness

Choose a community organization that is involved in health care or focused on improving the health and wellness of people who live in your community. Research the organization. Make a poster that illustrates the organization's mission and values. Describe the services provided by the organization and the types of people who work there and their job duties. Does the organization collaborate with area hospitals and health care workers? If so, how? Does the organization rely on volunteers? If so, describe the role of its volunteers and who is eligible to participate. How does the organization benefit the community? What might happen if the organization no longer existed?

Regardless of what job you have, your appearance, attitudes, and behaviors reflect the organization for which you work. **Front-line workers**, such as nurses, medical assistants, housekeepers, patient transporters, and cafeteria staff, have some of the greatest influence on their organization's reputation because they have the most frequent contact with patients, visitors, and guests. What might happen if you publicly criticized your employer, complained about a policy, or questioned how a physician treated a patient? By damaging the reputation of your employer, you're hurting yourself and countless other employees who strive to do a good job each day. If you take issue with something

front-line workers
(FRUHNT-lahyn WUR-kers)
Employees who have the most frequent contact with a company's customers

going on at work, speak with the appropriate person and communicate your concerns in a professional manner. Consider the following:

- Don't make negative remarks about your organization or its employees in public.
- Use discretion when offering opinions about your organization's policies.
- Give your employer and your coworkers the benefit of the doubt; assume that everyone is there to do their best.
- If you have serious doubts about your employer and the way your organization does business, it's probably best to look for employment elsewhere.

discretion
(dis-KRE-shen) Being careful about what one says and does

EVALUATING YOUR PERFORMANCE

performance evaluation
(per-FOR-muhns ih-val-yoo-EY-shuhn) Measurement of success in executing job duties

subjective
(suhb-JEK-tiv) Affected by a state of mind or feelings

objective
(uhb-JEK-tiv) What is real or actual; not affected by feelings

probationary period
(proh-BEY-shuhn PEER-ee-uhd) A testing or trial period to meet requirements

Now that you're familiar with what it takes to demonstrate a strong work ethic, let's examine how health care employers evaluate job performance. If you take your job seriously and apply everything you are learning in this book, you should have no problem when it comes time for your performance evaluation. However, if you lack the competence or the commitment required to perform your job effectively, your deficiencies will soon become apparent.

The process used to conduct performance evaluations varies from employer to employer. Sometimes it's called a *job evaluation* or *performance appraisal*. The purpose of a performance evaluation is not to determine how well an employee *is liked* or how his or her supervisor *feels* about the employee, as this would involve subjective criteria. Instead, employers evaluate job performance using objective criteria which is based on factors such as competence (knowledge and skills), behaviors (customer service and teamwork), and traits (appearance and attitude). Evaluating competence and behaviors using objective criteria is fairly straightforward. However, assessing traits such as *appearance* and *attitude* without becoming subjective can be difficult.

FIGURE 2.5
Employee undergoing a performance appraisal
Source: Ambrophoto/Shutterstock

It's not unusual for new employees to undergo a probationary period whereby their attendance and performance are closely monitored for the first few months to make sure they are a *good fit* for the organization and the position. New employees are evaluated at the end of their probationary period, and a supervisor makes a decision about whether or not to retain them. Having successfully completed their probationary period, employees are then subject to regular performance evaluations from that point forward, typically on an annual basis.

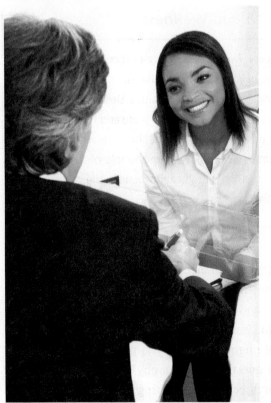

Small organizations may evaluate performance on an informal basis. The supervisor observes the employee's performance over a period of time and provides verbal feedback regarding strengths, weaknesses, and areas for improvement. Informal evaluations may or may not be documented in writing and kept in the employee's personnel file. Larger companies typically evaluate performance on a more formal basis. The supervisor observes the employee's performance during the year, completes a written performance evaluation form, and meets with the employee to discuss the results. The performance evaluation form and notes from the meeting are documented in writing and kept in the employee's personnel file.

Some companies give their employees the opportunity to do a self-evaluation. This can be very helpful in preparing for your evaluation meeting with your supervisor. Think about your performance over the past year and what you have accomplished. Jot down notes and bring them with you to the meeting.

RECENT DEVELOPMENTS

360 Degree Feedback

Many employers are now using **360-degree feedback** tools as part of performance evaluations. People who have worked with the employee during the past year are asked to provide input on the employee's evaluation. This could include **peers**, subordinates, team members, customers, and people from other departments or outside the organization. Obtaining feedback from people in addition to the employee's supervisor helps reduce subjectivity and provides a broader view of the employee's performance. When employees work on teams, getting performance feedback from other team members helps evaluate the employee's team skills as well as his or her individual performance.

360-degree feedback
(three-hundred-and-sixty dih-GREE FEED-bak) Feedback about an employee's job performance that is provided by peers, subordinates, team members, customers, and others who have worked with the employee who is undergoing evaluation

peers
(PEERS) People at the same rank

In addition to focusing on previous performance, the evaluation process also lays out plans for the coming year. Through discussions with supervisors, employees develop annual or monthly goals to help them progress from where they are to where they eventually want to be within the organization. The goal setting process helps employees overcome deficiencies, enhance skills, and work toward job promotions and career advancement.

Each employer has its own rating scale. Typically, a few employees will receive an *outstanding* evaluation; most will receive an *average* evaluation, and a few may receive a *poor* evaluation. Performance evaluations may result in more than just feedback about how well you're doing on the job. Many companies now tie the amount of an individual's pay increase to the score on his or her performance evaluation. This is called *performance-based pay*, *merit-based pay*, or *pay for performance*. Employees who receive high scores on their performance evaluations receive higher pay raises than employees who receive lower scores. Employees with poor scores may not receive any pay increase. When pay is tied to performance, it's even more important to focus on objective criteria rather than subjective criteria in the evaluation process.

When undergoing a performance evaluation, you should prepare yourself for some negative feedback. If you've done your best all year long, you should also hear lots of positive comments. Accept constructive criticism and learn from it. Compare the score on your self-evaluation with the score your supervisor gave you and discuss any differences. If you disagree with what your supervisor is saying during your evaluation, state your opinions clearly and objectively, but don't expect your score to change. If you're expected to make improvements during the coming year, make sure you know exactly what's expected of you and how these improvements will be measured. Work with your supervisor to develop your goals for the coming year. When your personal goals align with your employer's goals, your value to the organization becomes more apparent.

constructive criticism (kuhn-STRUCK-tiv KRIT-uh-siz-uhm) Offering positive input on another person's weaknesses with the goal of their improvement

THE MORE YOU KNOW

Personal Goals

Wanting or needing something can be a strong motivator, which encourages you to set goals and make decisions that will lead to happiness and success. A goal is something that you strive to attain. You might set a goal to obtain something specific, such as a passing grade in algebra. Or you might set a goal to achieve a position, such as president of your senior class. Goals help you focus on what is really important to you and what you are willing to work for.

Long-term goals are plans that help you focus on what you want in the future—at least a year from now, or even five or ten years from now. Short-term goals can be achieved in a shorter amount of time. For example, completing a first aid course is a short-term goal that will take just a few months. Becoming employed as a registered nurse will take years to achieve.

List two or three short-term goals for yourself. What steps will be necessary to achieve your goals?

Remember, no one is perfect, and everyone has more to learn. Even if your organization doesn't have a performance evaluation process, you can (and should) request periodic feedback from your supervisor. This can be as simple as asking, "How do you think I'm doing?" You don't have to wait until annual review time to ask. Solicit feedback from your supervisor and coworkers on a regular basis and then act upon what they've told you. If your performance becomes an issue, chances are your supervisor will let you know as soon as the problem becomes apparent. But don't subscribe to the *no news is good news* theory. Soliciting feedback from those most familiar with your performance is the best way to increase your value to the organization.

Which attitudes and behaviors result in outstanding evaluations? Keep reading this book because most everything you need to know to earn an outstanding evaluation is covered in these chapters. As you read, start evaluating your strengths and weaknesses. Think about what areas you need to improve and what steps you will take to do so. Understanding the elements of a strong work ethic and performing well on the job are vital to developing your reputation as a health care professional. The next step is examining your personal traits and how they impact your work.

REALITY CHECK

Perhaps you've already had one or more jobs where you've been held to certain performance standards and had to comply with employer policies and procedures. If you appeared for work every day and on time, demonstrated competence and a commitment to your job, and proved to be a reliable and enthusiastic employee, then you probably earned a satisfactory performance evaluation and perhaps a pay raise or job promotion. If so, this experience and what you learned from it will serve you well as you assume your new role in health care.

However, working in health care presents some unique challenges. More than likely, you'll be working in a complex, stressful environment where everything that you say and do will make an impact on other people. It's like throwing a pebble in a pond and watching the ripple effect. You can see some of the ripples created because they happen right in front of you. But other ripples occur off in the distance, too far away to observe.

Your attitude and behaviors at work cause ripples. Some ripples you will notice; others you will not. When you smile and project a friendly attitude, for example, you create positive ripples. When you complain and spread negativity, you create negative ripples. When you *go beyond the call of duty* to do something special for a patient or a coworker, you create positive ripples. When you get lazy and develop an *I don't care* attitude about your work, you create negative ripples. Like ripples in the pond, the full impact you've made, whether positive or negative, will be hard for you to observe directly.

It all comes back to being intentional about everything you say and do. Stop and think before you act, because the ripples *you* create should only be positive ones.

Key Points

- Focus on developing both hard skills (technical skills) and soft skills (people skills).
- Commit to your job and make it a high priority in your life.
- From a systems perspective, know where your role fits in.
- Be present in the moment.
- Stop and think before you act; everything you say and do should be intentional.
- Develop effective critical thinking and problem solving skills.
- Report for work when scheduled and arrive on time.
- Adopt an optimistic attitude and display enthusiasm at work.
- Maintain your competency and always work within your scope of practice.
- Pay attention to quality and submit suggestions to improve it.
- Fulfill the authority and responsibilities stated in your job description.
- Comply with all policies, laws, and rules that apply to your job.
- Avoid illegal, unethical, and inappropriate behavior.
- Represent your employer in a professional manner.
- Pay attention to feedback about your job performance.
- Make positive ripples with everything that you say and do.

Section Review Questions

Answer each of the following questions. Indicate which page in the textbook led you to your answer.

1. Explain the difference between *soft skills* and *hard skills* and discuss why health care workers need both types of skills.
2. Define *interdependence* and *systems perspective* and explain their importance in health care.
3. Define *critical thinking* and list three things that critical thinkers do to make good decisions.
4. What are *HIPAA* and *HITECH,* and why are they important?
5. Explain the purpose of performance evaluations.
6. What is the difference between objective and subjective evaluation criteria?
7. In your own words, explain what Abraham Lincoln meant when he said, "Character is like a tree and reputation like its shadow. The shadow is what we think of it; the tree is the real thing."

Learn By Doing

Complete Worksheets 1– 5 in Section 2.1 of your *Student Activity Guide.*

SECTION 2.2 Your Personal Traits and Professional Image

Background

How well you function at work depends greatly on who you are as a person. Your attitude and behavior are based largely on personal traits such as your character, personal values, and morals. Displaying a positive personal image at work is also important. The impression that you create is a result of your attire, grooming, hygiene, and posture. Your grammar, personal habits, and the language you use complete the personal image that you portray to other people. Aspects of your personal life can also have a major impact on your professional image. This includes the ability to manage your time, personal finances, and stress. Developing effective personal management skills and learning to adapt to change will help support your success at school, at home, and at work.

Objectives

After completing this section, you will be able to:

1. Define the key terms.
2. Define *character*, *personal values*, and *morals* and explain how they affect your reputation as a professional.
3. List four examples that demonstrate a lack of character in the workplace.
4. Explain how attire, grooming, hygiene, and posture impact a professional image.

5. Describe how grammar and vocabulary affect your professional image.
6. Discuss the importance of maintaining professionalism after hours.
7. Explain the importance of good time management skills and list three time management techniques.
8. Explain the importance of good personal financial management skills and list three financial management techniques.
9. Explain the importance of good stress management skills and list three stress management techniques.
10. Define *adaptive skills* and explain why the ability to manage change is important in health care.

YOUR CHARACTER AND PERSONAL VALUES

Professionalism brings together who you are as a person and how you contribute those traits in the workplace. Before you can achieve success by *doing* something, you have to *be* something, and being a health care professional depends greatly on who you are as a person. Much of this comes down to your character and personal values.

Employers are becoming increasingly concerned about a lack of character and positive personal values in the workplace. Each year in businesses throughout the country, employees are responsible for a variety of dishonest, illegal, and unethical behaviors, and this includes people working for health care organizations. Consider the following examples.

- Hidden video cameras in hospitals reveal employees stealing computers, office supplies, syringes, medications, and patients' personal possessions.
- Job seekers falsify information on employment applications and overstate their education and work records.
- Countless numbers of fraudulent workers' compensation claims are filed each year.
- Employees bring weapons to work, and incidences involving workplace violence and sexual harassment are becoming more frequent.

Many employers now run criminal history background checks, credit checks, and drug screens on job candidates before they start work. Employers are also placing more emphasis on the character of their employees to help reduce theft, absenteeism, dishonesty, substance abuse, safety infractions, and low productivity. For example, increasingly, employers are hiring, praising, and promoting for character. Character reflects a person's morals and influences their integrity and trustworthiness, two key factors in professionalism.

How do character, personal values, reputation, morals, integrity, and trustworthiness apply to you as a person? How do they affect the way you approach your work? Do you know the difference between right and wrong? Are you honest? Can you be trusted? If you make a bad decision, can you overcome it and get back on track?

character
(KAR-ik-ter) A person's moral behavior and qualities

personal values
(PUR-suh-nl VAL-yoos) Things of great worth and importance to a person

morals
(MAWR-uhls) The capability of differentiating between right and wrong

integrity
(in-TEG-ri-tee) Of sound moral principle

trustworthiness
(TRUHST-wur-thee-nus) Ability to have confidence in the honesty, integrity, and reliability of another person

Character Traits

Character traits lead to a person's behavior, thoughts, and emotions. Here are a couple of examples of positive and negative character traits:

- *Amiable* (good-humored and friendly) versus *ill-natured* (unpleasant and grumpy)

Would you like to work with an amiable person, one who is good-humored, friendly, and able to establish positive relationships with patients and coworkers? Or would you rather

FIGURE 2.6

Receptionist demonstrating positive character traits

Source: Somos Images/Corbis Images

work with a grumpy person who doesn't seem to like being around other people?

- *Ambitious* (having a strong desire to achieve) versus *shiftless* (lacking ambition and initiative)

Would you prefer to have an ambitious coworker, one who strives to exceed others' expectations? Or would you prefer a shiftless coworker who fails to take initiative and doesn't seem to care?

If you were choosing a new team member, which of these character traits would you look for?

Depending on the reference, you can find lengthy lists of character traits. Here are several examples to consider, each of which identifies both the positive and negative aspects of each trait. Think about each trait. Which of these describe you? How might each trait affect customer service, relationships, and morale in the workplace?

Character Traits

Appreciative/Ungrateful

- Feeling or expressing gratitude
- Feeling thankless or unappreciative

Caring/Callous

- Feeling concern and interest
- Being insensitive and emotionally hardened

Cheerful/Grumpy

- In good spirits
- Ill-tempered

Conscientious/Careless

- Taking extreme care and attention to details
- Lacking attention and forethought

Courteous/Impolite

- Being polite and using good manners
- Being rude and failing to demonstrate good manners

Dependable/Undependable

- Worthy of trust, reliable or can be counted on
- Unreliable, unworthy of trust

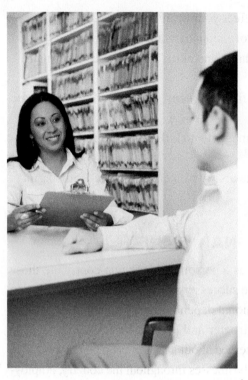

Diligent/Neglectful

- Careful in one's work
- Sloppy or failing to show care or attention

Generous/Selfish

- Willing to give and share with others
- Thinking of one's self to the detriment of others

Honest/Deceitful

- Marked by truth
- Deliberately false and fraudulent

Humble/Boastful

- Showing modesty and a lack of arrogance
- Exhibiting self-importance or arrogance

Impartial/Biased

- Free from favoritism and preconceived opinions
- Favoring one person or side over the other

Integrity/Immoral

- Showing sound moral principle
- Failing to differentiate between right and wrong

Loyal/Disloyal

- Remaining faithful to people whom one is under obligation to defend or support
- Deserting people whom one is under obligation to defend or support

Reliable/Unreliable

- Can be counted on, trustworthy
- Not worthy of reliance or trust

Respectful/Disrespectful

- Feeling or showing honor or esteem
- Showing lack of concern or disrespect; being rude and discourteous

Sincere/Hypocritical

- Being open, genuine, and honest
- Pretending to be or feel something that is false

FIGURE 2.7

Demonstrating reliability is a key character trait

Source: REDAV/Shutterstock

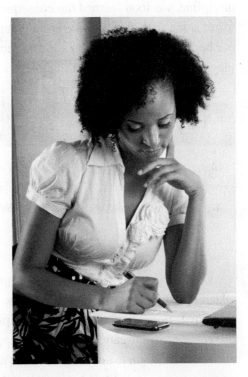

Self-disciplined/Indulgent

- Ability to control one's impulses; avoids temptations
- Inability to control one's impulses; gives in to temptations

Tolerant/Intolerant

- Showing respect for the rights, opinions, and practices of others
- Showing an unwillingness to respect the rights, opinions, and practices of others; being narrow-minded

Truthful/Untruthful

- Conforming to the truth; refraining from lying
- Lying intentionally and spreading false information

Reputation

No single factor is more important in being recognized as a professional than your reputation—your character, values, and behavior as viewed by other people. It takes a long time to develop a good reputation, but only a split second to lose it. After years of being an honest, law-abiding individual, all it takes is one dishonest act or a single incidence of unprofessional behavior to shake people's confidence in you and lose their trust. This is why professionals must work hard each and every day to do what's right and to maintain the trust and respect of others.

cheating
(CHEET-ing) Deceiving by trickery

If you've developed a pattern of behavior over the years based on lying, **cheating**, stealing, and taking advantage of other people, then changing your character at this point in your life is going to be quite a challenge, but it is possible. Our sense of acceptable behavior starts at a very young age when our parents and other influential people teach us the difference between right and wrong. As children, we experiment with different kinds of behavior to see what reactions we get. If those who raised us believed in discipline, we soon learned the consequences of *doing something bad*. We were taught to get along with other children, share our toys, wash our hands before we eat, and make our beds. Unacceptable behavior resulted in *getting grounded* and losing privileges like playing with friends or watching television.

APPLY IT CHEATING AND POOR CHARACTER

Make a list of five things that students might do that would involve cheating. List the negative character traits that are associated with cheaters. What positive character traits are missing in people who cheat? Why do you think people cheat? What might happen if they get caught?

judgment
(JUHJ-muhnt) Comparison of options to decide which is best

Over the years, we learn to make **judgment** calls, comparing our options and deciding which decision is best. We also learn the concept of self-control and the importance of avoiding temptation. Through relationships with other people, we learn about fairness and respect. We learn to care, to give, and to appreciate. And before long, our character, values, and priorities begin to define who we are as people and how we conduct our lives.

Judgment

As adults, we're faced with multiple decisions every day—what to do, why or why not to do it, how to do it, when to do it, where to do it, with whom to do it, and so on. Some of these decisions are small ones. But other decisions, especially those involving relationships with other people, require more thought and carry significant consequences, such as how to resolve a disagreement, when to say "no," and when to ask for help.

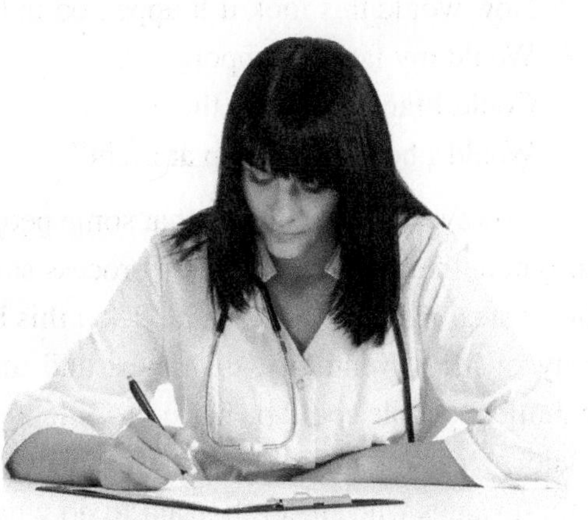

FIGURE 2.8

Listing options to determine the best course of action

Source: Aletia/Shutterstock

We consider several questions when we use judgment to make decisions; these include:

- What are my choices?
- How do the different options compare with one another?
- What might happen?
- Who might be affected?
- How would it make me feel?
- How would my decision be viewed by other people?

When the decisions you face involve your job, more questions arise. These include:

- What would my supervisor think?
- How would my coworkers feel?
- How would this decision affect patients?
- Could I lose my job?

BUILD YOUR SKILLS *Doing the Right Thing*

Do you always follow the rules? Or do you *bend* the rules when you think you won't get caught? For example, do you:

- Exceed the speed limit when no police are present?
- Park in a handicapped spot when no one is looking?
- Borrow another person's ID to get their discount on your purchase?
- Return a mail-order item that you broke, claiming it was damaged in shipment?
- Wear an item of clothing and then return it to the store for a refund?
- Sneak food into a movie theatre to save money?

According to Dr. Michele Borba, an educator on parenting and character education, "The best way to teach morality is by example." That's difficult to do when parents lie, cheat, steal, and perform other dishonest acts themselves.

When it comes to honesty in the health care workplace, keep this in mind—professionals don't do the right thing because they're afraid of getting caught. Professionals do the right thing because *it's the right thing to do.*

Conscience

conscience (KON-shuhns) Moral judgment that prohibits or opposes the violation of a previously recognized ethical principle

Most people have a conscience; it's that little voice that gnaws away at you, keeps you from sleeping at night, and constantly says, "You *know* this *isn't* the right thing to do!" Your conscience can be quite reliable in reminding you of the difference between right and wrong. When you're facing some difficult situations involving right versus wrong, you must answer even more questions. These include:

- How would this look if it appeared in the newspaper?
- Would my family support me?
- Could I face myself in the mirror?
- Would I be able to sleep at night?

However, the problem is that some people either have no conscience or have learned to ignore their conscience. This process starts with something minor, like telling a little lie or stealing something small. Then this behavior grows and grows until it becomes a way of life. Eventually, dishonest and unethical behavior will become obvious, but countless people could be harmed while it remains undetected. The good news is that the majority of Americans are honest, law-abiding people with good character and sound moral values who sincerely want to do what's right in their lives. For example, they:

- Face temptations, but summon up the courage to say "No!"
- Avoid engaging in dishonest behavior just because *everyone else does it.*
- Forgive people and move on, instead of harboring anger and resentment.
- Look out for themselves, yet treat other people with fairness and respect.
- Exercise good judgment and make the right decisions for the right reasons.

In the health care workplace, character, values, morals, integrity, and trustworthiness are absolutely vital. If you were sick or injured, what kind of people would you want caring for you? If you owned a health care business, what kind of people would you want working for you?

Consider This *Medicare Fraud*

Massive, nationwide arrests of doctors, nurses, physical therapists, and other health care providers for Medicare fraud are on the rise. Medicare fraud is estimated to cause an additional $60 to $90 billion per year in unnecessary government health care costs. Here are some examples:

- A proctologist earned $6.5 million for hemorrhoid removals, most of which never occurred.
- A podiatrist collected $700,000 for partial toenail removals which were actually toenail clippings.
- Physical therapists collected $57 million for providing little more than back rubs.
- Doctors and nurses from a home health care agency collected $25 million by writing fake prescriptions for expensive treatments for homebound patients.

The federal government is stepping up its efforts to uncover and stop these kinds of fraudulent practices.

Trust

Part of developing a professional reputation is convincing people that they can trust you and the quality of your decisions. In today's society, we've become increasingly suspicious of other people. "Don't trust anyone!" is common advice. Unfortunately, that perspective gets reinforced each time we set ourselves up to believe in someone or depend on someone, only to end up being disappointed or let down. It's important to be reliable and follow through when someone is counting on you. When your word is *as good as gold* your supervisor and coworkers know they can trust you keep your promises and meet your obligations. Remember the following:

- If you promised to give a coworker a ride to work, don't forget to pick him up.
- If you received training on a new procedure and your supervisor trusts you to perform it properly, make sure you apply what you learned.
- If you tell a patient you'll relay a message to her nurse, follow through.

If you want people to view you as a professional, make sure you can be trusted.

Honesty

Earning trust relies greatly on being viewed as an honest person. The cost of health care is high enough without employers having to pay for extra supplies, food, and equipment that were stolen by dishonest employees. Most health care workers would deny that they steal from their employers or patients. However, theft goes well beyond stealing a computer or a patient's wallet. Stealing also includes:

- Manipulating your time card or attendance record to get paid for more hours than you worked
- Sleeping on the job, taking unauthorized breaks, or leaving your work area without permission
- Taking food off of a dietary cart delivered for someone else's meeting
- Taking supplies from a patient's bedside table to use at home

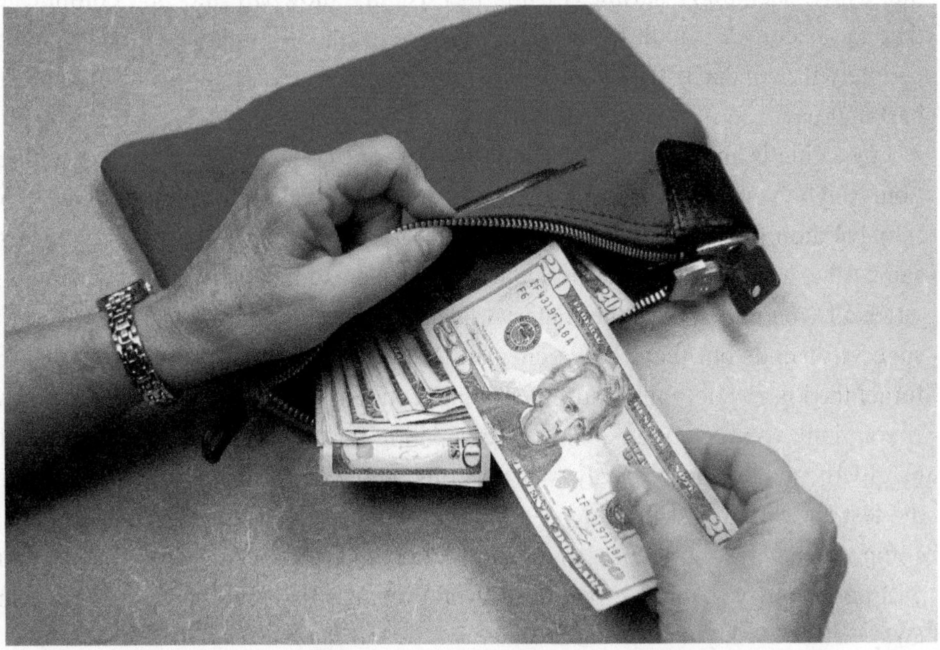

FIGURE 2.9

Counting cash for an accurate deposit

Source: Carmen Martin/Pearson Education

Anytime you take *anything* that doesn't belong to you without permission, it can be construed as theft. Is a free sandwich or box of cotton swabs worth losing your job? What about an extra hour of pay that you didn't really deserve? This is where both honesty and good judgment enter the picture. Even if taking something that doesn't belong to you appears harmless, what might be the consequences?

When employees spend time on-the-clock doing something other than their assigned job duties, they aren't just wasting time. They are stealing from their employer by collecting pay for non-productive time. Examples include texting friends, visiting social networking sites, viewing pornographic websites, gambling, shopping online, and using business computers for other inappropriate activities. Employees may also be caught watching television while on-the-job.

Language Arts Link — Portrayal of Health Care Workers on TV

The number of TV shows about hospitals and health care workers has increased significantly over the last several years. Many of the health care workers shown on TV appear as glamorous, hard-working, and dedicated professionals, while others appear less-than-professional. Select two television episodes. One should depict a health care worker with positive character, morals, integrity, and good judgment. The other should depict a health care worker who exhibits unprofessional behavior, such as creating a hostile environment, sexually harassing other workers, or ignoring policies and procedures.

Prepare a five minute oral presentation for your teacher and classmates. Explain why you chose the two episodes, and describe how the TV programs present both positive and negative character traits. Do you think these TV programs are realistic portrayals of the health care environment? Why or why not? Why do you think television networks produce these kinds of scripts and episodes? What impact do you think these shows have on patients and on people such as yourself who are considering careers in health care?

Lying and cheating are two more dishonest behaviors that can get you in big trouble. Little, seemingly harmless *white lies* usually snowball into big, complicated lies that can become difficult to manage. Lies are eventually uncovered and, before long, people will wonder if they can believe anything you say. Being truthful is always the best approach.

Cheating is an example of dishonest behavior that results from giving in to temptation. Maybe you have to pass a written test to prove your competency for a job promotion, but didn't have time to prepare for it. Dozens of people will be taking the test at the same time, and no one would notice if you sneaked some notes into the room with you. After all, you could learn the material later on after passing the test. However, if your supervisor finds out that you've cheated on the test, you'll be in big trouble. You can forget the job promotion because your main concern will be keeping the job you've got. If you think your coworkers, who are competing for the same job promotion, will stand by quietly and let you get away with cheating on the test, think again. They prepared for the test and you didn't. If you get a job promotion as a result of cheating, your lack of competence may quickly become obvious, and other people may suffer. Your reputation will be seriously damaged, perhaps beyond repair. Can you cheat just a little and get away with it? Ask your conscience.

A serious example of dishonest behavior is falsifying information, also known as fraud. Fraud isn't just dishonest, it's also illegal. A few examples of fraud include:

- Misrepresenting your education, credentials, or work experience on a job application, résumé, or other document
- Billing an insurance company for a patient procedure that never occurred
- Back-dating a legal document
- Entering incorrect data on equipment maintenance records
- Changing the results of a research study to reflect desired outcomes

As with stealing and cheating, there may be more to fraud than you realize. Fraud includes:

- Signing someone else's name without his or her permission (also called forgery)
- Turning in a time card that you know isn't accurate
- Telling your supervisor you renewed your professional license when you really didn't
- Pretending to be someone else to meet qualifications that you can't meet yourself

Because fraud is illegal, a fraud conviction can not only cost you your job, it can also cost you your freedom.

If it seems as if behaviors such as lying, cheating, stealing, and other forms of dishonesty overlap with one another, your observations are correct. It's hard to separate one type of dishonest and unprofessional behavior from another. The point is that every decision you make and every action you take can have a huge impact. One bad judgment call can erode someone's trust in you. One dishonest act can destroy your reputation. One incidence of fraud can result in job termination, or worse.

RECENT DEVELOPMENTS

Dishonesty at Work

Research shows that 70% of applicants overstate their qualifications on job applications. More than one third lie about their experience and achievements, and 12% fail to disclose criminal records. About a third of all job applicants admit to thinking about stealing from their employers. What happens when these applicants become employees? About half of all new hires don't work out, often as the result of dishonest behavior before and during employment. The result can be devastating to the companies that hire them. About 30% of all business failures in the U.S. are caused by employee theft. Employee theft is growing by 15% a year, and as much as 75% of internal theft is never detected. In addition to theft, work-related violent crimes affect about 2 million people every year.

According to a recent study, as many as 80% of group practice physicians could be victimized by embezzlers during their careers, mostly involving office personnel who handle cash before and after office hours. The problem is sometimes detected when workers refuse to take time off for fear their dishonest acts will be discovered while they're away from the office. To reduce the potential for theft, some physicians run periodic credit checks on employees who handle cash, and they rotate assignments so that more than one person is responsible for overseeing the finances in an office.

If you find yourself in a difficult situation, weighing one option against another, and you're not quite sure which course of action to pursue, consider the following questions about each option:

- Is it honest?
- Does it reflect character and good judgment?
- Is it based on sound moral values?
- How would it affect my reputation?
- Would it damage the trust others have in me?
- What impact would my actions have on other people?
- What does my conscience tell me to do?
- What would a professional do?

DISPLAYING A PROFESSIONAL IMAGE

Now that we've examined the importance of character, personal values, morals, and honesty in the workplace, it's time to explore the connections between your personal life and your professional life.

personal skills
(PUR-suh-nl skils) The ability to manage aspects of your life outside of work

personal image
(PUR-suh-nl IM-ij) The total impression created by a person

You're just one person, so it stands to reason that if your personal life is out of control, your professional life will also suffer. When you have good **personal skills**, you're able to manage aspects of your life outside of work. This frees you up to concentrate on your job and your career. Of course, many of your personal skills transfer to the workplace and influence your reputation as a professional. This includes your **personal image**, personal health and wellness, and the ability to manage your time, finances, and stress and adapt to change. What does it take to have a well-orchestrated personal life that puts you on the right path to success in your career? Let's start with your personal image.

Hygiene, Grooming, and Posture

Your personal image is especially important in health care. Patients need to have confidence in their caregivers. They want assurance that the people caring for them are competent and professional. How would *you* feel if *your* caregiver had a ripped uniform, dirty shoes, oily hair, grimy fingernails, body odor, or bad breath? Would you wonder if that person's unprofessional appearance might also indicate a lack of pride or competence in his or her work? Family members and friends who visit patients also need reassurance that their loved ones are being cared for by professionals. Vendors, guests, and other people who come into your workplace expect to see employees supporting a professional environment. Your coworkers and supervisor expect you to uphold the organization's professional standards as well.

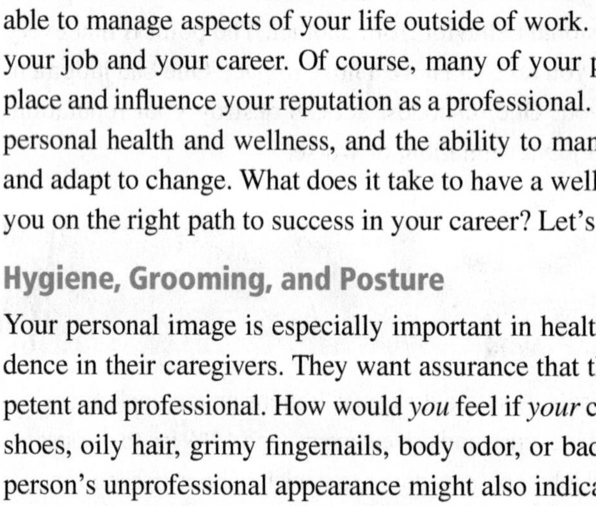

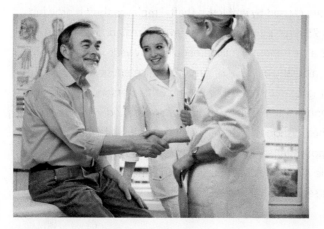

FIGURE 2.10
Displaying a professional image to gain the patient's trust
Source: Alexander Raths/Shutterstock

Then there's you. When you *look* good, you *feel* good. Setting high standards for your personal image not only conveys professionalism to other people, it also reinforces your pride and self-esteem. How can you expect others to view you as a professional if you don't look like or feel like a professional yourself?

One of the first things people notice about you is your personal appearance, which includes **hygiene**, **posture**, and how well you are **groomed**. Here are some tips to ensure good personal hygiene and grooming:

hygiene
(HIE-jeen) Body cleanliness

posture
(POS-cher) The position of the body or parts of the body

groomed
(GROOMD) Clean and neat

- Clean and trim your fingernails to avoid harboring bacteria beneath the nails.
- Brush and floss your teeth two to three times per day to prevent tooth decay, gum disease, and bad breath; use mouthwash.
- Wash your hands with antibacterial soap frequently throughout the day, and especially before preparing and eating food and after using the bathroom.
- Bathe with soap every day to wash off perspiration, dirt, and bacteria that can cause infection and body odor; use deodorant after bathing or showering.
- Shampoo your hair daily, treat dandruff, and style your hair with a comb or brush.

Good posture supports your personal image and your health. When growing up, you were probably encouraged to "Sit up straight and don't slouch". This is good advice. Poor posture puts extra strain on your muscles and ligaments and can cause neck and back pain. Poor posture can cause serious ailments for health care workers who stand on their feet all day or sit at a desk operating a computer. Good posture improves breathing and helps prevent fatigue. Here are some tips to ensure good posture:

- Sit with your back straight and your shoulders back, with your legs at a 90 degree angle with your body.
- Stand with your head up straight and your chin tucked in slightly; keep your shoulders back and your chest forward; balance your weight on the balls of your feet instead of your heels or toes.
- Keep your neck, back, and spine in alignment and as straight as possible.
- When lifting something, avoid straining your lower back; bend at the knees instead of at the waist, and use your leg muscles.

Dress Code and Attire

Most employers have a written **dress code** outlining appropriate and inappropriate attire. Dress code requirements vary from place to place, depending on where you work and your duties. Dietary workers, for example, have a different dress code than secretaries. People who work in respiratory therapy have a different dress code than pharmacists. One of the advantages of a dress code is that patients, visitors, and physicians can easily identify different types of workers (such as registered nurses) by their attire.

dress code
(DRES kohd) Standards for attire and appearance

Many health care workers wear uniforms. Consider the following as a general *rule of thumb,* whether you wear a uniform or street clothes appropriate for your job:

- Your clothes should be clean, pressed, and properly fitted. Avoid clothing that is wrinkled, frayed, too short, too tight, too baggy, or too revealing.
- Avoid clothes with wild colors and prints. Don't wear shirts or tops with messages printed on them unless approved by your employer.
- Avoid showing visible skin on your torso below the neckline of your blouse, shirt, or top. This means no visible tummies, breasts, or back skin. No short shirts, no

short skirts, no low rise pants, and no undergarments which are visible through your clothing.

- Shorts, capris, leggings, cropped pants, tight pants, tank tops, bare back tops, miniskirts, midriff tops, athletic attire, sweatshirts, sweatpants, T-shirts, painter pants, bib overalls, spaghetti strap dresses, reflective clothing, see-through fabrics, low or revealing necklines, spandex tops and pants, and untucked shirttails are not acceptable at work.
- Some health care employers ban any type of clothing that's made of denim, including scrubs, skirts, shirts, pants, dresses, and jeans, regardless of the color.
- Shoes should be clean, polished, and closed-toe. Wear socks or stockings; no bare feet, slippers, flip-flops, or open-toe shoes.
- Keep makeup, jewelry, and other accessories to a minimum and in good taste. (In some disciplines such as dental assisting, wearing jewelry is not allowed.)
- Avoid brightly polished fingernails and acrylic, artificial nails.
- Pull back long hair and secure it to avoid sanitary or safety problems.
- Groom and neatly style facial hair.
- Never wear perfume, aftershave, or scented lotions. Aromas may not be welcome among patients and coworkers, and could aggravate breathing difficulties.
- Wear your employee identification badge as prescribed in your dress code.
- Avoid non-traditional hairstyles and colors, cover up tattoos, and remove facial piercings.
- Don't wear sunglasses except for medical reasons.
- The use of head coverings is limited to religious customs or job-specific regulations.

You don't come to work to set fashion trends or compete in a beauty contest, so save your evening wear, party attire, sportswear, and the latest fashions for after hours. Your clothing and accessories should be geared to getting your work done safely and efficiently while instilling a feeling of confidence among those you serve. On *casual days*, remember that you're still in the workplace. If your job involves contact with patients and other customers, avoid wearing blue jeans, T-shirts, or other questionable attire even on casual days. If your duties include working off-site to represent your employer at health fairs, conferences, or other gatherings, dress code standards still apply.

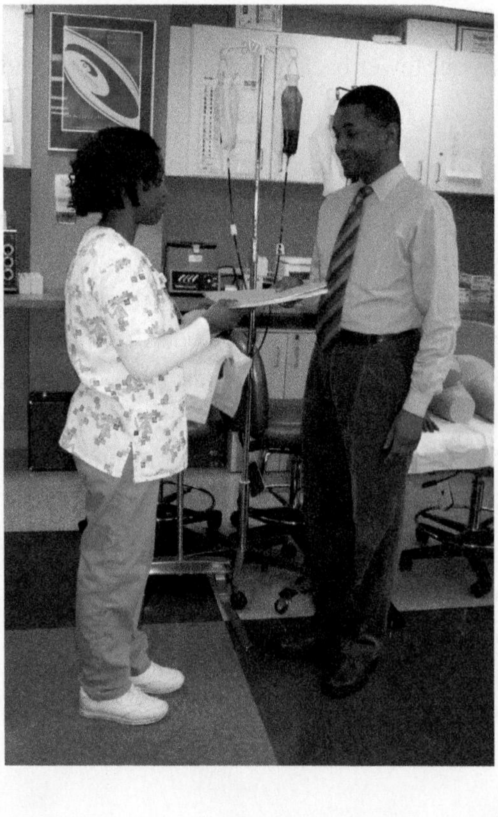

FIGURE 2.11

Complying with standards for professional attire

Source: Carmen Martin/Pearson Education

Keep in mind that what constitutes a professional image to one person might be quite different from that which constitutes a professional image to another person. In other words, professional image is *in the eye of the beholder*. Such

FIGURE 2.12
Wearing denim in the workplace may violate dress code
Source: Carmen Martin/Pearson Education

differences often relate to the age and generation of the beholder. Clothing and other appearance factors that seem appropriate for your age group may be disturbing to other people, especially those who are older than you. This includes such things as facial piercings, tattoos, and non-traditional hairstyles and hair colors.

Based on history, the dress codes of tomorrow may be less rigid than those of today. As younger generations enter the workforce in large numbers, dress code requirements will likely change. However, health care organizations tend to be conservative, and it can take a long time for dress codes to loosen up. Depending on where you work and what job you have, dress code requirements may limit opportunities to express your individuality. You may have to dress like everyone else in your department, practice, or office. You may have to comply with a dress code that was written by people much older than you. Adherence to dress code policies is a requirement of your job. Always think twice about attire, accessories, or other aspects of personal appearance that might make someone else feel uncomfortable or question your professionalism or competence. When you're at work, it's all about the patients and other customers, not your personal style or fashion.

Stereotypes

stereotypes (STER-ee-uh-tipes) Beliefs that are mainly false about a group of people

Stereotypes, which are often based on appearance, can affect your personal image at work. When older people, for example, see younger people with nose rings, tattoos, or purple hair, they form first impressions based on stereotypes. First impressions may not be accurate, but unfortunately they still occur. If someone stereotypes you in a negative manner, their opinion will improve once they get to know you. However, in the meantime, they may request to have a *different* worker take care of them, referring to someone who fits their stereotype of a professional-looking person.

Younger people may also form inaccurate first impressions of older people, again based on stereotypes. Stereotyping is a fact of life. Yet if you're aware of it, you can counteract its impact. Try to avoid stereotyping other people. Give everyone you

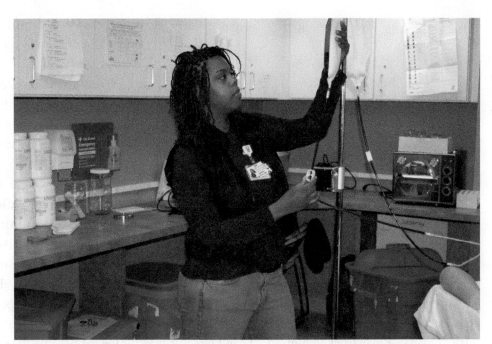

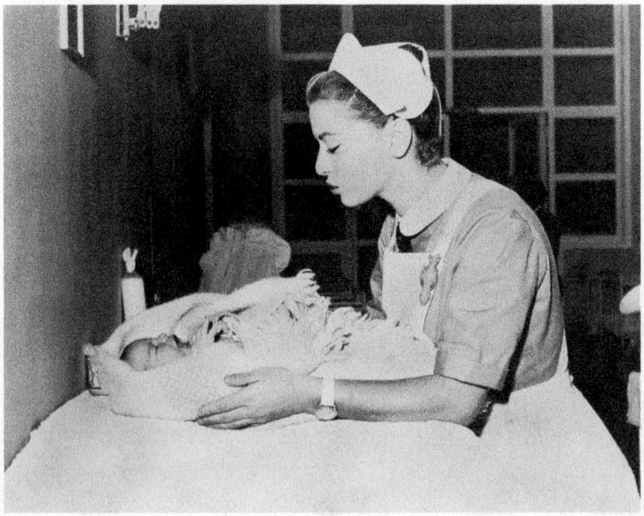

FIGURE 2.13

Not too long ago nurses wore starched white uniforms with caps

Source: Everett Collection/ Shutterstock

meet the benefit of the doubt and don't rely on first impressions.

When discussing stereotypes, the topic of body weight needs to be addressed. Although it's a sensitive issue, people who are extremely overweight may notice it adversely affects their job opportunities. Although we would like to believe that weight is not a factor in employment decisions, it does sometimes affect them. Overweight people may be unfairly stereotyped as lazy or unable to muster self-control. The issue of limited work space may come into play. A manager may think to himself, "I can't hire this man for the job because the space he has to work in would be too cramped for him to function properly." In surgery, others may have concerns about an obese nurse or surgical technologist contaminating a sterile field when working in a tight environment. In radiology, equipment controls may be housed in cubicles too confining for a large person. In jobs requiring heavy lifting or physical work, employers may feel that such activities could jeopardize the health and safety of an overweight employee.

Although it's unfortunate that a person's body weight could have a negative impact on his or her career, it is a fact of life. If you are seriously overweight and wish to do something about it, work closely with your family physician to plan a safe and healthy course of action. If you're content with your weight, or for medical reasons are unable to reduce your weight, be on the lookout for employment opportunities where weight is not a factor.

Personal Habits

Habits, which are part of your personal image, can sometimes be annoying to other people at work. Consider the following tips for minimizing potentially annoying habits:

- Don't wear noisy shoes or jewelry that jangles.
- Don't chew gum, pop your knuckles, or bite your fingernails.
- Don't play jokes and childish pranks on coworkers.
- If you must eat or drink in your work area, don't make a mess.
- If you have a hearing loss, get fitted for hearing aids; asking people to repeat things can become tiresome.
- Don't play music loudly enough for other people around you to hear it.
- Don't forward chain e-mail messages to coworkers.
- Don't use business computers for personal purposes.
- Don't make personal calls, use personal cell phones, or send text messages during work hours.
- Don't bring things to work to sell to your coworkers.
- Don't congregate with coworkers in patient or visitor areas before or after your shift.

FIGURE 2.14

Displaying unprofessional behavior by keeping a patient waiting while taking a personal telephone call

Source: Dylan Malone/Pearson Education

These are just a few examples of personal habits that can be irritating to other people. Always use common sense and ask yourself, how might my behavior affect the people around me?

Most health care organizations are smoke-free. If employees must smoke, they're directed to designated *smoking huts,* or they stand outside the building, huddled together on public sidewalks. As you might image, this doesn't present a very professional image to the public. Some health care employers have a total campus-wide ban on smoking and won't allow employees on-site if their clothing smells like smoke. If you must smoke, consider the following:

- Make sure you're familiar with your employer's smoking policies.
- Confine smoking to designated areas to protect others from secondhand smoke.
- Avoid taking too many smoking breaks or breaks that last too long.

Don't appear for work smelling of cigarette, cigar, or pipe smoke. Many people are allergic to smoke. Patients are ill, and the smell of smoke can be detrimental to their comfort.

An increasing number of health care employers require job applicants to undergo drug or nicotine screens, and they won't hire people who smoke. Some employers charge higher premiums on health insurance benefits for employees who smoke. Just as obesity may have an adverse affect on your job opportunities, so may smoking. It's hard to maintain your professional image when engulfed in a cloud of smoke or wearing clothing that reeks of cigarettes, cigars, or pipes. Employers may offer free smoking cessation classes for their employees. If you smoke and wish to quit, join a support group and get your doctor's advice.

Language and Grammar

Another habit that may annoy people at work is the language you use. Unless you have a close relationship with someone, don't refer to the person as *honey*, *sweetie*, or *dear*. While these may be terms of endearment to you, they're often annoying or demeaning to other people. Adult males are *men*, not *boys* or *guys*. Adult females are *women*, not *girls* or *gals*. Don't assume that an older female is a *Mrs*. It's best to refer to females as *Miss* or *Ms*.

Some language is totally unacceptable in the workplace. This includes obscene, cursing, vulgar language; sexually explicit or risqué comments; and terms that demean members of any racial, cultural, or ethnic group. *Street language* that might be acceptable after hours with your family or friends may be viewed as inappropriate by coworkers, patients, or visitors. If you're overheard using these words at work, chances are you'll be reprimanded and put on corrective action.

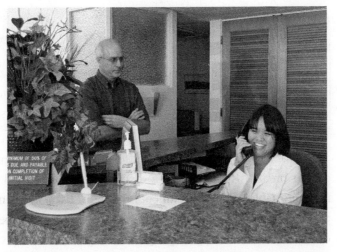

APPLY IT AVOIDING STREET LANGUAGE AT WORK

Watch for words that are used in *street language* that would not be acceptable at school or at work. When you hear someone use these words, notice the reaction by other people. What might happen if a patient, doctor, supervisor, or guest overhears these words in the workplace?

Telling jokes in poor taste and making *off-color* remarks is not a good idea, even during breaks. Remember the discussion about sexual harassment and creating an uncomfortable work environment for others? Even if you mean no harm, someone else's perception might be different than yours. Always be respectful of other people's points of view and avoid using language they might find offensive.

grammar
(GRA-mer) System of word structures and arrangements

Grammar also plays a role in your personal and professional image. Poor grammar is a warning signal, indicating a lack of education and refinement. It's not uncommon for people to mismatch the subject and verb in a sentence. Here are some examples:

- "We was there" should be, "We *were* there."
- "I seen you do that" should be, "I *saw* you do that."
- "Me and him" should be, "He and I."
- "She don't know" should be, "She *doesn't* know."
- "Her and I" should be "she and I."

Poor grammar is learned and then reinforced by the people with whom you associate. Poor grammar starts with your family as a child and expands to include your friends and coworkers. Contemporary music, advertisements, and the media also reinforce poor grammar (such as the lyric, "It don't matter to me"). If the people who are close to you use incorrect grammar, it's likely you will, too, without even realizing it. Just being aware of the need to use good grammar might help. If your grammar is weak, work towards improving it. You might be surprised by how much it can affect your personal and professional image.

Remember the old saying, "You only get one chance to make a good first impression"? In health care, *every* impression you make is important. *You* are the organization you work for. If you appear less than professional, so might your employer. Put together a total personal package that portrays a professional image. It's a big part of your job, and it can make or break your reputation as a professional.

APPLY IT REINFORCING POOR GRAMMAR

Find three examples of music lyrics and advertisements that intentionally include poor grammar. Share your examples with your classmates and discuss how music lyrics and advertisements promote poor grammar. Why do you think this occurs?

Professionalism After Hours

You might not realize it, but even when you're away from work your behavior can affect your professional image. For example, how do you answer your telephone? What kind of impression does your recorded telephone answering message make on people who call you? Don't assume that every caller is a friend, family member, or stranger trying to sell you something. What if your supervisor calls you, or a potential employer? Your telephone is an extension of your personal image, so think about who might be calling and the impression you want to make on them. Also ask yourself what impression your ring tone makes on people who hear it.

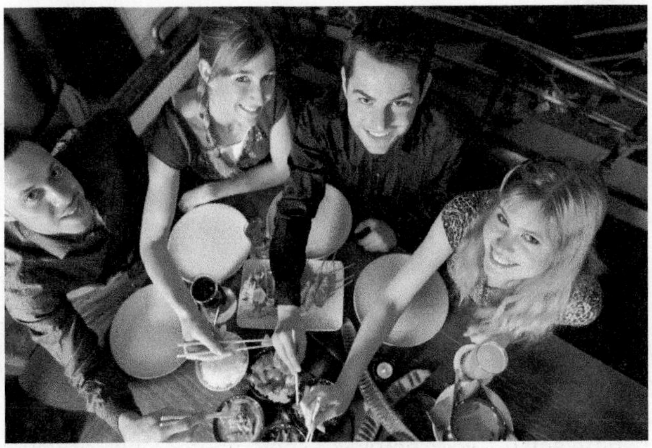

FIGURE 2.15

Keeping a professional image in mind, even after work hours

Source: Kzenon/Fotolia

Your relationships, both at work and outside of work, can also have a positive or negative effect on your image. The types of people with whom you associate are a reflection of your personal values and of who you are as a person. What impact do the people with whom *you* associate have on your reputation?

It's a small world. You never know when you might run into your supervisor, a coworker, or *someone who knows someone you know* after hours. "So what?" you might ask. "If I'm not at work, what difference does it make? What I do on my own time is no one's business." While it's true that you are off-the-clock, what you do after hours can make a huge difference. Your reputation goes with you *every place* you go. You never know who might be sitting across the room from you in a restaurant, concert, or another public place. If you call in sick when you really aren't and then go out in public, you never know whom you might run into. If someone sees you and word gets back to your supervisor, you wouldn't be the first person to get fired under such circumstances. If you're arrested and spend the night in jail, don't be surprised if your employer finds out.

If your work group, department, or organization has a special event after hours, the standards that govern acceptable behavior at work apply during those events, too. Always conduct yourself in a professional manner. It's hard to reestablish trust, respect, and your professional reputation after making some poor decisions the night before. Be very careful about what you post on Facebook, Twitter, and other Internet social networking sites and blogs. Sharing personal photographs and private information, posting complaints and gossip about coworkers and your employer, and making even casual comments about patients are easy ways to ruin your reputation and lead to corrective action or dismissal from your job.

Give serious thought to the pros and cons of dating someone with whom you work before you decide to do it. How might having a personal relationship outside of work affect both of you at work? What might happen when the relationship ends? Could the other person become your supervisor someday, or your subordinate? What issues related to sexual harassment might arise? If you're dating your supervisor and things go wrong, you may have to change jobs. If you *mix business with pleasure* with people who report to you, you may have difficulty supervising them later on. It's best to avoid these kinds of social relationships because they often lead to trouble.

The point of this discussion is to remember that you are just one person. You aren't one person at work and a different person after work, so do your best to maintain a positive image after hours, too. It is okay to *let your hair down* and have a good time, but don't let your guard down as well. Always think before you act.

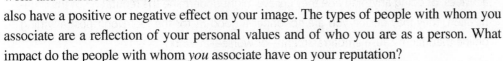

THE MORE YOU KNOW

When Your Personal Image Goes Public

Any content that you post on the Internet, or that other people post about you, is public information that can impact your professional reputation. Employers now visit social networking sites and review blogs to track down personal information about job applicants and current employees. New policies lead to corrective action or dismissal when employees display an unprofessional image online. This might seem unfair since your Facebook page or blog, for example, is your own private business. However, employers see things differently. If your employer spots photographs of you naked, drunk, engaged in illegal activities, or doing anything else they believe might undermine the reputation of the organization, they may decide you are no longer a good fit for the job. Don't post anything online that might cause embarrassment—or worse—at work.

PERSONAL MANAGEMENT SKILLS

personal management skills
(PUR-suh-nl MAN-ij-muhnt SKILS) The ability to manage time, finances, stress, and change

Personal management skills help you keep your personal life in order and support your success at work. Attendance and punctuality are good examples of how your personal life can affect your job. After all, does it really matter how professional you look or how competent you are if you can't get to work on time and be there when you're supposed to be? Your ability to show up for work on a daily basis and keep your appointments is one important aspect of your job. If you have trouble managing your time, handling your finances, dealing with your stress, or adapting to change, your personal life could have a negative impact on your job and your career. Let's take a closer look.

Time Management

time management
(tahym MA-nij-ment) The ability to organize and allocate one's time to increase productivity

When it seems like there are never enough hours in the day to get everything done that needs to get done, time management skills can be a big help. Here are some suggestions to help you use your time efficiently in order to balance school, work, family, and the many other priorities in your life:

- Use an electronic or pocket-sized calendar to record your work schedule, classes, appointments, and so on. Refer to your calendar every day and think about what's coming up tomorrow so you can be prepared. Don't schedule things too closely together, allow extra time for travel, and have contingency plans for unexpected complications.
- Make lists of things that need to get done. If you become overwhelmed, decide which are the most important and which you can let go. Eliminate activities that waste time and learn to say "no" when you're overbooked.
- Don't procrastinate. Letting things build up is a sure way to become overwhelmed, disorganized, and stressed out.

procrastinate
(proh-KRAS-tuh-neyt) To postpone or delay taking action

Identify your priorities and allocate your time accordingly. You can't create more hours in the day, but you can seize control of the time you have. After all, time is one of your most precious and most limited commodities. Learning how to manage it appropriately can have a huge impact on your personal and professional lives.

Personal Financial Management

How well you manage another precious and limited commodity, your personal finances, can have a big impact your personal and professional lives. Effective personal financial management skills can help you pay your bills on time and avoid financial problems that could cause embarrassment at work. Here are some suggestions to help you live within your means and avoid wasting money:

personal financial management
(PUR-suh-nl fi-NAN-shuh MAN-ij-muhnt) The ability to make sound decisions about personal finances

- Develop a budget, monitor your expenses, and know where your money is going. Have a checking and saving account and keep them balanced. Match up paydays with the dates you pay your bills to avoid getting charged late or overdraft fees.
- Read the fine print on loan and credit card applications. Avoid the high cost of doing business with companies that offer check cashing services, payday loans, rent-to-own furniture, and income tax refund anticipation loans.
- Limit credit card use to emergency situations or to make purchases that you already have the cash to cover. If you must rely on credit, look for the lowest interest rates. Always make the minimum monthly payment, and pay down and eliminate the balance as quickly as possible.
- Have a savings plan and stick with it. Put some money away for emergencies and other unexpected expenses. Start saving now for retirement. You'll be surprised how even small investments can grow over the years.
- Think twice before loaning someone money or cosigning their loan. If you must loan someone money, use a written and signed agreement detailing plans for repayment. Here's some good advice: don't loan someone money unless you can afford to never get it back. If you loan money to a friend, or if a friend loans you money, your friendship could suffer in the long-run.
- Ask if having liability insurance is recommended for people in your profession. This is especially important for some types of licensed professionals.

Managing personal finances can be quite a challenge in today's world. Establish priorities for how you want to allocate your resources and make your financial decisions accordingly.

Stress Management

Health care jobs are among the most stress-producing occupations in the nation. Stress can affect your physical health as well as your mental and emotional health. Physicians and researchers are convinced that stress is a contributing factor to several diseases and disorders. Stress can make you sick and cause symptoms such as headaches, fatigue, sleep problems, diarrhea, indigestion, ulcers, hypertension, dizziness, hives, teeth grinding, skin disorders, and stuttering. Stress has been linked with heart attacks, high blood pressure, alcoholism, depression, and drug abuse.

People with *Type A* personalities are among the most susceptible to stress-related disorders. They are highly competitive, impatient, high achievers with strong perfectionist tendencies. They rush from place to place, work long hours, have an intense drive to get things done, become frustrated easily, and have trouble relaxing. When Type A

FIGURE 2.16

A surgical professional experiencing stress and exhaustion

Source: stefanolunardi/Shutterstock

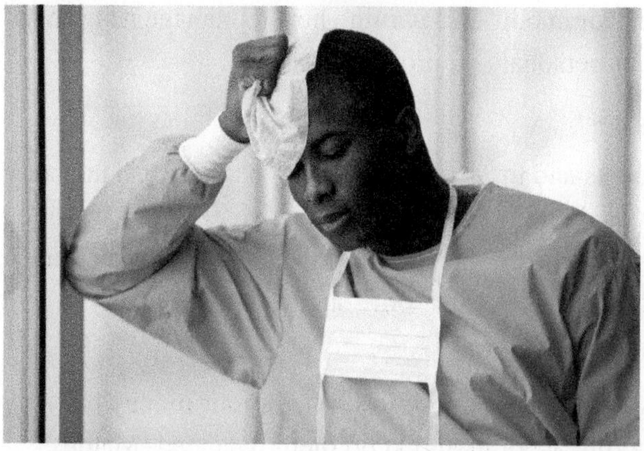

personalities have a lifestyle that includes smoking, drinking, poor diet, lack of exercise, and obesity, they become targets for stress-related illness. If you're a Type A personality yourself, or if the stress you experience tends to affect your health in any way, don't wait until it's too late. Watch for the warning signs and seek help in dealing with it.

stress management (STRES MA-nij-ment) The ability to deal with stress and overcome stressful situations

Effective **stress management** skills are valuable in both your personal and professional lives. Managing stress is a key factor in your image as a professional. If you *blow up*, *melt down*, or *run for the door* at the first sign of stress, you may be letting down your coworkers and patients. Your ability to perform your job duties may be affected and your personal health and wellness may suffer. Good stress management techniques can help you keep everything in balance and add more enjoyment to your life. Here are some suggestions:

- Become aware of when, how, and why stress is affecting you; identify the source of your stress and seek ways to reduce or eliminate the stress.
- Identify someone with whom you can talk, such as a person who can relate to what you're experiencing and help you think through it.
- Try to keep work-related stress from affecting your personal life, and try to keep stress in your personal life from affecting your job and your work. This is easier said than done because you are just one person.
- Maintain a healthy balance between school, work, recreation, and rest. Use your vacation time wisely. Learn to relax and schedule time for hobbies, sports, and other personal interests.
- Get plenty of sleep, and exercise and eat properly.
- Use conflict resolution skills and avoid keeping negative feelings bottled up inside you.

An important part of managing stress is being well adjusted and finding happiness in life. Professionals have a positive self-image. They have high levels of self-esteem and self-respect and they know they are worthy individuals. Let's face it—it's difficult for others to have confidence in you if you don't have confidence in yourself. Consider these strategies:

- Look for the good in yourself, know your limits, and work within them.
- Be patient with yourself and with others. Avoid being a perfectionist—no one is perfect. Setting unrealistic goals is counterproductive and leads to disappointment, low self-esteem, and unnecessary stress.
- Set high but realistic standards for yourself and feel good about your accomplishments.

Learn to manage your stress and find ways to achieve happiness at school, work, and home. Making the most of change is a good place to start.

Managing Change

If you're going to work in health care, one of the most important skills you'll need is the ability to adjust to change. Just when you think everything is arranged as it should be, something will change. You might acquire extra job duties, undergo cross-training, or be assigned to work in a different location. Your work schedule might get altered, your organization might merge with another organization, or you might get a new supervisor. At the same time you're affected by changes at work, you're probably facing changes in your personal life, too. Family responsibilities, relationships with friends, and pressures involving finances, housing, and personal health can all cause many changes over the course of our lives.

It's almost impossible to avoid change. If you're the type of person who resists change, you're going to face some difficult struggles working in health care. On the other hand, if you have effective adaptive skills you'll be well prepared for the many changes that life will throw your way.

adaptive skills
(uh-DAP-tiv SKILS) The ability to adjust to change

Years ago, health care workers were encouraged to *cope* with change. When the pace of change increased, people were encouraged to *manage* change. Now that change is occurring so rapidly, health care workers must *embrace* change and *lead* change from time to time. Change can be a positive influence in your life if you learn to accept it and let it open new doors for you. Having your job redesigned, for example, can be pretty scary. You might have to learn some new skills and take on new responsibilities. But the more new challenges you face, the more you will grow. The more you grow, the better your chances for advancement. View change as positive and learn to make it work *for* you instead of *against* you. After all, do you really want your personal life and your career to be exactly the same five years from now as they are today?

REALITY CHECK

What does your personal image say about you? Will your appearance, habits, language, and grammar lead people to view you as a professional? Or will patients, coworkers, and doctors question your competence because of your attire or the condition of the clothes you wear? Do you take into account how elderly people might react to your appearance? Or could your unsettling image lead patients to ask for *someone different* to take care of them? Are you careful about what you say at school and at work? Or is your use of *street language* offending people and damaging your reputation?

You might be amazed at how some people show up for work. They look like they just rolled out of bed, or never went to bed. It's obvious they either don't care what they look like, or they don't have a clue how people are supposed to dress in a business environment. Once you've made an unprofessional first impression, it might be difficult to change someone's opinion of you. Bare cleavage, visible undergarments, nose rings, or spandex clothes are enough to shock your supervisor into putting you on corrective action and sending you home without pay. If any of this describes you, it's time to cleanup your act and your appearance.

Key Points

- Remember that it takes a long time to develop a professional reputation, but only a split second to lose it.
- Review the list of positive character traits and decide which ones you need to improve upon.
- Use good judgment in making decisions.
- Listen to your conscience and avoid temptations to do the wrong thing.
- Make sure that your word is *as good as gold* and follow through on your commitments.
- Don't take anything that doesn't belong to you without proper authorization.
- Don't lie, cheat, steal, commit fraud, or engage in any other illegal or inappropriate behavior.
- Do your best to keep your personal life in balance so that personal problems don't negatively affect your professional reputation.
- Adhere to dress code policies to portray a positive personal image.
- Choose clothing and accessories that allow you to perform your work efficiently and safely.
- Practice good grooming and hygiene habits, and pay attention to your posture.
- Avoid stereotyping other people and forming inaccurate first impressions.
- Avoid personal habits that might annoy other people.
- Use proper language and grammar, and avoid *street language* at work.
- Don't let your guard down after-hours.
- Think twice before dating a coworker or your supervisor.
- Develop effective time management skills and don't procrastinate.
- Keep your personal finances in order and live within your means.
- Identify the sources of your stress and take steps to reduce or eliminate them.
- Sharpen your adaptive skills and be open to opportunities that come with change.

Section Review Questions

Answer each of the following questions. Indicate which page in the textbook led you to your answer.

1. Define *character*, *personal values*, and *morals* and explain how each affects your reputation as a professional.
2. List four examples of a lack of character in the workplace.
3. Explain why it's important to maintain professionalism after hours.
4. List three techniques to help manage your time and explain what might happen if these techniques aren't followed.
5. List three techniques to help manage your personal finances and explain what might happen if these techniques aren't followed.
6. List three techniques to help manage your stress and explain what might happen if these techniques aren't followed.
7. Define *adaptive skills* and explain why the ability to manage change is important in health care.

Learn By Doing

Complete Worksheets 1–5 in Section 2.2 of your *Student Activity Guide*.

Teamwork and Diversity

SECTION 2.3

Background

Forming effective relationships, functioning as part of a team, and developing competence in working with different groups of people are crucial elements in becoming a health care professional. Professionals devote a lot of energy to establishing and maintaining positive interpersonal relationships and treating each other in a caring, respectful manner. Focusing on courtesy, etiquette, and manners will go a long way in improving relationships with people in both your personal and professional lives. Chances are you'll serve on many teams over the course of your health career, and you'll need some special skills to collaborate with others and achieve the team's goals. We live in a world of diversity. Valuing diversity and learning about other cultures will help you better understand and respect your patients and provide quality care.

interpersonal relationships (in-ter-PUR-suh-nl ri-LEY-shuhn-ships) Connections between or among people

diversity (dih-VUR-si-tee) Differences, dissimilarities, variations

Objectives

After completing this section, you will be able to:

1. Define the key terms.
2. List three ways to strengthen relationships at work.
3. Explain the roles of courtesy, etiquette, and manners in the workplace.
4. Identify two types of workplace teams and give an example of each.
5. Discuss the roles and responsibilities of health care team members.
6. Define *consensus* and explain why it is important, but difficult, to achieve.
7. Explain the value of having a team mission statement and group norms.
8. Explain why health care workers need to be culturally competent.
9. Explain how culture influences behavior.
10. Identify culturally acceptable and effective gestures, terms, and behaviors.
11. Identify common folk medicine practices.
12. Explain how understanding cultural beliefs affects you as a health care worker.

INTERPERSONAL RELATIONSHIPS

Once you're employed on a full-time basis, you will probably spend as much time with your coworkers as you do with your family and friends. People want to feel good about coming to work so it's important to create a positive, enjoyable work environment. Nothing can make your job more pleasant or miserable than your relationships with your coworkers. Think about the relationships you've had in the past. Why did those relationships work well, or not work well? Effective relationships are based on many of the factors already discussed in this text—trust, honesty, and morals. But several other traits and skills are also necessary.

While it's obvious that patients, visitors, and guests are customers of health care organizations, it's important to realize that your coworkers are also customers. Although that might seem strange, coworkers are considered your *internal* customers, and they deserve to be treated with the same respect and compassion that you would give your patients and other *external* customers.

Much like tossing a pebble in a pond, your attitude at work creates ripples. Displaying a friendly, positive attitude, saying hello to people you pass in the hallway, and smiling every chance you get goes a long way toward creating a pleasant work environment. Always look for the best in people, give them the benefit of the doubt, and assume that everyone is there to do their best.

Professionals need to be viewed as *team players*. Cooperate with your coworkers, and avoid whining, complaining, and questioning authority. Complainers *poison* the workplace and stir up discontent. If you get labeled as a complainer or troublemaker, your opportunities for advancement could be limited. Colleagues may ask that you not be part of their professional team. As this chapter will show, health care is all about competent and compatible teamwork.

Inclusion and Friendliness

inclusive
(in-KLOO-siv) A tendency to include everyone

cliques
(KLIKS) Small, exclusive circles of people

When forming relationships with coworkers, it's best to be **inclusive**. Instead of excluding people and participating in **cliques**, you might invite your coworkers to join you for lunch and make them feel welcome. Don't leave people out of the group. Excluding people can hurt their feelings and undermine their self-esteem. Self-esteem results, at least in part, from the feedback that people get from other people. So how you treat coworkers can have a direct impact on how they feel about themselves. If you want your coworkers to feel confident and good about themselves, then include them in your activities at work, reinforce their strengths and abilities, and help support their growth and advancement.

You and your coworkers don't need to be friends outside of work. Relationships with coworkers can enrich your professional life, but friendship is not the goal of your work relationships. In fact, you might not even like some of the people with whom you need to work. Regardless of your feelings, you need to find ways to get along with them and respect the knowledge, skills, and talents they bring to the workplace.

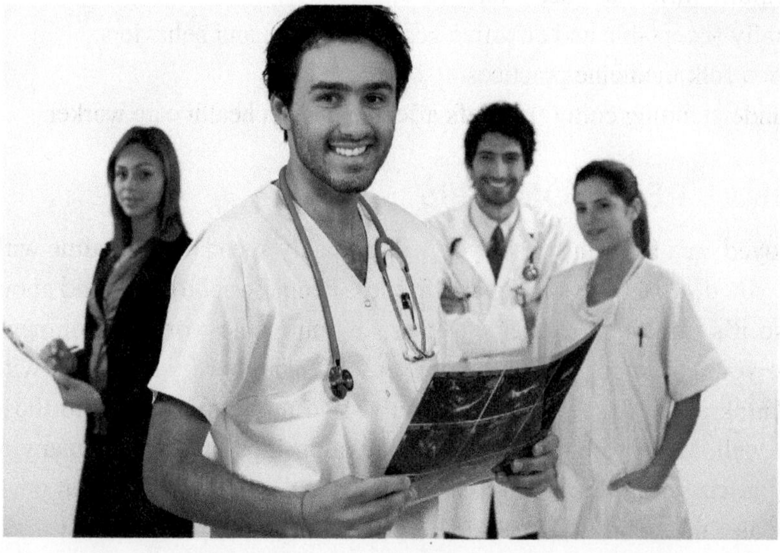

FIGURE 2.17
Building relationships through friendliness, inclusion, and loyalty
Source: auremar/Shutterstock

Because health care workers must depend on one another to get their work done, they must be willing to share work-related information openly. Unfortunately, some people hoard information because it gives them a sense of power. They know something that you don't know, and that makes them feel important. But such an attitude is counterproductive to relationships and teamwork. It's also important to share space, equipment, and supplies. After all, you're all there for the same purpose—to serve patients and other customers, so there's no need for competition.

Laugh at yourself, be a good sport, and maintain your sense of humor. Avoid arrogance and don't be a snob. When you accomplish a goal, take pride, but don't brag. Never *look down* on your coworkers or treat people in a demeaning way because they have less education, income, or *status* than you. There will always be people above and below you in your organization, and each person plays a critical **role** in fulfilling the organization's mission. Remember the **golden rule**—treat other people the way you want to be treated. Or better yet, treat other people the way *they* want to be treated.

role
(ROHL) A position, responsibility, or duty

golden rule
(GOHL-duhn ROOL) Treat other people the way you want to be treated

Building effective relationships doesn't happen overnight. It is hard work, and you have to be persistent. Be patient and forgiving with yourself and with your coworkers. No one is perfect—not even you! Get to know people better. You may discover a whole different side of someone's personality. Let your coworkers get to know you better, too. The better your relationships, the more likely your coworkers will be there for you when you need them, and vice versa.

Loyalty

Showing **loyalty** to the people who have helped you goes a long way in developing a professional reputation. One way to demonstrate loyalty to your coworkers is to be supportive when situations become stressful. Everyone who works in health care needs some encouragement and support from time to time. Getting the kind of emotional support that you need from people who don't work in health care themselves can be difficult. Even though family and friends may want to be helpful, it's hard to relate to the stress of working in health care unless you've experienced it yourself. This is especially true for employees who work on burn units and with critically ill children and patients facing death. Professionals need to *be there* for one another, to lend a helping hand or a shoulder to cry on. When someone you work with needs support, be ready to help. Most of the time it means just listening—and understanding.

loyalty
(loi-uhl-tee) Showing faith to people that one is under obligation to defend or support

The concept of loyalty also relates to your relationship with your employer. Remember the statement, "*You* are the organization you work for"? Stop and think about it. You don't actually work for an organization; you work for the *people* who manage the organization. Companies and organizations are just legal entities that own assets such as buildings, property, and equipment. You don't work for a building, you work for people. Professionals are able to make that distinction, and they feel a sense of loyalty to the people whom they *work for* as well as to the people whom they *work with.* You may not agree with management's policies, but don't forget that it's the people who manage your organization who are providing you with a job and an opportunity to earn a living.

How can you demonstrate loyalty to your employer? Here are some examples:

- Let management know you appreciate them and are proud to be part of the organization. Managers are people, too, and they appreciate being appreciated.

- Give management the benefit of the doubt. Until you've walked in their shoes, you can't fully appreciate the challenges they face every day.
- If your employer invests in your education and training, help pay back their investment by continuing to work there for a reasonable length of time. If a local competitor offers you extra pay to switch employers, remember who invested in your education and show your loyalty. Someday you may need a recommendation from your current employer. If management views you as a loyal employee, it can only help.
- Represent your employer in a professional manner. Always speak highly of management when in public and do your best to enhance your organization's reputation.

Cooperation

Cooperation is essential in maintaining effective relationships at work. Offer to help your coworkers even if they haven't asked for assistance. When you have a tough job to do or you're running late, isn't it a welcome relief to hear someone say, "Need a hand?" Offer to rotate shifts and holiday coverage—your coworkers will appreciate the consideration. Make personal sacrifices, such as coming in early or staying late, to help a coworker—sensitivity and kindness are rewarded many times over. Learn to rely on one another, especially in emergencies and other stressful situations. Gain an appreciation for the strengths, abilities, and personal traits that each coworker contributes. Volunteer to serve on committees and sign up for employer-sponsored recreational activities to meet people and establish more relationships. Join people during your meal break and widen your circle of colleagues. You'll find there's synergy in working with other people. Remember the saying, "Two heads are better than one"? A group of people can accomplish so much more working together than several individuals working on their own.

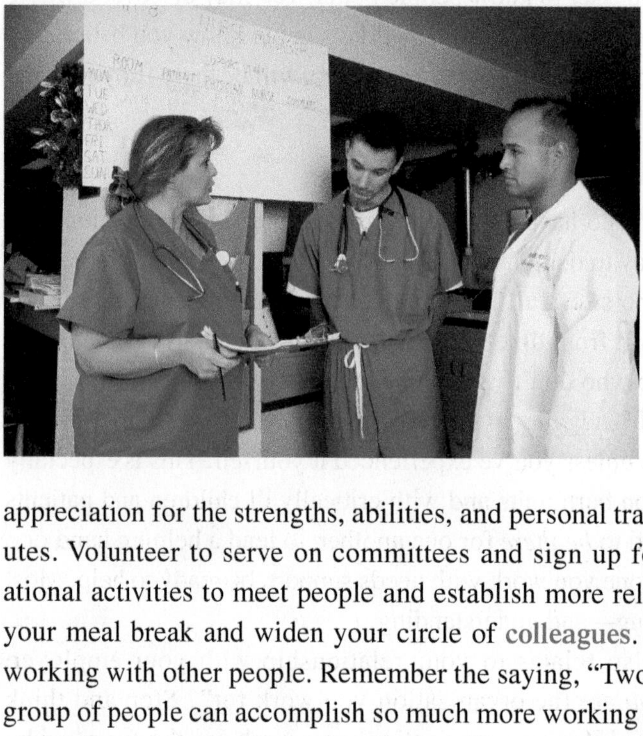

FIGURE 2.18

Coworkers functioning as a team based on effective interpersonal relationships, loyalty, and cooperation

Source: Michael Newman/PhotoEdit

colleagues
(KOL-eegs) Fellow workers in the same profession

synergy
(SIN-er-jee) People working together in a cooperative action

civility
(SIH-vil-i-tee) Politeness, consideration

polite
(puh-LITE) Courteous, having good manners

courtesy
(KUR-tuh-see) Polite behavior, gestures, and remarks

etiquette
(ET-i-kit) Acceptable standards of behavior in a polite society

manners
(MAN-ers) Standards of behavior based on thoughtfulness and consideration of other people

Etiquette and Manners

A growing number of Americans, especially employers, are expressing concerns about the erosion of civility in our society. The decline of polite behavior is especially problematic in health care where people must work together, often under stressful conditions, to meet customer needs. As a result, employers are increasingly emphasizing the roles that courtesy, etiquette, and manners play in forming and maintaining effective relationships.

If it seems like the definitions of courtesy, etiquette, and manners overlap with one another, that's okay. What's important is the role that polite behavior plays at work, at home, and in all aspects of your life. Here are just a few examples.

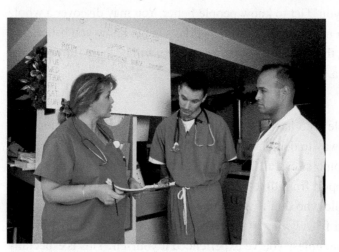

Courtesy

- Ask others before changing the room temperature, adjusting window blinds, turning on the TV, or playing music.
- Respect other people's possessions; return borrowed items quickly and, if you break something, repair it or replace it at your expense.
- Don't expect other people to clean up after you; keep your work area neat and orderly so it doesn't become an irritation for others.
- Don't display risqué calendars, posters, or other personal items that might offend someone else.
- Listen while other people are talking and don't interrupt them.
- When riding on an elevator with a patient on a cart or in a wheelchair, protect their privacy and don't stare at them.

Professional/Business Etiquette

- Shake hands with a firm grip when you meet someone; be aware that some people will resist a hand shake due to an injury or concern about spreading germs.
- Refer to an older person or a superior (such as your boss's boss) by his or her last name (Mr. Smith, rather than Bill).
- Respect other people's time and don't make them wait on you.
- When you put someone on hold on the telephone, check back frequently to let them know you haven't forgotten about them.
- When people arrive for a meeting, if possible, offer them a beverage.
- Don't text, check e-mail messages, or talk on your cell phone during work hours when you're in meetings, with patients, or with people who expect to have a conversation with you.
- Maintain eye contact when speaking with people; when speaking to a group, make eye contact with everyone, not just one person.
- When invited as a guest to eat with your supervisor or a coworker, follow the lead of the host and order in a similar price range.

Manners

- When you notice someone carrying a heavy or cumbersome package, offer to help.
- When in a crowded area, offer your seat to an elderly or handicapped person, a pregnant woman, or anyone else who needs the seat more than you do.
- Hold doors open for people who are entering or leaving the building right before or after you.
- If an elevator is crowded, step back and wait for the next one.
- When encountering a disfigured or handicapped person, don't stare or ignore the person; make eye contact and acknowledge their presence in a friendly manner.
- Always say "please" and "thank you" and acknowledge the kindness of other people.
- Cough or sneeze into your shoulder or elbow; wash you hands frequently to reduce the spread of germs.
- Acknowledge people when they walk into the room and make them feel welcome.

Far too many examples of polite behavior exist to list them all here. If you feel you need to learn more about courtesy, etiquette, and manners, many good books and other resources are available on the subject.

Consider This *Etiquette Outside of Work*

Etiquette in your personal life also affects your reputation. Here are some tips:

- RSVP to invitations in plenty of time to let the host know if you'll be attending.
- Don't bring children or other guests with you to an event unless they've been invited.
- Acknowledge gifts by sending the giver a written thank you note within two weeks.
- When seated for a meal, don't start eating until everyone at your table has been served; don't leave the table until everyone has finished eating.
- When going through a buffet line, leave enough food for those in line behind you.
- Refrain from texting and using a cell phone when socializing with friends in person.
- When speaking on the phone, lower your voice to avoid annoying the people around you.
- When walking down the street or up/down the stairs, stay to the right.

How can practicing good etiquette improve relationships in your personal life? What might happen if you don't?

TEAMS AND TEAMWORK

Relationships with coworkers become even more important when working on teams, and teamwork is *the name of the game* in health care. In fact, many health care providers now rely on *high performance work teams* to care for patients and complete other assignments. Depending on your profession and where you work, you'll probably participate on many teams during your career. Some teams will be composed of people from your department or **discipline**, while other teams will include a mixture of people. Some teams will meet on an on-going basis as part of their jobs, while other teams will meet for a specified period of time and disband when their work has been completed.

discipline
(DIS-uh-plin) A branch of knowledge or learning

High performance work teams often work independently with little direct supervision, so it's important that you and your teammates participate effectively. For example, teams may:

- Arrange their own work schedules and holiday coverage
- Select new equipment and medical supplies
- Monitor and improve quality outcomes
- Resolve budgetary and staffing issues
- Interview and select new team members

Team members may evaluate each other's performance and work collectively to **delegate** job duties. With responsibilities such as these, team members need effective skills in communicating, negotiating, and delegating as well as the ability to manage group dynamics and resolve disagreements. Team members also need skills in both *leading* and *following*. You'll probably find yourself in both roles from time to time, even within the same team. *Shared leadership* is becoming more common. Members rotate the leadership role from time to time, or each team member takes the lead when the task to be completed falls within his or her area of **expertise** or interest. *Leading*

delegate
(DEL-i-geyt) To give another person responsibility for doing a specific task

expertise
(ek-sper-TEEZ) High degree of skill or knowledge

team members is not the same thing as *supervising* team members. In many situations team members are peers, so no one on the team reports to someone else on the team. If one team member fails to complete his or her responsibilities, the whole team may suffer. In many health care settings, team performance is just as important (or more important) as individual performance. When the team performs well, each member is held in high regard. When the team fails, each member is held accountable.

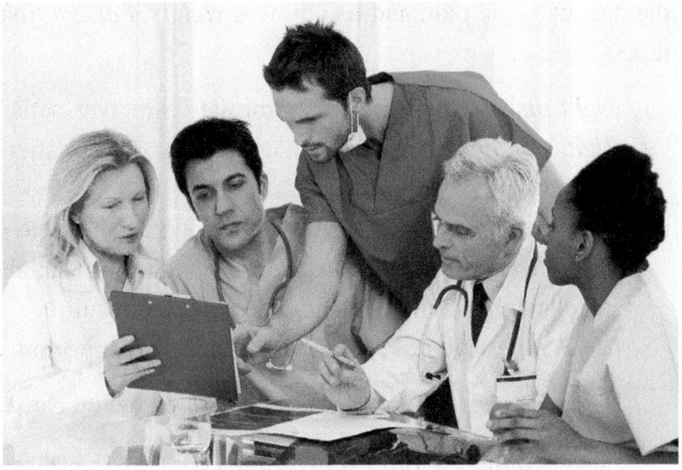

FIGURE 2.19

Team members collaborating to provide high quality patient care

Source: Yuri Acrcurs/Fotolia

Providing quality care for patients depends on every health care worker doing his or her part. Let's take a closer look at teams and how they function.

The Team Concept

A team is a group of more than two people who work together to achieve a common goal. Teamwork is quite helpful because an individual has only a limited amount of knowledge and experience. By bringing together different people with a variety of backgrounds, more ideas can be generated, and more problems can be solved.

A team's identity is formed by the nature and purpose of the work to be done by the team. Most teams develop through a series of stages. At first, members of the new team might feel nervous or uncomfortable. Individuals must interact with other members who they do not know well. They might also begin tasks that are new to them. As teammates begin to work together, members might misunderstand or misinterpret each others' behaviors. A teammate might disagree with another's opinion. This kind of **conflict** is natural and can actually strengthen a team as members learn to resolve their differences. Many teams will eventually achieve **cohesiveness**. The team will feel a sense of unity or team identity. Once groups establish this unity, they may become quite productive. This productive period lasts as long as the team dynamics do not change. Some teams might eventually break apart because team members move to new teams or leave the organization, or the team's work has been completed.

conflict
(KON-flikt) A contradiction, fight, or disagreement

cohesiveness
(koh-HEE-siv-nus) State of being well integrated or unified

Interdisciplinary teams are common in health care. These groups consist of people from two or more disciplines who work in the same setting. Professionals with different backgrounds, education levels, and areas of expertise (such as registered nurses, physical therapists, occupational therapists, and rehabilitation aides) all work together to provide appropriate quality care. Team members contribute their opinions about treatment plans and then collaborate to implement *one plan* based on *one set of goals*. Members of an interdisciplinary team must depend upon one another and communicate frequently.

interdisciplinary
(in-ter-DIS-uh-pluh-nair-ee) Involving two or more disciplines

In hospitals, registered nurses collaborate with interdisciplinary team members on patient care units (nursing units) to coordinate care provided for patients. RNs determine the patient's care plan and use the *five rights of delegation* to coordinate completion of tasks:

1. ***Right task:*** Identifying an appropriate caregiver-patient relationship.
2. ***Right circumstances:*** Verifying that the correct patient setting and resources are available.
3. ***Right person:*** Identifying who is trained and capable of doing the task.
4. ***Right direction/communication:*** Providing a clear, short description of the task and clarifying limitations and the expected result.
5. ***Right supervision:*** Providing appropriate monitoring, assistance, and feedback.

Here are some examples of other types of health care teams:

ad hoc
(AD-hoc) For a specific purpose

- Ad hoc teams are formed for a limited amount of time to address a specific problem. Members may be from the same department (such as surgery) or from several departments (such as patient registration, admitting, and surgery). Ad hoc teams may address issues such as remodeling surgery suites or improving patient check-in procedures. Once their work has been completed, the team disbands.
- Nominal care groups include a physician who refers a patient to different specialists. The specialists provide care independently, but the physician coordinates the flow of information among the specialists to facilitate a team approach in caring for the patient.
- Unidisciplinary groups are organized around a single discipline, such as nursing or respiratory care. These teams are relatively permanent and function on an ongoing basis. Hospital nursing units or critical care respiratory therapy teams are good examples of unidisciplinary teams.
- Multidisciplinary teams are composed of workers from different disciplines who work with a patient during the same time period. Each practitioner has his or her own goals and recommendations for the patient, but they communicate among themselves to provide a team approach to the patient's care.
- Emergency response teams are composed of several individuals with different experience and expertise that may include paramedics, rescue squads, medevac professionals, emergency department nurses, and doctors. These highly trained team members often attend to patients in life-threatening conditions, requiring efficient and responsive team interaction and performance.

Team Goals and Roles

mission statement
(MISH-uhn STAYT-muhnt) A summary describing aims, values, and an overall plan

short-term goals
(SHAWRT-term GOHLS) Aims that will take a relatively short time to achieve

long-term goals
(LONG-term GOHLS) Aims that will take a relatively long time to achieve

A team needs to decide early what goals it wants to accomplish. Goals might be assigned by management when the group is formed, or team members might have the opportunity to set their own goals based on the situation. Team goals might relate to patient needs, professional needs, or team needs. They may include ways of exchanging information or evaluating outcomes.

To develop meaningful goals, each member needs to communicate his or her individual goals so they can be incorporated into the group's shared goals. Teams may want to develop a broad mission statement that all members can support. Goals can then be developed from this mission statement. In order to create goals that everyone can understand, each goal should be clear and include an observable, measurable end point. Teams may set either or both short-term goals and long-term goals. Short-term goals can be accomplished within a day, week, month, or year depending on the overall timeline of the team's mission. Long-term goals, on the other hand, require significantly more time but often lead to the most desirable outcomes. When we apply this to patient care, a short-term goal might be helping an elderly patient learn to walk and move around steadily; the long-term goal might be helping him to live on his own. Teams may set priorities for their goals to help members stay focused and promote cohesiveness. In addition, team members may revise or add new goals based on changing needs.

Language Arts Link Teamwork and Mission Statements

It is vital in today's medical field to know how to work with others. To be able to work as a team, it's essential that everyone has the same end goal in mind. A mission statement, which is a brief statement of purpose, can ensure that all team members have the same intentions.

Work in a team to create a mission statement for this course. Be sure to include your team's responsibilities, values, and main objectives. Proofread your work to see if you can improve it by making it more clear, concise, or interesting to read. Check the spelling and grammar and correct any errors. Each team should prepare a presentation on their mission statement. Part of working as a team is determining who is best suited for a job. Each team member should practice delivering the mission statement; then, as a team, decide who your presenter will be.

An interdisciplinary team may consist of many different types of professionals, such as physicians, social workers, psychiatrists, physical therapists, massage therapists, medical assistants, nurses, radiographers, dietitians, and home health care workers. When serving on a team, these workers may find some overlap in their skills. Several professionals, for example, may have expertise in interacting with patients, forming care plans, and educating patients. Several providers might diagnose and treat illnesses. Therefore, health care teams must identify the role of each member. This starts by identifying the specific tasks that need to be done. A team's goals may help to define these tasks. Tasks may include activities such as ordering diagnostic tests, taking a patient's vital signs, contacting the patient, or writing prescriptions. Decisions about each teammate's role may depend on availability, level of training, or worker preferences. For example, a nurse's role on the health care team may be to coordinate patient care, protect the patient from illness, and provide instructions for the patient and/or family members. Another nursing role might be assisting with the patient's mobility. The team's physical therapist would prescribe the activity (such as assisting the patient in using a walker), the nursing staff would carry out the activity, and the physical therapist would evaluate the patient's progress.

Assigning roles to each team member helps eliminate conflict and establish expectations. One or more members of the patient care team may serve as the leader of the group, and the leader may change over time depending on the nature of the problem to be solved. In the past, physicians typically took the leadership role. But today, with an increased emphasis on caring for *the whole person,* non-physician professionals are acquiring

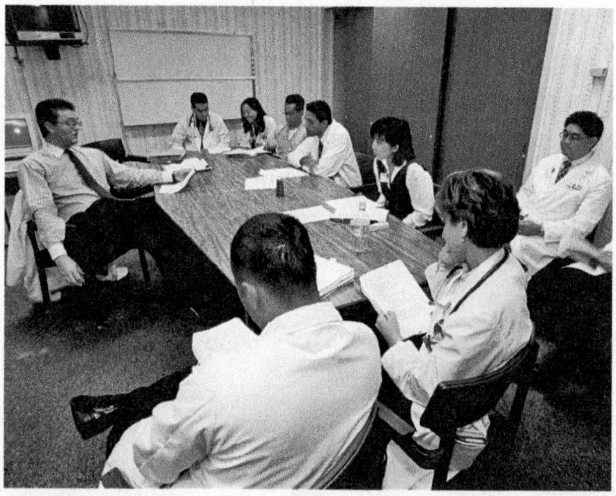

FIGURE 2.20
An interdisciplinary team meets to review progress in achieving patient safety goals
Source: Jonathan Nourok/PhotoEdit

more leadership responsibilities. Regardless of whether the team leader is a physician or another health professional, that person needs effective leadership skills to help guide the team in accomplishing its goals.

As *followers* rather than leaders, team members need some special skills as well. They must be committed to the group's **productivity** and demonstrate effective interpersonal skills. This includes being open-minded, respectful of other people's opinions, and willing to cooperate and **compromise**. Team members should:

productivity
(proh-duhk-TIV-i-tee) The power to reach goals and get results

compromise
(KOM-pruh-mize) A settlement of disagreement between parties by each party agreeing to give up something that it wants

- Understand and commit to team goals and objectives
- Practice good communication skills to share ideas, concepts, and knowledge
- Share thoughts and feelings openly and honestly
- Involve others in the decision-making process
- Trust other team members and be trustworthy themselves
- Provide encouragement, support, and help when needed
- Accept accountability for their actions, and avoid blaming others
- Listen carefully when other people are sharing ideas or beliefs
- Respect and value different opinions even when they don't agree with them
- Identify and work through interpersonal conflict
- Consider and use new ideas and suggestions from other people
- Encourage feedback about their own behavior
- Maintain a positive attitude and a good sense of humor
- Avoid criticizing other team members
- Perform duties to the best of their ability

Team Communication

Effective interpersonal communication is vital to the smooth functioning of any team. Team members should be skilled in active listening, giving and receiving feedback, and checking for comprehension. It is also important for a team to develop an effective communication network. For example, team members should establish who relays information to whom within the team. The team must work to share relevant information in the most efficient way possible. Some other important communication practices for a health care team include keeping accurate records of decisions that were made, scheduling meetings and follow-up activities, and developing a procedure for communicating with other groups inside or outside the health facility.

The goal of team communication is achieving **consensus** when decisions are needed. Coming up with a decision that all team members can support isn't quick or easy. Consensus involves much more than just *taking a vote* on the different options and declaring *majority rules*. With *majority rules*, there are winners and there are losers—

consensus
(kuhn-SEN-suhs) Reaching a decision that all members agree to support

the majority wins and the minority loses. The objective of consensus, however, is to arrive at a win–win solution where no one feels like a loser. Through group discussion, negotiation, and compromise, team members find an option that everyone can support even if it isn't their first choice. As you might imagine, achieving consensus takes time and is much more difficult than just counting votes. But operating by consensus to find win–win solutions is the foundation of good teamwork. Think about it. Wouldn't it be less enjoyable to win when some of your teammates are losing?

APPLY IT MEETING TO ACHIEVE A GOAL

Divide into groups of six to ten to practice having a meeting. Each group should decide on a health care topic to discuss and a goal to achieve through the team meeting. Appoint a leader for your meeting, and then conduct an orderly, business-like meeting. Change leaders at least once during your meeting. At the end of your meeting, discuss how successful the team was in achieving its meeting goal.

Interdisciplinary collaboration can be complex because team members bring a variety of skills, work experiences, and professional and personal opinions to the table. In these situations, conflict among team members is inevitable and consensus may be difficult to achieve. While conflict can cause problems in a group, it can also encourage problem-solving, trust, and understanding among team members once the conflict is resolved effectively. Conflict may occur because of disagreement about how to treat a patient for the best outcome. In some instances conflict occurs because of dominating, overbearing, or even reluctant team members. It may also occur as a result of personality clashes. Sometimes a misunderstanding of the roles, skills, or responsibilities of another team member may lead to disagreements. No matter what causes the conflict, teammates need to keep the lines of communication open and be willing to confront one another in a constructive, respectful manner. Sometimes, people will just need to *agree to disagree*. If you find yourself in a situation where you disagree with members of a group, it's best to resolve the problem within the group. Avoid forming a smaller group within the team, as this divides the team and undermines cohesiveness. Team members should stay focused on the overall mission of their team and the care of the patients. This helps to keep the conflict professional instead of personal.

One of the best ways to reduce conflict among team members is to establish **group norms**. Group norms are guidelines that team members develop themselves and agree to follow to help the team function smoothly over time. For example, team members may be expected to:

group norms
(GROOP nawrms)
Expectations or guidelines for group behavior

- Attend all meetings, arrive on time, and stay until the end
- Speak up, play an active role, and participate in decision-making
- Respect and value the ideas and opinions of others
- Follow through on obligations and complete assignments on time
- Carry their share of the workload
- Share information openly
- Cooperate and provide assistance when asked

- Focus on solutions instead of problems
- Put patient needs first
- Serve as both leader and follower as needed

Group norms are most helpful when they are:

- Developed at the beginning of the team's work
- Aligned with the team's mission statement
- Created through input from all members
- Put in writing and included in the team's meeting records
- Posted on the wall where team meetings take place

When issues and conflicts arise, members can refer back to their team's group norms for guidance. If disagreements can't be overcome within the team, a **facilitator** from outside the group might be called in to help resolve the conflict.

facilitator
(fuh-SIL-i-tey-ter) A person responsible for leading or coordinating a group or discussion

THE MORE YOU KNOW

Health Care Meetings

Meetings are important in the workplace. In a health care setting where patient care requires teamwork, meetings are an efficient way for team members to communicate with one another. There are different types of meetings: a team meeting for coworkers to communicate about job duties; a staff meeting for supervisors to communicate about policies and schedules; a status meeting for team members to report on how patients are doing; and so forth.

Effective meetings require leadership to make sure that goals are achieved without wasting people's valuable time. Meeting leaders should:

- ***Set goals.*** These goals are based on topics that need to be covered.
- ***Invite.*** Decide who should attend the meeting based on the goals.
- ***Schedule.*** Set a time and location for the meeting. Confirm that the key participants plan to attend. Prepare an agenda to share the objectives before, or at the start of, the meeting.
- ***Maintain control.*** Begin and end on time. Assign a note-taker. Introduce each topic, guiding the team to focus and make decisions. If something cannot be resolved, set a time to address the issue after the meeting. At the end of the meeting, make sure all attendees are aware of the next steps.
- ***Follow-up.*** After the meeting, send a brief written summary. List action steps and a timeline for the team to achieve required follow-up activities. Thank attendees for their time and attention.

Formal meetings require *parliamentary procedure*, typically following *Robert's Rules of Order*. Parliamentary procedure is used by professional organizations, government legislative bodies, and fraternal groups when debate and decision-making must be done through a highly detailed, well-established, structured process. The first edition of *Robert's Rules of Order* was published in 1876; the most recent revision (11th edition) was released in 2011. For more information, including a list of Frequently Asked Questions about proper procedure, visit www.robertsrules.com.

Teamwork will continue to play an important role in health care in the future. As a health care professional, you will likely serve on many different teams during your career. Developing effective team skills takes time, especially when you're working with groups of people with different backgrounds, personalities, and communication styles. But serving on a smooth-running, high performing team can be one of the most exhilarating experiences you'll have as a health care professional. Let's examine how developing your cultural competence can help.

FIGURE 2.21

Team members meet to share information, exchange ideas, and plan the next steps

Source: Konstantin Chagin/Shutterstock

DIVERSITY AND CULTURAL COMPETENCE

One of the challenges in forming effective relationships is the ability to work well with people who are different from you. You're probably familiar with the term diversity as it relates to racial differences. However, diversity includes other kinds of differences as well, based on factors such as gender, age (or the era in which you grew up), ethnic background, sexual orientation, religious beliefs, socioeconomic status, physical or mental conditions, and occupation, neighborhood, family size, language, and more.

Health care workers interact with people from many cultural backgrounds. This includes coworkers as well as patients, visitors, guests, and vendors. The ability to interact effectively with people from different cultures is called **cultural competence**. Cultural competence is a process of continually learning by being open to how their cultures influence people. It's important to know culturally acceptable and effective gestures, terms, and behaviors. This knowledge allows the health care worker to adapt his or her care and communication techniques to meet individual needs. Cultural competence supports teamwork, ensures that decisions about patient care are made in a fair and equitable manner, and leads to positive patient-caregiver interactions.

cultural competence (KUHL-cher-uhl KOM-pi-tuhns) The ability to interact effectively with people from different cultures

Community Service Culture and Health Care

Visit a local community service organization dedicated to the culture of a specific group (such as Latinos, Asian Americans, or Native Americans). Work with volunteers of that organization to better understand the way their members address health care issues. What problems do they have? What resources are available? What role do volunteers play? If no local organization exists, visit a senior day care center or nursing home and interview the residents. Create a list of concerns or issues and resources, compile your information as a class project, and discuss your findings. How might this information be of value to local health care providers?

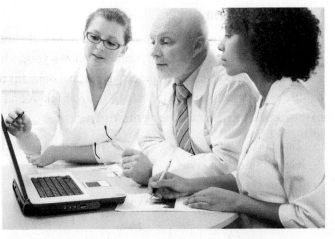

Culture and Behavior

When caring for and working with people from different cultures, you must understand their cultural background. Understanding allows you to have positive experiences and to communicate effectively. Our understanding and opinions of other cultures develop through our life experiences. Culture includes a shared background. This means that cultural groups have shared experiences. Among those experiences common to most groups are:

- Language
- Communication style
- Belief system
- Customs
- Attitudes
- Perceptions
- Values

Language and communication styles and some customs are visible to people outside of a specific cultural group. Belief systems, some customs, attitudes, perceptions, and values are less visible. Think of a tree. The trunk, branches, and leaves are all visible—like language, communication styles, and some customs are visible in people. The roots of a tree, however, grow deep underground and nourish it to keep it strong—but they are not visible. So it is with culture: belief systems, some customs, attitudes, perceptions, and values all come together to create a strong foundation that helps form a person. It is important to remember that concepts of right and wrong do not exist when comparing various cultures. Cultures are only different. Cultural differences do not weaken society, but in fact strengthen society if there is a sense of openness that allows mutual understanding. This does not mean changing one culture to adopt another cultural view. It only means that understanding and consideration reflect the value of dignity toward those from different cultures. Taking interest in different cultures broadens your thinking and opens doors to new adventures. Think for a moment about what life would be like if our ancestors were afraid to start a fire or go into the water. How different would your life be today without fire or an appreciation of the ocean? When we refuse to be open or seek understanding, we can easily **prejudge** and form prejudices. Some prejudices include:

prejudge
(pree-JUHJ) To decide or make a decision before having the facts

Age prejudice:	A person is too old or too young
National prejudice:	A person comes from a foreign country
Physical prejudice:	A person looks different from you
Mental prejudice:	A person knows less than you or processes information differently
Religious prejudice:	A person's religious beliefs are different from yours
Racial prejudice:	A person belongs to a different race from you

You can overcome prejudice by learning more about other people. Here are some suggestions:

- Keep an open mind.
- Look for additional information. Why do people think the way they think?

- Watch documentaries, read books, magazines, and newspapers for information.
- Look at several credible resources before you form an opinion.
- Evaluate all of the information. Ask yourself, is it true or false?

Some basic points to keep in mind when experiencing aspects of a different culture include:

- Values are an important part of every culture. Cultures have values and ideals that they believe, yet individual conduct may not always reflect those values. For example, a culture may value and honor their national flag, but not everyone in the cultural group may have a flag or display it.
- Behavior is not only the result of culture. Age, financial status, education, gender, experience, relationships, health, and many other factors influence behavior.
- It helps to look for the common characteristics of different cultures or to seek a common ground. For example, we are all part of the human race, so food is common to all of us. We can explore different flavors, which are created by spices, cooking techniques, and so on. We also all have seasons of the year that have special meaning and that are celebrated through traditions.

APPLY IT DIVERSITY IN ART

Work as a group to develop a piece of artwork. This could be a painting, drawing, quilt, tapestry, photo collage, mosaic, sculpture, and so on. Each student should contribute something that represents his or her culture or reflects a unique characteristic that makes the student *different* from his or her classmates. When the artwork is complete, each student should explain his or her contribution and why they chose it. Discuss how the artwork reflects the diversity of the group. Why is the artwork more interesting than it would have been if just one or two students had created it?

Ethnicity, Culture, Gender, and Race

We often refer to culture, ethnicity, and race interchangeably. Culture relates to the behaviors, beliefs, and actions characteristic of a particular social, ethnic, or age group. Ethnicity refers to identity with or membership in a particular racial, national, or cultural group and observance of that group's customs, beliefs, and language. The United States recognizes six main ethnicity groups: African American, Asian American, European American, Hispanic American, Middle Eastern/Arab American, and Native American. Race is a human population that is considered distinct based on physical characteristics, such as White, Black, or Latino.

In a *melting pot* country, we see a lot of cultural *assimilation*, the process of integration of members of an ethno-cultural group into an established, generally larger community. This can result in a loss of many characteristics of the absorbed group. So, second generation Asian American children may not be as likely to respond to the **traditional** family structure. In a *salad bowl* country, on the other hand, we see *acculturation*, the exchange of cultural features that results when groups come into continuous

traditional
(truh-DISH-uh-nl) Customary beliefs passed from generation to generation

firsthand contact. The original cultural patterns of either or both groups may be altered, but the groups remain distinct. So, for instance, we may see rap music appealing to youths of all backgrounds.

Workers must exhibit sensitivity—understanding the value of cultural differences and treating them with respect and dignity. For example, a traditional Muslim woman is not allowed to be examined by male members of the medical staff. It is always preferable that a female member of the medical staff is present.

bias
(BYE-uhs) Favoring one way over another, based in having had some experience

disparities
(dih-SPAR-ah-tees) Lack of similarity or equality; health disparities: unfair and misdiagnosis and treatment

Health care workers need to be objective; they should not be predisposed in favor or against an idea. Bias can impact diagnosis and treatment, lead to health disparities, and result in unfair and inappropriate care. For example, don't assume that all elderly patients cannot accurately describe their symptoms or make viable decisions about their care.

Health care workers must also be concerned about *ethnocentricity*, a belief in the superiority of one ethnic group. For example, western medicine is not necessarily superior to alternative Chinese treatments. Finally, health care workers must avoid stereotyping. You cannot assume, for example, that breast cancer will only occur in women.

Being open and willing to learn about others includes choosing your words carefully so they express your desire to learn. It is best to avoid saying things like:

- "We're all alike; we're all human." A statement like this ignores the important differences that bring depth and richness to life. Dignity could be diminished, causing people to feel as if they need to blend in more. People may change their names to fit in or avoid traditions that may draw attention to the differences.
- "We should stay with our own culture; we are too different." This statement may cause fear and separation. When fear causes separation, defensive attitudes and behavior often follow. Arguments or fights are often the result of such fear. Learning about other cultures is enriching and broadens our view about life. Understanding other cultures usually brings a more complete understanding of your own culture and helps you communicate better with others.

FIGURE 2.22
Diversity among coworkers reflects the diversity of their patient population
Source: Stephen Coburn/Shutterstock

Gestures and Body Language

body language
(bod-ee lang-gwij) Nonverbal messages communicated by posture, hand gestures, facial expressions, etc.

Gestures and body language play a role in working with diverse groups of people. This includes personal space and touching, greetings, hand gestures, eye contact, and the influence of family structure.

Personal Space and Touching

Personal space and touching are defined in different societies as *close-contact* and *more-distant contact.* Personal space is the space needed to feel comfortable when we are with

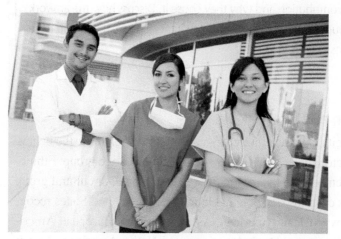

BUILD YOUR SKILLS *Occupational Cultures*

In health care, another type of culture is the occupation in which you work. Registered nurses, for example, have a culture based on their educational background, where they work, what functions they perform, and the knowledge and abilities they possess. Physicians have a culture, too, as do medical technologists, maintenance workers, and so forth. When workers are cross-trained, they function in more than one discipline and work in more than one area. They may encounter several occupational cultures and not feel totally accepted or comfortable in any one of them.

Health care teams often include multiple occupations, even in the same department. Surgical teams, for example, are composed of surgical technologists, surgical nurses, surgeons, and anesthesiologists. These teams are supported by schedulers, surgical attendants, instrument technicians, and others. Each type of worker has a different education level and scope of responsibility, but all of them must depend upon one another to care for surgery patients.

It's important to recognize the diversity among health occupations and learn to work well with everyone. Even though each occupation has its own culture, everyone is there for the same purpose—to provide high-quality health care. Focusing on the mission of patient care gives diverse groups of workers some common ground to build upon.

Ideally, the health care workforce should be as diverse as the patient population it serves, so that workers can view things through the eyes of their patients. This is why health care organizations try to recruit new employees who possess some of the same diverse characteristics as their patients.

other people. People in close-contact societies are comfortable with less space between them. Close-contact societies may be more likely to touch an arm or shoulder of the person they are talking with in the United States. It is important to use caution when touching. A touch can be easily misunderstood. Some Southeast Asian cultures believe that a person's spirit is on the head. Touching the head is often considered an insult.

TABLE 2.1 Close-Contact and Distant-Contact Regions

Close-Contact Regions	Distant-Contact Regions
Africa	Canada
Indonesia	Great Britain
Latin America	Northern Europe
Hispanic Americans	United States
Mediterranean	Native Americans
Southern Europe	Middle Eastern
French	Arabic Nationalities
	Asian Americans
Common Behavior:	
• Men hold hands with men and women hold hands with women.	• People greet one another with a handshake or hand gesture.
• Men and women greet one another by kissing on both cheeks.	• Close friends or family members may hug each other.

FIGURE 2.23

Regions of the world showing the location of close-contact and more-distant contact cultures

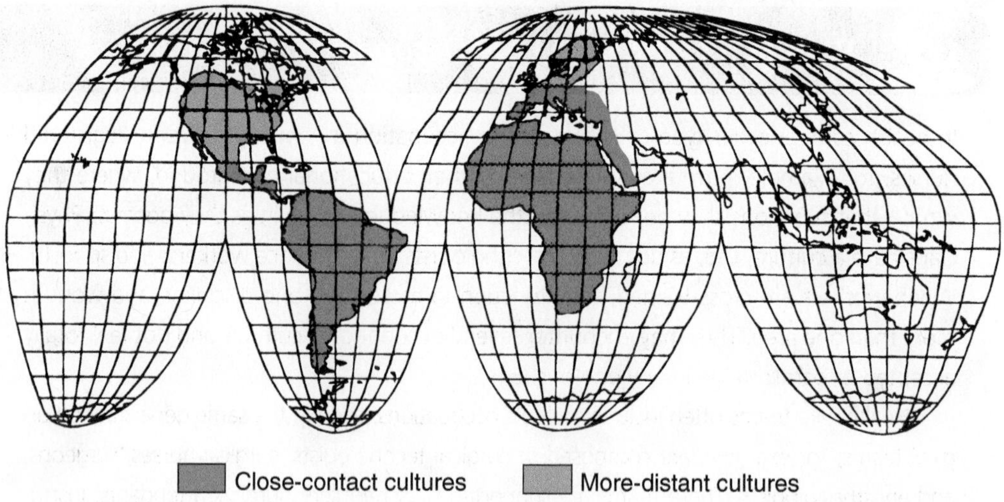

TABLE 2.2 Guidelines Restricting Touch and Physical Closeness in Southeast Asian Cultures

Cambodian	Vietnamese	Laotian
• Only a parent can touch the head of a child. • Members of the opposite sex never touch each other in public, not even brothers and sisters.	• Only elderly people can touch the head of a child.	• It is necessary to ask permission to move near another person.

Greetings

Greeting another person is important in all cultures. The way a greeting is given and received often determines how positive or negative the interaction is.

TABLE 2.3 Guidelines for Greeting People

Anglo-American	Latin American	Cambodian, Laotian	Vietnamese	Hmong
Shake hands if desired.	Shake hands or hug.	Do not shake hands. Instead, put hands together at different levels. 1. Equal status—hands must be at chest level. 2. Older person or stranger—hands must be at chin level. 3. Relative or teacher— hands must be at nose level.	Salute by joining both hands and moving them against the chest.	Bow head or shake hands.

Hand Gestures

Hand gestures help communicate many things. It is very important to use correct gestures so that others are not offended.

SAME GESTURE, SAME MEANING, BUT VERY DIFFERENT CONNOTATIONS

	American Culture	Asian Cultures
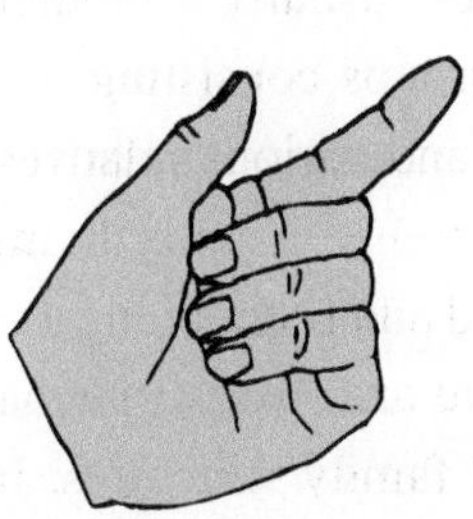	OK for "Come here."	Absolutely *taboo* for calling a person, even a child. It's the way to call an animal (a dog, in particular), especially when accompanied by a whistle. Considered *very insulting.*
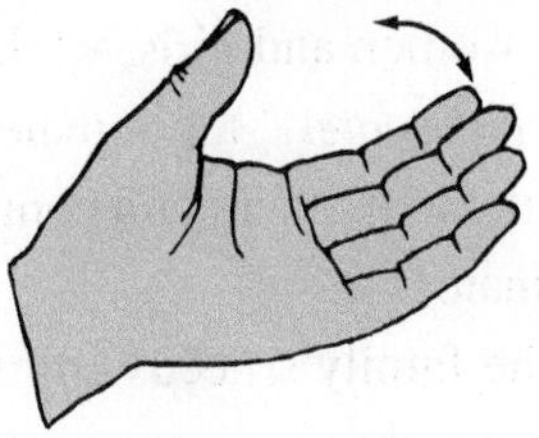	OK for "Come up here."	Never use. Only an inferior person would be summoned this way. Considered *insulting*, even to a child.
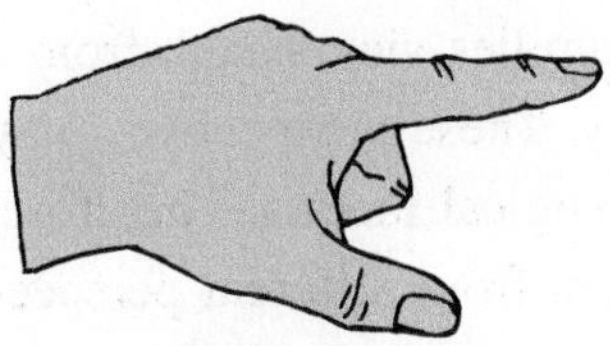	OK to point at someone or something.	OK to point at *something* but not at *someone*. Considered too direct a reference, amounting to confrontation, which the Indo-Chinese avoid by all means.
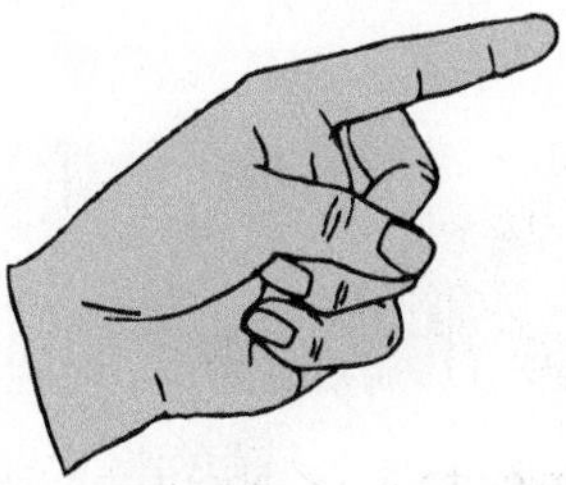	Slight threat (or warning) when making a point to someone.	Relatively strong threat made by a person of superior rank to an inferior (father to son, teacher to student). This is one step ahead of corporal punishment. (A parent would *never* use this gesture to a girl because it is considered too brutal.)

FIGURE 2.24

The same hand gestures, with the same meanings, result in different cultural implications.

Eye Contact

In some cultures, eye contact may indicate that a person is listening, sincere, or honest. In other cultures, direct eye contact is considered to be hostile or disrespectful.

TABLE 2.4 Eye-Contact Guidelines

Anglo-American	African Americans	Navajo	Japanese, Southeast Asian, Hispanic
• Eye contact is important; it indicates interest, honesty, and listening.	• Eye contact may not be important. Being in the same room indicates attentiveness.	• Direct eye contact is avoided. • Peripheral vision is used. • Direct stares are considered hostile or a way to scold children.	• Eye contact is avoided as a form of respect.

Family Organization

The structure of family is important in all cultures. There are *nuclear families*, a term developed in western society referring to the basic family group—usually a mother, father, and children. There are also *extended families*—kinship groups consisting of a family nucleus and various relatives, such as grandparents, usually living in one household and functioning as a larger unit. There are also patriarchal and matriarchal family structures. In a *patriarchal family*, the actions and ideas of men and boys are dominant over those of women and girls, while in a *matriarchal society*, the female, especially with the mothers of a community, dominate.

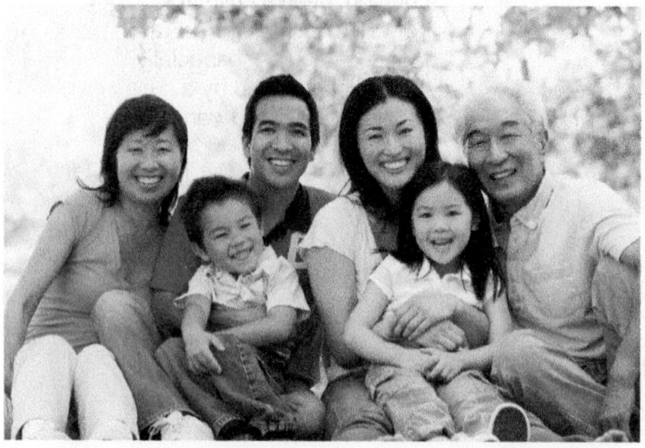

FIGURE 2.25

Extended family includes several generations

Source: Monkey Business Images/ Shutterstock

For example, in the traditional patriarchal Asian culture, the family's needs come before those of an individual's needs. Family members often live together as an extended family, including parents, children, grandparents, and families of paternal uncles. The extended family is involved in all major decisions. Asian families view health from a variety of different perspectives, sometimes simultaneously. These perspectives may involve spiritual factors, imbalance of vital forces, and biological factors. Therefore, Asian patients may want to combine diagnosis and treatment from different perspectives with the goal of getting maximum health benefits.

Each culture has its own set of beliefs and values that must be incorporated into any health care interaction.

RECENT DEVELOPMENTS

Demographics

Every ten years, the United States Census Bureau conducts a survey to learn about the demographics of the country. Demographics are statistical data summarizing the population via characteristics such as age, race, marital status, language spoken at home, location, and income level. The last major census took place in 2010. At that time, the data showed that 12.5 percent of the U.S. population consisted of people born in other countries. It also showed that more than 20 percent of the population over five years of age spoke a language other than English at home.

These statistics showed a continued increase in the everyday use of languages other than English since the 1990 census. In some states, the number of people not speaking English at home has risen even higher—43 percent in California, 36 percent in New Mexico, and 34 percent in Texas. These data suggest that the American population is continuing to undergo major changes that affect the way people understand and interact with each other. Health care workers need to be especially aware of the evolving population and take cultural differences into account when providing care.

How might the language spoken at home affect a person's health care in the U.S.?

Communicating Effectively with People from Other Cultures

When speaking with people from other cultures, the tone of your speaking voice is similar in importance to the gestures you use. Speaking tone includes voice quality, volume, and pitch. Voice tones cause positive or negative reactions from others. Clear pronunciations are more easily understood. When speaking to others who are learning English:

- Speak clearly; do not slur words.
- Speak so that they can hear you easily.
- Do not raise your voice or yell.
- Speak in moderate tones.
- Pronounce the entire word; do not draw it out or shorten sounds.
- Summarize often.
- Confirm their understanding.
- Clarify when necessary.
- Do not assume that they understand.

You gain greater interpersonal effectiveness when you strive to understand and respect people of a different culture and viewpoint. Making every effort to understand and to be understood is one way to treat others with dignity.

APPLY IT COMMUNICATION BARRIERS

You are a warm, outgoing pediatrician's assistant. Have four of your classmates represent a parent accompanying a small child. One is Cambodian; one is Laotian; one is African-American; one is Japanese. Conduct an initial interview with each to get the information you need. Do they respond to you? Why or why not?

Folk Medicine

Folk medicine is a collection of traditional beliefs and customs for treating pain or illness. Many who practice folk medicine believe that natural materials, such as herbs, spices, and spiritual prayers and rituals keep evil spirits away and allow the body to heal. The U.S., however, uses a biomedical or "Western" medical system that includes encouraging patients to learn about their own illness, informing patients about terminal illnesses, teaching self-care, using medications and technology to cure or treat diseases, and teaching preventive care.

It's important to respect the beliefs of other cultures. If you insult the patient, you will be ineffective in providing care. Some caregivers work with their patients' beliefs to create positive relationships. Then they can introduce other suggestions for care. Learn about the common practices in your patients' cultures. Read magazines and books about other cultures. Ask questions. Learn about ritual healing, folk medicine, and spiritual healing. Keep informed! Your understanding helps the patient get well faster and feel respected. The experience will be positive for both of you.

The following information is an overview of some common folk medicine practices in various cultures. Some practices that cause painful symptoms are not considered abusive because they are based on a belief of the culture. Not everyone from a particular culture practices some or even any of these folk beliefs.

prohibit
(proh-HIB-it) To not allow

Armenians

- Give the mother a party one week after a baby is born. The mother is served bread, which she dips into a paste of margarine, sugar, and flour. This is a celebration of the birth of the child.
- **Prohibit** a menstruating woman from attending church, taking a shower, or eating spicy foods.

Asians

- Think that health is balance of yin and yang
- Use treatments, such as herbal remedies and acupuncture
- Believe pain must be endured silently

Cambodians

- Use herbs as medicine
- Use cupping for headaches
- Use coining for pain
- Consider the color white to be a sign of bad luck

Central and South Americans

- Use herbal home remedies
- Teach a menstruating woman not to get her head wet and to avoid eating cucumbers, oranges, lemons, pork, lard, and deer meat

Chinese

- Use herbs as medicine
- Practice acupuncture and use herbs over puncture sites
- Use cupping with heated bamboo

Europeans

- Believe that illness is caused by outside sources
- Focus on treating with medication, surgery, diet, and exercise

Hispanics

- Believe that health is a reward from God
- Believe in good luck
- Use heat and cold remedies to restore balance
- Rely on prayers and massage

Hmong and Mien Tribes

- Perform spiritual ceremonies to please the spirits that cause illness
- Use herbal home remedies, including opium

Iranians

- Believe that poor health is predetermined (fatalism)
- Use herbs, foods, rituals, and magic formulas for healing
- Believe the "evil eye" (a person or animal that causes injury through a look) causes sudden illness

- When of the Islamic faith, require washing of the face and hands before prayer
- Require periodic baths for cleansing

Koreans

- Practice alchemy, a medieval practice of magic and natural herbal remedies
- Use acupuncture
- Go to hot springs for bath rituals and massage
- Use substances to stimulate energy and the brain

Middle Easterners

- Believe that health is spiritual, cleanliness is essential
- Believe males are dominant and should make decisions on health care
- Believe in spiritual causes of illness, such as the "evil eye"

Native Americans

- Use herbs and spices
- Use modern medical practices
- May rely on a healer/shaman (medicine man or woman) to remove pain and evil spirits
- Believe that health is harmony with nature
- Believe that a tolerance of pain signifies power and strength
- Believe that illness is caused by supernatural forces and evil spirits

South Africans

- Believe in maintaining harmony of body, mind, and spirit
- Believe the causes of ill health are spirits, demons, or punishment from God
- Use prayer or religious rituals as treatment

Vietnamese

- Commonly use herbal medicine
- Use cupping for head pain, cough, muscle pain, and motion sickness
- Use acupuncture for musculoskeletal problems, visual problems, and other ailments

When patients who don't speak English need to communicate with their caregivers, they use a variety of terms to describe their health problems.

TABLE 2.5 Typical terms used by non-English-speaking Asian cultures to describe health problems

Term	Condition
Weak heart	Palpitations, dizziness, faintness, feeling of panic
Weak kidney	Impotence, sexual dysfunction
Weak nervous system	Headache, malaise, inability to concentrate
Weak stomach or liver	Indigestion
I'm skinny.	Sickliness
Fire, hot	Dark urine, flatulence, constipation
Air/wind, cold	Illness was caused by too much air

Spiritual Beliefs and Family Traditions

When dealing with people from other cultures, it is important to demonstrate respect for a patient's spiritual beliefs and practices. You can uncover these beliefs by talking to the patient. In helping to meet these spiritual and religious needs, the health care professional has to relate to each patient as unique and distinctive. You must be willing to listen, and to respect any symbols or books on which the patient relies. It is important to maintain hope and explore the patient's fears and doubts. Sometimes, it can help to encourage the patient's religious community or clergy involvement for support. Finally, it is very important to refrain from imposing your own beliefs on to the patient.

There are differences between spirituality and religion. *Spirituality* refers to matters of the spirit or soul, as distinguished from material things. *Religion* is a belief in a supernatural power or powers regarded as the creator and governor of the universe, or beliefs based on the teachings of a spiritual leader. Some people are *agnostics*; they believe that it is impossible to know whether or not there is a God. You may also have patients who are *atheists*, who deny or do not believe in the existence of any supreme being.

Health care providers must be careful to be considerate of any patient's beliefs. They can make medical decisions that are consistent with the patient's spiritual and/or religious views. They should support the patient's use of spiritual coping during the illness, encouraging him/her to speak with their clergy or spiritual leader, or referring the patient to a hospital chaplain, appropriate religious leader, or support group that addresses spiritual issues during illness.

Language Arts Link — Cultural and Spiritual Beliefs

A person's cultural and spiritual beliefs may affect how they respond to different situations. Pretend that you have a pen pal in another country. Write a letter to your friend describing how your cultural and spiritual beliefs affect your attitudes towards health care. Or, write the letter based on the beliefs of another culture. Include at least three key points on your beliefs. Be sure to proofread your work to see if you can make it more clear, concise, or interesting.

Check spelling and grammar and correct any errors. When you've completed your letter, exchange it with a classmate. Provide feedback on your classmate's letter, and then exchange back. Read your classmate's comments and revise your letter as necessary.

Family Traditions

Family support is an important part of patient care. Some family traditions are unique to individual families. Other traditions are a blend of beliefs and traditions from cultures, as well as from spiritual and religious beliefs and practices. When dealing with patients and their families, their traditions, beliefs, and practices must be respected, just as you respect their culture, religion, or other beliefs. As with culture and spiritual beliefs, you will uncover family traditions while talking to the patient and observing interactions between the patient and his or her family.

As a health care provider, you must make it a priority to relate to family members in a positive and productive manner. Being aware of family traditions that can help nurture a patient will benefit everyone involved with a patient's care.

REALITY CHECK

How well you interact with other people is *where the rubber meets the road* in health care. From the first day you walk in the door, your people skills will be front and center. You might be the highest-skilled person in your entire organization when it comes to the hands-on, technical duties of your job. But if you fail to form and maintain effective working relationships with your coworkers, your high degree of competence will soon be overshadowed by your lack of interpersonal skills. If you get labeled as a loner, troublemaker, or complainer, other people won't want to work with you, and your supervisor will regret hiring you. Once this happens, you'll need to either change your ways or change your job and start over again.

Complying with etiquette standards, using good manners, and functioning as a team player isn't difficult. In fact, treating other people in a polite, considerate manner should just be common sense. But the problem is—common sense isn't common anymore. Too many people forgot the lessons they learned as children, and turned into adults totally focused on no one but themselves. If you want to succeed in health care, you have to put the needs of other people ahead of your own.

This chapter presents a wealth of information about participating on teams and working effectively with people who may be different from you. The terms and concepts associated with diversity and cultural competence (such as race, ethnicity, bias, disparities, ethnocentricity, and prejudice) may be somewhat confusing. Here's the bottom line—learning to interact effectively with diverse groups of people and patients from other cultures may require some extra effort on your part, but it's absolutely critical. This is especially true if you've lived in a *sheltered environment* most of your life. Learn all you can about other cultures, and remain open-minded to see things from other points of view. Most people enjoy talking about their background and the culture in which they grew up and live. Help people learn more about you and your culture, as well. Everyone has insights to share, and you might be surprised what you'll learn.

Key Points

- Work hard to develop and maintain positive relationships with other people.
- Consider coworkers your internal customers and treat them with kindness and respect.
- Display a friendly attitude, cooperate with people, and create a positive work environment.
- Show loyalty to your coworkers and your employer.
- Practice good etiquette and manners and treat everyone with courtesy.
- Develop effective team skills; use team mission statements and group norms.
- Strive to achieve consensus when making group decisions.
- Develop an appreciation for diversity and other cultures.
- Be aware of culturally acceptable gestures, terms, and behaviors.
- Show respect for folk medicine customs, spiritual beliefs, and family traditions.
- Avoid letting bias and prejudice govern your behavior.
- Learn about other cultures and share information about yours.

Section Review Questions

Answer each of the following questions, and indicate the page number in the textbook where the answer can be found.

1. List three ways to strengthen relationships at work.
2. Why are courtesy, etiquette, and manners important at work?
3. Give two examples of being inclusive with coworkers.
4. List two kinds of workplace teams and give an example of each.
5. Explain how consensus is different from, and better than, majority rules.
6. Explain why health care workers need to be culturally competent.
7. Identify culturally acceptable and effective gestures, terms, and behaviors.
8. Discuss how bias and prejudice can cause health care disparities.

Learn by Doing

Complete Worksheets 1–5 in Section 2.3 of your *Student Activity Guide*.

CHAPTER 2 Review

Chapter Review Questions

Answer each of the following questions. Indicate which page in the textbook led you to your answer.

1. Define *character* and *personal values* and explain how they affect your reputation as a professional.
2. List four examples of a lack of character in the workplace.
3. Give three examples of dishonest behaviors and describe the impact of dishonesty in the workplace.
4. List two ways to demonstrate loyalty to your coworkers and two ways to demonstrate loyalty to your employer.
5. Identify two types of workplace teams and give an example of each.
6. Give three examples of diversity in addition to age and gender.
7. Explain why health care workers need to be culturally competent.
8. List two types of prejudice and two ways to overcome prejudice.
9. Discuss why health care workers need to be aware of cultural preferences for personal space and touching.

Chapter Review Activities

1. Select an annual event, such as the beginning of a new year or a birthday. Ask people from five different cultures how they treat this event. Prepare a chart which includes the following information for each of the five people: age, country of origin or ancestors, native language, and description of the event.
2. Place sheets of paper on the classroom wall. Label each sheet with the name of a different culture. Walk around the room, and write on each sheet something that you have heard or believe about each culture. Discuss your beliefs. Are they accurate? Is it possible to make assumptions about a person based on his or her culture?
3. Work in teams of four to research a culture of your choice. Use *National Geographic*, the Internet, or other resources for your research. As a team, decide each team member's responsibility. Include the following in your report: language, religious beliefs, medical practices, and feasts and celebrations. Prepare a 5-minute presentation about the culture that your group researched and present it to the class.

What If? Scenarios

What would you do in each of the following situations? Record your answer, explain it, and indicate which page in the textbook led you to your decision.

1. A patient on your unit gets discharged. While cleaning the room for the next patient, you find an expensive watch in the drawer in the bedside table. It's a woman's watch, and the former patient was a man.
2. When it's time for your competency evaluation, your supervisor announces that you and your coworkers will be checking each other off. Your coworkers get together and decide just to give each other a satisfactory evaluation without actually checking each person's competency level.
3. A new person joins your work group. She's much older than everyone else, and no one seems to like her. It's time to go to lunch, and your coworkers leave her behind.
4. Several people from your unit, including you, have been cross-trained to work in three different areas. Since all of you rotate on a weekly basis, none of you feel as if you really fit in anywhere.

5. You need to have your time card signed by the end of the day. You know your supervisor would sign it, but she's tied up in a meeting and your shift ends in 10 minutes.
6. You were invited to participate on a new team in your department. The first meeting didn't go well because no one really knew why they were there, and everyone tried to speak at the same time.
7. Your patient is a female from the Middle East. You notice that she's reluctant to make decisions about the next steps in her treatment plan.

Media Connection

Use the companion website for additional interactive learning activities.

Portfolio Connection

Facing big decisions regarding your future, and starting to determine which career best matches your interests and strengths, can seem overwhelming. Before setting your career goals, it's a good idea to think about what you enjoy doing most, what you are *good at*, and how challenges that lie ahead might impact your future.

Understanding your basic personality is critical in helping you identify a career path. Are you methodical and detail-oriented or do you focus on the *big picture*? Do you prefer dealing with research or dealing with people? Are you interested in building relationships or working quietly in isolation? Are you a *doer* or a *thinker* … or both?

Some employers use personality assessments to help determine where a job candidate might best fit in the organization. One of the most common is the Myers-Briggs Type Indicator (MBTI). The MBTI personality questionnaire is designed to identify certain psychological preferences according to the theories of Carl Gustav Jung, a Swiss psychiatrist credited for founding analytical psychology. You can find information about this personality assessment and what it measures at www.myersbriggs.org.

In addition to the MBTI, several other assessments and tools are available that can help you choose the best health career for you. These resources will be discussed in detail later in this textbook. For the time being, let's focus on what *you* think are your strongest personality traits.

Create a list of your "Ten Strongest Personality Traits." Rank your list in order, with trait #1 being your strongest trait. For example, you may thoroughly enjoy nurturing or taking care of people and would rate it as #1. You may also dislike competitive behavior, but you still compete in sports. You would rate that as #2, and so forth.

Think about the health careers described in this textbook. It's still early in the process, but have you spotted a few careers that sound interesting? Make a list of these careers and the reasons why you think they might suit you. Keep the list of your ten strongest personality traits and your list of interesting health careers in your portfolio. These documents will become helpful later on.

CHAPTER 3

Communication in Health Care

Source: Monkey Business Images/Shutterstock

SECTIONS

"Think enthusiastically about everything, but especially about your job. If you do so, you'll put a touch of glory in your life. If you love your job with enthusiasm, you'll shake it to pieces."

NORMAN VINCENT PEALE, CLERGYMAN AND CHAMPION OF POSITIVE THINKING, 1898–1993

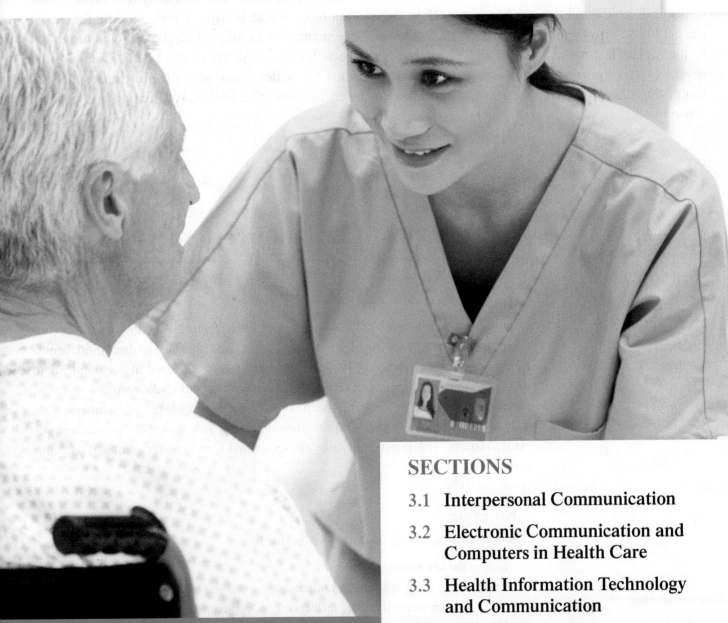

GETTING STARTED

Effective communications are essential to providing appropriate and accurate health care. One study by a large health care organization determined that on an average two-day stay in an acute care facility, patient information is shared among forty-seven different health care professionals. Clearly, if communications are not shared with care and accuracy, diagnosis and treatment can be inappropriate and even dangerous to the patient outcome.

To show how information must be shared accurately and appropriately and how easy it is for mistakes to occur, join your classmates in a circle. Have one person in the circle whisper a message into the ear of the person next to them until each person in the circle has shared the message with the person sitting next to them. The last person to hear the whispered message will share what he or she heard. Compare the results to the original message. As a group, discuss the results of patient treatment if the information is different than the original message. (*Example:* Mr. Johansen in room 222, bed B, isn't eating and appears disoriented.)

SECTION 3.1 Interpersonal Communication

Background

Communication is essential in the exchange of ideas, feelings, and thoughts. Communication helps us to understand the needs of others and how best to meet those needs. Health care workers should understand the many factors involved in communication, as well as types of communication, including written and spoken words, gestures, facial expressions, body posture, touch, and listening. Knowledge of communication techniques will increase your skills in communicating with coworkers, patients, physicians, visitors, and guests and your ability to make good observations about your patients.

Objectives

After completing this section, you will be able to:

1. Define the key terms.
2. Explain why communication is important.
3. Name four elements that may influence how you communicate with others.
4. List three barriers to communication.
5. List four elements necessary for communication to take place.
6. Describe three things that a good listener does.
7. Differentiate between verbal and nonverbal communication.
8. Describe the four styles of communication, and explain why assertive communication works best.
9. Discuss the importance of conflict resolution skills.

10. Explain the importance of anger management.
11. Describe the role that defense mechanisms play.

EFFECTIVE PATIENT RELATIONS

Effective patient relations are a necessity. To communicate effectively, we need to work through a process that includes engagement, understanding, education, and creating a sense of partnership.

engagement (en-GAGE-muhnt) Securing the attention of a person

Engagement is a connection between the health care professional and patient that sets the stage for establishing a partnership. Barriers to engagement by the health care professional might include things like not introducing yourself, pointed and critical questioning, and interrupting the patient. An understanding health care professional will make patients feel accepted. To exhibit understanding of a patient's needs, you might first introduce yourself to the patient while he or she is fully clothed and in a safe environment. You can allow the patient to share thoughts and feelings and respond by repeating them in your own words. Sharing anecdotes—without being too personal—can also help you create a positive bond between yourself and the patient.

Educating the patient includes helping to increase their knowledge and understanding and minimize their anxiety. Health care professionals should assume that all patients share many of the same questions, including:

- What is happening to me?
- What will I have to do?
- Will it hurt?
- When will I have the results?

To have good communication, you must be certain to answer all of the patient's questions. Avoid using complicated, clinical terms and be clear. Determine if you have answered the patient's questions by using statements such as "Have I answered your questions?" "Do you have questions about anything I have not covered?" or "Is there anything you want to add to the information I have obtained about you?"

Good communication helps create a partnership. The health care professional and patient work together regarding the problem and the treatment plan. Many times, a patient may think he or she knows the problem. You need to make sure the patient understands the diagnosis, plan, and treatment as expressed by his or her physician.

SENDING A CLEAR MESSAGE

Good communication means that you are sending a clear message—one that is understood by both your coworkers and your patients. In order to make sure you are doing so, you must:

- Use active listening skills.
- Use a positive tone.
- Watch your body language.
- Treat patients and coworkers with respect.
- Be precise and detailed about what you expect.

Consider This *Illiteracy and Health Literacy*

Even though health care professionals focus on their communication skills to provide quality care, a large percentage of their patients may not be getting the full benefit.

The term *health literacy* is gaining importance as efforts to improve the health and wellness of Americans continue to evolve. According to the U.S. Department of Health and Human Services, health literacy is defined as "the degree to which individuals have the capacity to obtain, process, and understand basic health information needed to make appropriate health decisions and services needed to prevent or treat illness."

However, according to an article by Ruth Parker of the Emory University School of Medicine (published in *Health Promotion International Journal*) a significant number of adult patients lack the literacy skills required to communicate effectively with their caregivers and understand the medical instructions and information they receive.

The National Literacy Act of 1991 defines *literacy* as "an individual's ability to read, write, and speak in English, and compute and solve problems at levels of proficiency necessary to function on the job and in society, to achieve one's goals, and develop one's knowledge and potential." A national survey conducted in 2008 found that about 20% of all American adults are functionally illiterate, and almost 50% have difficulties with reading, basic math skills, or English comprehension. Low literacy occurs most often among elderly, minority, poor, and medically underserved populations.

Many health care workers are either unaware of the problem or lack the skills required to overcome literacy-related communication issues. Patient education materials are available mostly in print, and written at a 10th grade or higher reading level. This means that millions of Americans struggle to understand the information they're given and apply it correctly. Patients have a limited knowledge of medicine and health care to begin with, and medical language can be especially confusing. Problems occur when patients must read and follow medication instructions, share their medical histories, prepare for exams and treatments, manage chronic conditions, and provide follow-up self-care in a safe and effective manner. Concerns arise when patients must complete medical applications, sign consent forms, review insurance claims, and arrive prepared for doctors' appointments. To make the situation more challenging, patients who are illiterate often hide their deficiencies from family members, friends, and health care providers out of shame or embarrassment.

It's not surprising that low literacy can result in less-than-optimum outcomes for patients. In fact, research shows that illiterate patients have higher rates of hospitalization than literate patients.

To improve patient-provider communication, health care workers should:

- Watch for signs of low-literacy, and take extra steps to make sure that patients understand the information they're given.
- Reduce the reading level of printed information and include illustrations to add clarity; provide video- and audiotapes for patients who can't read.
- Communicate verbally with patients; ask follow-up questions to make sure they comprehend instructions and know how to follow them.
- Demonstrate self-care techniques (such as using an inhaler or checking blood pressure), and then have patients demonstrate the technique themselves to make sure things are done correctly.
- Speak slowly, explain things carefully, and use terms that patients can understand.
- Ask for assistance from a coworker, or from a patient's family member or friend, when English isn't the patient's primary language; provide print, video, and audio materials in languages other than English when possible.

What would you need to do as a health care worker to reduce illiteracy-related barriers when communicating with patients? What steps could you take to improve your own health literacy?

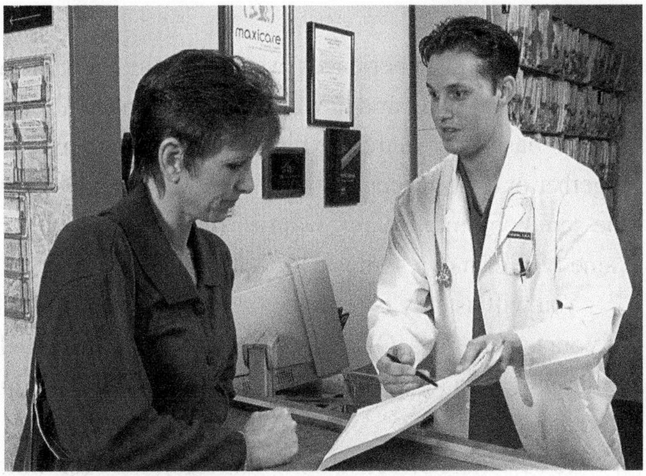

FIGURE 3.1

Medical assistant giving clear instructions to make sure the patient understands

Source: Michael Heron/Pearson Education

- Model the behavior you want others to follow.
- Explain your reasoning.
- Discuss any conflicts in a calm and rational way.

Communicating clearly is the key to creating a high functioning health care team and establishing a positive relationship with your patients.

ELEMENTS THAT INFLUENCE YOUR COMMUNICATION WITH OTHERS

Several factors influence your communication with other people. These include prejudices, frustrations, life experiences, and aging.

Prejudices

All people form opinions or biases as they are growing up. These prejudices affect how they feel about other people and how they relate to them. You may have very strong feelings about the backgrounds or the values of your patients or coworkers. Your feelings affect how you communicate. For instance, if you believe that certain people are lazy, overly emotional, or inferior, you need to think about your prejudices. When you understand your prejudices and feelings, you have an opportunity to overcome them.

inferior
(in-FEER-ee-or) Lower or less than

Frustrations

When you care for and work with others, you may experience impatience, annoyance, and even anger. Perhaps other people do not understand your directions, or they may move too slowly. You feel irritated. These feelings interfere with your ability to communicate. Take time to understand why you feel frustrated. Evaluate the situation, and then try to correct it. It is your responsibility to control your behavior and to understand that patients, families, and coworkers have problems that are the cause of their behavior.

impatience
(im-PEY-shuhns) Restlessness

annoyance
(uh-NOY-uhns) Irritation

How you act toward others and how they act toward you affect the quality of communication. If you are disinterested or bored, if you are in a bad mood, if you wish you were someplace else, your communication breaks down. However, if you show interest and concern for others, you will experience worthwhile communication, your job will become easier, and you will be more effective.

Life Experiences

People have new experiences every day. These experiences help us know what to expect in day-to-day living and how to act in certain situations. The most effective communication is based on shared experiences. These may be experiences you went through together or experiences that you each went though individually. Perhaps you grew up in the same community and went to the same school. It may be as simple as liking the same type of movies, music, or books.

You will usually communicate more effectively with someone who has shared some of your experiences. Of course, the reverse is true as well; less shared experiences causes communication to be more difficult and frustrating. This is especially true in the area of slang and dialect.

slang
(SLANG) The informal language of a particular group

dialect
(DIE-uh-lekt) A variety of language that is distinct to a culture

To be a more effective communicator, look for things that you have in common with the other person. You can do this by listening to what they say and how they say it, looking for something familiar and then focusing a bit more on that shared experience. As you find more and more areas in common, your communication with that person will become more effective.

Aging and Communication

What happens when a younger health care professional deals with an older patient, or vice versa? Certain physical issues may make communication with the elderly more difficult, such as hearing or vision problems. An older patient may have mental or emotional issues. For example, older people may be afraid of losing the ability to think, reason, or explain themselves. Certain cultural issues, such as believing the doctor is always right or being afraid to complain about aches and pains, may also make communication challenging. Finally, younger and older individuals may have fewer shared experiences which make it even more important to work on finding some common ground that you may share.

APPLY IT ESTABLISHING COMMUNICATION

Conduct a role play with one of your classmates. Initially, you are the health care professional, such as a nurse, for example. Your classmate is an elderly patient. What steps can you take—verbal and/or nonverbal—to establish successful communication with this patient? Then, reverse roles. This time, your classmate is a medical assistant, and you are a somewhat sullen teenager. What steps might the health care professional take in this situation to communicate effectively?

BARRIERS TO COMMUNICATION

Recognizing barriers to communication allows you to become an understanding health care worker. The following are four major communication barriers:

labeling
(LAY-buhl-ing) Describing a person with a word that limits them

- ***Labeling.*** Deciding the other person is mean, lazy, a complainer, or difficult causes a breakdown in communication. When labeling, you do not pay attention to the message being sent. If you listen, however, you might find out the reason for the behavior.

THE MORE YOU KNOW

Hearing Loss

The ability to hear plays a key role in interpersonal communication. The gradual hearing loss that occurs as you age (presbycusis) is a common condition. However, the number of people experiencing hearing loss at younger ages is gradually increasing.

Each day you are surrounded by a variety of sounds in your environment. Most sounds occur at safe levels that do not affect hearing. However, sounds that are too loud or last for a long time can damage sensitive structures called hair cells in the inner ear. The result is noise-induced hearing loss (NIHL).

Hair cells convert sound energy into electrical signals that travel to the brain. Once damaged, hair cells cannot grow back. Scientists once believed that the force of vibrations from loud sounds caused the damage to hair cells. Recent studies, however, have shown that exposure to harmful noise triggers the formation of molecules that can damage or kill hair cells.

NIHL can be caused by a single exposure to a quick, intense sound such as an explosion, or through long-term exposure to loud sounds over an extended period of time, such as noise generated in a woodworking shop. The loudness of sound is measured in decibels. Sources of noise that can cause NIHL range from 120 to 150 decibels. Examples include motorcycles, firecrackers, and small firearms.

Long-term or repeated exposure to sounds at or above 85 decibels can also cause hearing loss. The louder the sound, the shorter the time period before NIHL can occur. Sounds of less than 75 decibels, even after long exposure, are unlikely to cause hearing loss.

The good news is that NIHL is 100 percent preventable. In order to protect yourself, you must understand the hazards of noise and how to practice good hearing health in everyday life. To protect your hearing:

- Know which noises can cause damage.
- Wear earplugs or other hearing protective devices when involved in a loud activity.
- Be alert to hazardous noise in the environment.
- Protect the ears of children who are too young to protect themselves.
- Teach family, friends, and colleagues about the hazards of noise.

Exercise care when using headphones, earphones, and ear buds. Listening to loud music will have less of an impact on your hearing when you limit your exposure time and use higher quality earphones that block out background noise as compared with the stock ear buds or earphones that come with iPods and MP3 players.

If you suspect hearing loss, have a medical examination by an otolaryngologist, a physician who specializes in diseases of the ears, nose, throat, head, and neck. You may also have a hearing test by an audiologist, a health professional trained to measure and help individuals deal with hearing loss.

Why is the rate of hearing loss among younger people gradually increasing? What are some sources of loud sounds to which you are exposed? What should you do to reduce your potential hearing loss?

- ***Sensory impairment.*** Deafness or blindness can be a communication barrier. Always evaluate the people with whom you are communicating to be certain they do not have a sensory impairment.
- ***Talking too fast.*** Speaking slowly is especially important when you are working with elderly people. Communication can break down when the message is delivered too rapidly.
- ***Cognitive impairment.*** Cognitive impairment may affect memory, perception, problem solving, emotional reaction, and idea formulation. These types of impairments might result from autism, brain injury, Parkinson's disease, Alzheimer's disease, or the aging process. Be careful to make sure your patients understand what you are saying. You may ask them to tell you, in their own words, what you have just explained to them. Or, you may write down suggestions for them to follow.

Developing skills in communication helps you become a better health care worker. It is important always to be courteous and understanding. Take time to evaluate gestures, facial expressions, and tone of voice in order to understand what the other person is really saying. While you may feel frustrated, angry, or irritated, as a health care worker, it is your job to make every attempt to listen and to understand. Hearing accurately and then responding appropriately are essential. Remember to communicate your messages so that they can be understood easily.

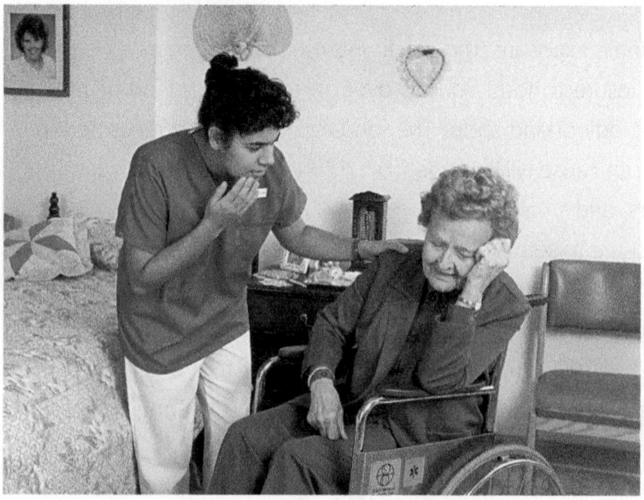

FIGURE 3.2

Home health aide consoling an elderly patient with a hearing loss

Source: Michael Heron/Pearson Education

ELEMENTS OF COMMUNICATION

Four essential elements are necessary for communication to take place:

- ***A message.*** This refers to the information you want to convey to another person. Perhaps the purpose of the message is to give information or to acquire information. Perhaps there is something you want another person to do.
- ***A sender.*** Unless there is someone who wants to send a message, there cannot be communication.
- ***A receiver.*** Even if there is a message and a sender, there must be a receiver. If there is no one to receive the message, communication is incomplete.
- ***Feedback.*** Capturing feedback is of critical importance. If you are not seen to be listening and acting on what you are told, why would people tell you anything?

Interference with any of these elements can disrupt communication. Remember that in order to ensure clear communication:

- The message must be clear.
- The sender must deliver the message in a clear and concise manner.

- The receiver must be able to hear and receive the message.
- The receiver must be able to understand the message.
- Interruptions or distractions must be avoided.

How can we ensure clear communication? We have to remember that communication is a two-way street. You must listen to others to make sure they listen to you. If you're interested in what the other person has to say, that person will more likely be interested in you. Remember to smile and maintain eye contact, so that the other person knows that you are interested in him or her. Use your voice and body language to show your enthusiasm.

On the other hand, many elements can disrupt communication. Don't be competitive or make it seem as if what you have to say is more important than what the other person is saying. Watch your body language. You don't want to appear bored or disinterested. Don't hunch your shoulders, fidget, tap your toes, or twiddle your hair. Finally, don't be too aggressive or pushy in your conversation.

Language Arts Link Effective Communication

Being able to communicate important information to a patient, a colleague, or your supervisor is an essential skill in any profession. Communication has many forms: written communication, oral communication, and nonverbal communication using body language.

Write a brief report on the importance of developing effective communication skills. Create a new document on the computer, or on a blank sheet of paper. Write a descriptive title for your report. In paragraph form, detail why communication skills are indispensable to anyone who wishes to work in a health care profession. Include a thesis statement, or a sentence stating your main ideas, in the opening paragraph. Be sure to proofread your work to see if you can improve it by making it more clear, concise, or interesting to read. Check the spelling and grammar and correct any errors. Exchange reports with a classmate. Provide feedback and corrections as necessary, and then exchange back. Read your classmate's comments and revise your report as necessary.

Verbal Communication

Verbal communication includes spoken and written messages.

- ***Spoken messages.*** When you speak to someone, you send a message. The tone of your voice, the language you use, and the message you send are interpreted by the receiver. Always speak clearly and concisely. This ensures that your message is understood.
- ***Written messages.*** You communicate frequently with the written word. You take messages and orders. You may write notes in the patient's chart, and you may need to leave instructions for fellow workers. It is important to spell correctly, use proper grammar, and write in a clear and concise manner.

Listening Skills

When you think of communication, you may not think of listening. However, listening is a very important element in all communication. If you do not receive the message

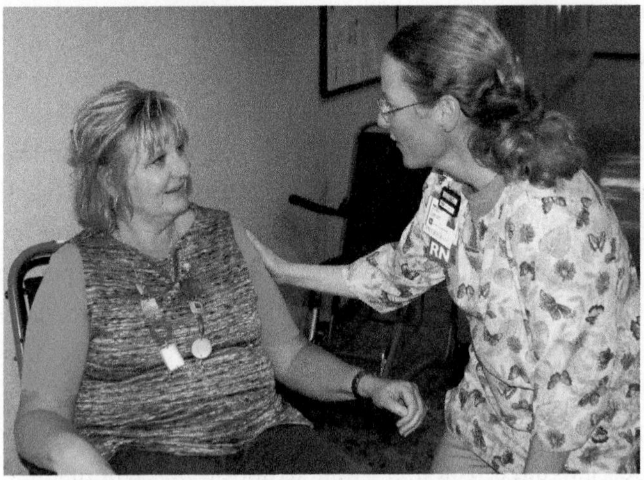

FIGURE 3.3

Registered nurse displaying good listening skills and body language that conveys caring and concern

Source: Carmen Martin/Pearson Education

that is being sent, communication has not taken place. Your understanding of how to be a good listener makes you a better health care worker. Here are some helpful tips:

- ***Show interest.*** It is important for you to show interest in the person who is sending you a message. If you follow all of the other rules of being a good listener but tune out the message because you are not interested, communication will not take place.
- ***Hear the message.*** Health care workers frequently think that they understand what is being said to them when they really do not. It is important to repeat what you believe you heard to be certain you heard correctly. It is not necessary to repeat exactly what was said, but check to see that you have understood the general message. Watch the speaker closely to observe actions that may contradict what the person is saying. Evaluate how well you listen, and if you are using all of the above skills during and after each conversation with patients and peers.
- ***Do not interrupt.*** Have you ever tried to send a message and been frustrated by the receiver interrupting you? Allow the sender to give you the entire message without interruptions. If you need to ask a question to clarify the meaning, be patient and wait until the sender is finished. She or he may give you the information you need without your questions.
- ***Pay attention.*** This is critical. Eliminate distractions by moving to a quiet area for the conversations. Avoid thinking about how you are going to respond. Try to eliminate your own prejudices and see the other person's point of view.
- ***Maintain a positive attitude.*** Keep your temper under control, even if you become irritated.

Being a good listener takes patience. You need to concentrate on being a good listener until the skills become easy for you. As a health care worker, you require good

APPLY IT IMPROVING LISTENING SKILLS

Have a conversation about career goals with a partner. Each of you should share your thoughts and ideas for two to three minutes. As you listen to your partner, observe your listening skills. Are you showing interest? Do you find yourself interrupting, or wanting to interrupt? After you finish with the listening exercise, take a few minutes to write down observations about your own listening skills. Note any personal barriers to listening that you notice. Review the guidelines for good listening skills and make a plan for how you can improve your listening skills.

listening as an essential skill. Good listening skills also help you follow directions, make good observations of patients, and understand your fellow workers.

Nonverbal Communication

Communication also takes place in nonverbal ways. It is not necessary to speak in order to send a message. You send messages with your eye contact, facial expressions, gestures, and touch. Remember to keep cultural differences in mind when communicating nonverbally.

- ***Eye contact.*** Making eye contact with the person with whom you are communicating is important in the Anglo-American culture. Eye contact lets others know that you are paying attention. When you do not make eye contact, you send others a message that you are not interested or that you wish to avoid them.
- ***Facial expressions.*** A smile sends a different message than a frown does. It is possible to say something very kind and still send a message of anger with your eyes. Try to think of an instance when you knew that what was being said was not what was meant. How did you know? The expression on the sender's face probably sent you a different message.
- ***Gestures.*** Shrugging your shoulders, turning your back, and leaving the room while someone is talking to you certainly convey a lack of interest in the sender's message. You need not say "I am not interested" because you have effectively sent that message through your gestures.
- ***Touch.*** Touch can convey great caring, warmth, concern, and tenderness. It can also convey anger, rejection, and distaste. Touch is a very important part of your communication. It is important that your nonverbal communication be supportive and positive.

Science Link — Communication Differences Between Men and Women

Studies have shown that men and women vary in the way they use nonverbal communication.

Differences between men and women are found in their body movements, eye contact, and use of space.

Women tend to use facial expressions to express more emotion than men. They are more likely to smile and use facial and body expressions to show friendliness. In contrast, men smile less often and are more likely to interrupt a person who is smiling. While women may show some friendly nonverbal cues, their posture tends to be more tense than men's posture. Men are more relaxed and more likely to use gestures.

While women do not often stare, men may use staring to challenge power. This nonverbal cue for power is also seen when observing the behavior of a man during an initial gaze. Men will wait for the other person to turn away, while women are more likely to avert their eyes on initial gaze. Men also use staring to signal interest. Instead of staring, women signal interest by maintaining eye contact.

Men and women also differ in their use of personal space. Women tend to approach others more closely, while men want more personal space. However, men are more likely to invade another's personal space than women, if necessary. While these differences are not always the case with every man or woman, they add to the complexity of communication.

How might these differences between men and women affect communication in the workplace? What could you do to take advantage of these differences or overcome them?

To summarize, communication requires a sender, a receiver, and a message. The message may be verbal or nonverbal, and many factors influence the effectiveness of communication. These factors include prejudices, frustrations, attitudes, and life experiences. Good listening skills are important to ensure successful communication, and an awareness of barriers to good communication is important.

SYMBOLIC LANGUAGE

People with sensory impairment may participate in an alternative way of communicating called symbolic language. People who are hearing impaired (sometimes referred to as *deaf)* or vocally impaired (unable to speak) may use sign language for communication. (Note: vocally impaired people are sometimes referred to as *dumb.* This term shows a lack of respect and should not be used.)

American Sign Language (ASL) is a formal method of communication that involves hand gestures, movements, and facial expressions. Many people with hearing impairment can hear minimal sounds and read lips to some degree. Written communication is also effective with hearing impaired people.

FIGURE 3.4

The American Sign Language Alphabet

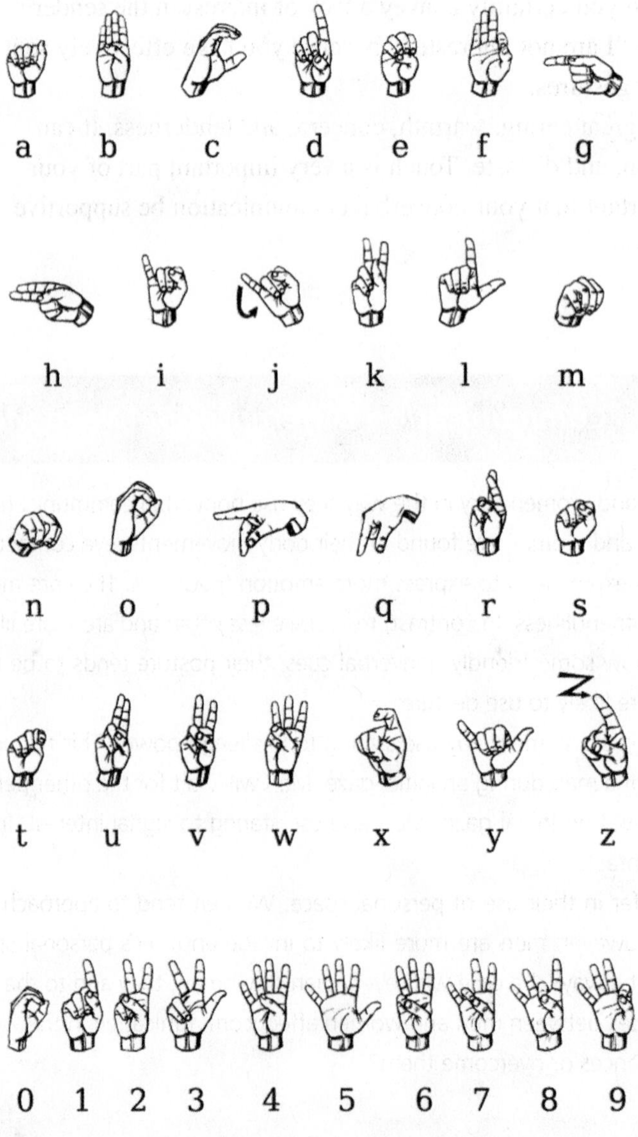

When communicating with hearing impaired people, use your normal tone of voice. Face the person so that he or she can read your lips and see your facial expressions, even when an interpreter is assisting. Avoid trying to just spell out letters of the alphabet, because sign language is a much more complex system of grammar rules and signs. Instead, learn some basic phrases such as "good morning" and "thank you" in sign language.

FIGURE 3.5

Interpreter using sign language to facilitate communication between a patient and a receptionist

Source: Dylan Malone/Pearson Education

People who are vision impaired (blind) use a system of writing called Braille. Letters of the alphabet are presented in patterns of raised dots on paper. Blind people can read these words and numbers by touching the dots with their fingertips. Blind people are not hard of hearing, so there's no need to raise your voice when speaking with them.

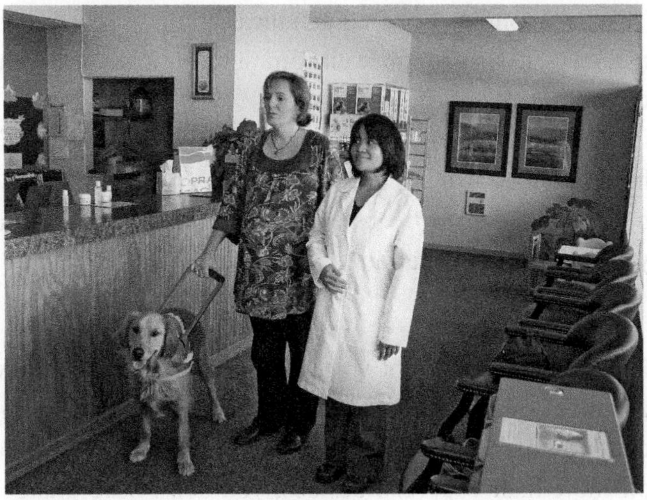

FIGURE 3.6

Receptionist assisting a vision impaired patient and her service animal

Source: Dylan Malone/Pearson Education

Depending on the health occupation you choose, and the types of patients with which you will work, you may need to become proficient in the use of symbolic language.

RECENT DEVELOPMENTS

Communicating via Social Media

Communicating via social media is growing rapidly and becoming an integral part of people's lives around the world. Social media is the number one activity on the web. Half of the world's population is under thirty years of age, and 96% of them use social media. About half of all baby boomers belong to at least one social media network. Recently, Facebook added 2 million users in less than one year. If Facebook were a country, it would be the third largest in the world. More than 1.5 million pieces of content are shared and 60 million status updates occur on Facebook each day. The fastest growing segment of Facebook users is 55- to 65-year-old women. YouTube is the one of the largest websites in the world with more than 100 million videos.

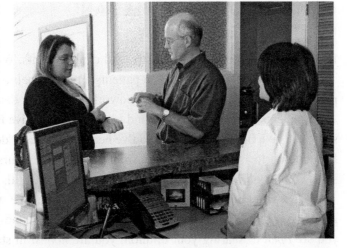

COMMUNICATION STYLES AND CONFLICT RESOLUTION

Health care workers function in stressful environments. When workers are under pressure and feeling rushed, and when patients are overwhelmed and feeling anxious, interpersonal conflict may occur. When coworkers strongly disagree with one another, and when patients express their anger and frustration, effective interpersonal communication skills can be a big help. Perhaps you've heard the phrase "dealing with difficult people." Responding to **confrontation**, confronting someone yourself, and resolving interpersonal conflict all require some special communication skills in **conflict resolution**.

confrontation (kon-fruhn-TAY-shuhn) To face boldly, defiantly, or antagonistically

conflict resolution (KON-flikt rez-uh-LOO-shuhn) Overcoming disagreements between two or more people

aggressive (uh-GRES-iv) Behavior aimed at causing harm or pain

passive (PAS-iv) Accepting or allowing an action without response

passive-aggressive (PAS-iv uh-GRES-iv) Appearing passive, but aggressive in behavior

assertive (uh-SUR-tiv) Bold, confident, self-assured

When you confront someone or respond to someone who has confronted you, the goal is to communicate your point of view in an open, honest, direct manner. This means you are *open* to sharing your opinion, you are *honest* in stating your opinion, and you state your opinion in a *direct* manner to make sure the other person gets your point. There are four styles of communication: **aggressive**, **passive**, **passive-aggressive**, and **assertive**. Let's see how well communication goals are met when using each of the four different styles of communication.

Here's the scenario. You and a coworker both want Christmas day off. Both of you have relatives arriving in town and wish to spend time with them. After discussing the holiday schedule, it becomes obvious that one of you must work on Christmas day, so you start the conversation.

Aggressive Style

In a loud, angry tone of voice you say, "I've worked here longer than you, so I get the day off! Besides, my kids are coming, and they live farther away than your kids!" Your coworker replies, "You got Thanksgiving off, and I had to work! So I deserve Christmas off more than you! And besides, you don't have grandchildren, and I do!" You reply, "Why do you always have to insist on getting your own way? Every time we do the schedule, you complain!" "I complain?" your coworker responds. "You're the one who always refuses to work overtime!"

You can imagine where the conversation goes from here. With aggressive communication, the conflict usually gets worse. You've expressed your opinion in an open, honest, direct manner, so why didn't the aggressive style of communication work? The answer is that you failed to show respect or consideration for your coworker, so he became defensive and fought back. Before long, anger took over, other issues entered the conversation, and the conflict escalated into an argument. Situations involving aggressive communication can turn violent, and shouting or fistfights might result. The conversation might be overheard by other people including supervisors and patients. Did anyone *win* in this situation? Was the conflict resolved? It's clear the answer is "no." Let's try a different approach.

Passive Style

In a meek, quiet tone of voice you say, "Well, I guess if you want Christmas off, I'll have to work. Maybe my kids can come back for Easter." That was a pretty short conversation. Using passive communication, you failed to express your opinion in an open, honest, direct manner. You turned into a floor mat to be walked on. Your coworker won; he got his needs met. But you lost, and came off looking (and feeling) weak and pitiful.

Was the conflict resolved? Yes. But in the long run you'll resent your coworker and feel disappointed in yourself for not standing up for something that was important to you. Let's try again.

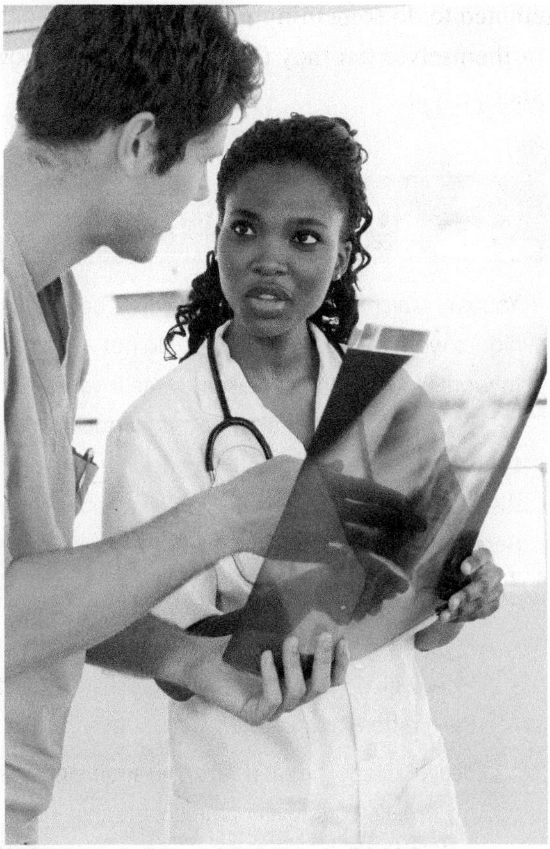

FIGURE 3.7

Communicating assertively to resolve a disagreement

Source: wavebreakmedia/Shutterstock

Passive-Aggressive Style

You say, "Well, I guess if you want Christmas off, I'll just go ahead and work. Maybe my kids can come back for Easter." Then, as soon as you get the chance, you do something sneaky to *get even* with him. You send your supervisor an anonymous note saying your coworker takes long, unauthorized breaks. You spread malicious gossip about him behind his back. Or you call in sick on a busy day when the two of you are assigned to work together. After all, there are lots of ways to get even. Maybe getting even will make you feel better, and maybe not. Using passive-aggressive communication, you still failed to express your opinion in an open, honest, direct manner. To make matters worse, you did something sneaky and dishonest. Was the conflict resolved? No. Let's try one more time.

Assertive Style

In a normal tone of voice you say, "Well, we both want Christmas off. I'm sure you'd like to spend Christmas with your grandchildren. After all, you had to work Thanksgiving, didn't you? On the other hand, I've worked here twice as long as you, so I have seniority. And my children are really looking forward to spending the day together as a family. So let's figure out a way to work this out so we can both get our needs met." Maybe you could split the holiday shift. Maybe you could arrange a long weekend off to make up for one of you having to work the holiday itself. Maybe you could work together to find a third person who's willing to cover the holiday in exchange for a different day off. There's almost always a workable solution to any problem. However, if you're arguing with the other person, your energy is spent on the conflict, not the solution. Using assertive communication, you stated your opinion in an open, honest, direct manner, and you did so in a way that showed respect and consideration for your coworker. Did it solve the problem? Maybe, and maybe not. Yet assertive communication represents the best opportunity for you to work together, compromise, and come up with a solution that's acceptable to both of you. It's a win-win solution which is the goal of conflict resolution.

It should be obvious that assertive communication is the only acceptable communication style to employ at work. You must have enough self-respect to state your needs openly and honestly. You must not allow yourself to be *walked on*, pitied, or tempted to do something underhanded and sneaky to get even. Professionals look out for themselves but they do it in a way that shows respect for the needs and desires of other people.

BUILD YOUR SKILLS *Learning to Communicate through Observation*

You can learn a lot by watching other people and noticing which communication techniques work for them, and which do not. Once you've observed an approach that appears to work, you can try it yourself to see if you get the same results.

Here's an example that occurs frequently. You notice a male customer and his companions seated at a table near yours in a restaurant. It's obvious that he isn't pleased with the food he was just served. You're wondering how he will react and what will happen. Here are four options:

Reaction #1: In a loud and angry tone of voice, he says to the waiter, "This isn't what I ordered! Either get it right, or I'm not going to pay one dime for this food!"

How well do you think this aggressive style of communication worked? Let's imagine a different approach.

Reaction #2: The man says to his table companions, "I don't like this place. They get my order wrong every time I come here. Let's go someplace else." While the waiter isn't looking, he sneaks out of the restaurant, takes the other members of his party with him, and leaves nothing to pay for the food that's already been served.

Is this *get-even* approach any better? Let's try again.

Reaction #3: In a pitiful, whining tone of voice, the man says to his companions, "This isn't what I ordered. But I don't want to make a scene, so I guess I'll just eat it anyway."

Did this passive approach meet his needs? Let's try one more time.

Reaction #4: The man signals for the waiter to come over to the table. In a calm tone of voice he says, "I hate to complain, but I ordered French fries and got a baked potato instead. I was really looking forward to the fries. Could you take the baked potato back and switch it to fries for me? Thank you."

How well do you think this assertive approach worked?

Consider each of the different approaches.

- How might the waiter have responded to the man's reactions?
- How might his table companions have responded to the man's reactions?
- Were the man's needs met? Why or why not?
- Which approach worked best, and why?
- Which approach worked the least, and why?
- What could you learn by observing these interactions?
- Which approach would you use if you were in this situation?

By sharpening your observation skills, you can improve your assertive communication skills. Notice what works best for other people and try it yourself. The more you practice, the more skilled you will become.

Assertive communication doesn't come easily—it takes practice. Maybe you're not used to standing up for yourself when someone confronts you or disagrees with you. Maybe aggressive or passive-aggressive communication has been your style up until now. If so, it's time to start working on a different approach that's more appropriate in the workplace. Put some effort into developing your assertive communication skills. Observe how other people deal with conflicts and the results they get. Then keep practicing your skills. The more you practice, the easier assertive communication will become.

Learn to *choose your battles wisely*. Decide which conflicts are really worth tackling and which ones you should just *let go*. Some battles aren't worth the effort. Be careful! Just because you're taking an assertive approach doesn't guarantee the other person will as well. Someone could turn aggressive on you. When communicating with a *difficult person*, make sure you can get out of the area quickly if necessary. If you have any concern about your physical safety, make sure someone else is nearby who can come to your aid if necessary. Remember, it can be an unsafe world. You never know when someone might be carrying a weapon or behaving in an aggressive or passive-aggressive manner. Here are some things to think about when confronting another person:

- Treat the other person with respect. Give him or her the benefit of the doubt until you've fully investigated the matter.
- Make sure you have complete, accurate information before confronting someone. Don't proceed on assumptions or unverified, third-hand information that might not be true.
- Stay calm and keep your anger and tone of voice in check.
- Arrange a suitable time and place to discuss differences; never conduct this type of conversation in a public area. If you are concerned about safety, don't choose a secluded area either.
- Don't say or do something that you might regret later.
- Listen carefully and make sure you understand the other person's point of view.
- Aim for a win-win solution.
- Take safety precautions. You may be able to control your own behavior but you cannot control the behavior of the other person.

Once you fully understand the other person's point of view and he or she understands yours, you both should find a middle ground where you can each compromise and feel like your needs have been met.

When you have a conflict with a coworker, resolve it quickly. Procrastination only makes things worse. But calm down first and

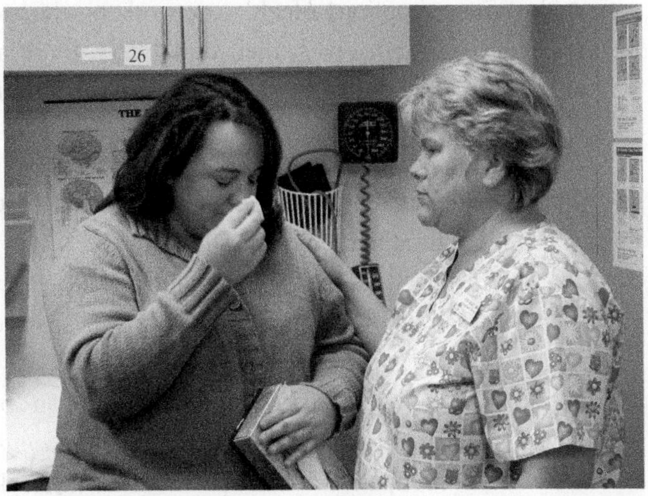

FIGURE 3.8

Coworkers showing mutual respect as they resolve a disagreement

Source: Dylan Malone/Pearson Education

make some rational decisions about how to handle the matter. Attack the issue, not the person. Remember that you cannot change other people; only they can change themselves. All you can do is make your best effort at communicating appropriately. If necessary, ask another person with good conflict resolution skills to serve as a facilitator.

If your supervisor is the *difficult person*, proceed cautiously! Remember to respect his or her position of authority. Weigh the pros and cons of addressing the situation head-on or just learning to live with it. If you decide to discuss the matter with your superior:

- Plan in advance what you're going to say, how you're going to say it, and what response you'll give to how he or she might react.
- Practice delivering the message in advance and consider role-playing the situation first with someone you trust.
- Listen carefully, watch for a win-win resolution, and be open to receiving some constructive feedback that might help you form a more positive relationship with your supervisor in the future.
- If the matter is still unresolved and you cannot move forward, speak with a human resources representative or another person in authority in your department.
- If the situation is serious and cannot be resolved, you may need to transfer into another position.

If the *difficult person* is a patient, visitor, or guest, stop and think about what it takes to deliver good customer service. Apply your listening and assertive communication skills. Find a resolution that meets everyone's needs in a respectful and professional manner.

Defense Mechanisms

Assertive communicators show respect for the other person's feelings and needs. This is the primary reason that assertive communication provides the best opportunity for resolving conflict. When people are confronted, they feel as if they're under attack. They become defensive and their **defense mechanisms** kick in. Once someone becomes defensive, he or she *fights back* instead of calmly working together to solve the disagreement.

defense mechanisms
(dih-FENS MEK-uh-niz-uhms)
Mental devices that help people cope with various situations

All people use defense mechanisms to help feel more comfortable and to make their behavior seem reasonable. Defense mechanisms are mental devices that help people cope with various situations. Health care workers who are aware of defense mechanisms better understand themselves, their coworkers, their supervisors, and their patients' behavior. The following are some examples of key defense mechanisms:

- ***Rationalization:*** Finding good reasons to replace the real reason for behavior in order to maintain self-esteem. *Example:* Mark did poorly on a test and explained it by saying, "I'd rather be popular than smart."
- ***Compensation:*** Substituting one goal for another. *Example:* Mary really wanted to be on the track team but wasn't good enough. Instead, she joined the choir and became a soloist.
- ***Projection:*** Placing the blame for your actions on someone or something else because you cannot accept the responsibility. *Example:* "I didn't get a good grade in my health occupations class because the teacher doesn't like me."

- ***Sublimation:*** Redirecting feelings toward a constructive objective. *Example:* You enjoy playing tennis, and you use the game to work out aggressiveness and hostility instead of directing those feelings toward others.
- ***Identification:*** Idolizing someone you would like to be like. *Example:* Margaret especially admired her music teacher. She began to walk and dress like her.

When you are aware that everyone uses defense mechanisms, and when you know what they are, you are better able to understand your behavior and the behavior of others. As a health care worker, it is important for you to realize that a defense mechanism may be involved in certain behavior. This allows you to give better care. Your knowledge of defense mechanisms also helps you understand the behavior of the people with whom you work.

Anger Management and Workplace Bullies

Effective communication and conflict resolution skills will serve you well in all aspects of your life. Avoid letting other people *press your buttons*. When you hear yourself saying, "She makes me so angry!" stop and think about that statement. You have a choice as to whether to be angry or not. Allowing other people to *make you* angry means you are handing over control of your behavior to someone else. Is that really what you want to do? If you have issues managing your anger, get some help from an anger management specialist. An inability to control your anger at work is a sure way to get fired. An inability to control your anger in your personal life can only lead to one problem after another. Find ways to maintain control of your behavior and don't allow other people to push you into doing things or saying things that you would rather not do or say.

People who use an aggressive or a passive-aggressive style of communication at work may be viewed as **workplace bullies**. These rude and unprofessional workers use verbal and nonverbal language to demean and intimidate other people. They rarely show respect,

workplace bullies (WURK-pleys BULL-ees) Employees who intimidate and belittle their coworkers

REALITY CHECK

Becoming an effective communicator is essential in developing and maintaining a professional reputation. You must be able to engage people in conversations in order to obtain and share vital information. Whether you are the sender or the receiver of a message, how well you communicate will have an impact on your relationships with other people and on your overall job performance. Keep the lines of communication open, become a good listener, and watch for nonverbal body language. Avoid the aggressive, passive, and passive-aggressive styles of communication, and devote as much energy as it takes to becoming skilled in assertive communication. Assertive communication is the key to standing up for yourself and making sure that your needs get met while showing respect for the feelings and the needs of other people. This is where your communication skills intersect with your character and personal values. Treating other people with respect is absolutely vital to your success in health care. If you are the type of person who gets angry easily, becomes defensive quickly, or harasses and intimidates people to feel more powerful yourself, it's time to make some major changes in your life. It should be obvious by now that these types of behavior are not tolerated in health care.

good manners, or civil behavior. Bullies create a hostile work environment and may be guilty of sexual harassment and various forms of workplace violence. If you encounter a workplace bully, using conflict resolution skills probably won't help much. Document the aggressive behaviors in writing, and file a report with the appropriate person.

Key Points

- Apply good communication skills to engage patients and create a sense of partnership.
- Introduce yourself and make people feel welcome and accepted.
- Be prepared to answer your patients' questions using terms they can understand.
- Send clear messages and avoid barriers to communication.
- Don't allow prejudice, bias, impatience, or annoyance to undermine communication.
- Look for shared experiences and things you have in common to improve communication.
- Develop your listening skills; use feedback to make sure understanding has occurred.
- Watch for nonverbal messages related to eye contact, facial expressions, gestures, and touch.
- Develop conflict resolution skills, and use the assertive style of communication to overcome disagreements.
- Understand defense mechanisms and how they affect people's behavior.
- Manage your anger, and don't let other people control your behavior.
- Never intimidate or harass people.

Section Review Questions

Answer each of the following questions. Indicate which page in the textbook led you to your answer.

1. Name four barriers to communication.
2. List the four essential elements of communication.
3. Give two examples of nonverbal communication.
4. Explain why good listening skills are so important.
5. List the four styles of communication and describe each style.
6. Explain how observing others can help you learn to communicate assertively.
7. List three steps in resolving interpersonal conflict.
8. What are defense mechanisms?
9. In your own words, explain what Norman Vincent Peale meant when he said, "Think enthusiastically about everything, but especially about your job. If you do so, you'll put a touch of glory in your life. If you love your job with enthusiasm, you'll shake it to pieces."

Learn By Doing

Complete Worksheets 1–5 in Section 3.1 of your *Student Activity Guide*.

Electronic Communication and Computers in Health Care

SECTION 3.2

Background

Communication between health care providers is vital to patient care. Today's technology has helped to improve the efficiency and the speed at which a message or file can be sent to another person. A worker in the health care environment needs to know how to use common software programs in order to access and record important patient information. In addition, workers need to be well-trained to use telephones, fax machines, e-mail, and the **Internet** to complete daily tasks.

Internet
(IN-ter-net) The worldwide computer network with information on many subjects

Computers are essential in health care. Health care agencies use computers in most departments to help save time, improve accuracy, increase productivity, and reduce costs. Computers are used for record keeping, diagnostic tests, education, research, and many other tasks. Health care workers must have a basic understanding of how computers work and how they are used in health care in order to be employable.

Objectives

After completing this section, you will be able to:

1. Define the key terms.
2. List key factors in the appropriate use of telephones, fax machines, e-mail, and the Internet at work.
3. Describe *texting* and explain why texting abbreviations should not be used at work.
4. List five potential mistakes when communicating electronically and explain how to prevent them.
5. Explain why computer security at work is important and list two ways to protect computer security.
6. Describe the roles of web browsers, Internet search engines, and domain names.
7. Describe the basic components and functions of computers.
8. List two examples of how computers are used in therapeutic and diagnostic services.
9. Discuss computer security issues related to the use of laptops, PDAs and flash drives.
10. Explain why people need computer skills to work in health care.

COMMUNICATION TECHNOLOGIES

Using communication technology at work requires some special skills which are focused on meeting customer service expectations and exchanging information in a professional and appropriate manner. Everyone uses a telephone; however, using a telephone at work requires some additional considerations.

Telephone Communication

The telephone is an important communication tool between you and those you serve. All departments in the health care setting require good telephone communication skills. For example, you may be asked to answer the telephone, take a message, or respond to a request. Always follow good communication standards when answering an incoming or placing an outgoing call. Telephones at workstations are for communication of health care issues pertinent to those you serve. Personal calls and socializing must be done on your break or outside of your assignment or work time.

When communicating by telephone:

- Demonstrate open, honest, and respectful communication.
- Present ideas, information, and viewpoints clearly.
- Listen actively and seek to understand others.
- Use good telephone manners.
- Screen calls as required. For example, if a doctor asks you to screen calls at an office or clinic, answer the phone and identify the caller, or use caller ID, and then politely notify the caller that the doctor is unable to speak at the moment. Offer to take a message so the doctor can return the call.

Demonstrate the following behaviors when on the telephone:

- Answer the telephone cheerfully.
- Use a pleasant, caring, and sincere tone of voice.
- Answer the telephone on the first ring, if possible.
- Speak clearly and courteously.
- Thank the caller for calling, or for returning a call.
- Identify yourself and give your title (such as, "This is Monica, nurse assistant").
- Identify your department or doctor's office (such as, "Dr. Smith's office").
- Allow the caller to hang up first to ensure that the caller has said everything he or she wanted to say.

Use appropriate words and phrases, such as:

- May I have your name, please?
- Would you repeat that, please?
- How may I assist you?
- I'm sorry; I didn't understand.

Avoid inappropriate words and phrases, such as:

- What's your name?
- What did you say?
- What do you want?
- Huh?

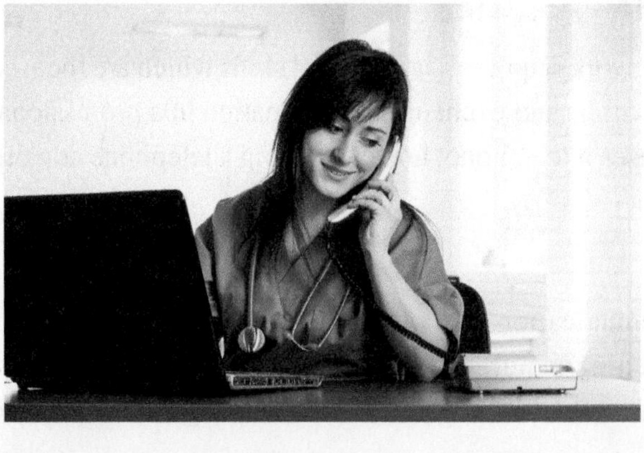

FIGURE 3.9
Communicating by telephone to coordinate patient care
Source: Minerva Studio/Fotolia LLC

Tips for being prepared:

- Have the necessary materials handy (pencil, message pad, and telephone directories).
- Before placing a call, prepare questions, gather the information you'll need, and determine the appropriate action to take.

When placing a caller on hold:

- Ask the caller if he or she can hold, and wait for the response.
- Check every thirty seconds to see if the caller wants to continue to hold.
- Ask if you may take a message.
- Transfer the call as soon as possible.

When transferring a caller:

- Explain where you are transferring the caller and to whom.
- Give the caller the number to which you are transferring them.
- If possible, stay on the telephone and introduce the caller to the person receiving the call.

When writing a phone message:

- Record time and date.
- Clearly write the caller's name (verify spelling) and the telephone number (read back the number).
- Summarize information with the caller by repeating the message.
- Sign or initial the message.
- Record the action you take to deliver the message.

When leaving a message:

- State for whom you are calling, your name, from where you are calling, your message (remembering to follow confidentiality guidelines), and the times that you will be available for a return call.
- Document date, time, and message left.

APPLY IT TELEPHONE COMMUNICATION

Role-play with a classmate. One of you will be the patient, calling his or her doctor's office to discuss the results of a lab test. The other student will be the receptionist, answering the telephone. The patient should ask several questions. Notice how the receptionist responds, no matter how the patient acts. Is the patient angry or annoyed? Does the patient keep repeating his or her questions? Is the receptionist listening and responding in a clear, understandable manner? Have the patient's needs been met? Switch roles and repeat the role-play.

Fax Communication

If a health care employee needs to send a patient's record to another provider, the worker may use a **facsimile** or **fax machine**. A fax transmission is a way to send or receive printed pages or images over telephone lines by converting them to and from electronic signals. You may work on a computer, or have access to a printer, that is connected to a phone line so that you can send and receive faxes directly from your computer or printer. In order to send a fax, you need a fax number, or a telephone number used for faxes, for the person to whom you want to send the documents.

facsimile or **fax machine** (fak-SIM-uh-lee) A device that sends and receives printed pages or images as electronic signals over telephone lines

Remember the following when sending a fax:

- Use a **cover page**. This is the first page of a fax that gives the receiver important information about the fax. It should include your name, contact number, number of pages being sent, name of the intended recipient, and any other important information.

cover page
(KUV-er payj) The first page of a fax or a written report

- Confirm that the intended **recipient** received the fax. Because a fax often contains important patient information, call or e-mail the recipient to ensure that he or she has received it.

recipient
(ri-SIH-pee-ent) A person or thing that receives

- Remember that you may be dealing with confidential information. If you are sending confidential or potentially sensitive information, call ahead and let the recipient know to be ready. Using an online fax may help avoid security issues, as it lets users send and receive faxes from the privacy of their own computers.

E-mail Communication

E-mail is an important method of communication in the health care business. However, health workers sending e-mails should choose their words carefully. A person cannot hear vocal inflections in an e-mail; therefore, do not use sarcasm and humor in a business e-mail because they may lead to miscommunication or misunderstandings.

Remember that any message you send is permanent and may be forwarded to others. Do not use a business e-mail address to send trivial or highly sensitive information. Before you hit *send*, follow these guidelines to write a professional e-mail:

- Begin with a greeting.
- Include short, simple, and straight-forward information. If a message is long, discuss the topic in a short e-mail, and use an **attachment** to provide details. An attachment is a file linked to an e-mail message. You may also break up a longer e-mail that has many topics into multiple, shorter e-mails that discuss each topic separately.

attachment
(uh-TACH-ment) A file linked to an e-mail message

- Read your e-mail aloud to check the tone of your message. Using *please* and *thank you* with requests ensures a polite tone.
- Proof the content for spelling and grammar mistakes. Use upper and lower case when writing. (Use of all capital letters implies yelling.)
- Include important contact information at the end of your e-mail, such as your name, position, organization, telephone number, e-mail address, and perhaps fax number.
- Include a subject on the subject line of the e-mail.
- Use features, such as **blind carbon copy** and **carbon copy**, when appropriate. Carbon copy (cc) is used to send a copy of your e-mail to another recipient. For example, you may send an e-mail to a patient, but carbon copy a doctor on the e-mail so that he or she knows what was sent to the patient. Blind carbon copy (bcc) is used when an e-mail is sent to multiple people. Blind carbon copy allows a recipient to read the message; however, the recipient cannot see the other e-mail addresses to which the message was sent. This is beneficial because it protects the recipients' e-mail addresses and eliminates clutter in the e-mail.

blind carbon copy
(BLINED CAR-buhn kah-PEE) An e-mail feature that allows a person to send an e-mail to multiple people without them seeing the other receivers' e-mail addresses

carbon copy
(CAR-buhn kah-PEE) An e-mail feature that allows a person to send a copy of an e-mail to another person

- When replying to an e-mail message, be careful with *reply* and *reply all* functions. Don't select *reply all* unless it is really necessary for everyone who was included in the original message to receive your reply.

Respond to incoming e-mails within twenty-four hours. If you need more time to respond, call or e-mail that you are looking into the matter and will get back to the person as soon as possible. Also be sure to answer all questions when responding to an e-mail. When sending an e-mail with questions, allow one or two days for a response. If you need an immediate response, you may want to call the person.

In health care, **memorandums** (memos) are used as reminders, to persuade an action, to issue a directive or to provide a report. Memorandums can be delivered via e-mail. When sending a memorandum via e-mail, be sure to:

memorandum
(mem-uh-RAN-duhm) A short note written to help a person remember something, or to remind a person to do something; also known as a memo

- Confirm the memorandum looks as intended in print and on the screen.
- Use fonts and graphics that are clear on all recipients' computers.
- Ensure attachments are readable by all recipients.

As an alternative to e-mailing and speaking by telephone, millions of people now rely on **texting**, or text messaging, for communication. Texting is sending real-time, short text messages between cell phones or other handheld devices using sites such as Facebook and Twitter. Because text messages are limited to about 140 characters, users insert abbreviations (such as BTW for *by the way*, and LOL for *laughing out loud*) to convey their messages. Although texting abbreviations are becoming a common form of language, do not use them in your e-mail or written communication at work unless approved by your employer. Many health care workers are not familiar with texting abbreviations. The use of unauthorized abbreviations in health care can cause serious problems related to patient care and medical records.

texting
(TEKST-ing) Sending real-time, short text messages between cell phones or other handheld devices; also known as text messaging

THE MORE YOU KNOW

Cell Phones at Work

For safety reasons, the health care facility where you work will probably have restrictions on the use of your personal cell phone in the workplace. Cell phones can cause interference with medical equipment, including ventilators and pacemakers. Cell phones may also set off alarms on medical machines. You need to be aware of a facility's policy on how, where, and when employees, patients, and guests can use their cell phones. You may have to ask a patient or family member to turn off their phone. If so, politely explain the facility's policy and the need for it.

Despite the problems associated with using cell phones in health care environments, advancing technologies offer beneficial uses for cell phones in regard to health care. For example, Twitter, a website that offers social networking and microblogging services, enables doctors and other medical personnel to send and receive **tweets** about health care issues and questions.

Health care **apps** (or applications) are available, as well. Remember that patients are accessing health care information via these technological sources. Remind them that, like the medical information they find online, health care information they receive in a tweet or with an app should be discussed in greater depth with their doctors.

What other health care related benefits might cell phones offer for workers and patients?

tweets
(TWEETS) Text-based messages of up to 140 characters

apps
(APPS) Software applications for smartphones and computerized hand-held devices

username
(YOO-zer-naym) A unique identifier composed of letters and numbers used as a means of initial identification to gain access to a computer system or Internet service provider

The Internet

Many health care positions may require a worker to find or access information online. In order to gain access, employees usually need to have a username. Usernames are names used to gain access to a computer system. Once on the computer, employees may research and access information on the Internet. The Internet is a worldwide computer network that provides information on many subjects.

When researching information, it is important to choose a website that is credible. Not every medical website is supported by research or written by experts in the medical field.

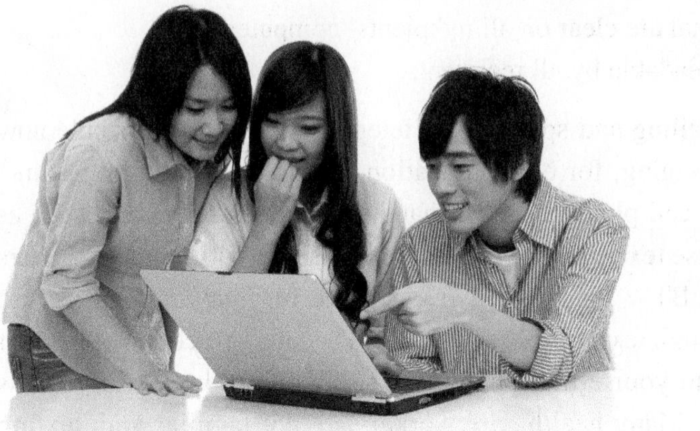

FIGURE 3.10
Viewing a website to find helpful information
Source: East/Shutterstock

Some examples of credible sources on the Internet include organizations such as the American Cancer Society or the Leukemia and Lymphoma Society. Websites sponsored by the government, such as the Food and Drug Administration (FDA) website, are reliable as well as those sites posted by educational institutions such as Johns Hopkin's University.

website
(WEB-sahyt) A group of pages on the Internet developed by a person or organization about a topic

Web browser
(web BROW-zer) A software application that allows users to locate and access Internet web pages

Internet search engines
(IN-ter-net SURCH EN-jens) Programs that search documents for keywords and produce lists where the keywords were found

Web browsers are software applications that allow users to locate and access Internet web pages. Browsers convert basic computer code into image, text, and audio formats and provide hyperlinks to help users move among different web pages. Several kinds of web browsers exist, such as Microsoft Internet Explorer, Firefox, Safari, and Netscape Navigator, based on their differing functions. However all browsers provide a toolbar that lets users find web pages, save favorite websites, print content, store web history, and move forward and backward among the websites they have visited. Internet search engines (such as Google, Yahoo, Bing, and Ask.com) are programs that search documents for keywords and then produce a list of the documents where the keywords were found. When users enter a keyword or phrase such as "health career planning," a list of websites that provide information on health career planning will appear.

Language Arts Link Reliance on the Internet

Make a list of the things you do that involve use of the Internet. For one week, keep track of how much time you spend doing each of these activities. Include time spent surfing websites, researching information, making online purchases, downloading music and movies, playing games, communicating with family and friends, and so forth. Think about how different your life would be without the Internet. Identify the top three advantages of the Internet from your personal point of view. Then identify the top three reasons why you should be careful when using the Internet.

Write a brief report to present what you have learned from this exercise. Be sure to proofread your work to see if you can make it more clear, concise, or interesting to read. Check the spelling and grammar and make necessary revisions. Exchange reports with a classmate and share what you have learned.

A **domain name** is used as an Internet address to identify the location of a particular web page. For example, the URL (Uniform Resource Locator) for the American Cancer Society is http://www.cancer.org. The domain name in this address is "cancer." Many health care providers create Internet websites that provide important information for patients and the community. These websites are open to the public and may include directions to the facility, office hours, contact phone numbers and e-mail addresses, as well as other helpful information about the provider's organization. Some health care providers also post **intranet** websites which are private computer networks open only to people within the organization. Intranet websites help employees share information and computing resources while protecting the organization's privacy and confidentiality.

domain name
(doh-MAYN naym) The Internet address for a web page

intranet
(IN-truh-net) A private computer network with limited access

E-mail and Internet Policies

With the current use of technology in the workplace, most employers have policies regarding use of the Internet and e-mail for personal business while at work. Employees may be required to read and sign a policy concerning Internet and e-mail use. While some employers allow employees to use the Internet and e-mail for personal use on a limited basis, most policies prohibit employees from sending disruptive or offensive e-mail. This may include forwarding jokes or pictures that have been e-mailed to an employee. In addition, employees may not access websites that contain pornographic material or discriminatory messages. E-mail and Internet access should always be used in a manner that is accurate, appropriate, ethical, and lawful.

In order to ensure that workers are following these policies, many employers monitor employees' e-mail and Internet usage. Software programs help employers identify e-mails or website visits that may be inappropriate. Some employers block access to certain types of websites. Employees should always remember that any e-mail or file they have stored on a business computer may be read by someone in the organization's technology department or a manager. If an employee notices a violation of the organization's policy, the employee is expected to notify a supervisor. Policy violations typically result in disciplinary action and may cause a person to lose his or her job.

Tips for Using Electronic Communication

In addition to the information presented previously, here are some more general tips to remember when communicating electronically at work:

- Slow down and think about what you are saying. Draft your message and read it later before sending it, time permitting. Once a message has been sent electronically, it cannot be cancelled. Anyone who receives your message can forward it on to someone else without your knowledge or permission.
- Keep your messages short and to the point. Omit information that could be embarrassing if it falls into the wrong hands, or result in a violation of confidentiality and privacy standards.
- Be especially careful when forwarding messages. Before you click on *send,* double-check the content of the *entire message* and confirm to whom it is being sent.
- Avoid using fancy fonts, smiley faces, and **emoticons**.
- Electronic communication isn't foolproof. You cannot be certain your message was received and read without following up. People receive scores of e-mail messages

emoticons
(ih-MOH-ti-kons) Use of punctuation marks and letters in an e-mail message to convey the sender's emotions

at work every day. Sometimes a message is accidentally deleted or ends up in junk mail or a Spam filter before it has been read. People may become overwhelmed with too many messages and never open some of them. Some people who are assigned e-mail accounts at work never use them.

- Every time you prepare to send a message, ask yourself how you would feel if your message appeared in the newspaper or showed up on your supervisor's computer screen. Never send an electronic message when you are angry or emotionally upset.

Community Service Communicating Safely Online

Work with students in a local elementary school computer class. Create a poster that lists the do's and don'ts of safe online communication. Include how to act in blogs, chat rooms, or on sites such as Facebook, Twitter, and so on. Participate in a discussion about the benefits of online communication and its risks.

Computer Security

Computer security is a major issue in today's world where **hacking** has become common. Hackers are computer experts. Some hackers just enjoy computer programming and push the limits of what they can accomplish. Other hackers have malicious intent. They can steal passwords, gain access to someone's computer, and make modifications without permission. Hackers look for weaknesses in computer systems and exploit them. They may obtain and use someone's private and personal information for their own benefit. They may send e-mail messages from another person's account, insert a virus, damage files and software, and commit other acts intended to take advantage of people and cause harm.

password
(PAS-wurd) A secret series of numbers and letters that identifies the person who should have access to a computer, file, or program

Unauthorized access to business computers can cause major problems in health care when privacy and confidentiality are crucial. Be sure to follow your employer's policies and procedures governing computer security. Protect the secrecy of your passwords, don't share your passwords with anyone, and avoid using the same passwords at work that you use at home. Change your passwords on a regular basis, and don't write them down or store them in places where security could be breached.

COMPUTERS AND HEALTH CARE

During the past fifty years, computer technology has grown and changed at an unbelievable rate. The early computers were made of vacuum tubes and required large, environmentally controlled rooms. They often overheated and became inoperable for many hours. Repairing them was time consuming. Large systems were very expensive, and only the largest organizations were able to afford them. Today's computer technology allows computers to be smaller, more powerful, and less expensive. Today's computer equipment is the result of a development process. Models and devices continue to change frequently as new technology becomes usable and marketable. Computers have basic components and functions that you need to learn about in order to understand computer terminology. All computers allow users to input information, process information, and provide ways to output information.

Basic Computer Components and Functions

Basic computer functions include inputting, processing, and outputting.

Inputting

The most common device used to **input** data into a computer is a keyboard. In addition to alphanumeric keys, a keyboard has function keys, punctuation keys, arrow keys, and conjunction keys. Function keys have different purposes, depending on the software that is running on the computer. Arrow keys, along with a mouse, can be used to move the cursor around on the computer screen to control where you input information. Conjunction keys are used in combinations that are specific to the software that is running. For example, in some programs, when the Alt key is pressed in conjunction with the Shift key and the letter t, the current time is entered.

input
(IN-put) To enter data into a computer for processing

With advances in mobile-device technology, touch screens are becoming a frequently used data input method. Touch screens, or touch pads, are common inputting devices for tablet or handheld computers. They are also used on computers in places where many people can access information, such as at a kiosk that gives directions in a medical facility. Uses for touch-screen technology in health care are growing. For example, touch screens have been developed that allow cancer patients to accurately show the location and intensity of their pain at times when they may have trouble communicating this information to their caregivers.

Some types of computer systems used in health care facilities may utilize tablet computers that require a stylus for inputting data. A stylus looks like a pen or pencil, but using it on a tablet computer that is designed for this type of inputting allows a user to write information that can be digitally interpreted and stored. For example, some hospitals and medical offices may have patients enter their personal information directly into tablet computers; the information is digitally input into the computer system and does not need to be transcribed by a person in order to be added to the patient's medical record.

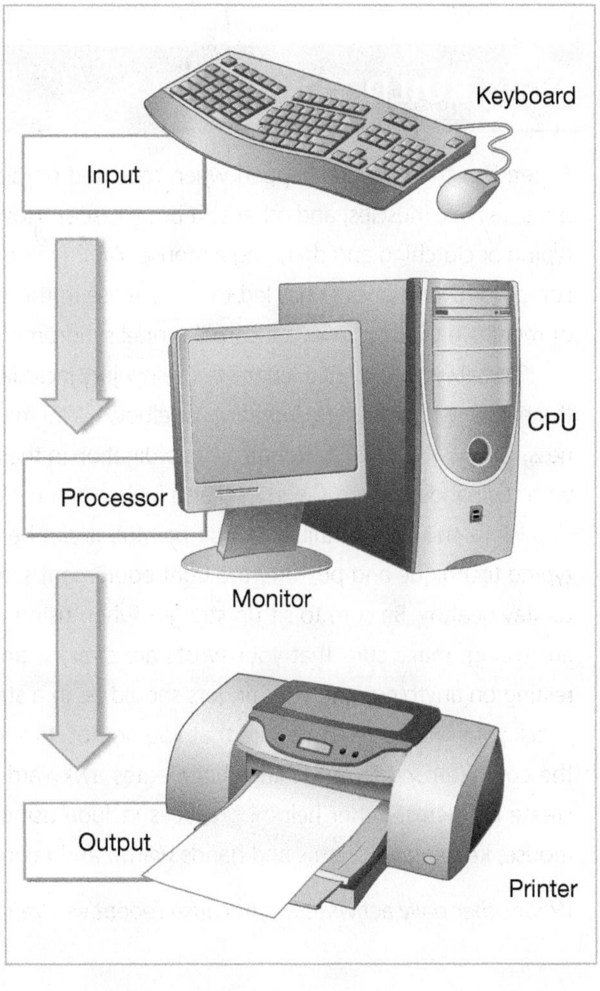

FIGURE 3.11
Components of a computer system

Other input devices include external hard-disk drives, CD-ROMs, DVD-ROMs, USB flash drives, optical drives, and magnetic disks. These devices are used for inputting and storing data or information.

Processing

central processing unit (SEN-truhl PRAH-sess-ing YOO-nit) The part of a computer that interprets and carries out instructions; also known as the CPU

A computer processes the information that is input and returns the information to the person who input it or to someone in another department. The **central processing unit** (CPU) is the working unit of the computer. The CPU consists of many electronic components and microchips. The CPU can process only the information it receives. If it receives incorrect information, it processes incorrect information. (Remember the phrase, "Garbage in, garbage out".) The information that you enter must be accurate if you expect accurate results.

Outputting

output (OUT-put) To produce information; turn out

Just as there are multiple devices for inputting information into a computer, there are several devices for outputting. The two most common items used to **output** are the monitor and the printer. The monitor, or display screen, of a computer allows a user to see what is happening. Monitors may be monochrome, grayscale, or color. Monochrome monitors display one color for the background and one color for the foreground—black and white, green and black, or amber and black. As its name suggests, a grayscale monitor is a monochrome monitor that displays in different shades of gray. Color monitors, sometimes called RGB monitors, combine the colors *red*, *green*, and *blue* to display anywhere from sixteen to more than a million colors. A printer is used to print the processed information on paper. Information printed on paper is called *hard copy* and can be filed with the patient's records. In most work environments, you will use the same printer as a group of your coworkers.

BUILD YOUR SKILLS *Preventing Computer-Related Repetitive Strain Injury*

Repetitive strain injuries happen when repeated physical movements do damage to tendons, nerves, muscles, and other soft body tissues. Nowadays, you may spend hours a day typing or clutching and dragging a mouse. An increase in the amount of time spent at the computer over the years has led to an increase in this type of injury. Some common types of repetitive strain injuries are carpal tunnel syndrome, bursitis, and tendonitis.

Typical symptoms of a repetitive strain injury include a tightness, soreness, or burning in the hands, wrists, fingers, forearms, or elbows. You may also experience tingling or numbness, coldness, or loss of strength or coordination in the hands. While most symptoms occur with the hands and arms, you may also feel pain in the upper back, shoulders, or neck.

While this type of injury can be painful, it can be prevented. You should use correct typing technique and posture, the right equipment setup, and good work habits in order to stay healthy. Be sure to sit up straight when using a computer. In addition, when you are typing, make sure that your wrists are straight and level. Your wrists should not be resting on anything, and your fingers should be in a straight line with your forearm. Also, check your work area to be sure that you do not have to stretch to reach the keys or read the computer screen. Anything that creates awkward reaches or angles in the body will create problems. Other helpful practices include using a light touch on the keyboard or mouse, keeping your arms and hands warm, and taking breaks to stretch and relax.

What other daily activities might cause repetitive strain injury?

Using Computers in Health Care

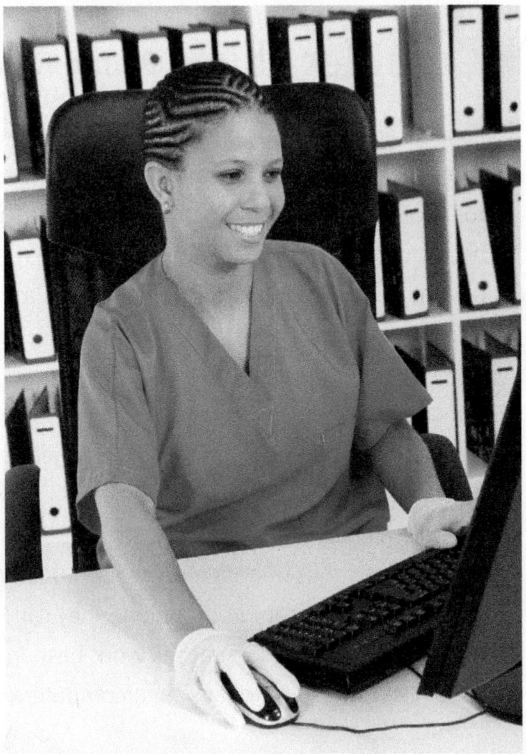

FIGURE 3.12

Using a computer to track patient data for research

Source: michaeljung/Shutterstock

Computers are processors of information. They process large amounts of information at incredible speeds, accurately, and consistently. Computers are used to communicate standards of care and to guide the practitioners in making patient care decisions. Wherever your career path in the health field takes you, you will do a portion of your work on a computer. Hospitals and medical and dental offices are converting their methods of keeping medical records, as well as accounting, and purchasing functions to storage and processes that use computers. Some health care agencies have computer diagnostic services where a complete physical examination is analyzed by a computer.

In the hospital, a computer performs many functions. The following are some of the procedures computers assist with:

- Recording physicians' notes and orders
- Creating a nursing treatment/work sheet based on physician orders (updates automatically with each additional physician order)
- Creating templates for interventional protocols
- Charting at the patient's bedside
- Monitoring patients
- Ordering or changing patients' diets
- Ordering unit supplies
- Processing charges for patient care equipment
- Ordering lab work, receiving lab results, and recording lab results in patient records
- Scheduling x-rays, special tests, and surgeries
- Processing patient discharges
- Performing diagnostic testing
- Processing medical billing
- Performing emergency dispatch
- Researching via the Internet

In medical and dental offices, computers can be used to schedule appointments, set up a recall system, bill patients, schedule lab work, dial the telephone, manage the security system, and keep the inventory. Computers are an important part of the search for correct specific patient data that meets the **HEDIS** requirements.

One of the most exciting and promising use of computers in health care involves **electronic health records** (EHRs), also know as electronic medical records (EMRs). The advent of electronic health records will be covered in the next section of this chapter.

HEDIS
(HEDIS) Health Plan Employer Data and Information System, an organization that provides quality care guidelines

electronic health records
(ih-lek-TRON-ik helth REK-erds) Medical records kept via computer; also known as EHRs

mortality rate
(mawr-TAL-i-tee RAYT) The ratio of deaths in an area to the population of that area, over a one-year period

comparative data
(kuhm-PAIR-uh-tiv DEY-tuh) Information gathered from multiple sources that is analyzed to identify similarities and differences

transparency
(trans-PARE-uhn-see) Open, clear, and capable of being seen

first responders
(FURST ri-SPON-ders) The first people to appear and take action in emergency situations

smartphones
(SMART-fohns) Mobile telephones that have advanced computing and connectivity features

data mining
(DEY-tuh MINE-ing) Sifting through large amounts of data to find significant information

homeostasis
(hoh-mee-oh-STAY-sis) Constant balance within the body; balance is maintained by the heartbeat, blood-making mechanisms, electrolytes, and hormone secretions

tomography
(TOE-muh-graf-ee) Radiographic technique that produces a scan showing detailed cross-sections of tissue

Consider This *Online Resources and Supercomputers*

Patients are taking advantage of online resources to learn about medical conditions and compare prices and outcome statistics such as **mortality rates** and readmission rates for local hospitals. This **comparative data** allows patients/consumers to *shop* for health care services, providing more **transparency** among health care providers. As patients become more informed, they're playing a larger role in making decisions about their health care.

First responders such as EMTs, paramedics, and flight doctors and nurses are using **smartphones** with apps to access volumes of medical information on drugs, drug interactions, and treatment options wherever needed to speed up the care process before the patient arrives at the emergency department.

Researchers are using large computerized databases to store and analyze information on thousands of patients. Through **data mining** (sifting through large amounts of data to find significant information), they can follow patients before and after treatment to determine which approaches work best. In the past, this type of research could take years. However, with today's supercomputers, the analysis can be done in just minutes.

Therapeutic Services

If you choose to enter an occupation in the therapeutic services, you'll have opportunities to work with a computer every day. In the pharmacy, drugs are inventoried using a computer. A computer also assists the pharmacist in keeping track of the medications that a person receives. The computer can alert the pharmacist when one medication acts against another medication or contains a substance that may cause an allergic reaction. In physical and occupational therapy, a computer assists paralyzed patients to walk. In respiratory therapy, a computer keeps critically ill patients in **homeostasis**. In emergency services and intensive care units, computers monitor patients and warn caregivers, via special programming, when a potentially dangerous condition occurs.

Diagnostic Services

In diagnostic services, highly sophisticated computers are being used. In the past, patients required surgery and other invasive procedures to help providers reach a diagnosis. Today, computerized diagnostic equipment helps providers diagnose many illnesses without the risk of surgery and the pain and discomfort of invasive tests.

The following are examples of computerized tests.

- The *CT scanner* performs computerized **tomography**. This test allows for the "dissection" of an organ via radiographic imaging to help find abnormalities (such as tumors) without surgery. CT scans provide the radiologist and the patient's physician with a permanent record for future use.
- The *Coulter counter* completes multiple examinations of many blood specimens in seconds.
- The *electrocardiogram computer* creates pictures on a computer screen. It also prints out the electrical activity of the heart. This helps the physician diagnose heart disease correctly.

- The *magnetic resonance imaging* (MRI) computer scans the body, producing a cross-sectional body image. This helps the radiologist and the patient's physician find tumors, see the results of medication and treatment, and diagnose the cause of an illness or disease.

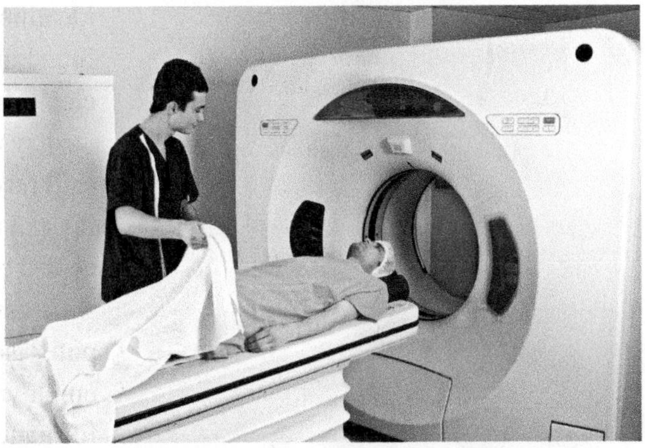

FIGURE 3.13

Patient undergoing a magnetic resonance imaging (MRI) computer scan

Source: Hakan Kiziltan/Fotolia LLC

- The *positron emission tomography* (PET) computer is also a scanner. It produces a three-dimensional image that shows an organ or bone from all sides.
- The *ultrasound imager* computer produces a picture of internal organs, tumors, aneurysms, and other abnormalities. It also produces pictures of the fetus developing in the uterus to help with fetal monitoring. These pictures can be seen on the monitor or can be processed on photographic film.

The latest electronic technology scans an organ and not only provides pictures, but also creates a three-dimensional object out of plastic. This object is an exact replica of the organ scanned in the patient's body. It allows the physician to practice difficult or experimental surgical procedures on the plastic replica before performing the procedure on the patient.

telemedicine (TEL-uh-MEH-duh-sin) The use of telecommunications technology to provide patient care in remote areas where patients and caregivers cannot meet in person

Science Link — Telemedicine and Computer Technology

One of the biggest challenges in health care is providing medical services for patients who live in remote parts of the country without direct access to hospitals, nurses, or physicians. Thanks to computers and sophisticated telecommunication systems, **telemedicine** (also known as *telehealth* or *e-health*) now enables health care professionals to diagnose and treat patients without actually meeting with them. Medical specialists can evaluate patients and "see" them electronically, eliminating the need for long-distance travel.

Research the topic of telemedicine and identify a situation where telemedicine was used to care for a patient. Prepare a brief oral report that describes its history and benefits of telemedicine for both patients and caregivers. Briefly describe the science behind the technology and how telemedicine was used to care for a patient. Predict some potential scientific breakthroughs related to telemedicine that might occur in the near future. Present your report to your classmates and teacher, and ask for feedback.

How widespread has telemedicine become in the U.S? Is telemedicine improving access to health care in other countries of the world? If so, how?

Other Computer Applications

In addition to therapeutic and diagnostic services, many other areas within health care rely on computers for everyday functions. Medical records workers manage and process records on computers. With diagnostic-related groupings, the computer is used to help categorize and track patients in the medical system. Health unit coordinators/unit secretaries use computers to process many of the orders or transmit requests to other departments. Central supply services (also known as central processing services) are computerized for tracking and reordering inventory and for billing. Supplies are even categorized and

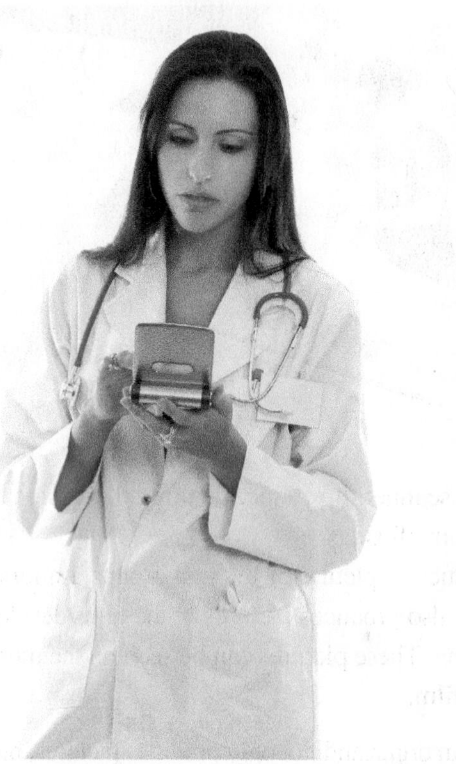

FIGURE 3.14

Physician using a personal digital assistant (PDA)

Source: Leah-Anne Thompson/ Shutterstock

identified by bar scanners similar to those found in the grocery store. Wall-hung time clocks have been replaced with computerized systems that produce electronic time card records. Purchase orders and invoices for payment are entered into, and processed by, computers. Work schedules and shift assignments are managed by computer software. Job vacancy postings, employment applications, employee performance reviews, and job descriptions and compensation information are often computerized. In large, urban hospitals, most of the day-to-day operations now rely on computers.

The use of small, mobile, hand-held devices called **personal digital assistants** (PDAs) is on the rise in health care. PDAs can be used to access medical information quickly, such as medication doses or information about potential drug interactions. Health care workers may manage their schedules and calendars on PDAs and store contact information, such as telephone numbers and e-mail addresses. PDAs connect with laptop and desktop computers, so information and data can be transferred back and forth. Physicians, for example, can download patient information from their office computers to their PDAs. They can review and update the information off-site, and then transfer the updated files back to their office computers when they return to work.

personal digital assistant (PUR-suh-nl DIJ-i-tl uh-SIS-tuhnt) A small, mobile, hand-held computerized device; also known as a PDA

RECENT DEVELOPMENTS

Less Invasive Surgery

Surgery is becoming less invasive due to laser procedures and miniature cameras that allow surgeons to perform operations with very small incisions. Less invasive procedures are leading to less scarring, shorter recovery times, less hospitalization, and more patients eligible for the treatments. Surgical robots, such as Da Vinci, are becoming more routine.

Using **telerobotics**, scientists are now developing tiny robots that can be inserted into the patient to help perform surgical procedures without making an incision. Robots crawl and swim, taking pictures as they move around. For example, with the Assembling Reconfigurable Endoluminal Surgical System (ARES), after the patient swallows fifteen separate parts, the robot self-assembles the parts inside the patient's body to help surgeons complete the procedure. With SpineAssist, a tiny robotic fly controlled by a magnet outside the patient's body travels through arteries and veins, detecting blockages and delivering drugs directly to tumors. More of these amazing new devices are on the way.

telerobotics (tele-roh-BOT-iks) Robots controlled from a distance using wireless connections; used in conducting remote surgery

Contingency Planning

Whenever human beings depend on machines, contingency plans are necessary just in case the machine stops functioning. When a computer is not functioning, it is said to be *down*. Downtime can be scheduled to allow a new program to be entered into the computer's memory or to make changes. Downtime can also be unexpected due to a power failure or an equipment malfunction. Health care providers have back-up plans in place so that patient care and business processes can continue to function if and when their computers go down.

Security and Confidentiality

Now that you're aware of the extensive use of computers in health care, you can appreciate that computer security is a major issue. The ability to download large amounts of patient information onto laptop computers, PDAs, and **flash drives** creates significant security concerns. Laptops can be stolen; flash drives are small enough to fit into your pocket and get lost; and PDAs are easily misplaced. When highly sensitive, private information is taken from the workplace on devices such as these, extra effort must be made to protect security and confidentiality. Never take confidential information away from your worksite without proper authorization. When transporting sensitive information is part of your job, always follow your employer's policies and procedures to avoid a breach of confidentiality.

flash drive
(FLASH drive) A small memory device used to store and transport files among computers; also known as a thumb drive or jump drive

APPLY IT BREACH OF CONFIDENTIALITY

Conduct some online research or visit a library to find an example of confidential files being lost or stolen because someone took the files away from their workplace. Find answers to the following questions. Who was involved? Why were the files taken from the workplace? How were the files transported (such as a laptop computer, PDA, or flash drive)? What kind of information was contained in the files? Did the information fall into the hands of the wrong people? If so, was anyone harmed? What happened as a result of this breach of confidentiality? What else might have happened? How could this situation have been prevented?

REALITY CHECK

Learning to communicate in an effective, professional manner is the basis of your reputation as a health care professional. Whether you're communicating with someone in person or by telephone, fax, e-mail, or texting, the words that you use and the nonverbal messages that you send reveal aspects of your personality, personal values, and the training you've undergone. While technology certainly facilitates communication, electronic communication also provides many opportunities for things to go wrong. The miscommunication of important information, or the failure to convey messages that are concise, accurate, timely, and courteous, can lead to major problems in health care. While the emergence of the Internet is a wondrous breakthrough that provides an amazing array of information and resources, you can't believe everything you find online. Learn to use good judgment in deciding which online information is accurate and which is not. Misuse of the Internet at work can get you in big trouble. You wouldn't be the first employee to get fired from his or her job for visiting inappropriate sites or wasting time surfing the Net during work hours.

Computerization has swept through the health care industry, providing state-of-the-art therapeutic, diagnostic, and business tools to support patient care. But computers are just that—tools. They enable health care workers and their patients to tackle medical challenges in ways that couldn't even be imagined in years past. But the *high tech* provided by computers will never replace the value of *high touch* provided by competent and caring professionals.

If you plan to become a health care professional yourself, start sharpening your interpersonal communication skills and your computer skills right now, while you're still in school. The information in this book, the assignments you're completing, and the guidance your teachers are offering all help in laying the foundation.

Key Points

- Develop effective skills in using electronic communication devices at work.
- Convey concise information, apply good listening skills, record accurate messages, and provide superior customer service when speaking on the telephone.
- Follow your employer's policies regarding personal telephone calls, texting, and Internet use at work.
- When you need to be certain that someone has received your message in an accurate manner, either meet with the person face-to-face or have a telephone conversation.
- Exercise care when sending and replying to e-mail messages.
- Examine the credibility of a website before believing and using the information found there.
- Familiarize yourself with the components of computers and how they function; keep this knowledge up-to-date as computers continue to evolve.
- Learn some basic computer skills now, and expect to continue developing new skills over the course of your career.
- Many of the therapeutic and diagnostic services provided by hospitals and other health care facilities rely heavily on computers.
- Computer-based tests and treatments improve the quality of care and reduce risks, pain, and discomfort for patients.
- Many of the business functions performed by health care employers are computer-based.
- Maintain the security of your organization's computers; don't share your passwords with anyone and change them frequently.
- Avoid downloading sensitive and private information on a laptop, PDA, or flash drive and removing the device from your worksite unless doing so is part of your job.
- Computers provide amazing tools for health care workers, but *high tech* can never replace the value of *high touch* provided by competent and caring health care professionals.

Section Review Questions

Answer each of the following questions. Indicate which page in the textbook led you to your answer.

1. Name two things you can do to promote customer service when speaking on the telephone.
2. List three things you should do when taking a telephone message.
3. What should you do when sending someone a fax containing confidential information?
4. Explain how the Internet is a useful tool in health care.
5. Why should you avoid sarcasm and humor in e-mail messages?
6. Name two devices for inputting.
7. Which part of a computer processes information?
8. List two examples of how computers are used in therapeutic and diagnostic services.
9. Explain why contingency plans are necessary when using computers.
10. List two ways to protect the security of computers at work.

Learn By Doing

Complete Worksheets 1–5 in Section 3.2 of your *Student Activity Guide*.

Health Information Technology and Communication

SECTION 3.3

Background

As you might imagine, the most important communication in health care involves patient information and the patients' medical records. Health care workers must be skilled in collecting, organizing, managing, storing, and using medical information. The information contained in patient records needs to be accessed by, and shared with, the people and organizations who are involved in providing the care.

Hospitals and provider networks are increasingly moving from paper medical records to computerized electronic records. Observing patients, documenting information in medical records, using data via charts and graphs, and sharing information with others through medical terminology and written and oral communication are important responsibilities for health care workers. Depending on the occupation you choose, you may be involved in some or all of these activities.

Objectives

After completing this section, you will be able to:

1. Define the key terms.
2. List two functions and two benefits of health information technology.
3. List the four types of information contained in patient records.
4. Differentiate between subjective and objective observations.
5. List two advantages and two disadvantages of electronic health records.

6. Explain the roles of the root word, prefix, and suffix in medical terminology.
7. Describe why correct spelling is so important when using medical terms.
8. List four elements of effective written communication.
9. Explain the benefit of using charts, graphs, and tables in written documents.
10. List four elements of effective oral presentations.

HEALTH INFORMATION TECHNOLOGY AND MANAGEMENT

Information technology (IT) is spreading rapidly throughout the health care industry to improve the quality of patient care, reduce mistakes and errors, increase efficiency, reduce costs, and expand access to health care services. Health information technology (HIT) uses computer-based hardware and software systems and communication systems to acquire, store, transmit, and use medical and health information. Health informatics is the field of study that uses information technology to store, retrieve, and manage biomedical information, data, and knowledge to aid in patient care, problem-solving, and decision-making. As health information is stored and shared electronically, special care must be taken to protect the privacy and security of confidential medical information.

Let's begin by examining the types of information that need to be included in patient records.

Consider This *Careers in Health Information Technology*

If you like working with information and computers, you might consider a career in health information technology. Employment in this field is expected to increase by twenty percent by the year 2018. This above-average employment outlook is based on the rise of electronic health records and the growing need to keep patient information secure and confidential. Job openings can be found in hospitals, outpatient centers, physician practices, and so forth. Unlike many other health occupations, health information professionals have no direct, hands-on contact with patients. Most enter the field with at least an associate's degree, and all health information workers must have good computer skills.

Health information technicians, also known as medical records technicians, assemble and organize patient records. They manage health information data to ensure accuracy and security, and they communicate with other health care workers to clarify information and gather additional details. Health information technicians interact with software programs and computer systems and provide support for health information networks.

Health information technicians may specialize to become medical coders. Medical coders examine patient records to identify the patient's diagnosis and the procedures he or she has undergone. Using several classification systems, they assign a *code* that determines how much reimbursement the hospital, physician, or organization will receive for providing the patient's care.

Several professional credentials are available for health information technicians and medical coders. With more education and additional certifications, health information technicians and medical coders may specialize and advance into health information management roles.

PATIENT RECORDS

Patient records provide a detailed history of the "who, what, when, where, why, and how" regarding a patient's receipt of health care services. Who provided the care? What type of care was rendered? When and where was the care provided, and why and how was the patient treated, or not treated? These records must be accurate, complete, clear, and current. Because patient records may be needed for legal purposes, they must be well organized and based on facts instead of the personal opinions of caregivers. When legal questions arise, attorneys and medical experts use patient records to determine if the standard of care was met.

standard of care (STAN-derd ov KAIR) The type of care that would be reasonably expected under similar situations

Medical records typically contain four kinds of information:

1. ***Patient information.*** This includes personal information, such as the patient's name, address, date of birth, gender, and other details about the patient's identification.
2. ***Medical information.*** This includes a medical history of the patient and his or her family, physical examination results, diagnostic test results (e.g., lab tests, radiographs), prescribed medications, treatment details, and so forth. Medical information includes the patient's chief complaint, which is the primary reason why the patient sought medical care, and his or her diagnosis, when applicable. Records for hospitalized patients may include discharge plans, social worker reports, and treatment records from specialists.

chief complaint (CHEEF kuhm-PLAYNT) The primary reason why a patient seeks medical care

RECENT DEVELOPMENTS
Digital Paperwork

Health care providers rely on information from admittance forms, patient histories, lab forms, insurance forms, and much more to make both the medical and business parts of the organization successful. Currently, most of these forms are completed by using a paper form and pen. Information on paper forms has limited usefulness, however, so, in many cases, someone transcribes, or copies, the written information to a computer.

Periodically, new forms are completed on patients, and that information must also be entered into the computer system. Transcribing all this information represents an enormous amount of staff time that might be better spent on patient care. It also increases the possibility of errors being introduced as the information is copied. New digitalized systems are emerging to simplify and streamline the process. Some of it is already being seen in many facilities.

Tablet PCs, for example, have special light-weight and portable slate display screens. The forms appear on the screens and can be written on with a special pen, or stylus. Handwriting recognition software reads the handwriting. Information is instantly digitalized and can be transferred to the computer system without the need for separate transcribing. Another new technology even eliminates the display screen with special paper and digital pens. Patients simply fill out the medical forms as they normally do. The digital pens record the information as patients write. Again, the laborious manual transcription from paper forms to computer is eliminated.

How can a digitalized system like one of these improve the quality of patient care?

Victory Medical Center
4100 SW Highway 6
Victorville, WA 12345
(509) 555-9832

Patient Name: ____________________
Last Name First Name Middle Initial

Address: ____________________
Street City State Zip

Home Phone: __________ Work Phone: __________

Mobile Phone: __________ Birthdate: __________

Social Security Number: __________ Age:

Sex: ______ Marital Status: S M D W Children: __________

How do you prefer to be addressed? __________

Spouse's Name: __________

Primary Care Physician: __________ Phone No.: __________

Name of Person Responsible for Bill: __________

Relationship to Patient: __________ Phone No.: __________

Address of Person Responsible for Bill: __________

Patient's Employer: __________ Phone No.: __________

Occupation: __________

Spouse's Employer: __________ Phone No.: __________

Occupation: __________

INSURANCE INFORMATION

Primary Insurance: __________ Policy No.: __________

Name of Policyholder: __________ Birthdate: __________

SS#: __________ Relationship to Insured: __________

Secondary Insurance: __________ Policy No.: __________

Name of Policyholder: __________ Birthdate: __________

If Injured: Date: __________ Place: __________

Claim Number: __________ Nature or Cause of Injury: __________

Employer at Time of Injury: __________ Phone No.: __________

EMERGENCY INFORMATION

In case of emergency, local friend or relative to be notified (not living at same address)

Name: __________ Relationship to Patient: __________

Address: __________ Phone No.: __________

I hereby authorize the healthcare professionals in this clinic to diagnose and treat my condition. I clearly understand and agree that all services rendered me are charged directly to me and that I am personally responsible for payment. I agree that I am responsible for all bills incurred at this clinic. I hereby authorize assignment of my insurance rights and benefits directly to the provider for services rendered. I also authorize the healthcare professionals to discuss my care with other healthcare providers who I am currently treating with.

__________ __________

Patient's Signature Date Parent or Guardian Signature Date

FIGURE 3.15

Sample patient medical history form

Martin County Medical Clinic
2413 NW Greenlake Ave.
Westford, CA 12745

AUTHORIZATION TO RELEASE INFORMATION

ACKNOWLEDGMENT OF RECEIPT of the Notice of Privacy Practices of the Martin County Medical Clinic (MCMC)

I acknowledge that I have received or been offered the Notice of Privacy Practices of the Martin County Medical Clinic. I understand that the Notice describes the uses and disclosures of my protected health information by the Covered Entities and informs me of my rights with respect to my protected health information.

____

Name of Patient

____

Patient Date of Birth

____

Signature of Patient or Personal Representative

____

Printed Name of Patient or Personal Representative

____

Date

If Personal Representative, indicate relationship:

____

Declinations

_______ The Individual declined to accept a copy of the Notice of Privacy Practices.

_______ The Individual received a copy of the Notice of Privacy Practices but declined to sign an Acknowledgment of Receipt.

____

Signature of MCMC Healthcare Representative

____

Name of MCMC Healthcare Representative

FIGURE 3.16
Sample HIPAA Release of Information Authorization Form

3. ***Social information.*** This includes personal information, such as race and ethnicity, hobbies and sports activities, and lifestyle factors such as sexual habits, smoking, and the use of drugs and alcohol.
4. ***Financial information.*** This includes health insurance details, correspondence about billing and insurance payments, and the history and status of the patient's financial transactions with the provider. (Financial information and medical information are often stored in separate records.)

documentation
(DAH-cue-men-TAY-shuhn) A record of something

observations
(ob-ser-VAY-shuhns) Something that is noted

chart
(CHAHRT) To write observations or records of patient care

legible
(LE-je-buhl) Handwriting that can be read and accurately interpreted by another person

concise
(kuhn-SISE) Expressed in few words

Several forms may also be filed in patient records. These include verification that patients have been informed of, and agree to, the provider's policies regarding confidentiality and the release of patient information (HIPAA form).

When adding medical information to patient records, health care professionals must take great care with their **documentation** to ensure that **observations** about the patient are noted correctly. Any unusual event or change in a patient must be reported verbally and then documented in the patient's record. There are two types of observations:

1. ***Subjective.*** Subjective observations cannot be seen. They are ideas, thoughts, or opinions. If you cannot see it, feel it, hear it, or smell it, it is a subjective observation. (*Example:* If the patient complains of pain, you cannot see the pain, nor feel it, hear it, nor smell it.)
2. ***Objective.*** Objective observations can be seen. If you can see it, feel it, hear it, or smell it, it is an objective observation. (*Example:* If the patient has a cut, you can see the cut.)

When you document, or **chart**, information consider the following:

- Note the care or treatment given.
- Identify the time of the treatment.
- Indicate how the patient tolerated the care or treatment.
- Include observations that might be helpful to other caregivers.
- Include relevant information that was provided by the patient.
- Entries must be **legible**; it's best to print the information.
- Use short phrases rather than complete sentences; entries should be **concise**, clear, and meaningful.
- Remember, if the care provided was not documented, then (legally) it was presumed not done.

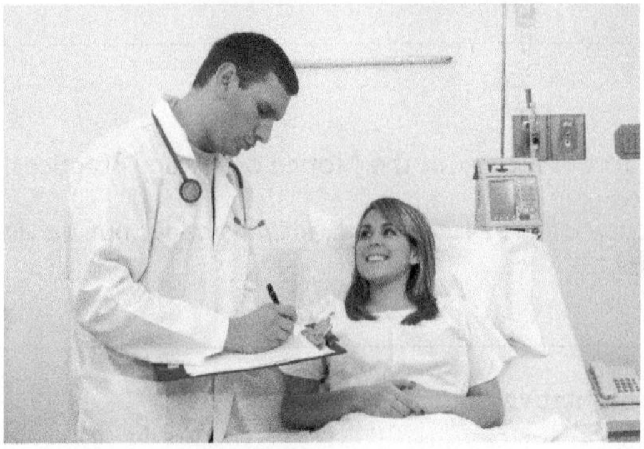

FIGURE 3.17
Doctor documenting patient observations
Source: Reflekta/Shutterstock

confidential
(kon-fi-DEN-shuhl) Limited to persons authorized to use information or documents

Workers must comply with a wide range of policies and procedures that govern the storage, use, and disposal of patient records. Patient records are private and **confidential**. The information contained in a patient's medical record, and the medical record itself, cannot be shared with other people without the patient's permission. This includes sharing information with *third parties*, such as the patient's health insurance company. The patient and his or her physician will decide when, and if, the patient's family can have access to the patient's medical information.

Many health care providers, including small and rural facilities and independent physician practices, continue to use patient charts recorded on paper and stored in files. However, this practice is changing due to incentives and penalties that encourage electronic records. Other providers, especially urban hospitals and their networks, are increasingly transferring to electronic records.

APPLY IT MEDICAL TERMS ON TV

Health care practices and procedures require a special vocabulary that could be considered another language. Watch a health care related television program and jot down some of the medical terms you hear. Try to guess the definitions and write them down next to each term. Then find the terms in a medical dictionary and record their real definitions. Were you able to correctly guess some of the meanings? Were you close to spelling the terms correctly? Do you think the terms were used accurately in the television program?

ELECTRONIC HEALTH RECORDS

Electronic health records (EHRs), also known as electronic medical records (EMRs), have been in limited use since the 1960s. In the U.S., the push is now on to convert paper files to computer files by the year 2014. EHRs are becoming increasingly common in hospitals, doctors' offices, and clinics where patient information needs to be shared quickly and frequently among providers at several different locations.

When patients move among doctors' offices, specialists, clinics, and hospitals, their medical information needs to travel with them. This mobility is only possible through the use of technology. When providers can access comprehensive, up-to-date information on each patient, the quality and continuity of care increases, and the cost associated with unnecessary duplication of tests (lab tests and radiographs, for example) decreases. Several advantages of EHRs include that they:

- ***Save paper and space.*** Instead of keeping paper files on patients, health care providers maintain patients' medical records in computer files, which save space and reduce the cost of paper.

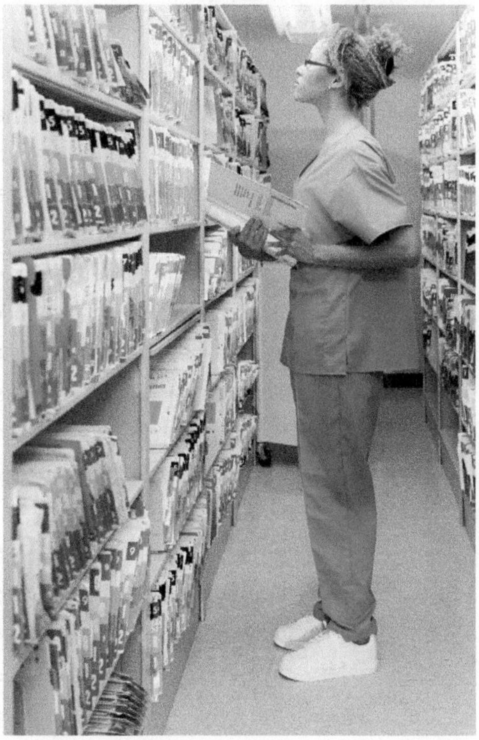

FIGURE 3.18

Filing and retrieving paper medical records

Source: Getty Images USA, Inc.

- ***Enhance coordination.*** All members of the patient's health care team, regardless of their locations, have access to the same medical information. They can see what other team members are doing to care for the patient as they develop their own treatment plans.
- ***Improve quality.*** When patients are being treated by several specialists at the same time, there's a risk that one doctor might prescribe a drug that is incompatible with the drugs prescribed by another doctor. Using EHRs, each doctor can see what the patient's other doctors are prescribing. This is just one example of quality improvement via EHRs.
- ***Reduce delays.*** When doctors need to review a patient's paper medical records, someone must first copy, mail, and fax or scan and e-mail those pages to other locations. This takes time and can delay the patient's tests and treatments. But when

THE MORE YOU KNOW

Metric Units in the United States

Patient records and other medical information often contain measurements that are documented via the metric system. Health care workers need a basic understanding of the metric system in order to complete daily tasks. Similar to learning a new language, it takes some practice to become comfortable converting to metric units.

Most nations around the world use metric units every day. In these countries, distances are measured in kilometers; lengths are measured in centimeters and millimeters, and volumes are measured in liters and milliliters. In the United States, we use standard units, such as miles, feet, inches, and ounces. If the metric system is so widely used, why doesn't the U.S. use it?

In fact, the 1970s saw a large push in the U.S. to change over to metric measurements. The government sponsored research studies that indicated the U.S. would eventually join the rest of the world in using metric measurements. However, this change still hasn't occurred, and fewer people are interested in making it happen. The metric system is only regularly used by people in science and medicine, mathematics, industry, and the military.

Part of the reason the U.S. has not converted to the metric system is that the public simply doesn't use these measurements regularly. Also, the transition would be expensive. For example, any sign indicating distance in miles along a highway would need to be replaced. Because the U.S. has not converted to the metric system, we have occasionally run into problems. For example, the Mars Climate Orbiter project failed because one of the contractors on the project used standard measurements. Everyone else who was working on the project used metric measurements. Because of the error, the orbiter burned up in the atmosphere of Mars.

Even though metric measurements are not always used in the U.S., they can still be found on everyday items such as food labels. Many cosmetics, drinks, and nutritional supplements rely on the metric system. Several sports events, such as track and field, are measured in kilometers and meters rather than miles and feet. Some organizations are still lobbying for the U.S. to use the metric system. It remains to be seen if we will ever make the transition.

What is a benefit of using the metric system?

doctors use technology to gain immediate access to records, tests and treatments can begin much sooner. This is especially important in emergency situations when response time is critical.

- ***Ensure legibility.*** Hand-written doctors' orders and treatment notes can be difficult to read, sometimes leading to confusion or mistakes. When orders and treatment notes are typed into an electronic record, illegible hand-writing is no longer a concern, but typos can still occur.

As with most technologic advancements, EHRs also have some disadvantages; these include:

- ***Training time and anxiety.*** Doctors, nurses, and other health care workers must be trained to use computerized records. Undergoing training and mastering new skills take time and this can cause a backlog in caring for patients until the staff is up-to-speed with the new technology. Some people, especially older workers, may resist having to learn new skills and this can lead to anxiety and frustration.
- ***System incompatibility.*** Currently, no universal EHR exist, and the different systems won't interact with one another. This is one reason why health care providers are joining networks, so that all members within the network can use the same electronic systems.
- ***Security concerns.*** Having medical information stored on computers raises concerns about potential security issues and the accidental release of private information. When storing, transmitting, and transporting medical records electronically, strict security measures must be followed to avoid a breach in confidentiality.

Not all medical facilities have the funds and training available to implement electronic medical data systems; however, the systems will gradually become more affordable and, therefore, more accessible over time. The long-term benefits of electronic health records will most likely be worth the investment.

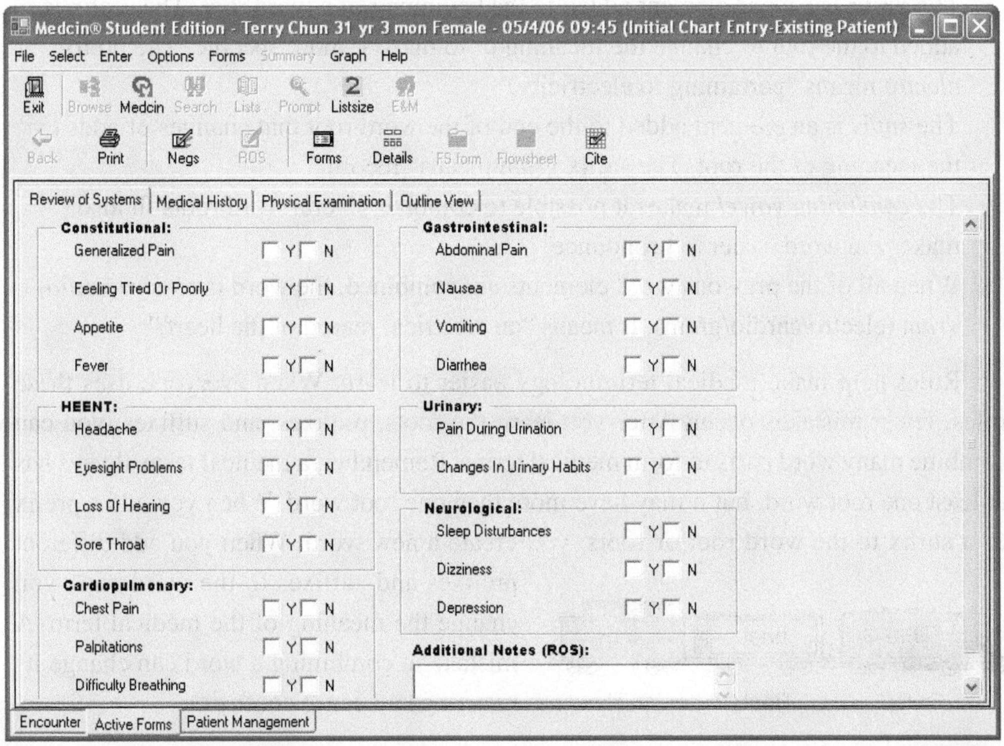

FIGURE 3.19

An intake screen in an electronic medical record

Language Arts Link Health Terms Dictionary

Sometimes a step towards learning a new vocabulary term is to write it out yourself, rather than just reading its definition in a textbook or looking it up in the dictionary. As you work through this course, you may find it beneficial to create your own dictionary of terms and definitions. If you have access to a computer, you can sort the terms alphabetically as you enter them. This will make looking up terms easier later. If you do not have computer access, you can use a small notebook to make your dictionary. Go back through the first chapters in this text and enter the key terms and definitions in your dictionary. Continue making entries as you complete the course. After you've completed your dictionary, you will have that as a reference tool as you continue your health care studies.

MEDICAL TERMINOLOGY

When you examine patient records and other types of medical information, you'll find that health care workers communicate in a different language called medical terminology. Caregivers use medical terminology every day to communicate effectively and quickly, and to record physician orders, write instructions, take notes, and document in patient charts.

Medical terminology can be interesting and challenging. At first, medical terminology may seem difficult to learn; however, with practice it becomes easier and easier. You'll need to learn how to build a medical term, how to pronounce it, and what it means. If you've never heard medical terms pronounced, they may seem very difficult to say out loud. But once you realize that medical terms are just words composed of several parts, you'll be on your way to learning the parts and how to combine them. Consider the following:

- All medical terms have a *word root.* The word root is the main part of the word and tells what the word is about. For instance, *cardio* is the root word that means "heart." This is the subject of the word you are going to build.
- The *prefix* is a word element added to the beginning of a word root. The prefix is added to the root to change the meaning or to make it more specific. The prefix *electro* means "pertaining to electricity."
- The *suffix* is an element added to the end of the word root that changes or adds to the meaning of the root. The suffix *gram* means "record."
- The *combining vowel* makes it possible to combine several word roots. It also makes the word easier to pronounce.
- When all of the previous word elements are combined, the word is *electrocardiogram* (electro/cardio/gram). It means "an electrical record of the heart."

Rules help make medical terminology easier to learn. When everyone uses these rules, fewer mistakes occur. After you learn the roots, prefixes, and suffixes, you can combine many word parts to form medical terms. Remember, a medical term always has at least one root word, but it may have more than one root word. When you add a prefix or a suffix to the word root or roots, you create a new word. When you add different prefixes and suffixes to the word root, you change the meaning of the medical term. A mistake in combining a word can change its meaning and cause confusion.

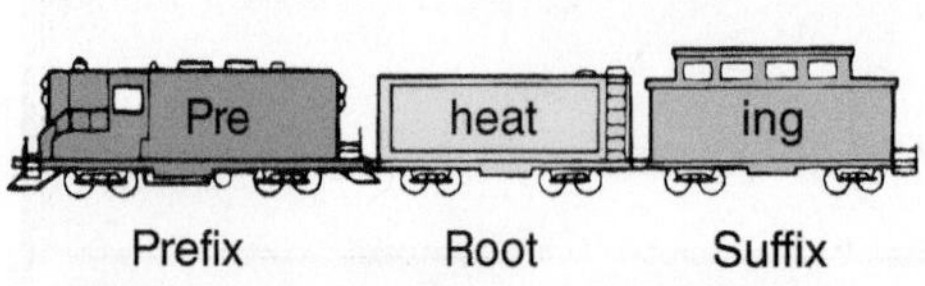

FIGURE 3.20
Combining word parts to form a medical term

Maria Fernandez-Raul, MD

Woodway Family Practice
2413 NW Greenlake Ave.
Milford, CA 12345

OPERATION DATE: 8/11/08
PATIENT: ADAM PARCHER
SURGEON: MARIA FERNANDEZ-RAUL, MD

PREOPERATIVE DIAGNOSIS:

Congenital external nasal deformity.

POSTOPERATIVE DIAGNOSIS:

Congenital external nasal deformity.

PROCEDURE:

Aesthetic rhinoplasty

DESCRIPTION OF PROCEDURE:

The patient is a 33-year-old male who presented with concerns for nasal airway obstruction and discontent with the external appearance of his nose. Examination confirms the above-noted concerns with a widened nasal base, palpable and visible dorsal cartilage and nasal bones.

Correction of the external deformity by open rhinoplasty, lowering of the dorsum, lowering of the cartilaginous dorsum, narrowing of the nasal bones, resection and narrowing of the nasal tip, excision of caudal septum and nasal spine were discussed. The nature of the procedures and risks, including bleeding, hematoma, infection, poor wound healing, scarring, asymmetry, airway difficulties, palpable or visible nasal structures, and possible need for secondary procedures were all discussed. The patient understands and wishes to proceed as outlined.

FINDINGS:

The patient underwent open rhinoplasty through a columellar chevron incision. The nose was copiously infiltrated with 1% lidocaine with epinephrine prior to incision. The chevron incision was incised and carried to bilateral rim incisions. The nasal skin was then degloved using sharp dissecting scissors. This was opened over the nose up to the root of the nose to allow full exposure. The irregular nasal bones were initially smoothed with a rasp. Excision of the dorsal nasal bone was then carried out using a straight guarded osteotome. Approximately 1 mm thickness of bone was removed. After osteotomy was completed from a low to high position, infracture of the nasal bones was carried out. This provided good narrowing of the nasal base. A small piece of septal cartilage was crushed and flattened using the cartilage crusher and this was placed over the nasal dorsum. Hemostasis was assured. The skin was redraped and closure was carried out using interrupted 6-0 Prolene for the columellar and stab incisions. Interrupted 5-0 plain gut sutures were used to close the rim incisions and the septal transfixion incision. Xeroform packs were removed and nasal splints were placed. A second set of Xeroform packs was placed lateral to the nasal splints. The dorsum of the nose was taped and a dorsal thermoplast splint was also placed. The procedure was well tolerated. The posterior throat was suctioned and a throat pack that had been placed at the beginning of the procedure was removed. The patient was awakened and extubated and discharged to the recovery room in stable condition.

Maria Fernandez-Raul, MD

FIGURE 3.21
Sample operative report using medical terminology

Knowing prefixes, roots, and suffixes makes it possible to write and decipher common medical and dental terms. For example, if you come across the term *tendonitis*, you can identify the root as *tendon* and the suffix *-itis*. Because this suffix means inflammation, *tendonitis* must describe an inflammation of a tendon. Now consider the term *arthroscope*. The root is *arthro*, meaning "joint," and the suffix is *-scope*, meaning "picture." An arthroscope is a diagnostic tool that gives physicians a way to take a picture, or form an image, of a structure inside the body, such as a knee. You can interpret a related term, *osteoarthritis*, in a similar way. To break this term into parts, find the prefix, root, and suffix. The root is *arthro*, meaning "joint." The prefix is *osteo-*, meaning "bone," and the suffix is *-itis*, meaning "inflammation." By putting the parts of the term together, you can figure out that *osteoarthritis* is an inflammation of the bone's joint.

Correct spelling is extremely important in medical terminology. Changing just one or two letters in a medical term can completely change its meaning. *Ileum* and *ilium* is a classic example. The pronunciation is the same, but ileum is part of the small intestine, and ilium is part of the hip. Just one single letter makes a huge difference in this example. Another example of the need for accurate spelling is the difference between *atherosclerosis* and *arteriosclerosis*. Atherosclerosis is the accumulation of fatty plaque in blood vessels. Arteriosclerosis is hardening of the walls of arteries. Based on the spelling and pronunciation, it's easy to understand how these two terms could be confused. But the two medical conditions are different and require unique treatment plans. As with other languages, it's important to communicate in a clear and accurate manner when using medical terminology. Otherwise, patient care and patient safety may suffer.

Depending on the occupation you choose, you may need to demonstrate mastery of medical terminology. It's never too early to learn some word parts and combine them to expand your vocabulary.

APPLY IT CREATING MEDICAL TERMS

Divide into teams of two to three students. Organize a word game in which one team creates a medical term using a prefix, root word, and a suffix. The other team has to break down the term into its component parts, guess what the term means, and decide if it's a real medical term. Use a medical dictionary to check the accuracy of your answers. Then reverse the roles and play again.

MEDICAL WRITING

Health care workers must be able to communicate effectively in writing. Some jobs rely more on written communication than others, but almost everyone can benefit from improving their writing skills. In addition to jotting down telephone messages, communicating by e-mail, and documenting patient information in charts and other records, health care workers need effective writing skills in order to compose:

- Memos, letters, and other correspondence
- Patient education materials
- Business reports

- Meeting agendas and notes
- Technical information
- Financial proposals
- Planning documents
- Research findings

There are several elements of effective written communication to keep in mind; these include:

- ***Appearance.*** Documents should be professional in appearance and easy to read.
- ***Content.*** Information should be accurate, up-to-date, and appropriate for intended readers.
- ***Professionalism.*** The appearance and content of the document should reflect the professionalism of the writer and his or her employer.
- ***Relevance:*** Documents should convey material that is interesting, meaningful, and of value to readers.
- ***Sources.*** Content should be factual and based on credible sources of information; when appropriate, sources should be referenced.
- ***Organization.*** Information should be concise, well organized, and include a brief introduction and summary.
- ***Terminology.*** Documents should use language and terminology that readers can easily understand and interpret.
- ***Mechanics.*** Writing should reflect proper spelling, grammar, and punctuation.
- ***Illustrations.*** Documents may include drawings, photographs, graphs, charts, tables, and so forth to help describe or explain the content.
- ***Compliance.*** Content must follow guidelines and meet legal requirements.
- ***Distribution/Access.*** Access to documents that contain confidential and private information should be limited to authorized readers.

Language Arts Link — Writing at Work

Your first job may not require much written communication, but if you expect to advance in your health career, you'll need effective writing skills. Choose a health care subject that's of interest to you, and do some research to learn more about it. Identify an aspect of your subject that you would like to explain to someone else via a written report.

Write your objective—a brief statement that describes what you want to communicate or accomplish. (For example, the objective of this paragraph is to "create an activity to help students improve their writing skills.") Think about your objective and the information you will need to cover to accomplish it. What is the *core message* that you want to convey? Think about your readers. How much do they know about the subject? What's the best way to engage their interest and help them learn more?

Before you start writing your report, compose an outline that lists each topic you want to cover, and list your topics in a logical order. Using your outline, write a report to accomplish your objective. Refer to the guidelines for effective written communication provided in this section of your textbook. Check for proper spelling, grammar, and punctuation. Print your report on 8.5″ × 11″ white paper and make sure it presents a professional image.

Exchange your report with a classmate, ask for feedback, and make revisions to improve the accuracy, clarity, completeness, and appearance of your document.

Did you accomplish your objective? Why, or why not? How can you tell?

subject line
(SUB-jekt line) A statement describing the subject of a letter

salutation
(sal-yuh-TAY-shuhn) Greeting

body
(BOD-ee) The main part of a letter or other written document

closing
(KLOH-zing) The ending portion of letter

font
(FONT) Style of type

letterhead
(LEH-ter-hed) Professional stationery imprinted with business contact information

logo
(LOE-go) Graphic image that represents a company or organization

proofread
(PROOF-reed) Reviewing a document for errors

spell check
(SPELL-chec) Software that verifies the correct spelling of words

thesaurus
(thi-SAWR-uhs) Reference source for locating alternate words with similar meanings

PDR
(pee-dee-are) *Physician's Desk Reference*; contains information on medical diseases, conditions, and drugs

executive summary
(ig-ZEH-cue-tiv SUM-uh-ree) A brief overview listing the major points of a business document

Here are some tips to improve your written communication:

- Keep your goals in mind. Know what you're trying to accomplish, and the reason why.
- Know your audience. Identify whom you want to reach, the best way to reach them, and the reactions you are hoping to receive.
- Create an outline. Organize your thoughts, identify the topics, and list your information in the proper sequence.
- Use complete sentences. Use words for numbers one through ten (such as *five*). Use numbers for quantities of 11 or more (such as *25).*
- For letters, include all of the proper components. This includes the date, **subject line**, **salutation**, **body** of the letter, **closing**, signature, and the sender's contact information.
- Use plain white paper and a standard black **font**.
- Print your document, such as a letter, on company or organization **letterhead** when appropriate.
- Follow company or organization policies when using a **logo** in a document.
- **Proofread** your work. Have another person review your document before sending or submitting it in case you missed something.
- Use **spell check**, but don't rely on it. Spell check won't catch words that are spelled correctly but used incorrectly. For example, the words *to*, *too*, and *two* will all pass as correctly spelled, however each word has a different meaning. Spell check may not work when it comes to medical terms.
- Use references such as a regular dictionary, a medical dictionary, a **thesaurus**, and a **Physician's Desk Reference (PDR)**.
- Use only standard medical abbreviations to avoid confusion.
- Do not use texting (text messaging) abbreviations.
- For long documents, include an **executive summary** and one or more separate attachments to reduce the length of the body.
- Include contact information and *next steps* to assist the reader in following up, if appropriate.

Depending on your job, your written documents may include charts, graphs, or tables. These illustrations help readers better understand the relationships between numbers and other data, and give meaning to information. Pie charts are a classic example. A pie chart provides a visual picture showing how different percentages, for example, compare with one another. The whole pie represents 100 percent. If the pie is split into two equal amounts, each portion represents 50 percent. When the pie is split into several sections, each representing a different percentage, the reader can quickly interpret the information. Printing each section in a different color would lead to an even quicker analysis. Charts, graphs, and tables can be constructed on paper or via computer software. Health care workers should not only be familiar with how to create charts, graphs, and tables but also how to use and interpret them.

PUBLIC SPEAKING

No discussion about communication in health care would be complete without addressing the topic of public speaking. Few challenges in life are more anxiety-producing than having to get up in front of a group of people and make a presentation. But public speaking

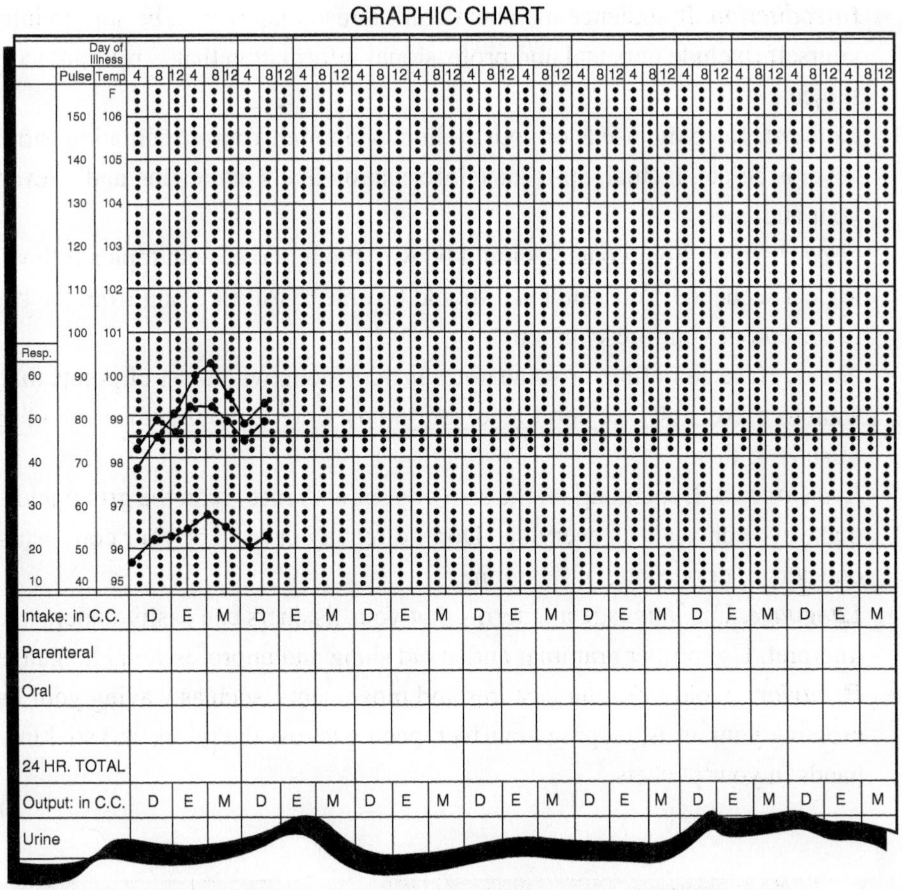

FIGURE 3.22
Graphic chart tracking patient information

skills are important, especially if your job requires you to give updates at meetings, make announcements to the rest of the staff, or teach coworkers something new. You may be invited to speak at a workshop or conference as a representative of your organization or your professional group, so developing your oral communication skills is important.

Becoming comfortable with public speaking is like facing any other fear—the more you do it, the better you'll get, and the more comfortable you will become. Start out small, with a group of supportive people, and build from there. Make sure you're well prepared, organized, and familiar with your subject matter. Learn as much about your audience in advance as you can and tailor your presentation to meet their needs. Expect questions and comments; have your responses in mind. It's okay to admit that you're nervous. Most of the people in the audience will be glad it's you up in front of the group instead of them.

Here's some helpful information about the elements of effective oral presentations:

- ***Room set-up.*** Arrange the room so that audience members can easily see you, hear you, and view any visual aids that you might be using.
- ***Goals.*** Keep your goals in mind and make sure your audience knows what they are. If you want your audience to focus on something specific, make your intent clear.
- ***Handouts.*** If you're using an agenda and/or handouts, provide them in advance or at the beginning of your presentation. Allow space on the pages for people to take notes if they wish to do so. Depending on the setting, you might want to provide notepads and pens.

- ***Introduction.*** If audience members don't already know you, be sure to introduce yourself. Include personal and professional information that is relevant to your subject.
- ***Content.*** Keep the needs of your audience in mind. Your presentation should cover accurate, factual, up-to-date information that's interesting and relevant to your audience.
- ***Organization.*** Your content should be well thought out, with topics following a logical sequence. Your audience should be able to follow along from the beginning to the end of your presentation.
- ***Notes.*** Have an outline or some notes handy, along with a list of points that you want to make, however don't read your notes. Look at your audience and speak directly to them.
- ***Eye Contact.*** Depending on the size of your audience, scan the group and try to make eye contact with everyone. Don't direct all or most of your comments to just one person or one side of the room.
- ***Language.*** Use language and terms that your listeners can easily understand and interpret. Use proper grammar and avoid slang and unprofessional language.
- ***Behavior.*** Avoid irritating gestures and movements, such as waving your hands, crossing your arms, tapping your feet, pacing across the room, and sticking your hands in your pockets.

BUILD YOUR SKILLS *Public Speaking*

Based on surveys, people fear public speaking even more than getting cancer or dying! Learning to give effective oral presentations is just like developing any other skill—you need practice and more practice to become competent and confident.

Many opportunities exist to help you develop your skills. The formal route would be to join an organization such as Toastmasters International. In operation since 1924, Toastmasters has 13,000 clubs in 116 countries. Clubs hold sixty to ninety minute meetings weekly, biweekly, or monthly depending on the location. Instead of listening to lectures by an instructor, Toastmaster participants complete a series of "speaking assignments" to improve their public speaking skills.

Members give presentations and lead meetings in a "no-pressure atmosphere" and receive helpful feedback from other members. To learn more about Toastmasters International, go to www.toastmasters.org.

Other options for developing your public speaking skills include volunteering to serve on committees at school and in your community. Committee work often includes leading discussions, facilitating meetings, and giving informal reports. You could join a student organization or a health care professional group. Several activities in this text and in your *Student Activity Guide* include giving brief reports to your classmates and teacher.

If the thought of public speaking scares you, there's no time like the present to start building your skills. Who knows? You may one day become a highly-paid, in-demand public speaker yourself.

- ***Visuals.*** Use PowerPoint slides, handouts, or other visual aids that will help audience members understand your comments.
- ***Participation.*** Encourage audience participation whenever possible. Engaging people will help you hold their attention, and they will be more likely to remember what happened during the session.
- ***Group dynamics.*** Manage questions and comments by audience members; don't let a few people control the discussion or consume too much time.
- ***Rules.*** Stay within your allotted amount of time. If you end your presentation too early, you'll look unprepared. If you run too long, you'll inconvenience other speakers and your audience members. If your presentation is sponsored by a company or organization that has guidelines for its speakers, make sure you follow them.

Here are some tips to improve your oral presentation skills:

- Practice your presentation ahead of time. Ask family members or friends to serve as audience members and give you some helpful feedback.
- A few days before your presentation, stop by the room where you will be speaking. Familiarize yourself with the layout of the room and the location of light switches and other controls. If possible, practice using the microphone, projection equipment, and audio controls.
- Provide a comfortable environment for your audience. Make sure the room isn't too hot or too cold. If your presentation is scheduled during meal time, consider offering refreshments or encouraging people to bring their own.
- Arrange seating so that everyone may comfortably face the speaker. If people are seated at round tables, encourage them to turn their chairs around to face the front of the room.
- If you're using visual aids that appear on a screen at the front of the room, don't turn your back on your audience. Have a copy of your visuals in front of you so you may continue to face your listeners.
- Make sure that handouts and visual aids are professional in appearance and content.
- When considering what to wear, remember these two statements: "When you look good, you feel good" and "Professional image is in the eye of the beholder." Dress comfortably and select clothing that's appropriate for the setting and the audience. What might the audience expect in terms of a professional image? Don't over-dress or under-dress for the occasion.
- Avoid over-used words and phrases such as "um," "uh," "like," and "you know."
- If you don't know the answer to an audience member's question, admit it. Offer to follow up with the person after the session.

FIGURE 3.23

Health care professional using her public speaking skills

Source: Carmen Martin/Pearson Education

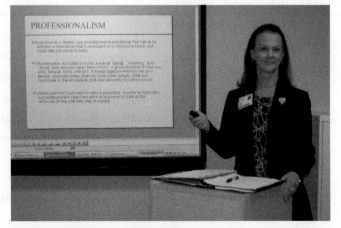

- Take advantage of the expertise within the audience. Members may have some good ideas and experience to share.
- Show your sense of humor. If you make a mistake, admit it and laugh at yourself.
- Keep the session moving. If you lose your place or forget what you were going to say, just move on. Chances are your audience won't realize what happened.

Some people are *born speakers*, while others are not. If you fall into the "not a born speaker" category, then expect sweaty palms, wobbly knees, shaky voice, and a stomach *tied in knots* until you become comfortable speaking in front of a group of people. A fear of public speaking can be detrimental to your career, so the sooner you start honing your public speaking skills, the better.

REALITY CHECK

When you are the patient, you want to be sure that your medical records are accurate and up-to-date. When you're seeing more than one doctor for the same illness or condition, you want all of your doctors to communicate and coordinate your care. This can be quite a challenge when doctors work in different locations and you have to travel from site to site. If your doctors and the organizations where they work have transitioned to electronic health records, communication and coordination become less challenging. When providers document their observations, enter information, and update your medical records in a timely manner, each of your caregivers can easily see what the others are doing to treat you. This speeds up your treatment plan and hopefully improves your outcomes.

If your job involves working with patient information, charts, and medical records you have to be very careful. Losing information, entering the wrong data, and misspelling medical terms are just a few examples of how your poor performance could have a major impact on patient care. The ability to concentrate and pay attention to details is crucial.

If you have the opportunity, take a medical terminology course. There's no better way to start *getting your feet wet* in health care than learning the language. Also work on strengthening your written and oral communication skills, as both will have an impact on your career, your opportunities for advancement, and your reputation as a health care professional.

Key Points

- Health information technology is spreading rapidly to improve quality of care, increase efficiency and access to services, and reduce errors and expense.
- Health informatics helps convert information into knowledge, leading to improvements in patient care, problem-solving, and decision-making.
- Medical/health records contain patient information, medical information, social information, and financial information.
- Workers document both subjective and objective observations in patient records.
- Patient records must be accurate, factual, and up-to-date, and may be used in legal cases to determine if the standard of care was met.

- Patient records are private and confidential; the release of information requires the patient's permission.
- Organizations are transitioning to electronic health records; EHRs provide benefits for patients, but create some challenges for providers.
- Medical terminology is the language of medicine; medical terms are formed by combining root words, prefixes, and suffixes. Correctly spelling medical terms is critical.
- Health care workers need effective written communication skills to compose correspondence, business reports, patient education materials, and other documents.
- The need to speak in front of a group often leads to anxiety and fear, but health care workers need public speaking skills to give reports at staff meetings, make presentations at workshops and conferences, and so forth.

Section Review Questions

Answer each of the following questions. Indicate which page in the textbook led you to your answer.

1. Describe the role of health information technology.
2. List the four types of information contained in patient records.
3. List two advantages of electronic health records.
4. Explain why electronic health records raise concerns about confidentiality.
5. Describe why correct spelling is so important in medical terminology.
6. Give two reasons why health care workers need effective written communication skills.
7. List three things to remember when making oral presentations.

Learn By Doing

Complete Worksheets 1–5 in Section 3.3 of your *Student Activity Guide*.

CHAPTER 3 Review

Chapter Review Questions

Answer each of the following questions. Indicate which page in the textbook led you to your answer.

1. List the four elements required for communication to occur.
2. List three barriers to communication.
3. Explain why assertive communication is the best approach to resolving conflict.
4. List two ways to protect the security of computers at work.
5. Explain how laptop computers, PDAs, and flash drives could jeopardize the privacy of patient information.
6. List two disadvantages of electronic health records.
7. Explain how patient health records can help determine if the standard of care was met.
8. Name three things you could do to meet your audience's needs when giving an oral presentation.
9. Describe how charts, graphs, and tables can enhance the content of written documents.
10. Explain the role that health information technicians play in health care.

Chapter Review Activities

1. Think about why patient health records include *social information*. Develop a list of at least five examples that illustrate the connection between a patient's lifestyle factors and his or her health. Include factors such as hobbies and sports activities, sexual habits, smoking, and the use of drugs and alcohol.
2. How would you explain to a new employee the legal importance of clear and complete documentation? Create a bulleted list of points you would use in your explanation.
3. You are describing the functions of the telephone, fax, e-mail system, and the Internet to a new employee. How would you illustrate the proper use of each of these communication tools? Develop a list of do's and don'ts to share with your coworker.
4. Share some medical terms with someone who is not familiar with medical terminology. Show him or her how the terms combine root words, prefixes, and suffixes.

What If? Scenarios

What would you do in each of the following situations? Record your answer, explain it, and indicate which page in the textbook led you to your decision.

1. While providing care for an elderly patient in your clinic, you have explained three times the proper way for him to take his prescription drugs, but the patient just doesn't seem to understand.
2. You're beginning to get the impression that your performance at work isn't meeting expectations, but you aren't sure why. You met with your manager this morning, but all you could think about during the meeting was possibly getting fired.
3. One of your coworkers is hearing impaired. Although he's a highly skilled professional, it's difficult to communicate with him.
4. Your coworker has started leaving early without permission. You could finish your work and his if you had to, but you don't think it's fair.
5. Trying to remember all of your usernames and passwords for work and home is becoming a

chore. Keeping a written list in your wallet, or using the same passwords at work that you use at home, would make things easier.

6. As a research assistant, you need to create some graphs to include in a report that's due on Monday. It's already noon on Friday, and you still have some patient information to collect. You could copy all of the patient records on a flash drive and work at home over the weekend to finish your report.
7. Your manager just announced that your clinic will be converting to electronic health records within the next few months. Some of your coworkers are voicing their concerns about having to learn new equipment and software and are questioning management's decision.
8. You have been asked to give a presentation at next month's staff meeting to describe a new procedure in your department, but the thought of speaking in front of the group is keeping you awake at night.

Media Connection

Use the companion website for additional interactive learning activities.

Portfolio Connection

By now, your career portfolio should be taking shape. To organize your samples, use a three-ring notebook, three-ring pocket inserts, and tab dividers. This will enable you to add and exchange documents as you complete them. Keeping your file current shows your organizational skills and provides you immediate access to materials that reflect the positive results of your learning.

Create a tab with each of the following labels:

- Portfolio Introduction
- Résumé
- Project
- Writing sample
- Workplace Learning or Supervised Practical Experience
- Oral presentation
- Community Service or Service Learning
- CPR and First Aid
- Internet Application
- Leadership
- Journaling
- Other Content

Once your portfolio file is organized, start adding your samples. Include samples of your written documents and other assignments that you complete for this course and for other health care related courses. Add performance evaluations from current or previous jobs. Include any advice or insights that will help you in your career. When it comes time to share your portfolio with a prospective employer, you'll be using just certain documents. Other documents will be helpful solely for your personal use.

Keep your portfolio in a place that is easy to access. File portfolio items as soon as you complete them. If you have access to a computer, consider keeping an electronic portfolio as well as a hard copy version. You may create computer folders for different topics and save the portfolio to a flash drive if you are not using your own personal computer. Computerizing your portfolio will save space and paper and give you important practice in using a computer.

CHAPTER **4**

The Health Care Industry

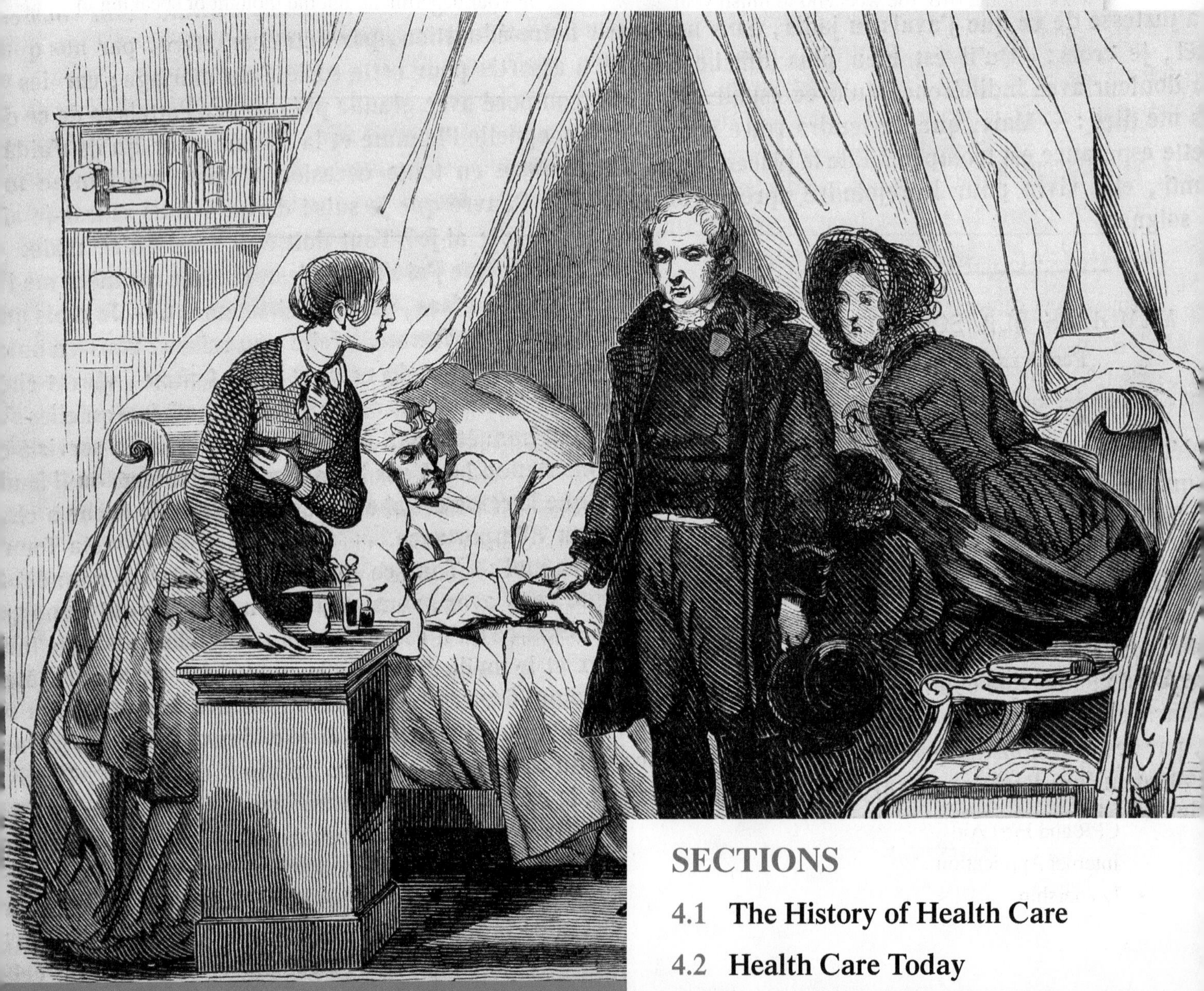

SECTIONS

Source: Antonio Abrignani/Shutterstock

"The joy of discovery is certainly the liveliest that the mind of man can ever feel."

CLAUDE BERNARD, FRENCH PHYSIOLOGIST, 1813–1878

GETTING STARTED

As you will learn in this chapter, many people have contributed to finding the causes and cures of illnesses, injuries, and other disabling conditions. Others have identified different body parts and their functions. Some notable discoveries include Louis Pasteur's identification of the process that makes milk safe for human consumption. This process is called pasteurization, in honor of its inventor. Bartolommeo Eustachio discovered the tube leading from the ear to the throat, an important finding that was named the Eustachian tube after its discoverer. Other discoveries include the Salk vaccine to prevent polio (named after Dr. Jonas Salk) and the Roentgen Ray (now called x-ray) after Wilhelm Roentgen, its discoverer. Imagine you could find a cure for, or identify a cause of, a disease or illness such as cancer, juvenile arthritis, hepatitis C, autism, or asthma. Write the condition and your cure (or its cause) on a 3″ × 5″ card. Name and share your discovery with the class. Why did you choose this particular disease or condition?

The History of Health Care

SECTION 4.1

Background

Health care has developed and changed throughout history. Knowing the history of health care helps you understand current procedures, practices, and philosophies. The experiences and discoveries of the past led to the advances of today. Today's achievements could not have occurred without the trials and errors of the past. When you understand the primitive beginnings of medicine, you appreciate the advances made during the past 5,000 years.

Objectives

After completing this section, you will be able to:

1. Define the key terms.
2. Identify three scientists and explain what they contributed to medicine.
3. Choose one era in the history of health care and explain how medical knowledge and technology changed during that time.
4. Describe the role of Florence Nightingale in advancing the role of nursing.
5. List two trends that led to the emergence of the allied health professions.
6. Give two examples of allied health professions.
7. Name two advances in medicine in the twentieth century.
8. Identify a possible advancement in medicine for the twenty-first century.
9. List two ethical questions or problems resulting from medical advancements.

EARLY BEGINNINGS

Primitive human beings had no electricity, few tools, and poor shelter. Their time was spent protecting themselves against **predators** and finding food. They were **superstitious** and believed that illness and disease were caused by supernatural spirits. In an attempt to

primitive
(PRI-meh-tiv) Ancient or prehistoric

predators
(PREH-de-ters) Organisms or beings that destroy

superstitious
(SUE-per-STI-shus) Trusting in magic or chance

exorcise
(ECK-sore-size) To force out evil spirits

heal, tribal doctors performed ceremonies to exorcise evil spirits. One such ceremony involved an early form of trephining, whereby the tribal doctor would remove part of the cranium with a primitive tool to exorcise demons. Primitive people also used herbs and plants as medicines. Some of the same medicines are still used today. Here are some examples:

intravenously
(in-tra-VEE-nus) Directly into a vein

- Digitalis comes from the foxglove plant. Today it is given as a pill, intravenously, or by injection to treat heart conditions. In early times, people chewed the leaves of the foxglove plant to strengthen and slow the heartbeat.
- Quinine comes from the bark of the cinchona tree. It controls fever, relieves muscle spasms, and helps prevent malaria.
- Belladonna and atropine are made from the poisonous nightshade plant. They relieve muscle spasms, especially those associated with gastrointestinal (GI) pain.
- Morphine is made from the opium poppy. It is an effective medication for treating severe pain. It is addictive and used only when nothing else will help.

APPLY IT PLANTS AS MEDICINE

Identify one medicine derived from a plant that was used in primitive times and is still in use today. (Choose a medicine not discussed in this section.) Research information to answer the following questions: Who first used the plant as medicine? What medical condition was the plant used to treat? Was the early use of the plant effective? Why or why not? How is the medicine used today?

MEDICINE IN ANCIENT TIMES

accurate
(AA-cue-ret) Exact, correct, or precise

The Egyptians were the earliest people to keep accurate health records. They were superstitious and called upon the gods to heal them. They also learned to identify certain diseases. In the Egyptian culture, the priests acted as physicians. They used medicines to heal disease, learned the art of splinting fractures, and treated disorders by bloodletting with the use of leeches. Interestingly, leeches are being used today as a treatment to help heal skin grafts and restore blood circulation. Their primary function is to drain blood because pooled blood around a wound can threaten the healing of tissue.

The ancient Chinese, from as early as the Stone Age, were first to use primitive acupuncture therapies. These early medical pioneers learned to treat a variety of illnesses and diseases with stone tools. Their methods eventually developed into the advanced practice of Chinese acupuncture, still in common use today.

The ancient Greeks considered medicine an art, not just a profession. Greek physicians had a noble and sacred mission, and were often housed in sacred temples of healing. They were the first to study the causes of disease and to determine that illnesses may have natural, rather than spiritual, causes. They kept records on their observations and ideas about the possible cause of illness. The Greeks understood the importance of searching for new information about disease. This research helped eliminate superstition. In addition, Greeks further developed the use of massage and herbal therapies.

During ancient times, religious custom did not permit the **dissection** of human bodies. The father of medicine, Hippocrates (c. 469–377 BC), based his knowledge of **anatomy** and **physiology** on observation of the external body. He kept careful notes of the signs and **symptoms** of many diseases. With these records he found that disease was not caused by supernatural forces. Hippocrates wrote the standard of ethics called the "Oath of Hippocrates." This standard is the basis for today's medical ethics. Physicians still take this oath.

The Greeks observed and measured the effects of disease. They found that some disease was caused by lack of sanitation. The Romans learned from the Greeks and developed a sanitation system. They brought clean water into their cities by way of aqueducts (waterways). They built sewers to carry off waste. They also built public baths with filtering systems. This was the beginning of public health and sanitation.

The Romans were the first to organize medical care. They sent medical equipment and physicians with their armies to care for wounded soldiers. Roman physicians kept a room in their houses for the ill. This was the beginning of hospitals. Public buildings for the care of the sick were established. Physicians were paid by the Roman government. It is interesting to note that the Roman physician wore a death mask. This mask had a spice-filled beak, which the Romans believed protected them from infection and bad odors.

dissection
(die-SEK-shun) Act or process of dividing, taking apart

anatomy
(ah-NAH-tu-mee) The science of dealing with the structure of animals and plants

physiology
(fih-zee-AH-leh-gee) The branch of biology dealing with the functions and activities of living organisms and their parts

symptoms
(SIM-tums) A sign or indication of something

THE DARK AGES (A.D. 400–800) AND THE MIDDLE AGES (A.D. 800–1400)

When the Roman Empire was conquered by the Huns (nomads from the north), the study of medical science stopped. For a period of 1,000 years, medicine was practiced only in **convents** and **monasteries**. Because the Church believed that life and death were in God's hands, the monks and priests had no interest in how the body functioned. The primary treatment was prayer.

Medication consisted of herbal mixtures, and care was **custodial**. Monks collected and translated the writings of the Greek and Roman physicians. Terrible **epidemics** caused millions of deaths during this period. Bubonic plague (the Black Death) alone killed 60 million people. Other uncontrolled diseases included smallpox, diphtheria, syphilis, and tuberculosis. Today, these illnesses are not always life threatening. Scientists have discovered **vaccines** and medications to control them. It is important to remember that some diseases can become epidemic if people are not vaccinated.

convents
(CON-vents) Establishments of nuns

monasteries
(MA-neh-stare-ees) Homes for men following religious standards

custodial
(cus-TOE-dee-al) Marked by watching and protecting rather than seeking to cure

epidemics
(eh-peh-DEH-mik) Diseases affecting many people at the same time

vaccine
(vak-SEE) A weakened bacteria or virus given to a person to build immunity against a disease

THE RENAISSANCE (A.D. 1350–1650)

The Renaissance period saw the rebirth of learning. During this period, new scientific progress began. There were many developments during this period:

- The building of universities and medical schools for research.
- The search for new ideas about disease rather than the unquestioning acceptance of disease as the will of God.
- The acceptance of dissection of the body for study.
- The development of the printing press and the publishing of books, allowing greater access to knowledge from research.

These changes influenced the future of medical science.

THE SIXTEENTH AND SEVENTEENTH CENTURIES

The desire for learning that began during the Renaissance continued through the next two centuries. During this time, several outstanding scientists added new knowledge. Here are some examples:

- Leonardo da Vinci studied and recorded the anatomy of the body.
- William Harvey used da Vinci's information to understand physiology, and he was able to describe the circulation of blood and the pumping of the heart.
- Gabriele Fallopius discovered the fallopian tubes of the female anatomy.
- Bartolommeo Eustachio discovered the tube leading from the ear to the throat (Eustachian tube).

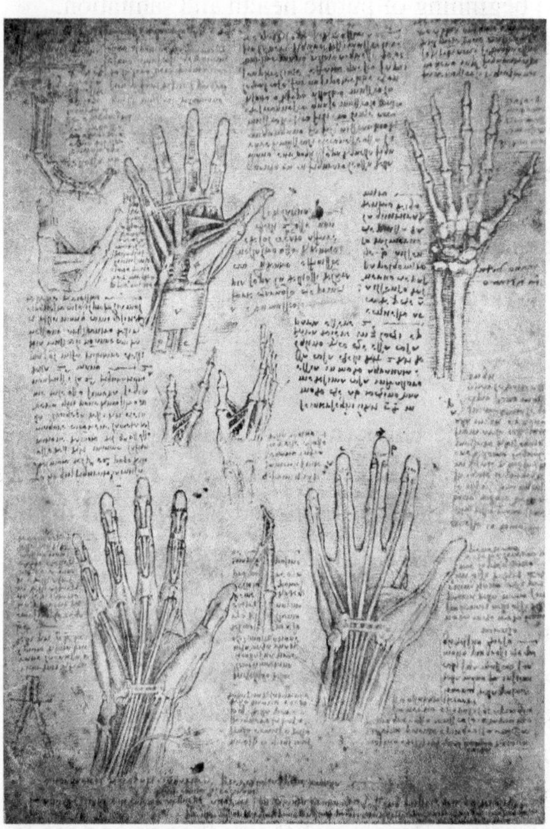

FIGURE 4.1

Leonardo da Vinci's anatomy of the hand

Source: lolloj/Shutterstock

- Antonie van Leeuwenhoek invented the microscope, establishing the existence of life smaller than the human eye can see. Van Leeuwenhoek scraped his teeth and found the bacteria that cause tooth decay. Although it was not yet realized, the germs that cause disease were now visible.
- Apothecaries, early pharmacies, started in this time. In medieval England, these apothecaries engaged in a flourishing trade in drugs and spices from the East.

Unfortunately **quackery**, mass death from childbed fever, and disease continued. The causes of infection and disease were still not understood. Interestingly, infections are, even today, one of the leading causes of death.

quackery
(QUACK-er-ee) The practice of pretending to cure disease

Language Arts Link Historical Contributions

Today we would never expect a doctor to examine us with a wooden stethoscope or to perform surgery without anesthesia. However, as you are learning, medical equipment and procedures evolve over time. Select a medical device or procedure that made an important contribution to health care. (Choose a device or procedure not discussed in this section.) Begin your task by searching library resources or the Internet to learn more about your topic. Record the details and facts that you discover about the history of your topic and the impact it made. Be sure to cite any sources that you use in the format required by your teacher.

Create a new document on the computer, or use a blank sheet of paper. Write a descriptive title for your report. In paragraph form detail what you learned about your subject. Be sure to proofread your work to see if you can improve it by making it more clear, concise, or interesting to read. Check the spelling and grammar and correct any errors. Exchange reports with a classmate. Provide feedback and corrections as necessary, and then exchange back. Read your classmate's comments and revise your report as necessary.

THE EIGHTEENTH CENTURY

Many discoveries were made in the eighteenth century that required a new way of teaching medicine. Students not only attended lectures in the classroom and laboratory, but also observed patients at the bedside. When a patient died, if they dissected the body, they were able to observe the disease process. This led to a better understanding of the causes of illness and death. Also, in the eighteenth century a wider range of students was studying medicine. In 1849, Elizabeth Blackwell (1821–1910) became the first female physician in the United States.

The study of physiology continued, and more new discoveries were made; these included:

- René Laënnec (1781–1826) invented the **stethoscope**. The first stethoscope was made of wood. It increased the physician's ability to hear the patient's heart and lungs, allowing doctors to determine if disease was present.
- Joseph Priestley (1733–1804) discovered the element oxygen. He also observed that plants refresh air that has lost its oxygen, making it usable for **respiration**.
- Benjamin Franklin's (1706–1790) numerous discoveries affect us in many ways. His discoveries include bifocals, and he found that colds could be passed from person to person.
- Edward Jenner (1749–1823) discovered a method of vaccination for smallpox. Smallpox killed many people in epidemics. His discovery saved millions of lives and led to immunization and preventive medicine in public health.

stethoscope
(STEH-the-scope) An instrument used to hear sound in the body, such as heartbeat, lung sounds, and bowel sounds

respiration
(res-peh-RAY-shun) The inhaling and exhaling of air, or breathing

APPLY IT MAKE YOUR OWN STETHOSCOPE

The first stethoscope was made in 1816 by Rene Laennec. You can make your own stethoscope using common, everyday items. In small groups, use the Internet or library resources to find the directions for making a stethoscope. Two websites are www.sciencebuddies.org and www.sciencefairadventure.com. Select a model and work together as a team to construct the device. Use the finished product to listen to each other's heartbeats.

THE NINETEENTH AND TWENTIETH CENTURIES

Medicine continued to progress rapidly, and the nineteenth century was the beginning of the organized advancement of medical science, which continued throughout the twentieth and twenty-first centuries. Important events during the nineteenth and twentieth centuries include the following:

- Ignaz Semmelweis (1818–1865) identified the cause of childbed fever (puerperal fever). Large numbers of women died from this fever after giving birth. Semmelweis noted that the patients of **midwives** had fewer deaths than those of doctors. One of the differences in the care given by the physicians and that of midwives was that the physicians went to the "dead room" in the hospitals where they dissected dead bodies. These physicians did not wash their hands or change their aprons before they delivered babies. Their hands were dirty, and they infected the women. Although Semmelweis realized what was happening, other physicians

midwives
(mid-WIVES) Non-physician women who deliver babies

laughed at him. Eventually, his studies were proved correct by others, and handwashing and cleanliness became an accepted practice. Today, handwashing is still one of the most important ways that we control the spread of infection.

microbiology
(MY-crow-bye-ol-oe-gee) The branch of biology dealing with the structure, function, uses, and modes of existence of microscopic organisms

microorganisms
(MY-crow-or-gan-izms) Organisms so small that they can only be seen through a microscope

pasteurization
(pas-che-reh-ZAY-shen) To heat food for a period of time to destroy certain microorganisms

antiseptic
(an-the-SEP-tik) Substance that slows or stops the growth of microorganisms

pathogens
(PAA-the-jens) Microorganisms or viruses that can cause disease

anesthesia
(aa-nes-THEE-zea) Loss of feeling or sensation

- Louis Pasteur (1822–1895), known as the "Father of **Microbiology**," discovered that tiny **microorganisms** were everywhere. Through his experiments and studies, he proved that microorganisms cause disease. Before this discovery, doctors thought that microorganisms were *created by* disease. He also discovered that heating milk prevented the growth of bacteria. **Pasteurization** kills bacteria in milk. We still use this method to treat milk today. He created a vaccine for rabies in 1885.
- Joseph Lister (1827–1912) learned about Pasteur's discovery that microorganisms cause infection. He used carbolic acid on wounds to kill germs that cause infection. He became the first doctor to use an **antiseptic** during surgery. Using an antiseptic during surgery helped prevent infection in the incision.
- Ernst von Bergmann (1836–1907) developed aseptic technique. He knew from Lister's and Pasteur's research that germs caused infections in wounds. He developed a method to keep an area germ-free before and during surgery. This was the beginning of asepsis.
- Robert Koch (1843–1910) discovered many disease-causing organisms. He developed the culture plate method to identify **pathogens** and also isolated the bacterium that causes tuberculosis. He also introduced the importance of cleanliness and sanitation in preventing the spread of disease.
- Wilhelm Roentgen (1845–1923) discovered x-rays in 1895. He took the very first picture using x-rays of his wife's hand. His discovery allowed doctors to see inside the body and helped them discover what was wrong with the patient.
- Paul Ehrlich (1854–1915) discovered the effect of medicine on disease-causing microorganisms. His treatment was effective against some microorganisms, but was not effective in killing other bacteria. His discoveries brought about the use of chemicals to fight disease. In his search to find a chemical to treat syphilis, he completed 606 experiments. On the 606th experiment, he found a treatment that worked.

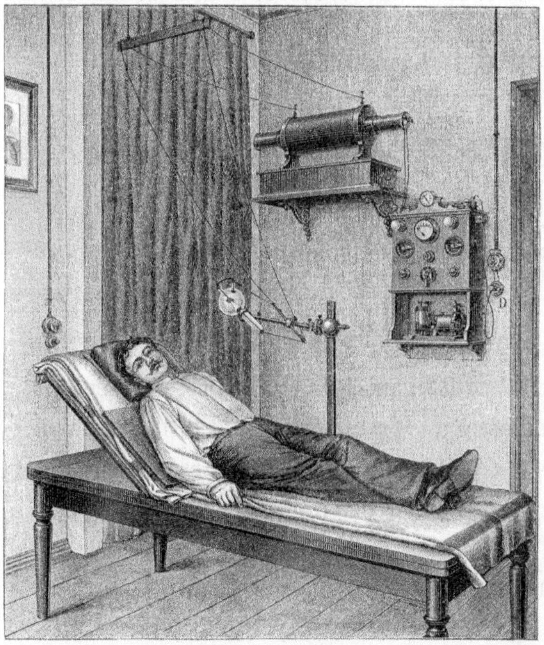

FIGURE 4.2
Undergoing an x-ray exam in 1897
Source: Hein Nouwens/Shutterstock

Before the nineteenth century, pain was a serious problem for patients. Surgery was performed on patients without **anesthesia**. Early physicians used herbs, hashish, and alcohol to help relieve the pain of surgery. They even choked patients to cause unconsciousness to stop pain. Many patients died from shock and pain. During the nineteenth and twentieth centuries, nitrous oxide (for dental care), ether, and chloroform were discovered. These drugs have the ability to put people into a deep sleep so that they do not experience pain during surgery. The knowledge of asepsis and the ability to prevent pain during surgery are the basis of safe, painless surgery today.

Scientists and physicians kept learning from the discoveries of the past. They continued to study and research new ways to treat diseases, illnesses, and injuries. Some of the most important discoveries in the late 19th and 20th centuries included:

- In 1932 Gerhard Domagk discovered sulfonamide compounds. These compounds were the first medications effective in killing bacteria. Until his discovery, the only treatment effective in stopping infections was amputation of a limb.
- In 1892 in Russia, Dmitri Ivanovski discovered that some diseases are caused by microorganisms that cannot be seen with a microscope. They are called viruses. These viruses were not studied until the electron microscope was invented in Germany. These are some of the diseases caused by viruses:
  - Poliomyelitis
  - Rabies
  - Measles
  - Influenza
  - Chicken pox
  - German measles
  - Herpes zoster
  - Mumps

APPLY IT VIRUSES AND DISEASE

Working in small groups, select a disease that is caused by a virus, and research it using the Internet and library resources. Create a presentation about the disease, including historical information, symptoms, outbreaks, and any other important facts you can find. Deliver your presentation to the class.

- Sigmund Freud (1836–1939) discovered the conscious and unconscious parts of the mind. He studied the effects of the unconscious mind on the body. He determined that the mind and body work together. This led to an understanding of psychosomatic illness (physical illness caused by emotional conflict). His studies were the basis of **psychology** and **psychiatry**.
- Sir Alexander Fleming (1881–1955) found that penicillin killed life-threatening bacteria. The discovery of penicillin is considered one of the most important discoveries of the twentieth century. Before penicillin, people died of illnesses that we consider curable today, including pneumonia, gonorrhea, and blood poisoning.
- Jonas Salk (1914–1995) discovered that a dead polio virus would cause immunity to poliomyelitis. This virus paralyzed thousands of adults and children every year. It seemed to attack the most active and athletic people. It was a feared disease, and the discovery of the vaccine saved many people from death or disability.
- In contrast to Salk's vaccine, Albert Sabin (1906–1993) used a live polio virus in his vaccine, which is more effective than the dead polio virus. This vaccine is used today to immunize babies against this dreaded disease.
- In 1953, Francis Crick and James Watson discovered the molecular structure of DNA, based on its known double helix. Their model served to explain how DNA **replicates** and how hereditary information is coded on it. This set the stage for the

psychology
(sie-KOL-eh-jee) The science of the mind or mental states and processes

psychiatry
(sie-KIE-eh-tree) The practice or science of diagnosing and treating mental disorders

replicate
(reh-pli-CATE) To reproduce or make an exact copy

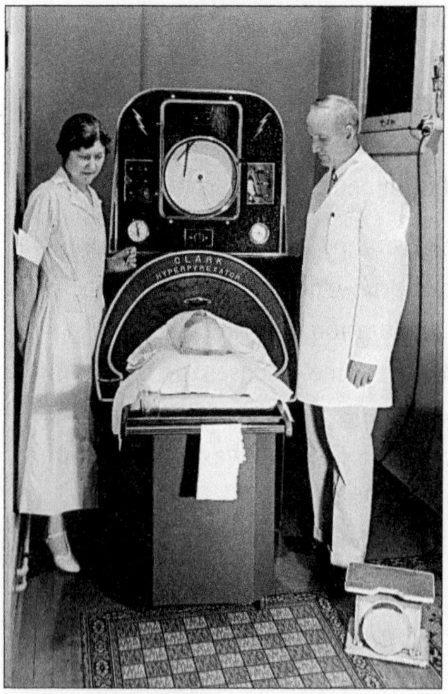

FIGURE 4.3
Receiving therapy in an iron lung
Source: ChipPix/Shutterstock

rapid advances in molecular biology that continue to this day. In 1962, they won the Nobel Prize in Medicine for this discovery.

- Christian Barnard performed the first successful heart transplant in 1968.
- Born in 1951, Ben Carson continues to be a pioneer in separating Siamese twins and performing hemispherectomies, surgeries on the brain to stop seizures.

The discovery of methods to control whooping cough, diphtheria, measles, tetanus, and smallpox saved many lives. These diseases kill unprotected children and adults. It is important for everyone to be immunized. Immunizations are available from doctors, clinics, hospitals, and public health services.

THE MORE YOU KNOW

New Therapies for Patients with Alzheimer's Disease

Finding a cure for Alzheimer's disease is a high priority for today's research scientists. Alzheimer's disease is a form of dementia, a sustained loss of brain functions and memory severe enough to cause dysfunction in daily living activities. Although it can occur at any time during the adult years, dementia most frequently affects the elderly population. Close to 66 percent of all dementias in the geriatric population can be attributed to Alzheimer's disease. Family history, increasing age, genetics, and a previous head injury are primary risk factors. About five percent of Americans between the ages of 65 to 74, and almost half of those 85 years and older, suffer from Alzheimer's disease.

Alzheimer's disease is a mental illness that causes the death of cells in the brain. Because of this cell death, parts of the brain become disconnected. As a result, some messages cannot be sent from one part of the brain to another. This interferes with brain functions, such as memory, and impairs thinking. Eventually people lose their ability to solve problems. For example, they may become lost while out driving in areas they are familiar with and cannot find their way back home. They may forget how to conduct activities of daily living, such as preparing a meal or even how to eat. Eventually, they may lose their ability to walk or communicate.

Unlike most other mental illnesses, the effects of Alzheimer's disease cannot be reversed. If caught early, the disease can be treated with medications that slow its progress. However, the symptoms will continue to worsen, and the disease cannot be cured. In addition to memory problems, the patient will experience depression and anger. A patient may eventually forget basic skills, such as hygiene and the ability to read. Eventually, an Alzheimer's patient will need full-time care. He or she will need home care or will need to be placed in a care facility.

Once people develop Alzheimer's disease, the disease cannot be cured. Most of the drugs currently used to treat Alzheimer's slow the course of the disease, but they do not stop it. According to the Mayo Clinic, the focus of future Alzheimer's treatments will be on preventing it in people who have a risk for the disease, but do not yet have it.

New Alzheimer's disease therapies are on the way. Scientists are working on the following preventive measures:

- ***Alzheimer's vaccine:*** A vaccine was developed and tested, but it caused dangerous side effects. Scientists continue to look for a vaccine that won't cause these side effects.
- ***Secretase inhibitors:*** Secretase is an enzyme, or protein, that causes the formation of plaques in the brain. These plaques have been thought to be the cause of Alzheimer's disease. Secretase inhibitors will prevent the formation of secretase and, thus, plaques. Unfortunately, the inhibitors are large molecules that do not easily pass from the blood to the brain. Scientists are working to fix this problem. In addition, new research is indicating that the role of plaques is more complex than originally thought, which is prompting other ideas in the hunt for a drug treatment for Alzheimer's disease.
- ***Cardiovascular therapies:*** The term *cardiovascular* refers to the heart and blood vessels. Cardiovascular diseases include high blood pressure and high cholesterol. These diseases often result from poor eating habits and lack of exercise. In some people, genetics plays a role in high blood pressure and high cholesterol. Some evidence indicates that controlling these diseases may also reduce the risk of Alzheimer's disease.
- ***Anti-inflammatory drugs:*** Some drugs, such as ibuprofen, may reduce the risk of Alzheimer's disease. However, these drugs have caused stomach and intestinal problems.

How might these therapies improve the quality of life for millions of Americans?

THE TWENTY-FIRST CENTURY

Our society is discovering new approaches to medical care every year. Patients are being taught more about wellness, and they are learning more about self-care. The word *healthy* no longer just refers to a person's physical health. It also refers to a person's emotional, social, mental, and spiritual wellness. To help patients achieve this kind of holistic health, the medical community has become more open to alternative and complementary methods of care. People now go to ayurvedic practitioners, Chinese medicine practitioners, chiropractors, homeopaths, hypnotists, and naturopaths to help meet their medical needs.

Family and friends are learning patient care skills, including how to perform detailed procedures. Nurses and technicians are visiting patients at home or caring for them in an ambulatory care setting. Just a few years ago, patients were admitted to the hospital for surgery and recovered in the hospital over a period of several days. Today, many patients enter the hospital, have surgery, and are sent home the same day.

Doctors are now practicing telemedicine. Health care providers may now e-mail, fax, or telephone important medical information to a patient or another health care provider.

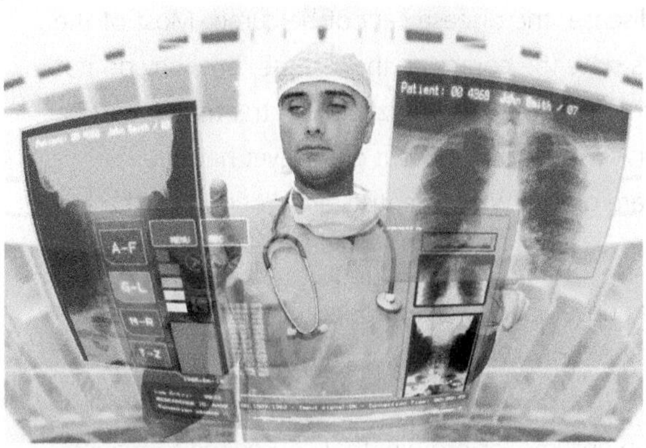

FIGURE 4.4

Using a high-tech computer to diagnose a medical condition

Source: Luis Louro/Shutterstock

This has improved patient care by supplying health providers and patients with quicker access to information and greater opportunities for communication. Telemedicine includes consultative, diagnostic, and treatment services.

People are living longer and are usually healthier than those in the past. New inventions and procedures have changed medicine as we once knew it. For example, consider the:

- Possibility of eliminating disabling disease through genetic research.
- Ability to transplant organs from a donor to a recipient.
- Ability to reattach severed body parts.
- Use of computers to aid in diagnosis, accurate record keeping, and research.
- Ability to use noninvasive techniques for diagnosis.
- Advancement in caring for the unborn fetus.
- Rediscovery and the medical profession's greater acceptance of alternative medicine and complementary medical practices, including acupuncture, acupressure, herbal therapy, and healing touch.

noninvasive
(non-IN-vay-siv) Not involving penetration of the skin

Every day, science makes new progress. We are living in a time of great advancement and new understanding in medicine. People are living longer, creating a need to better understand geriatric medicine. In addition, new types of facilities, such as assisted living centers, are being developed to better meet the physical, emotional, and mental needs of senior citizens. Frontiers in medical science include hope for treatment and cures for diabetes, cancer, AIDS, multiple sclerosis, arthritis, and muscular dystrophy.

Science Link Lyme Disease

If not for modern day medicine and scientific research, the United States may have experienced an epidemic situation with Lyme disease. The first case of Lyme disease was reported in Old Lyme, Connecticut in 1975. Since then, cases of Lyme disease have been reported in most parts of the United States. However, this disease can be detected by a blood test and treated with antibiotics. If caught early enough, Lyme disease may cause little or no complications.

Lyme disease is caused by a bacteria carried by ticks. The ticks contract the bacteria by biting a mouse or deer infected with Lyme disease. Humans contract the disease if bitten by an infected tick. Initial symptoms may include a rash around the area of the bite and flu-like symptoms, including, chills, fever, fatigue, and body aches. If the infection is not treated, it can cause severe joint pain and neurological deficiencies and even heart related problems. Meningitis (inflammation of the tissues around the brain and spinal chord), Bell's palsy (loss of muscle tone in the face), and numbness in limbs are some of the more severe effects of Lyme disease. In the most severe cases, paralysis can occur.

Why is it beneficial to study the history of health care and how it has progressed into modern day medicine and health care practices?

THE ADVANCEMENT OF NURSING

In the nineteenth century, nursing became an important part of medical care. In 1860, Florence Nightingale (1820–1910) attracted well-educated, dedicated women to the Nightingale School of Nursing. The graduates from this school raised the standards of nursing, and nursing became a respectable profession. Before this time, nursing was considered unsuitable for a respectable lady. The people giving care to patients were among the lowest in society—"too old, too weak, too drunken, too dirty, or too bad to do anything else."

Florence Nightingale came from a cultured, middle-class family who opposed her interest in caring for the ill. However, she convinced her father to give her financial support, and she gained experience by volunteering in hospitals. During the Crimean War, she took a group of thirty-eight women to care for soldiers dying from cholera. More soldiers were dying from cholera than from war injuries. She became a legend while she was there because of her dedication to nursing.

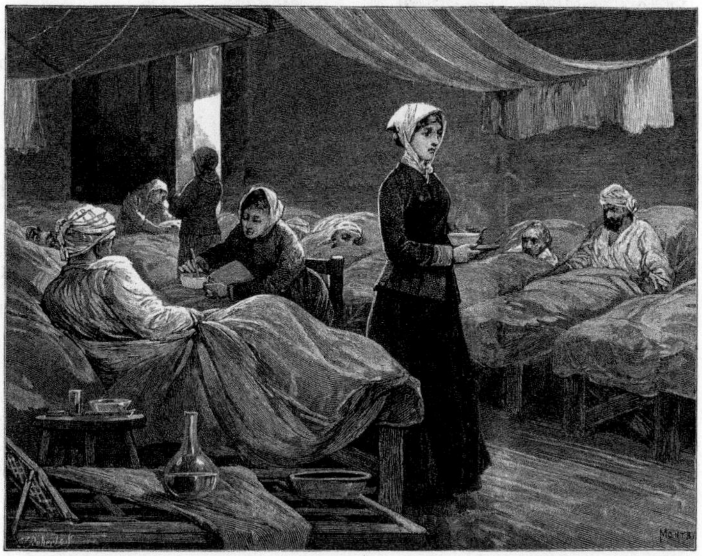

FIGURE 4.5

Florence Nightingale caring for patients

Source: 19th era/Alamy

After the war Nightingale devoted much of her life to preparing reports on the need for better sanitation and construction and management of hospitals. Her primary goal was to gain effective training for nurses. The public established a Nightingale fund to pay for the training, protection, and living costs of nurses. This was established in recognition of her services to the military during the Crimean War.

She also designed a hospital ward that improved the environment and care of the patients. Prior to this time, patients were crowded into small areas that were often dirty. The ward that she designed allowed for a limited number of beds, permitted circulation of air, had windows on three sides, and was clean.

During this time, Clara Barton (1821–1912) served as a volunteer nurse in the American Civil War. After the war, she established a bureau of records to help search for missing men. She also assisted in the organization of military hospitals in Europe during the Franco-Prussian War. Barton campaigned for the United Sates to sign the Treaty of Geneva, which produced relief for sick and wounded soldiers. These experiences led her to establish the American Red Cross in 1881 and to serve as its first president.

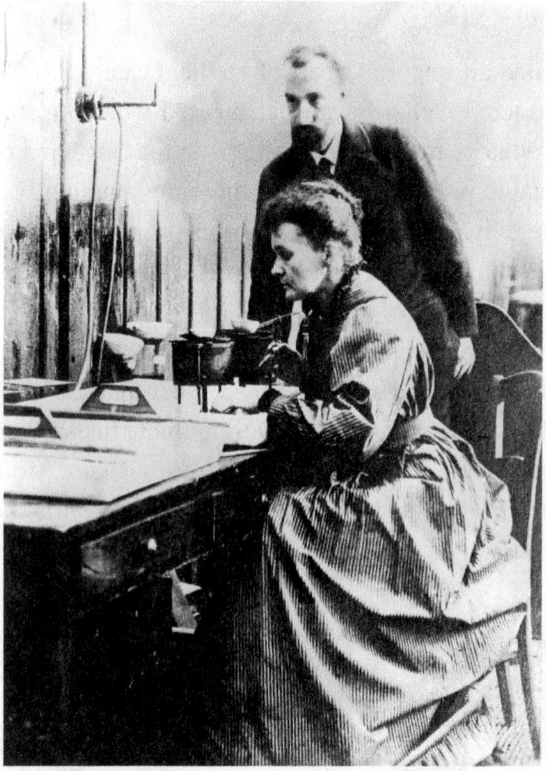

FIGURE 4.6

Marie and Pierre Curie working in their Paris laboratory in 1904

Source: CSU Archives/Everett Collection/Alamy

Another step forward in the field of nursing was contributed by Lillian Wald (1867–1940). She was an American public health nurse and social reformer who established the Henry Street Settlement in New York to bring nursing care into the homes of the poor. This led to the Visiting Nurse Service of New York. Today, visiting nurse services are found in most communities.

Nursing care has changed many times throughout the years. In the past, patients have been cared for by teams that included a registered nurse as team leader, a licensed vocational nurse (LVN) or practical nurse (LPN) as a medication nurse, and a nursing assistant who provided personal care. In primary care nursing, which followed team nursing, a registered nurse provided all patient care. Today, unlicensed assistive caregivers are part of the patient caregiver team. There are many titles and new job descriptions for these positions, including clinical partner, service partner, nurse extender, health care assistant, and patient care assistant. These new positions extend the role of entry-level employees. The nurse assistant performs additional tasks, such as **phlebotomy** and recording an electrocardiogram (EKG). Employees from departments other than nursing learn patient care skills. Environmental service workers and food service workers

phlebotomy (fli-BAA-the-mee) The practice of opening a vein by incision or puncture to remove blood

Language Arts Link — Women in Medicine

Over the centuries, male scientists led the way in discovering and inventing many of the medical beliefs, procedures, and equipment that changed the way health care was delivered. However, many women played important roles in improving health care practices and medical education.

Create a report highlighting a woman who helped advance health care and medicine. Do some research on the Internet or in a library and use only credible sources. Create a new document on the computer, or use a blank sheet of paper. Include a title for your report and a thesis statement (a sentence stating your main ideas) in the opening paragraph. Include information about who she was, when she lived, and where she worked. What role did she play? How was her work received at the time? What impact did she make?

Proofread your work to see if you can improve it by making it clearer, more concise, or more interesting to read. Check the spelling and grammar and correct any errors. Be sure to cite any sources that you use in the format required by your teacher. Exchange reports with a classmate. Provide feedback and corrections as necessary, and then exchange back. Read your classmate's comments and revise your report as necessary.

may help with serving food and providing some routine patient care. The registered nurse delegates patient care tasks according to the training and expertise of the assistive personnel.

Because of the scientific advances in health care, the role of the nurse has evolved into a more technological role. This has created a need for a complex mix of the technological nurse and the holistic caregiver. Never before has it been more important to maintain the art of nursing, which includes compassion, comfort, and the ability to see the patient as an individual and a member of a family and a community.

THE EVOLUTION OF THE ALLIED HEALTH PROFESSIONS

After World War II and 1945, the rapid expansion of scientific knowledge led to new types of medical equipment and diagnostic and therapeutic treatments for patients. These advancements called for health care workers who could operate complex medical equipment and perform sophisticated procedures. Health care services were expanding beyond the walls of hospitals into community-based care settings. Jobs were opening up in medical clinics, ambulatory care centers, emergency care facilities, and physician practices. The trend towards outpatient care, combined with the demand for people with technical knowledge and skills, led to the emergence of a variety of new health occupations and new health care workers. Examples include: medical technologists, radiographers, respiratory therapists, occupational therapists, physical therapists, and dental hygienists, to name just a few.

Today, these occupations, collectively known as the allied health professions, compose about 60 percent of the health care workforce. Professionals function in all aspects of health care, playing key roles in clerical, administrative, research, education, and support areas as well as in direct patient care. Although allied health professionals are considered

RECENT DEVELOPMENTS

New Vaccines

In the eighteenth century, Edward Jenner discovered a method of vaccination for smallpox that helped to end the epidemic. In the twenty-first century, doctors and scientists continue to do research to develop vaccines for diseases and illnesses.

While today's adults received only a few vaccines for illnesses, such as measles, mumps, and rubella, as children, today's children are offered a variety of vaccines. One such vaccine is Varivax. This vaccine helps to prevent, or at least lessen, the effects of chicken pox. In previous generations, children had to suffer the uncomfortable symptoms of this virus. The vaccine gives today's children some degree of protection.

Other new vaccines now offered to children are Gardasil, a vaccine developed to protect against cervical cancer and genital warts, and Menactra, a vaccine developed to prevent children from getting meningitis.

How might these new vaccines affect people's lives and the cost of health care?

separate from nurses, physicians, and dentists, they serve together on teams and work closely to provide patient care. Current trends in medicine and technology will continue to drive the demand for this large segment of the U.S. health care workforce.

THE PAST AND THE FUTURE OF HEALTH CARE

In the twentieth and twenty-first centuries, medicine has made great strides in improving health care. During these centuries, we have experienced many changes, including these:

life expectancy (LIFE ex-PECK-ten-see) The number of years of life remaining at any given age

- Antibiotics for bacterial diseases
- Improved life expectancy
- Organ transplants
- Healthier hearts (through reduced smoking, better diets)
- Dentistry without pain
- Noninvasive diagnosis with computers (CT, MRI)
- End of smallpox
- Childhood immunizations
- New understanding of DNA and genetics
- Control of diabetes with the discovery of insulin
- Decline in polio
- Medical machines, such as those for kidney dialysis and the heart-lung machine
- Test tube babies
- HMOs as an alternative to private insurance
- Hospice

Consider This: *Sigmund Freud and Modern Day Mental Health*

While other scientists were studying aspects of science related to the physical body, Sigmund Freud was studying the parts of the mind. Having decided that the mind and the body work together, he laid the foundation for what we know today about mental health and the study of psychology and psychiatry.

Mental health is all about how we think, feel, and interact with others as we manage the pressures of daily life. Everyone experiences some stress, sadness, or anxiety from time to time, but for a person with mental illness, these feelings do not go away. Health care professionals help people with mental illnesses. There are many types of health care professionals including psychiatrists, psychologists, social workers, and counselors.

Many people have the misconception that those with mental illnesses are *crazy* or *nuts*. This is simply not true, and using such words to describe people with mental illness is highly disrespectful. Most cases of mental illness are not severe. These cases can be treated, often with a combination of medication and regular meetings with a medical professional who specializes in treating mental illness. When caught early, the symptoms of most mental illnesses can be reduced or even reversed. In very severe cases, a patient may be dangerous to himself or herself or to other people and require hospitalization.

Most people will go to the doctor for an illness such as the flu, asthma, diabetes, or heart disease. But many people hesitate to see a doctor about mental illnesses. Teenagers, especially, do not want to be labeled with a mental illness and have their peers or teachers find out. Not seeking treatment may result in more advanced symptoms of the mental illness. Untreated mental illness can lead to increased physical illness. A person may think about or attempt suicide. Some mental illnesses cause violent thoughts or actions. In children, untreated mental illness has lead to both learning and social problems.

Medicines are often used to treat mental illness. Medicines can be prescribed to treat anxiety disorders, mood disorders, attention disorders, and personality disorders. Medicines can also help some people overcome drug addictions and help treat eating disorders. Many of these medicines need to be taken for several days or weeks. Sometimes, people need the medicines for longer periods. A doctor must carefully monitor mental illness medications. Some of these medicines have uncomfortable side effects. A doctor can adjust medications or dosages to make a patient more comfortable. Because of the uncomfortable side effects, some patients may decide to stop taking their medicines.

In addition to advancing the science of mental health, how did Sigmund Freud's work lead to psychotherapy and the practice of psychiatry?

The future of medicine holds many promises for better health. Current and future research will provide us with many new advances, including these:

- Finding a cure for AIDS.
- Decreasing the cases of malaria, influenza, leprosy, and African sleeping sickness.
- Finding a cure for genetically transferred diseases (such as Tay-Sachs, muscular dystrophy, multiple sclerosis, cerebral palsy, Alzheimer's, and lupus).
- Improving treatments for arthritis and the common cold.
- Isolating the gene that causes depression.
- Using electronics to allow disabled persons to walk.
- Using nutritional therapy to decrease the number of cases of schizophrenia.

Advancement in medicine raises ethical questions and creates new problems such as:

- How will the recipient of an organ be chosen?
- Who will be allowed to receive experimental drugs?
- How will the creation of in vitro embryos be ethically managed?
- Is it ethical to provide continuing confidentiality about AIDS patients, or should they be required to report their condition?
- Does a terminally ill patient have the right to euthanasia?

There are many questions now, and there will be more questions in the future as health care continues to evolve.

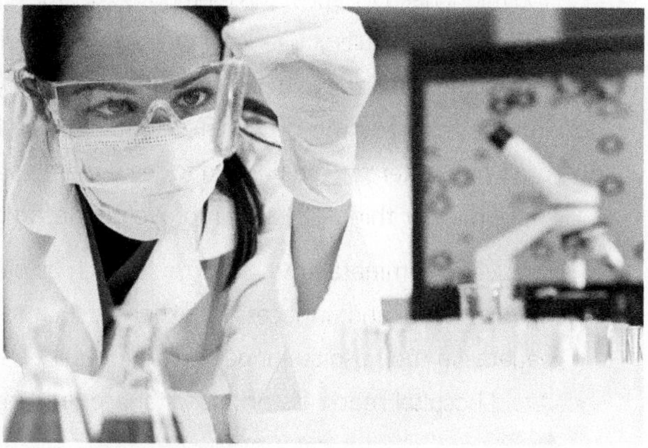

FIGURE 4.7

Conducting research to advance the science of medicine

Source: Darren Baker/Shutterstock

BUILD YOUR SKILLS *Using the Scientific Method to Improve Patient Care*

As a health care professional, understanding the scientific method can help you appreciate the discoveries and inventions of the past while contributing to the advancement of health care in the present. The scientific method has six steps that can be used to solve many different types of problems, in health care and at school and home. The six steps are:

1. State a problem or ask a question.
2. Gather background information.
3. Form a hypothesis.
4. Design and perform an experiment.
5. Draw a conclusion.
6. Report the results.

Let's take a look at how the scientific method is used among health care organizations to achieve better patient outcomes through continuous quality improvement (CQI).

Continuous quality improvement uses methods and tools to help identify, prevent, and reduce problems. It starts by examining the process by which work gets done—looking at each action or step in the work flow that must be accomplished correctly and in the proper order. By studying the process, you can determine if there's a better way to do things. This is especially important when something goes wrong. When something goes wrong, workers have to figure out what happened and implement a better process to prevent the same thing from happening again. They continually evaluate their processes and make the necessary adjustments. They also make sure that a quality improvement effort in one area doesn't cause problems for other areas.

When starting a quality improvement project, you ask:

1. What are we trying to accomplish?
2. How will we know if we are successful?

Once you have answered these questions, you are ready to identify options and figure out which ones work best. You can use the following steps to try different approaches:

Plan: Create a plan or a test to see how a different approach would work.

Do: Implement the plan to see what happens.

Study: Review the results to determine what was learned.

Act: Take action based on what was learned.

You might need to repeat this method, sometimes called the PDSA approach, several times before you get the results you're seeking. Using metrics is the key. In most quality improvement projects, you must be able to measure things to know if your approach was an improvement or not. You gather baseline data before you start and compare those statistics with your outcome data after you are finished to see if there's been any change and, if so, how much.

Among other things, quality improvement efforts can help to:

- Reduce or eliminate adverse effects, such as patient falls and bed sores.
- Reduce waste and unnecessary expense, such as duplicating blood tests or keeping patients in the hospital longer than necessary.
- Avoid hospital readmission, hospital-acquired infections, and medication overdoses.

hypothesis
(high-PAH-the-sis) An explanation for an observation that is based on scientific research and can be tested

continuous quality improvement
(con-TIN-you-us KWA-leh-tee im-PROOV-ment) The regular use of methods and tools to identify, prevent, and reduce the impact of process failures; also known as CQI

process
(PRAH-sess) Set of actions or steps that must be accomplished correctly and in the proper order

metrics
(MEH-triks) A set of measurements that quantify results

baseline data
BASE-line DAY-ta) Gathering information before a change begins to better understand the current situation

outcome data
(OUT-come DAY-ta) Information gathered after a change has occurred to examine the impact or results

adverse effects
(AD-verse EE-fekts) Unfavorable or harmful outcomes

readmission
(re-ad-MIH-shen) A quick return to the hospital after discharge

Another quality improvement strategy used in the health care industry is called Six Sigma. Six Sigma has been used successfully for many years in the manufacturing industry. Now it's helping health care organizations improve their existing processes and develop new processes to meet quality goals. When Six Sigma's *lean concepts* are applied throughout an entire organization, the organization can improve work flow, productivity, and the timely delivery of services while reducing waste and costs. Teams from different areas work together to examine each step in the process. When the process breaks down, the team looks for the root cause of the problem instead of just blaming someone. By openly sharing information across the different areas, Six Sigma teams try to develop a perfect process where each step creates value for the customer.

When a health care provider develops a best practice that improves quality of care, the practice often becomes a benchmark that other organizations aim to achieve. Sharing information about best practices helps *raise the bar* in the quality of care for all patients.

How could today's quality improvement methods have helped the scientists who were conducting research many years ago?

Six Sigma
(SIX SIG-ma) A strategy that uses data and statistical analysis to measure and improve an organization's operational performance

root cause
(RUTE CAW-zhe) The factor that, when fixed, will solve a problem and prevent it from happening again

best practice
(BEST PRAC-tis) A method or technique that has consistently shown superior results through research and experience as compared with other methods and techniques

benchmark
(BENCH-mark) A standard by which something can be measured or compared

REALITY CHECK

The science of medicine and health care has grown and developed over the last 5,000 years with amazing results. These changes have increased our average life expectancy and enhanced our standards of living. The dedication of the many scientists discussed in this section has led to the health care improvements we enjoy today. Their research has provided the foundation for the rapid growth in medical knowledge and technology, which is sure to continue well into the future.

For centuries, countless men and women have worked hard to improve the quality of life, health, and wellness for others. The advancement of health care in the near future will depend upon the continuing dedication and commitment of Americans, especially young people who are just now preparing for the health professions. What could be more exciting than watching new technology revolutionize health care yet again? Maybe you will play a role in discovering a new drug, treatment option, or medical breakthrough at some point in your health career.

Key Points

- Knowledge of the history of health care can help you better understand current practices.
- Primitive human beings were superstitious, believing that exorcism would help protect and heal people from the evils of supernatural spirits.

- The early Egyptians used medicine, leeches, and help from the gods to heal them.
- The Ancient Chinese used acupuncture and stone tools to treat illness and disease.
- The Ancient Greeks housed physicians in sacred temples and studied the causes of disease.
- Hippocrates noted signs and symptoms of disease, basing his knowledge of anatomy and physiology on observations of the external body. Realizing that supernatural forces did not cause disease, he wrote the Oath of Hippocrates (the Hippocratic Oath), which is still in use today.
- During the Dark Ages and Middle Ages, the study of medicine stopped and epidemics caused millions of deaths.
- The rebirth of learning occurred during the Renaissance period, leading to universities and medical schools for research.
- Scientists in the sixteenth and seventeenth centuries contributed new knowledge and inventions, but quackery continued.
- Major discoveries occurred during the eighteenth century, and medical education included dissection and bedside observations.
- The nineteenth and twentieth centuries saw rapid progress, including the discovery of microorganisms that cause disease. The ability to eliminate germs and treat infections led to many techniques still in use today. Sigmund Freud studied the mind and Francis Crick and James Watson discovered the molecular structure of DNA.
- Research, discoveries, and inventions from the past have led to today's twenty-first century approach to medicine and health care.
- Florence Nightingale, Clara Barton, and others devoted their lives to improving sanitation, hospital care, and quality of life and brought respect and high regard to the profession of nursing.
- The explosion of medical technology and the advent of community-based health care services resulted in a host of new occupations, which today are collectively called the allied health professions.
- Many changes have occurred in the past and the future holds yet more promise, but issues relating to medical ethics will need to be addressed.

Section Review Questions

Answer each of the following questions. Indicate which page in the textbook led you to your answer.

1. What did early human beings believe caused illness and disease?
2. Who were the first people to organize medical care?
3. Name two ways that medical progress was made during the Renaissance period.
4. Which discoveries in the nineteenth and twentieth centuries led to safer surgeries?
5. How does technology continue to improve medical care today?
6. Explain how society's view of women in medicine has changed over the years.
7. Who was the founder of modern nursing?
8. What role did Sigmund Freud play in modern-day mental health?

Learn By Doing

Complete Worksheets 1–5 in Section 4.1 of your *Student Activity Guide*.

Health Care Today

SECTION 4.2

Background

Today's health care industry is composed of a wide array of providers and delivery systems. Future health care workers need to have a basic understanding of the structure and function of the health care system, and the roles played by government agencies, not-for-profit organizations, and health care regulatory agencies. Health care **facilities** offer many different services and must be well organized to function effectively. When you understand how facilities operate, you gain an appreciation of how all components of the health care system must work together to meet the needs of the community.

facilities
(fa-SIH-lih-tees) Places designed or built to serve a special function, such as a hospital, clinic, or doctor's office

The cost of health care has increased significantly over the years. It is important to understand the causes for these increases as well as the methods that providers, employers, and government agencies use to help contain these costs. Reforming health insurance and the health care industry is a hot topic in the U.S. today. When workers are aware of the trends and issues involved in health care reform, they're in a better position to know how potential changes might affect their patients, their employer, their family members, and themselves.

Objectives

After completing this section, you will be able to:

1. Define the key terms.
2. List five types of health care facilities and describe their roles.
3. List four government agencies involved in health care and describe their roles.
4. Explain how not-for-profit organizations provide support for health care, and list two examples.
5. Discuss the difference between the service side and the business side of health care.
6. List three reasons for the rising cost of health care.
7. Describe the impact on patients and health care providers when people don't have health insurance or a family doctor.
8. Explain the concept of managed care and how it is different from fee-for-service.
9. Give three examples of how providers have modified their practices to provide quality health care at a lower cost.
10. Describe three types of health insurance organizations and programs.
11. Explain the purpose of HEDIS.
12. Discuss health care reform efforts, including two strategies and two issues of concern.

HEALTH CARE PROVIDERS AND DELIVERY SYSTEMS

Several facilities and agencies provide (deliver) and support medical care. Some are familiar, and others will be new to you. The following descriptions will help you understand the differences among the many providers of medical care.

General hospitals are facilities where patients are hospitalized for a short time, from a few days to a few weeks. They do not specialize in any one type of medical treatment; rather, they provide a wide range of diagnostic, medical, **surgical**, and emergency care services. General hospitals are staffed by physicians, surgeons, nurses, allied health professionals, and support staff to provide inpatient care to those who need close monitoring and outpatient care to those who need treatment but not constant monitoring.

surgical
(SER-jih-cull) Repairing or removing a body part by cutting

continuity
(con-teh-NEW-eh-tee) Continuous, connected, and coordinated

rehabilitation
(ree-ah-BIH-leh-tay-shun) Process that helps people who have been disabled by sickness or injury to recover as many of their original abilities for activities of daily living as possible

convalescence
(con-veh-LESS-ens) The gradual recovery of health and strength after illness

Specialty hospitals provide inpatient **continuity** of care for patients with persistent, recurring diseases or complex medical conditions that require long-term stays (often over a month) in an acute care environment. These may include chronic diseases, pulmonary or physical **rehabilitation**, wound care, and psychiatric problems. Specialty hospitals are not nursing home facilities or transitional units. One example of a specialty hospital is St. Jude's Children's Hospital.

Convalescent care (such as a nursing home or long-term care) facilities generally engage in geriatric care for elderly people needing nursing services and assistance with personal care and daily living activities. These facilities also care for physically ill or injured people of all ages who require an extended **convalescence** for recovery. Many of these facilities focus on rehabilitation, or optimizing the functional status of patients so that they may return to the community. The staff includes nurses; nursing aides and assistants; physical, occupational, and speech therapists; and recreational assistants and social workers.

Nursing homes can differ from extended care facilities. These facilities are places of residence for people who require constant nursing care and have significant problems with activities of daily living.

Extended care facilities are designed to care for those who need assistance with activities of daily living or with medical needs. An extended care facility is needed when someone has a condition that is likely to last for a long period of time or for the rest of his or her life, like moderate Alzheimer's disease.

Independent living and *assisted living facilities* are also available. For older individuals with an active lifestyle, independent living offers the opportunity to remain independent in a home of their own, yet close to health care professionals and facilities—people needing some assistance with activities of daily living, but who want to live as independently as possible for as long as possible. Assisted living bridges the gap between independent living and extended care or nursing homes.

ambulatory
(AM-bue-leh-tore-ee) Able to walk

specialties
(SPEH-shul-tees) Fields of study or professional work, such as pediatrics, orthopedics, obstetrics

Ambulatory care/clinics are facilities where several physicians with different **specialties** combine their practices. This allows the patient to have immediate care for a variety of illnesses. Ambulatory care can be delivered at a physician's office, in an area of a hospital designated for short stay care, and in urgent care centers. Patients do not spend the night in ambulatory facilities; these are outpatient services.

Physician and dental facilities provide care that promotes wellness and diagnosis of illness. Simple surgery, bone setting, counseling, and administration of drugs take place here. Diagnostic services, such as laboratory tests and x-rays, might also take place. Physicians and dentists may provide care in an ambulatory care setting.

Rehabilitation centers provide outpatient care for patients who require physical or occupational therapy, recreational therapy, hydrotherapy, and other therapies (such as speech or hearing therapy) for loss of function in mobility or the activities of daily living. They may receive prosthetics and learn how to use adaptive devices. Patients come from the community and will return to the community after a therapy session is completed.

Industrial health care centers are located in large companies and industrial facilities such as manufacturing plants. They provide health care for the employees of the business, including basic examinations and emergency care. In addition, many industrial health care centers teach accident prevention and safety.

occupational therapy
(ah-cue-PAY-shun-el THAIR-ah-pee) Helps to give people skills for everyday activities in order to lead satisfying lives

recreational therapy
(reh-kree-AY-shun-al THAIR-ah-pee) Uses play, recreation, and leisure activities to improve physical, cognitive, social, and emotional functioning; the primary goal is to develop lifetime leisure skills

hydrotherapy
(HIE-droe ther-eh-PEE) Treatment that uses water therapy for disease or injury

mobility
(MOE-bill-ih-tee) The ability to move from place to place without restriction

prosthetics
(prass-THE-tik) Artificial parts made for the body, such as teeth, feet, legs, arms, hands, eyes, and breasts

THE MORE YOU KNOW

The Rise of the Baby Boomers

The elderly population in the United States is growing rapidly due to the aging of the baby boomer population— the 78 million people born between 1946 and 1964. Here are some things to consider about this large population:

- Every eight seconds another baby boomer turns fifty years of age; the over-65 population will almost double in the coming years.
- The first baby boomer reached sixty-four in 2010; it will take another twenty-one years for the last one to reach that milestone.
- When compared with previous generations, baby boomers have higher education levels, use more online resources, and are more directly involved in their health care.
- Almost 20% of baby boomers are minorities, requiring more attention to cultural differences.
- Baby boomers possess 75% of the nation's disposable income but worry about covering their health care and retirement expenses.
- Thanks to joint replacements and other medical advancements, baby boomers are more physically active than seniors in the past and suffer from fewer disabilities.
- 70% of baby boomers subscribe to alternative or complementary medicine, such as massage therapy, chiropractic care, meditation, and acupuncture.

Efforts are already underway to prepare for the impact of this large patient population on the health care system. New medicines, monitoring equipment, and surgical techniques are in development. With new technology, seniors will be able to monitor more of their conditions from home and communicate remotely with physicians and specialists. Hospitals are remodeling to offer the more personalized care and convenience that baby boomers expect, including more private rooms with sound-reduction materials and in-room computers for patient use. These are just a few examples of how health care providers are preparing for the arrival of this large population of elderly patients.

complementary medicine
(com-pleh-MEN-the-ree) Combining alternative medical approaches with traditional medical practices

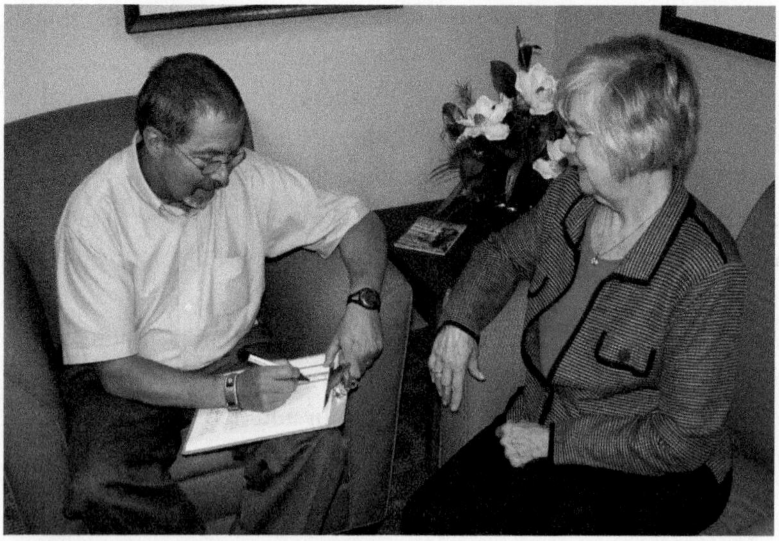

FIGURE 4.8

Baby boomers completing health care paperwork

Source: Carmen Martin/Pearson Education

School health services are found in educational institutions. They provide emergency care in case of accidents or sudden illnesses. School nurses also provide medication dosing, and monitor children with chronic childhood diseases and problems such as diabetes, asthma, and cognitive impairment.

Health Maintenance Organizations (HMOs) are a type of **managed care** organization. HMOs stress wellness (preventive health care). This avoids unnecessary major medical expenses. They provide health services that include hospitalization, basic medical services, **immunizations**, basic checkups, and education.

managed care
(MAH-nij-ed CAIR) A health care system where primary care doctors act as gatekeepers to manage each patient's care in a cost-effective manner

immunizations
(IH-mue-nie-ZAY-shun) Substances given to make disease organisms harmless to the patient; may be given orally or by injection, such as for tetanus and polio

Home health care agencies provide care in the home for patients who need health services but not hospitalization. Services include nursing, physical therapy, personal care (bathing, dressing, and so on), and homemaking (such as housecleaning, food shopping, and cooking). Home health care workers provide care for all ages, from infants to the elderly.

Telemedicine offers medical services through interactive audiovisual media, such as computers or close-circuit television. It is a way to provide health care, including consultations, procedures, and examinations, to remote areas or communities that do not have full time health care providers.

Senior day care provides for elderly people who are able to live at home with their families, but need care when the family is away. These centers are a place where the elderly can be cared for during the day with activities, rehabilitation, and contact with others. The elderly are given their medications and are aided in mobility.

The *World Health Organization (WHO),* an agency funded by the United Nations, was founded in 1948. It is concerned with world health problems and publishes health information, compiles statistics, and investigates serious health problems.

Hospices are important in our health care system. Hospices provide end-of-life care to those patients expected to live six months or less. The main diagnosis for hospice patients is cancer. Health professionals and volunteers provide medical services and psychological and spiritual support to both the patient and their family. The goal of hospice is to make the patient as comfortable as possible by controlling pain and providing comfort.

Language Arts Link Investigating Health Care Facilities

As you've learned in this chapter, many different types of health care facilities exist. Working with a partner, select two different types of health care facilities that are available where you live. Research the two facilities by using the Internet, calling the facility, or reviewing any available print information. Find key information on each, such as the facility's services, specialty areas, patient eligibility requirements, and designation as a provider of long-term or outpatient care.

With your partner, create a brochure or a booklet on the computer with information on both facilities that can be used by local school counselors, community centers, etc. Be sure to proofread your work and cite any sources that you used. Check spelling and grammar and correct any errors.

Government Agencies

The federal, state, and local governments provide health services that are funded by taxes. They are responsible for providing direct health care, safeguarding our food and water supplies, and promoting health education.

Veterans Administration hospitals are federally supported and provide care for veterans who served in the armed forces.

The *U.S. Public Health Department* is a federal agency that has six major responsibilities:

- Performing research on diseases that kill or handicap.
- Preventing and treating alcohol and drug abuse.
- Preventing and controlling diseases that are transmitted by insects, animals, air, water, and people.
- Checking the safety of food and drugs that **consumers** purchase.
- Planning more effective ways to deliver health services.
- Making quality care available and affordable by encouraging health personnel to work in underserved areas.

consumers
(con-SUE-mers) People who purchase or use a product or service

State psychiatric hospitals serve the mentally ill.

State university medical centers provide training for health workers, give medical care, and conduct medical research.

State public health services provide health education materials. They are responsible for water and food purity, **communicable** disease control, alcohol and drug abuse control, **maternal** health, and licensing of various health agencies.

communicable
(kuh-MEW-ni-keh-bul) Capable of being passed directly or indirectly from one person or thing to another

maternal
(meh-TER-nel) Relating to the mother or from the mother

The *U.S. Department of Health and Human Services (USDHHS)* protects the health of all Americans by providing vital human services, especially to those least able to help themselves. For example, WomensHealth.gov provides resources for domestic violence against women.

The *National Institute of Health (NIH)* is the world's leading agency for conducting and supporting medical research.

The *Centers for Disease Control and Prevention (CDC)* monitors and prevents disease outbreaks, including bioterrorism. The CDC implements disease prevention strategies and maintains national health statistics.

RECENT DEVELOPMENTS

Impact of the Baby Boomers

Baby boomers are predicted to have an unprecedented long-term impact on the health care industry, consuming far more medical services than any elderly population in the past. Baby boomers will live longer than their predecessors. In fact, half of all of the people who have ever lived to age sixty-five are alive today. By the year 2030, six out of ten seniors will have at least one chronic condition, one out of three will be considered obese, one out of four will have diabetes, and one out of two will be living with arthritis.

More than 25% of the total health care spending for each patient occurs in the final years of his or her life. By the year 2030, four out of ten adult visits to doctors' offices will be baby boomers; 55 million lab tests per year will be needed for diabetic seniors, eight times more knee replacements will be performed than today, and 4 million more Emergency Department visits will be logged than today.

obese
(oh-BEESE) Weighing more than 20% over a person's ideal weight

The *Food and Drug Administration (FDA)* assures the safety of foods, cosmetics, pharmaceuticals, biological products, and medical devices.

The *Occupational Safety and Health Administration (OSHA)* imposes safety and health legislation to prevent injury, illness, and death in the workplace.

The *Agency for Health Care Policy and Research (AHCPR)* works to improve the quality, safety, efficiency, and effectiveness of health care for all Americans by using research and technology to promote the delivery of the best possible care.

County hospitals provide care for the ill and injured, especially those patients who require financial help in order to receive care.

A *laboratory* is a government or private facility that provides controlled conditions in which scientific research, experiments, and measurements can be performed. Laboratories are found in hospitals, dental offices, schools, universities, industries, government, and military facilities.

Local *public health departments* provide services to local communities—focusing on the reporting of communicable diseases, public health nursing, health education, environmental sanitation, maternal and child health services, and public health clinics.

Senior centers have clinics that provide special services for geriatric patients, such as a podiatry clinic, hypertension clinic, and general medical care.

environmental sanitation
(en-VIE-row-men-tal sa-ne-TAY-shun) Methods used to keep the environment clean and to promote health

podiatry
(poe-DIE-ah-tree) The diagnosis and treatment of foot disorders

hypertension
(HIE-per TEN-shun) Elevation of the blood pressure

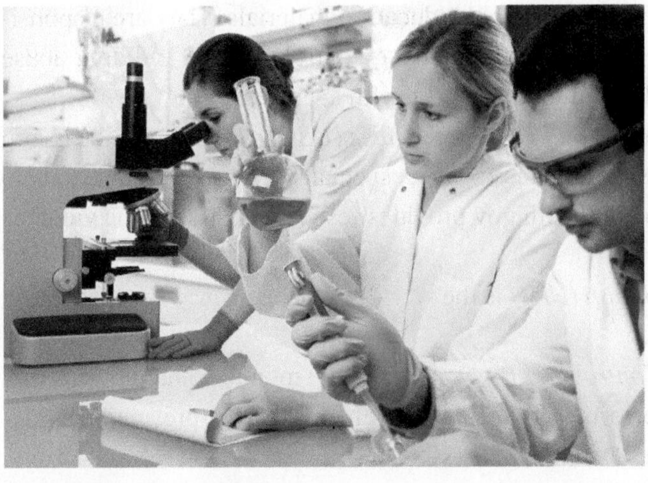

FIGURE 4.9
Conducting laboratory procedures
Source: Alexander Raths/Shutterstock

APPLY IT HIV/AIDS RESOURCES

The National Institutes of Health (NIH) and the Centers for Disease Control and Prevention (CDC) provide a wealth of information on current topics such as HIV/AIDS. Visit their websites (www.aidsinfo.nih.gov and www.cdc.gov/HIV). Locate resources regarding treatment and prevention for these conditions. Find the guidelines for people living with HIV/AIDS, as well as for their families and friends and health care providers.

Not-for-Profit Organizations

Not-for-profit organizations receive support from donations, gifts, membership fees, fund-raisers, and endowments. They are not supported by the government, and many of the people who work for them are unpaid volunteers. They raise funds for medical research and for public education about various health problems.

endowments (en-DOW-ments) Gifts of property or money given to a group or an organization

Many of them focus on a particular disease or medical condition, such as the:

- American Cancer Society
- National Foundation of the March of Dimes
- American Red Cross
- American Heart Association
- American Diabetes Association
- National Association of Mental Health
- National Association of People with AIDS
- National Coalition Against Domestic Violence
- American Respiratory Disease Association

All of these agencies and facilities help bring good health to individuals and communities.

Health Care Regulatory Agencies

State and federal regulatory agencies for the health care industry set standards for health care, keep health care workers informed, and monitor facilities' and workers' compliance with laws that pertain to health care.

The Joint Commission, for example, evaluates and accredits hospitals and health care organizations to make sure they meet quality and performance standards. State health departments inspect health care facilities to make sure they comply with laws and regulations. The Nuclear Regulatory Agency ensures the safe use of radioactive materials and ionizing radiation equipment in hospitals and diagnostic imaging centers. The Occupational Safety and Health Administration (OSHA) inspects health care facilities to ensure they are safe places to work. These are just a few examples of regulatory agencies involved in health care.

As a health care worker, one of your first encounters with a health care regulatory agency will be for certification or licensure. Based on your chosen profession, you will need to meet specific requirements set forth by the federal or state board that regulates that profession.

APPLY IT REGULATORY AGENCIES

Select an agency that regulates health care providers or health care workplaces. Do some research to find out when and why the agency was created and how it fulfills its mission. Identify what might happen if the agency did not exist.

Organization and Services

system
(SIS-tem) A coordinated body of methods or plans of procedure

Each health care organization operates as a **system**. Any kind of system has input and output, along with a feedback loop. This is referred to as *systems theory.* In a system such as a health care facility, the input is information, materials, and human effort or energy. The output is the services provided to patients. Both positive and negative feedback affect the input that occurs next. For a system to work, it requires goals and feedback that governs what continues to happen within the system. The ability to adapt based on feedback is important in achieving system goals.

To be efficient, a health care facility must be well organized. Organization improves the performance of health care workers at a facility and ensures that the facility delivers high quality health care to patients. An organizational chart shows how each department of a health care facility fits into the system and identifies the line of authority. When you look at an organizational chart, you can see who your immediate supervisor is. It tells you the areas of responsibility for all of the employees. The organizational chart also establishes the chain of command. The chain of command tells you to whom you take questions, reports, and problems.

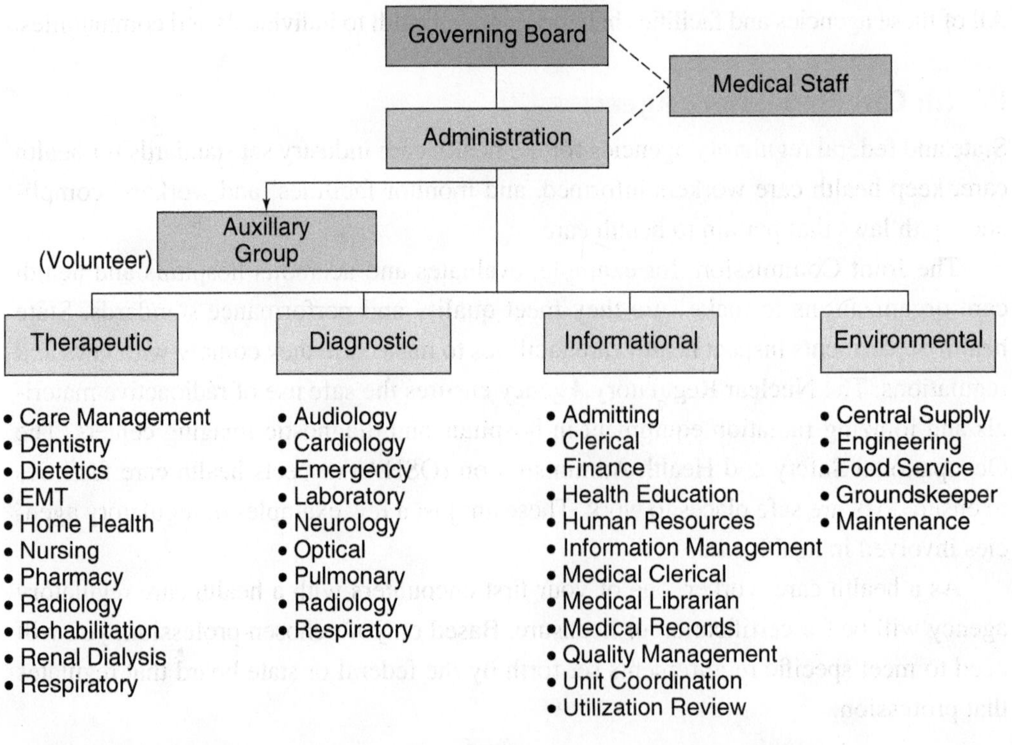

FIGURE 4.10
Sample organizational chart showing hospital services

Each of the four major services in health care has specialized departments. These departments are determined by the type of service they provide:

- ***Therapeutic services*** provide care over time.
- ***Diagnostic services*** provide tests to identify a particular condition or disease, such as radiographs or blood tests.
- ***Informational services*** document and process information.
- ***Environmental services*** help to create a clean, safe, healing, and supportive environment for patients, employees, visitors, and guests.

Services can be organized in several different ways. Your facility's organizational chart is your guideline to understanding its organization.

Language Arts Link — Global Health Care

This text focuses on the U.S. health care industry. But the United States is closely aligned with other countries in tackling global health issues such as HIV/AIDS, malaria, tuberculosis, and malnutrition. One billion people world-wide have no access to health care. Thirty-six million people die each year from heart disease, cancer, diabetes, and lung disease. More than 7.5 million children under the age of five die annually due to malnutrition and preventable diseases. More than 35 million people are living with HIV.

Select one global health issue and conduct some research to learn more about it. Prepare an oral presentation for your classmates and teacher that answers these questions: What causes the problem? Who does it affect, and how are they affected? What is being done to improve the situation? What role is the United States playing? What other countries are involved?

HEALTH CARE AS A BUSINESS

As you prepare for your career in health care, most of what you will learn relates to working in the patient care environment—the service side of the health care industry. But understanding the business side of health care is very important, too.

Health care providers are business organizations. Businesses provide goods and services to consumers. A business may function for profit or not-for-profit. A health care provider may be a corporation, such as a hospital, or a sole proprietor, such as a doctor who practices alone. Some health care providers are privately owned. Others are public corporations, owned by shareholders and managed by a board of directors. Some health care providers are part of larger networks that manage many health care providers. Hospitals that receive no financial support from taxpayers are called *private* hospitals. Hospitals that are subsidized with tax dollars are called *public* hospitals. Like other businesses, health care organizations have responsibilities to the community.

Many hospitals are not-for-profit, which means they are exempt from paying taxes. Their tax exempt status is based in part on the community benefits they provide. One of those community benefits is providing charity care for patients who lack health insurance and the financial resources to pay their medical bills. Hospitals also offer free health screenings to check for abnormalities such as high blood pressure and high cholesterol. They offer classes and groups to educate patients and promote personal wellness. The instructional sessions cover a range of topics. For example, some classes help patients understand their diseases. Classes about cancer, diabetes, and arthritis can help patients anticipate symptoms and explore types of care. Hospitals offer emotional support in the form of support groups for bereavement, cancer patients, and caregivers. These groups help patients and families deal with the mental and emotional stress that often comes with disease.

Not only do hospitals help with the difficulties associated with disease, they also offer classes on topics of daily health. Classes on exercise, men's and women's health, stress management, and nutrition are available. Expectant mothers can learn about pregnancy and parenthood through weekly classes. Hospitals reach out to communities to educate people and help keep them well. Some hospitals conduct training programs to prepare future health care workers, and these programs are often open to the public.

Consider This *Workforce Supply and Demand*

Millions of baby boomers work in health care, serving as doctors, nurses, and other health care professionals. As they age, they will retire from their health care jobs in large numbers. These rising retirement rates could lead to significant labor shortages during the same period of time when baby boomers are increasing the demand for health care services.

Consider the following:

- About one third of all registered nurses are currently fifty years of age or older.
- About 55% of RNs plan to retire in the next ten years.
- By 2020 there will be a shortage of one million nurses in the U.S.
- While 50% of nurses currently work in hospitals, the demand in other care settings is growing.
- The number of new RNs graduating from college is not sufficient to replace all of the retiring nurses.
- To meet the demand, new nursing graduates would have to increase by 90% a year.
- As the demand for RNs increases world-wide, there will be fewer foreign-trained nurses to work in the U.S.

Labor shortages are also predicted for other types of health care professionals, including doctors:

- About 40% of U.S. doctors are fifty-five or older.
- By 2020, there will be at least 100,000 fewer doctors in the workplace than today.

When you match these labor forecasts with the expected health care demands of the baby boomer population, you can easily understand some of the major challenges facing the American health care system. Keep this sobering fact in mind—these forecasts do not include the additional patients who will require health care services if and/or when health care reform expands access to millions of more patients.

How can health care employers and colleges prepare for this impending shortage of workers?

Health care is expensive, it's a necessity of life, and it affects everyone including consumers, taxpayers, employers, businesses, government, and other **stakeholders**. Consider the following:

stakeholders
(STAKE-hol-ders) People with a keen interest in a project or organization; may be end-users of a product or service

- As patients, everyone is a consumer of health care. When the need arises, consumers want the best health care available regardless of the cost.
- As taxpayers, everyone pays for health care through programs such as **Medicare** and **Medicaid**.
- The United States spends about $2.5 trillion per year (about $8,500 per person) on health care, significantly more than any other developed nation, and the cost is rising about 8% a year.
- Unpaid medical bills are a leading cause of bankruptcy in the United States.
- Health care costs account for about 18% of the nation's **gross domestic product**, and this number is rising.

Medicare
(MED-ih-CAIR) A government program that provides health care primarily for people 65 and older

Medicaid
(MED-ih-caid) A government program that provides health care for low-income people and families and for people with certain disabilities

gross domestic product
(GDP) (GROWS DOE-mess-tik PRAH-duct) The total market value of all good and services produced in one year

So when it comes to health care, everyone is a stakeholder with concerns and opinions to voice.

Providing health care for everyone who needs it at a reasonable expense is an enormous challenge. The cost of health care in the United States is growing faster than the cost of most other goods and services. Cost increases are a result of:

- Recruitment, payment, and retention of highly competent doctors and health professionals.
- Medical research to develop new drugs, devices, and medical procedures.
- Rising cost of medical equipment, supplies, and utilities.
- Building construction, remodeling, and maintenance.
- Training future doctors, nurses, and other health professionals.
- Expanding services, and increasing access to services, in order to care for more patients.

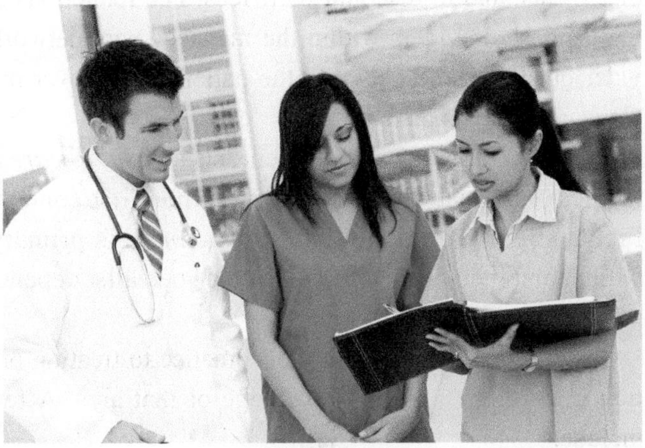

FIGURE 4.11
Training future medical professionals contributes to the rising cost of health care

Source: Stephen Coburn/Shutterstock

Millions of Americans don't have health insurance or a doctor. They go without medical care and prescription drugs, which makes their conditions more difficult, and expensive to treat in the long run. Pregnant women may have to forego prenatal care, which can lead to major problems, and high expenses, later on. Patients without health insurance often turn to expensive hospital emergency departments for basic health care services. When patients are unable (or unwilling) to pay their medical bills, the providers must write-off the loss as charity care or unreimbursed services. Since hospitals and doctors have to cover their expenses to remain in business, this loss of income drives up the cost for other patients who do have health insurance and who do pay their bills.

APPLY IT THE GREEN MOVEMENT

Health care organizations are joining the green movement, incorporating recycling and waste management programs. New buildings are designed with energy efficiency in mind, using recycled and natural building materials, natural lighting, and energy-efficient windows and utility plants. Retired computers and electronics are scrubbed clean of private information and disposed of safely. Environmentally friendly construction materials are helping to reduce the risk of bacterial infections. Building materials and landscaping plants are sourced locally to reduce transportation costs and fuel use. Sensors on public toilets and lavatories are conserving water.

Identify one health care organization that has *gone green*. Investigate the green projects they have undertaken, the reasons for the projects, and the results they are experiencing.

Managed Care

In the 1980s, health care providers received payment based on *fee-for-service* insurance plans. These plans allowed patients to select any physician and other providers without having to stay within a pre-established network. Fees were not arranged in advance, and the insurance plan routinely reimbursed providers for the fees they charged. These plans were among the most expensive because they didn't impose cost-control measures. Fee-for-service plans are rare today. They're used mostly by patients who are willing to pay extra for the freedom to choose their provider and to receive care when and where they wish to, without limitations.

Today, managed care plans cover most patients. Managed care is an approach to controlling the cost of health care while maintaining its quality. Managed care organizations enter into contracts with providers. The providers agree to care for a specific group of patients, and to discount their fees. Fee reductions are passed on to patients when they choose providers within the managed care network. If the patient chooses a provider outside of the network, the patient must cover more of the expense or, in some plans, all of the expense.

In managed care, each patient has a *primary care doctor* who provides the basic medical care that a person receives upon first contact with the health care system. Frequently known as the *family doctor*, this primary care physician will see the patient and then **refer** him or her to a specialist depending on the additional services needed.

Specialists usually limit their practice to treating one type of problem. Specialization gives them a broad knowledge of that area. A few examples of specialty areas include:

- Surgery
- **Orthopedics**
- Podiatry
- **Chiropractic**
- **Audiology**
- **Urology**
- **Obstetrics**

refer
(REE-fer) To send to

orthopedics
(or-theh-PEE-dik) The medical specialty concerned with correcting problems with the skeletal system

chiropractic
(KIE-reh-prak-tik) The method of adjusting the segments of the spinal column

audiology
(aw-dee-ALL-leh-jee) The study of hearing disorders

urology
(yu-ROL-leh-jee) The study of the urine and urinary organs in health and disease

obstetrics
(ob-STEH-trik) The branch of medical science concerned with childbirth

In managed care, primary care doctors act as gatekeepers to manage the patient's care. Their goal is to:

- Encourage preventive services such as vaccinations, flu shots, and health screenings.
- Provide medical care in the least expensive settings such as doctors' offices, outpatient clinics, and the patient's home.
- Avoid unnecessary or duplicate tests and treatments.
- Coordinate services from different providers to ensure continuity in care and the best outcomes for the patient.

gatekeepers
(GATE-keep-ers) People who monitor the actions of other people and who control access to something

One of the most effective ways to reduce the cost of health care is to encourage health and wellness. Preventive care, such as routine physicals, well-baby care, immunizations, screenings for patients with specific risk factors, and wellness education, helps keep patients healthy. Wellness education stresses the importance of good nutrition, weight control, exercise, and healthy living practices. Health education programs, wellness centers, weight-control programs, fitness centers, health food distributors, and health care organizations all promote wellness and preventive care. Being healthy helps prevent serious illness and lowers medical costs.

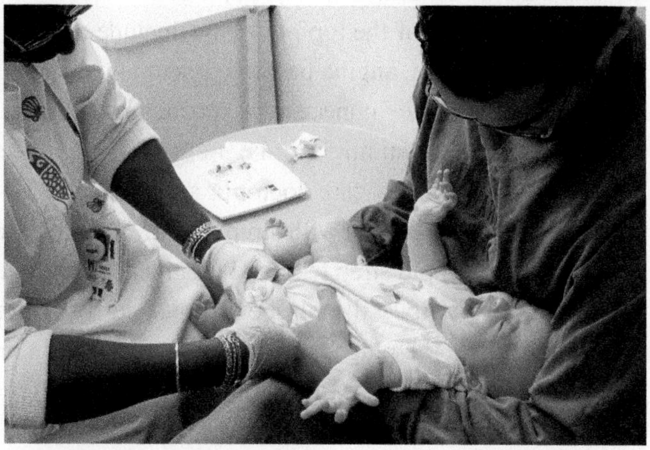

FIGURE 4.12
Infant receiving a vaccination
Source: George Dodson/Pearson Education

Using the appropriate level of emergency care also reduces costs. *Emergency care* and *urgent care* provide different services. Emergency care is for life-threatening conditions that require hospitalization. These might include ambulance services, rescue squads, and helicopter or airplane rescue vehicles. Urgent care is for non-emergencies that require prompt treatment, such as high fevers and moderate cuts and wounds. Hospital emergency departments deliver the most expensive care. Excellent care is available in the urgent care setting, and costs are much lower.

Outpatient care is much less expensive than hospitalization, and patients prefer to remain at home because it's more comfortable and familiar. The goal is to avoid hospitalization and to use outpatient care to the extent possible. As a result, only the very ill and severely injured are hospitalized. When hospitalization is necessary, patients must undergo *preadmission authorization* first. Outpatient services are provided in ambulatory care settings such as these:

- Physicians' offices
- Outpatient surgery centers
- Outpatient clinics and medical centers
- Rehabilitation centers
- Senior day care facilities

With ambulatory care, the patient goes to a facility for care and returns home afterward. Ambulatory care provides employment opportunities for multiskilled workers (radiographers who perform EKGs and phlebotomy, for example) and convenience for patients since multiple services are offered in the same location.

Some patients also need home health care to help with bathing, range of motion, dressing changes, intravenous therapy, and special treatments. Home health services are much less expensive than costly hospitalization.

Health care providers and the government are working to lower the cost of health care. The federal government passed **legislation** in 1983, originally developed for Medicare payment systems and then modified for the general population, to regulate the price of medical care. The system ensures that the health care provider will have to pick up any extra costs after the government and patient have paid their portions. This legislation approved the grouping of medical conditions, the reasonable cost for each condition, and its standard treatment. These groupings are known as *diagnostic-related groupings* (DRGs). Examples of the top groupings include normal newborn, heart failure, psychoses, cesarean section, angina pectoris, pneumonia, and hip/knee replacement.

legislation
(leh-jes-LAY-shun) A law or body of laws

DRGs help reduce unnecessary procedures and encourage self-care and home care. For example, a woman might wake up with a fever, sore throat, and ringing in her ears. She goes to her primary care doctor or an urgent care facility where she can be seen that morning, and is diagnosed with strep throat. The standard diagnosis for strep is based on a throat culture (rapid strep test) and treatment is about ten days of antibiotics. Based on the DRG, the facility will only be reimbursed by insurance or Medicare for a fee that falls within a specific range. The facility would not, on the other hand, be reimbursed for x-rays or a CT scan for this condition.

Health care providers also promote lower health care costs by combining services, offering outpatient services, purchasing supplies in **bulk**, and emphasizing early **intervention** and preventative care.

bulk
(BULK) A greater amount

intervention
(in-ter-VEN-shun) The act of interfering to change an outcome

Community Service Interacting with the Elderly Population

Spend some time volunteering in a nursing home or a senior day care center to interact with elderly people. Find answers to the following questions.

- What types of care and medical services are provided in this setting?
- Who is eligible to receive services?
- What age-related health conditions do the elderly experience, and how are their conditions diagnosed and treated?
- What types of health care workers are employed there?
- What training and credentialing requirements must be met?
- What regulatory agencies are involved, and what role do they play in the operation of the facility?
- What can you learn about geriatrics and the aging of the baby boomers from this experience?

Health Insurance

Health insurance has been offered in the United States since the mid-1800s. In 1929, hospital coverage was created by a group of Texas school teachers who contracted with a local hospital. The hospital agreed to provide up to twenty-one days of care for a cost of $6.00 per year per teacher. During World War II, employers began offering group health insurance as a benefit for workers to help offset the burden of frozen wages. The practice of offering employee benefit plans grew during the 1940s and 1950s to the point where labor unions began pushing for better benefit packages in contract negotiations with employers. Government programs started covering health care costs during the 1950s and 1960s. In 1954, social security began disability coverage, and the Medicare and Medicaid programs were created by the federal government in 1965. As the cost of health care started climbing rapidly in the 1980s, employers looked for ways to reduce their health insurance expenses. The result was an array of new kinds of insurance plans, with limitations and cost-controls.

Health care costs, including dental, are so high today that most people have some type of insurance plan. People with health insurance usually receive coverage through their employer, a government program such as Medicare or Medicaid, or an individual or group policy.

Insurance plans are called third-party payers. Insurance companies require the subscriber to pay a fee for insurance coverage and in return agree to pay for specific medical and dental care. Each insurance company determines what it will and will not pay for and how much it will pay. For example, many third-party payers require a **co-payment**. A co-payment is a set amount the subscriber pays for each medical service. This may be from $10 to $40 that a subscriber pays to the provider on the day that he or she visits a medical office or picks up a prescription. Most insurance companies also have a **deductible**, an amount the subscriber must pay before the insurance begins to pay. For example, a subscriber may have to pay the first $250 of medical bills in a given year. Even after a subscriber pays the co-payment and the deductible, he or she may still have to pay a **co-insurance**. For example, a subscriber may be required to

co-payment
(co-PAY-ment) A set amount the subscriber pays for each medical service

deductible
(di-DECK-teh-bil) An amount the subscriber must pay before the insurance begins to pay

co-insurance
(coe-IN-sure-ence) A percentage the subscriber is required to pay of every medical bill

Math Link: Finding Health Care Costs Using Percentages

When trying to figure out how much you or a patient will have to pay when dealing with a third-party payer, knowing how to work with percentages can help. A third-party payer may require the subscriber to pay a certain percentage of every medical bill. In order to figure out how much a subscriber will have to pay, follow these steps:

Step 1: Convert the percentage to a decimal. You can do this by moving the decimal point to the left two spaces. For example, 10% would be .10 and 20% would be .20.

Step 2: Multiply the decimal by the amount of the medical bill.

Example 1

Mike is having surgery on his arm. The total cost of the procedure is $1,982. Mike's insurance requires a 15% coinsurance.

Step 1: 15% = .15

Step 2: $1,982 × .15 = $297.30

Mike would have to pay $297.30 for the surgery.

Example 2

Kelly needs to have a cavity filled. The total cost of the procedure is $350. Kelly's insurance pays 30% of the cost of any dental procedure.

Step 1: In this instance, first you need to find out how much Kelly is required to pay.

100% minus 30% equals 70%.

70% = .70

Step 2: $350 × .70 = $245

Kelly would have to pay $245 to have the cavity filled.

Calculate percentages to solve this example. Andrew needs to have a mole removed from his back. The total cost of the procedure is $235. Andrew's insurance pays 65% of the cost of a medical procedure. How much would Andrew have to pay?

Why is it important to know how to figure out how much money an insurance company will pay for a medical procedure?

pay twenty percent of every medical bill. The subscriber must pay any fees that the insurance company does not pay.

Several different types of health insurance organizations and programs exist.

Health Maintenance Organizations

Health maintenance organizations (HMOs) require members to pay a co-payment, or co-pay, for medical services. The member must get medical care from the physicians, labs, hospitals, and so on that agree to the fee the HMO is willing to pay. If the member gets medical care outside the HMO, he or she will have to pay for the care.

Preferred Provider Organizations

In PPOs, physician groups and hospitals work together to give comprehensive health care at a reduced cost to various large companies and corporations. Employees of these companies contract with a preferred provider organization (PPO) and agree to see providers on the PPO list. If they see other providers, they pay a larger fee.

Medicaid

Health insurance is provided by the state and federal government. **Benefits** and **eligibility** are different in each state. People who are blind, disabled, or of low income are generally able to get Medicaid insurance.

benefits
(BEH-neh-fit) Payments and assistance based on an agreement

eligibility
(EH-leh-ji-bul) The quality or state of being qualified

premium
(PREE-me-um) The periodic payment to Medicare, an insurance company, or a health care plan for health care or prescription drug coverage

Medicare

Health insurance is provided to people over the age of sixty-five. Subscribers pay a monthly payment to the Social Security Administration. Medicare consists of two parts. Part A covers inpatient care at hospitals, hospice care, and home health care. Part B helps cover medical services like doctors' services, outpatient care, and other medical services that Part A does not cover. In addition, Part B covers some preventive services. While most people get Part A without paying a monthly payment, Part B requires a **premium** each month. Some health care providers accept Medicare payments, or reimbursements, as payment in full for services; others charge more than Medicare pays. To cover the extra costs, many people buy a third-party payer insurance to cover all of their medical costs. There are many programs for Medicare recipients that provide care for a small co-payment.

FIGURE 4.13
Senior citizens learning about Medicare coverage
Source: Rob/Fotolia LLC

Tricare

TRICARE is a health care program for active duty service members, retirees, and their families. One part of TRICARE is called TFL (TRICARE for Life). This medical care is for Medicare-eligible uniformed services retirees age sixty-five or older. The plan also covers family members and survivors. This health program works with Medicare to provide service members additional health benefits.

Workers' Compensation

Another example of a health care program is the workers' **compensation** program. Employees who are injured or die at work are covered by state workers' compensation laws. Workers' compensation also includes any illness that may result from the workplace. Employers are required to have workers' compensation insurance. Benefits include payment for lost wages and payment of medical bills.

compensation (com-pen-SAY-shun) Payment

Health Plan Employer Data Information Set

Under the direction of the National Committee for Quality Assurance (NCQA), the Health Plan Employer Data and Information Set (HEDIS) establishes guidelines and gives a report card to stakeholders that:

- Measures health plan performance.
- Identifies physicians who give high-quality medical care to their patients.
- Identifies physicians who do not meet the quality care guidelines.

These HEDIS report cards are used by almost all of America's health plans to measure their performance on important aspects of care and service. Quality health care can be defined as the extent to which patients get the care they need in a manner that most effectively protects or restores their health. This means having timely access to care, getting treatment that medical evidence has found to be effective, and getting appropriate preventive care.

RECENT DEVELOPMENTS

Geriatric Specialists in High Demand

By the year 2030, one in five Americans will be eligible for Medicare. Twenty percent of the population will be sixty-five years of age or older. This aging of America's population is driving the demand for doctors, nurses, pharmacists, physician assistants, counselors, and psychiatrists who specialize in caring for geriatric patients.

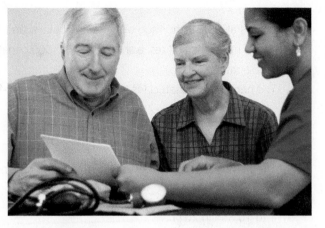

There's already a shortage of geriatric doctors, and the supply continues to decline. Even if the number stabilizes, a shortage of 20,000 geriatricians will occur by 2015. Consider these ratios:

The number of geriatricians to patients age seventy-five or older:

1 to 2,620 in 2011

1 to 3,798 in 2030

The number of geriatric psychiatrists (geropsychiatrists) to patients age seventy-five or older:

1 to 10,865 in 2011

1 to 12,557 in 2030

Of all U.S. registered nurses, pharmacists, and physician assistants, only one percent is certified in caring for geriatric patients. Only three percent of psychologists and four percent of social workers specialize in the geriatric population.

After graduating from medical school, most doctors don't continue their education into geriatrics because other specialty areas are more financially rewarding. In 2009, less than one percent of internal medicine and family medicine residents (just eighty-six people!) enrolled in geriatric medicine fellowship programs. Internal medicine, family medicine, and geriatric doctors earn less than other specialists and their work schedules aren't as predictable.

If the shortage of health care workers who specialize in geriatric care isn't addressed soon, older Americans may lack access to the medical care they need.

Health Care Reform

infant mortality rate (IN-fent mor-tah-leh-tee RATE) The number of infants that die during the first year of life

There's no question that the United States has one of the best health care systems in the world. Yet Americans lag behind other countries in life expectancy, **infant mortality rate**, preventive care, and other common measures of health and well-being. Studies indicate that as much as one-third of what is spent in the U.S. on health care is unnecessary. Almost everyone agrees that ample opportunities exist for improvement, and many are calling for extensive reform.

Since Congress first debated health care reform in 1994, the cost of health insurance has doubled and millions of Americans remain uninsured or underinsured. Many people agree that something must be done to control costs and increase access to health care. But there is little agreement about how to reform the system. Years ago the American Medical Association (AMA) was against any effort to regulate the health care system. More recently, however, even some doctors— Physicians for a National Health Program—were interested in a *single-payer* health system for all Americans. They claim that eliminating private insurance bureaucracy and paperwork could save enough to provide comprehensive, high quality coverage for all Americans.

After many months of heated debate and negotiation, the Patient Protection and Affordable Care Act (PPACA) became law in 2010. But the law is being challenged and debated. Some stakeholders believe the laws went too far in involving the government in the health insurance industry, while others think the laws didn't go far enough to control costs and overhaul the health care system. The intent of health care reform is to: 1) provide more comprehensive care to more Americans at an affordable cost, and 2) focus on preventive health care, immunizations, education, and behavior modification (such as encouraging people to stop smoking) to help lower health care costs.

It is important for consumers to pay attention to **trends** in reform efforts. Here are some of the terms and issues involved to help you *speak the language* of health care reform.

trends
(TREN-ds) General direction or movement

- ***Preexisting condition:*** A medical condition the patient knows about prior to applying for health insurance
- ***Individual mandate:*** A requirement that everyone must have health insurance coverage or pay a penalty
- ***Out-of-pocket expense:*** Expenses that patients with health insurance have to pay themselves
- ***Donut hole:*** The gap in insurance coverage for prescription drugs that Medicare patients must pay themselves
- ***Defensive medicine:*** When doctors order tests and treatments for patients to avoid potential lawsuits

Issues such as the following are part of the debate:

- ***Standard benefits:*** Which health care services should be included as a standard part of insurance coverage?
- ***Eligibility:*** Should people with medical conditions have to pay more for their health insurance than healthy people?
- ***Dependents:*** What is the maximum age that children could be covered under their parent's health insurance?
- ***Prevention:*** Should insurance companies be required to cover preventive services? If so, which services?
- ***Benefit limitations:*** What limits should be placed on annual and lifetime insurance benefits?
- ***Cancellation:*** Under what conditions could an insurance company cancel a policy?
- ***Waiting period:*** How long should a person have to wait for new health insurance coverage to take effect?

Much of the controversy surrounding health care reform centers on how to pay for health care services. The following terms represent some of the options under discussion:

- ***Capitation:*** When a doctor, hospital, or clinic receives a fixed amount of money per person to provide all of the health care services needed by the person
- ***Single-payer system:*** When the government collects taxes for health care from all citizens and then uses the money to pay for the citizens' health care
- ***Universal health care:*** An organized health care system where everyone has health care insurance coverage

health care exchanges (HELTH CARE icks-CHAINJ) Open marketplaces where buyers and sellers of health insurance come together to help consumers compare and shop for coverage

medical homes (MEH-di-cull) Organizations that deliver primary care through a comprehensive team approach that ensures quality outcomes

accountable care organizations (ah-COUN-the-bil) Networks where hospitals and doctors work together and share accountability to manage all of the health care needs of a large group of Medicare patients for an extended period of time

New types of health care organizations are under discussion as part of health care reform. **Health care exchanges** are open marketplaces where buyers and sellers of health insurance come together to help consumers compare and shop for coverage. **Medical homes** are organizations that deliver primary care (including acute, chronic, and preventive services) through a comprehensive team approach that ensures quality outcomes.

Another concept, **accountable care organizations (ACOs)**, is growing as one of the most talked about strategies in health care reform. ACOs are networks of providers that work together and share responsibility and **accountability** for managing all health care services for at least 5,000 Medicare patients over a minimum of three years. Primary care doctors, specialists, home health organizations, rehabilitation centers, and hospitals collaborate to eliminate duplicative tests and procedures, focus on prevention, manage diseases, share medical information, care for patients in the least expensive settings (outpatient clinics and doctor's offices as opposed to emergency departments), and reduce medical errors.

Under the new plan, accountable care organizations would receive financial incentives to reduce costs while achieving quality outcomes, thereby getting paid more to keep their patients healthy and out of the hospital. ACOs that fail to meet performance and financial expectations could face financial penalties. This plan is quite different from the current fee-for-service approach where providers receive payment based on hospitalized patients and the number and types of diagnostic tests and treatments they order and perform.

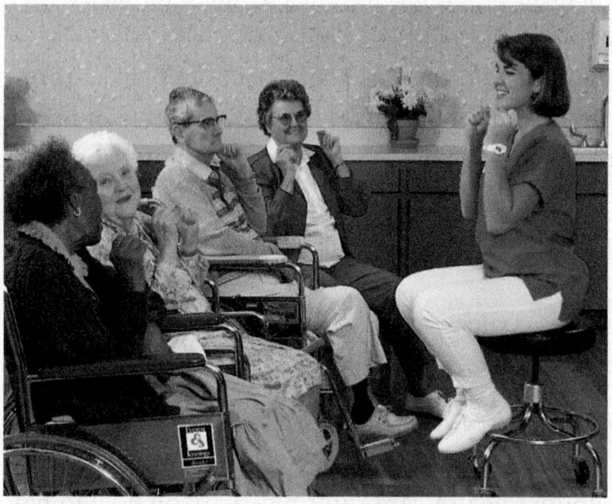

FIGURE 4.14

Geriatric patients participating in activities designed to enhance their health and wellness

Source: Michal Heron/Pearson Education

accountability (ah-coun-teh-BI-leh-tee) Willing to accept responsibility and the consequences of one's actions

malpractice (mal-PRAK-tiss) Negligence, failure to meet the standard of care or conduct prescribed by a profession

defensive medicine (di-FEN-sive MED-ih-sin) Medical practices aimed at avoiding lawsuits rather than benefitting the patient

The advent of ACOs is already having an impact on the American health care system as providers rush to form or enlarge their networks and adopt strategies to become integrated systems. Patient satisfaction is expected to play a major role in health care reform and how providers are paid.

As stakeholders consider options to reform Medicare and Medicaid, revisit medical **malpractice** laws to reduce **defensive medicine**, and create new ways for people to purchase affordable health insurance, it's clear that health care reform continues to be a work in progress.

BUILD YOUR SKILLS *Current Trends and Issues*

People who are considering a career in health care and those who already work in health care need to be familiar with current trends and issues. The health care industry is facing a period of unprecedented change with several major questions to be answered. As a consumer of health care yourself, it's important to read articles and view programs that feature information about health care reform and the various issues under debate. When you're part of the health care industry, your family and friends will assume that you know what's going on and have well informed opinions to share.

Where do you stand on efforts to reform the nation's health care system?

- What role, if any, should the government play in health care, health insurance, and health care reform?
- Should taxpayers cover the cost of health care for people who can't afford it?
- What changes, if any, should be made to Medicare and Medicaid to reduce the cost to taxpayers and ensure long-term viability?
- Should people be required to have health insurance or pay a penalty if they don't want the insurance, believe they don't need it, or can't afford it?
- Should employers have to provide health insurance for their employees or pay a penalty?
- Which health care services should be, and should not be, a standard part of health insurance benefits?

THE BIG PICTURE AND WHERE YOU FIT IN

Now that you are aware of *the big picture* in health care and its history, trends, and issues, it should be obvious that you have your work cut out for you. You must be able to view the health care industry from both the service side and the business side and keep both in balance.

You'll wear at least three different hats—as a patient, a taxpayer, and a health care professional. Each time you change a hat, your **perspective** will change along with it. Some of your perspectives might conflict with the others. Here are a few examples:

perspective (per-SPECK-tiv) The manner in which a person views something

- What's best for you as a patient might not be what's best for you as a taxpayer. As a patient, you want the very best health care that money can buy, no matter what the cost. But as a taxpayer, you know that resources to fund medical care are limited.
- What's best for you as a health care professional might not be what's best for you as a patient. As a health care professional, you want to leave work on time to get on with your busy personal life. But as a patient, you want your caregiver to stay as late as necessary to finish your procedure without handing you off to the next shift.
- What's best for you as a taxpayer might not be what's best for you as a health care professional. As a taxpayer, you want to reduce the cost of health care to avoid tax increases. But as a health care professional, you want the government to fund medical research to help develop new treatments and cures.

In order to make the best decisions, you must keep all of these perspectives in mind as you move through the day. Always try to see things through the eyes of your patients. Because, when you are at work and wearing your professional hat, your patients must always come first.

REALITY CHECK

Up to this point, you've learned a great deal about the health care industry. Here's a quick recap:

- You've examined why health care needs professionals and what it takes to develop a professional reputation.
- You've learned about the major services in health care and the wide variety of occupational choices available.
- You've read what it takes to develop a strong work ethic and meet performance standards related to character, attitude, behavior, and appearance.
- You've learned how to develop strong interpersonal relationships and function effectively on teams.
- You've explored the elements of interpersonal communication and how electronic communication, computers, and information technology are used in health care.
- You've become familiar with the history of health care and today's efforts to reform and improve the industry.

Now it's time to ask the question: "Is there a place for you in the health care industry?"

- Can you see yourself working in a health care facility, serving as a caregiver or working behind the scenes to support patient care?
- Do you have the motivation and commitment it takes to complete training and meet employment requirements?
- Are you committed to meeting performance and quality standards and complying with policies and regulations?
- Do you have the character and personal values required to be seen by others as honest and trustworthy?
- Can you work well with other people and treat them with respect?
- Do you appreciate the differences among cultures and value diversity?
- Do you communicate effectively and support teamwork and a spirit of cooperation?
- Can you put what's best for other people ahead of yourself?

By now, you should know enough about what it's like to work in health care to know whether or not you're cut-out for a career in this industry. Not everyone can achieve success working in health care. The work is stressful and tiring. It can be frustrating and demanding. Just when you think you have everything figured out and in place, something changes and you have to readjust again. The only constant in health care is change. If you don't like change, you'll probably struggle working in this industry. If you don't like people, and serving the needs of people, then health care probably isn't the best place for you.

constant
(CON-stent) Fixed, unchanging

On the other hand, if you are a *people person* and have been inspired and challenged by what you've read so far, perhaps health care might be the perfect place for you. There are few things in life more exhilarating than knowing you've made a positive difference in someone else's life.

Some health care workers are like *renters*, while others are like *owners*. Renters have a short-term outlook. They don't feel a sense of ownership, so they avoid investing their time, money, and energy in taking care of things and making improvements. Owners, on the other hand, are in it for the long run. They not only take care of things and make improvements; they also take pride in the results.

The health care industry needs owners—people who are in it for the long-run and for more than just a paycheck. Health care needs people who take pride in their work and make positive ripples with everything they say and do.

If you're willing to study hard, work hard, and dedicate your career to improving the lives of other people, then please keep reading. Health care needs people just like you. It's time to figure out where *you* fit in and what role *you* will play in the health care industry of the future.

Key Points

- The health care industry includes many types of providers and delivery systems to help people with health problems.
- Health care facilities offer a variety of services, including therapeutic, diagnostic, information, and environmental/support services.
- Many agencies—some private, some funded by federal, state, or local governments—meet special needs.
- Regulatory agencies develop and enforce standards to ensure safety and the appropriate delivery of health care services.
- Facilities have an organizational chart to help them be more efficient and to establish a chain of command.
- Health care has become very expensive in recent years; several programs have been put into place to help control and reduce costs.
- The current trend in health care is managed care, where primary care doctors serve as gatekeepers to help reduce costs while maintaining quality and continuity in care; outpatient care, wellness, and preventive care are emphasized.
- Efforts are underway to reform the health care system with a focus on new types of health insurance programs; examples are health care exchanges and accountable care organizations.
- The Patient Protection and Affordable Care Act, signed into law in 2010, is controversial and under debate.
- Health care workers wear at least three different hats—as a patient, a taxpayer, and a health care professional, but they must always put their patients first.

Section Review Questions

Answer each of the following questions. Indicate which page in the textbook led you to your answer.

1. What is the difference between the service-side and the business-side of health care?
2. Explain the purpose of HEDIS.
3. What is managed care and how is it different from fee-for-service?
4. How do primary care doctors function as gatekeepers?
5. List three reasons for the rising cost of health care.
6. List three ways that providers have modified their practices to provide quality health care at a lower cost.
7. Why are patients encouraged to seek outpatient care rather than inpatient care?

Learn By Doing

Complete Worksheets 1–5 in Section 4.2 of your *Student Activity Guide*.

Chapter Review Questions

Answer each of the following questions. Indicate which page in the textbook led you to your answer.

1. How do best practices and benchmarks improve the quality of care?
2. Who was the founder of the Red Cross?
3. What is PDSA and for what is it used?
4. Why might someone hesitate to seek help for mental illness?
5. What is a health care exchange?
6. Explain the statement, "The only constant in health care is change."
7. What is driving the need for more geriatric specialists?

Chapter Review Activities

1. Investigate Leonardo da Vinci to find out how his work combined medicine, science, and art. How and why did this happen, and what impact did his work make on health care overall? Identify another person whose work combined science, medicine, and art and answer the same question.
2. Think about the role that superstition played in the early days of medicine and health care. Make a list of three examples and discuss the impact of each. Do you think that superstition still plays a role in health care? Consider "An apple a day keeps the doctor away." Is this true? Can you think of another current example?
3. Find out how the United States compares with other countries in terms of life expectancy, infant mortality rate, and other measurements of health and wellness. Where does the United States exceed other countries, and where does it lag behind? What causes these differences? Do other countries get better health outcomes than the United States even though we spend more money per person on health care? If so, why?

What If? Scenarios

What would you do in each of the following situations? Record your answer, explain it, and indicate which page in the textbook led you to your decision.

1. You've been invited to participate on a panel next month to discuss options for health care reform. You really want to accept the invitation but you don't feel prepared. You've heard just enough about health care reform on TV to know it's a controversial topic. You read a newspaper article stating that health insurance is changing. And you overheard a heated conversation last week between your father and uncle, arguing about taxes, Medicare, and something called an individual mandate.
2. Your neighbor has paid you a visit, very upset about the bill he just received for having some blood tests run at a local clinic. He said the cost this year was 25% higher than what he was charged for the same tests a year ago. Since you are preparing to work in health care, he wants you to explain why the cost has gone up so much and what, if anything, is being done to reduce the expense.
3. An outpatient surgery center in your town is experiencing an increase in adverse effects. No one knows for sure what's causing the problem. The surgeons and staff are highly concerned that the situation might continue and even get worse unless the cause can be identified and fixed.
4. You need to select a new health insurance plan and you have two choices. Plan #1 is the least expensive, but you have to choose a doctor from the insurance company's list. Your family doctor, who

has cared for you and your family for many years, isn't on the list. Plan #2 is significantly more expensive, but you and your family can continue to receive care from your current family doctor. There also appear to be differences in the two plans with regards to premiums, co-pays, and deductibles.

5. Your parents are aging and about to the point where they need help with daily activities. You are wondering if they should think about selling their home and moving to a community or facility that can provide the extra support they need, but you aren't sure what types of options are available.
6. Your aunt has just been diagnosed with diabetes. You would like to connect her with an organization that can help her understand and manage her condition.
7. Your sister just had surgery and needs convalescent care, but you have no idea which health care facilities offer this type of care.

Media Connection

Use the companion website for additional interactive learning activities.

Portfolio Connection

Keep copies of your written assignments in your portfolio. These will serve as samples of your writing skills and your ability to conduct research and identify credible sources of information. Also keep copies of the outlines of the oral presentations that you've given. These will serve as samples of your ability to organize material and present topics in a well thought-out manner.

Start compiling a list of Health Care Trends and Issues to keep in your portfolio. Include a short description of each trend or issue to explain why it's a hot topic. As time passes, keep your list and descriptions up-to-date. This list will be helpful as you continue your studies and participate in conversations about your future industry.

CHAPTER 5

Finding the Right Occupation for You

Source: auremar/Shutterstock

SECTIONS

5.1 Career Planning and Self-Discovery

5.2 Career Exploration and Preparation

"In a world that is constantly changing, there is no one subject or set of subjects that will serve you for the foreseeable future, let alone for the rest of your life. The most important skill to acquire now is learning how to learn."

JOHN NAISBITT, INTERNATIONAL BEST-SELLING AUTHOR, 1929–PRESENT

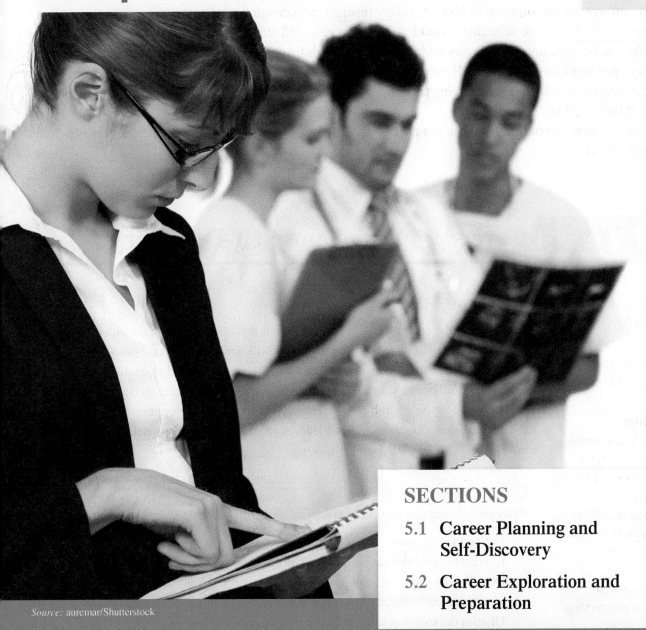

GETTING STARTED

Write a description of what an ideal day would be like for you once you've started working in health care. Let your imagination *run wild.* If you have already chosen a health occupation to pursue, include it in your description. If you haven't chosen your health occupation yet, that's okay. By the end of this chapter, you should be several steps closer to making some decisions.

In what type of health care facility would you be working? Where would the facility be located? Would you be working directly with patients or functioning behind the scenes? Would you be working in a diagnostic, therapeutic, informational, support, or biotechnology research and development service?

Describe your ideal work schedule. Would you be working full-time, part-time, or supplemental? What hours would you be working (such as day shift Monday through Friday, evening shift on weekends only, four 10-hour days per week, and so forth)? How much money would you be earning per hour, or per year? What employment benefits would you be receiving (health, dental, or vision insurance; retirement plan; paid holidays and vacation time, and so forth)?

Once you've written your description, list at least five factors that led you to come up with this ideal-day employment situation.

SECTION 5.1 Career Planning and Self-Discovery

occupation
(aa-cue-PAY-shen) A person's job to earn a living

part-time
(PART time) Working approximately 20 hours a week

supplemental
(suh-ple-MEN-tul) Flexible work schedule with no guaranteed hours or benefits

motivations
(MOE-the-vay-shuns) Forces that move you to set goals and achieve them

values
(VAL-yews) Important elements in a person's life

preferences
(PREH-fer-ens) Giving priority or advantage to some things over other things

interests
(in-TER-ests) Things that draw the attention of a person

Background

Having to make career decisions can be quite a challenge. When considering occupations in health care, it's important to focus on your motivations, values, personality preferences, priorities, and interests as well as your knowledge, skills, and abilities. When you understand yourself, you are better prepared to select an occupation that's a good match for you. Health care offers many different career opportunities from which to choose. Taking assessments and learning more about yourself will provide valuable information to help with decision making.

Objectives

After completing this section, you will be able to:

1. Define the key terms.
2. Explain the role that dreaming plays in career planning.
3. Describe the importance of having a career plan and a vision statement.
4. List the characteristics of SMART goals and explain why goals are necessary.
5. Discuss the role that self-discovery plays in career planning.
6. List three types of career assessments and explain their value.
7. Discuss how identifying your motivations, values, personality type, and interests can help you select a career that matches your needs and preferences.
8. List three skills included in the Framework for 21st Century Learning.
9. Discuss the importance of identifying your knowledge, skills, and abilities when considering career options.

CAREER PLANNING

Let's dream a little. Right now, your whole life is ahead of you, and you have the time and space to dream. You may not have a dream right now, but don't let anything hold you back at this point. Every person deserves the opportunity to shape his or her own future.

Once you have a dream, you need a plan to make your dream a reality. It's okay if you have to change your plan later on, because you ran into road blocks, discovered limitations, or decided to head in a different direction. Even though things might change, you still need a plan to get started.

Your dreams are essential in the career planning and decision making process. When you close your eyes and envision the future, what do you see yourself doing? What do you want to be? Deciding *what you want to be* isn't easy. In fact, many people in their thirties and forties are still asking that same question. Even if you know right now *what you want to be,* things will probably change in the future.

In today's world, people change jobs and occupations several times during their lives. Just when they think they have it all figured out, something changes. Perhaps they get married, move to a new town, start a family, lose their job, deal with a health issue, or become caretakers for aging parents. Changes such as these often take people away from their **career plan** for awhile, but they can usually get back on track later on.

In 2010, the U.S. Bureau of Labor Statistics reported that the average employee remains in his or her job for about 4.4 years. That means that as a working adult, you may have seven to ten different jobs within your lifetime. Some of these job changes will be promotions or even career changes. While no studies currently exist that suggest the number of actual career changes within a lifetime, having a long-term career plan that you update frequently will help you navigate the vision you design for yourself.

skills
(SKILS) Capabilities that can be acquired and developed through a learning, practice, and repetition

abilities
(aa-BIL-ih-tees) Underlying enduring traits useful in performing tasks

assessments
(aa-SES-ments) Tools or processes to gather information

career plan
(kuh-reer plan) Strategy for a person's professional growth and development

APPLY IT CHANGING JOBS

Do some research to find out why people change jobs, and make a list of the top ten reasons. Consider workers who are *forced out* of their jobs as well as workers who leave their jobs *voluntarily*. Think about these job-change factors as you begin developing your own career plan.

Author Ralph Waldo Emerson (1803–1882) said, "Life is a journey, not a destination." Think about that. It's not the *end point* that makes life worth living. It's the *journey* along the way. Where will *your* journey take *you*? Planning for your future involves taking some risks, pushing yourself, and stretching your limits to find out what you're really capable of accomplishing. There are no guarantees in life, just opportunities waiting to be seized.

Journalist Edgar Ansel Mowrer (1892–1977) said, "Life is unsafe at any speed, and therein lies much of its fascination." Which **capabilities** have *you* yet to discover?

capabilities
(kay-peh-BIH-la-tee) Potential abilities

Your journey starts with developing a plan, because *thinking ahead* is an important step in preparing for your future. If you skip the planning process and move directly into a job or an educational program right after high school, things might work out just fine. Or, they might turn out to be a big disappointment and a waste of your time, energy, and resources. A plan will ensure that you have the *right information* and are doing the *right things* at the *right time*. A well thought-out plan will guide your journey so you don't get lost.

You have your whole life ahead of you. You have time to make some mistakes and wish you had done things differently. But if you pause right now and spend some time thinking, planning, and researching, you'll likely make better decisions. As an adult, you will probably spend as much time at work as you will at home. It's important to choose an occupation that will lead to a satisfying and rewarding career. If you want to work in health care, you have lots of choices to consider.

Writing SMART Goals

SMART goals
(SMART goles) Goals that are specific, measurable, attainable, relevant, and time bound

Before you start developing your career plan, you need to know how to write goals. A goal is something that you strive to achieve. Goals help identify the steps that you'll need to take as you move through your career plan. Your goals should be SMART—specific, measurable, attainable, realistic, and time bound. **SMART goals** will bring awareness to what you need to be doing in order to make progress on your plan. Let's explore each aspect of a SMART goal.

- ***Specific.*** Specific goals are clear and include more details than general goals. "I want to work in a hospital" is a general goal. A specific goal would be, "I want to work in a pediatric unit caring for sick children." To be very specific, your goal should address these factors: who, what, when, where, why, and how. The more specific your goal, the more clear your approach can be to achieving it.
- ***Measurable.*** Measurable goals will answer the questions "how much, how many and/or how long." When a goal is measurable, you'll know for sure if you've achieved it. Using the example above, a measurable goal would be to "work in a pediatric unit caring for sick children by December of 2016."
- ***Attainable.*** Attainable goals are realistic. These are goals that you are willing and able to accomplish, and believe *can be* accomplished. "I want to become a physician by the time I'm twenty" isn't an attainable, realistic goal given the amount of education and training this requires. "I want to become a physician by the time I'm thirty" would be more attainable. When you believe a goal is attainable, you're in a better position to figure out how to accomplish it.
- ***Relevant.*** Relevant goals align well with your other goals and your overall career plan. For example, if your career plan is to become a surgical technologist, then "I want to learn to speak French fluently" would not be a relevant goal. "I want to learn medical terminology" would be, however.
- ***Time bound.*** Time bound goals have deadlines. "I will graduate from high school" for example, doesn't have a timeline. "I will graduate from high school by the time I reach 18 years of age" has a specific date in mind. When your goals have deadlines far into the future, it's hard to stick with them. If your deadlines come up too quickly, your goals might be unrealistic. Either way, you might become discouraged and fail to accomplish what you've set out to do.

FIGURE 5.1

Writing SMART goals for career planning

Source: Carmen Martin/Pearson Education

Short- and Long-Term Goals

Your career plan will contain both short-term and long-term SMART goals. Short-term goals can be accomplished within a day, week, month, or year depending on the overall timeline of your career plan. Long-term goals, on the other hand, require significantly more time to achieve, but often lead to your ultimate outcome. For example, if your long-term goal is "to become a registered nurse working in a rural clinic providing health care for families living in poverty," you would need to accomplish several short-term goals along the way. These goals might include:

- Graduating from high school.
- Becoming a Certified Nursing Assistant (CNA).
- Working as a CNA to earn money for college tuition and textbooks.
- Applying for financial aid to obtain a loan and college scholarship.
- Gaining admission into a four-year nursing program.
- Earning a bachelor's degree in nursing.
- Passing the nursing board exam to become a registered nurse.
- Obtaining employment in the rural clinic of choice.

Once you graduate from high school or earn your GED and move through a career plan such as this one without delays, your long-term goal will take at least four or five years to accomplish. By setting and achieving short-term SMART goals along the way, you'll be more likely to stay on track and reach your destination. Five years might sound like a long time to you right now, and it is. But as you work on your short-term goals, those five years will pass by faster than you can imagine.

Developing a career plan involves several steps. Let's get started.

Writing Your Vision Statement

Start with the end in mind. As mentioned, an important part of career planning is having a dream or a **vision** for your future. When you put your vision in writing, it becomes a **vision statement**, or a vivid and idealized picture of the future you desire. Your vision

vision
(VIH-zhun) A mental image to imagine what the future could be

vision statement
(VIH-zhun STATE-ment) A vivid and idealized picture of the future

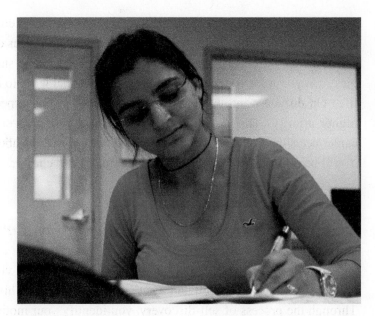

statement should be so *real* that you can feel it, taste it, smell it, and hear it when you close your eyes. It should inspire, energize, and help you focus on where you're headed.

What do you want your future to look like? What role should your job and career play? Do you want your career and your professional work to be a high priority in your life? Or, do you want an occupation that supports other aspects of your life that take higher priority? This is a key question because your answer will influence the other career decisions you need to make. Take some time to think about your vision statement. You'll be referring to it several times throughout this chapter.

UNDERGOING SELF-DISCOVERY

Before you can answer the question, "*What do I want to be?*" you need to know more about *who you already are*.

self-discovery
(SELF dis-KE-veh-ree) The process of learning about one's self

In order to develop a career plan that will support your vision statement, you need to know more about yourself and what's important to you. This is called self-discovery. Through the process of self-discovery, you identify your motivations, values, interests, personality preferences, and priorities. You also learn more about your knowledge, skills, and abilities. This information will help you understand yourself better so that you can choose the occupation that best fits you.

You can learn more about yourself in several ways; for example, you can:

- Answer the questions posed in this chapter and make some lists.
- Ask people who know you well to help you identify your strengths and abilities.
- Observe your own attitudes and behaviors and notice what works for you and what doesn't.
- Take some assessments to help you work through the self-discovery process.

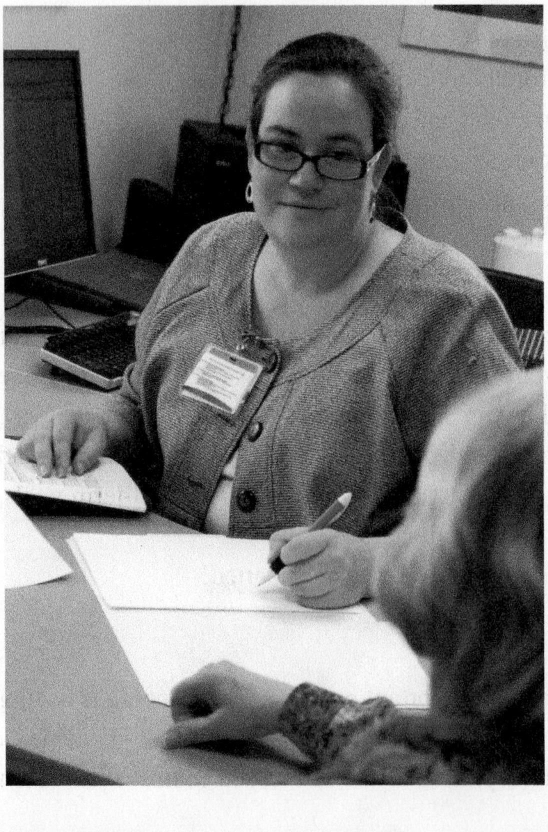

FIGURE 5.2

Career counselor explaining the benefits of assessments

Source: Carmen Martin/Pearson Education

Taking Advantage of Assessments

A variety of assessments are available to help with career planning. These are tools to help you learn more about yourself. Taking assessments can:

- Help you focus your time and effort on career planning.
- Improve your ability to make good decisions.
- Help you identify which careers fit you best.

Some assessments are free; others require a small fee. Some are paper and pencil; others are online. Some provide a self-report; others require assistance to interpret the results. Meeting with a career counselor can also be a big help. Career counselors administer and interpret a variety of assessments. They also combine the results from several assessments to help you *put the pieces together*.

Here are some examples of helpful types of assessments:

- ***Values assessments,*** such as the Values Inventory or the Work Values Profiler, can help you identify things that are important to you and motivate you.
- ***Personality assessments,*** such as the Myer's Briggs Type Indicator, the Keirsey Self-Directed Search, and the Golden Personality Type Profiler, can help you identify preferences based on your personality type. You can learn more about how you take in information and make decisions, how you reenergize yourself, and how you might react to stress at work.
- ***Interest assessments,*** such as the Strong Interest Inventory and the Self-Directed Search, can help you identify those things that are most interesting to you. You can expand or narrow your occupational search by identifying careers that match your interests.

Assessments are not tests. There are no *right* or *wrong* answers, or *good* or *bad* results. Assessments are just another way to learn more about yourself in order to make good career decisions.

Consider This *O*NET Online*

The U.S. Department of Labor's Employment and Training Administration resources are especially helpful in career planning. O*NET Online (http://www.onetonline.org/) is a comprehensive source of occupational information on hundreds of different jobs. At O*NET, you can enter a keyword in *Occupational Search* or browse under *Find Occupations* to locate a wealth of information about specific jobs. You can also use assessment results to search occupations that align with your work values, interests, skills, or abilities.

O*NET job profiles include:

- Occupational descriptions
- Job tasks
- Tools and technology used
- Knowledge, skills, and abilities required
- Job zone (extent of preparation, education/training needed)
- Education requirements
- Related occupations
- Wages and employment trends (national and state)
- Sources of additional information
- Details about **basic skills**, general work activities, personal interests, work styles, and work context

Spend some time exploring this site and become familiar with how to locate helpful information. You will be using O*NET resources several times in this chapter.

basic skills (BAY-sik SKILS) Fundamental aptitudes in reading, language, and math

Finding Out What Motivates You

extrinsic
(eck-STRIN-zik) Motivated by external influences

intrinsic
(in-TRIN-sik) Motivated by internal influences

Motivations are the forces in your life that move you to set goals and achieve them. Motivations may be something **extrinsic** or external, such as grades, money, or getting the keys to the car for the weekend. Or, motivations may be something **intrinsic** or internal, such as knowing you're *the best* at something, or gaining a sense of satisfaction by knowing you've helped someone. Not everyone is motivated by the same forces or to the same extent. Some people have a hard time becoming motivated to perform the simplest of tasks, while others will drive themselves to exhaustion to achieve a goal. Regardless, most everyone is motivated by something.

A lot of what drives us is psychological and cultural. Abraham Maslow, a noted psychologist, developed a model that describes how a person's *needs* influence his or her motivations. Maslow's Hierarchy of Needs describes what moves people to behave in certain ways. This hierarchy is often portrayed as a triangle. A person must meet *basic needs* (survival, safety/security, love and belongingness, and esteem) before the individual will focus his or her motivation on *higher needs* and strive for *betterment* in self-actualization and transcendence.

Maslow's Hierarchy of Needs includes:

- ***Survival:*** Includes breathing, food, water, and sleep.
- ***Safety/Security:*** Security of employment, resources, family, health, and property.
- ***Love and Belongingness:*** Friendship, family, and romantic love.
- ***Self-Esteem:*** Confidence, achievement, and the respect of others.
- ***Self-Actualization:*** Creativity, spontaneity, problem solving, and acceptance of facts.
- ***Transcendence:*** Connecting with something beyond yourself to help others.

Take a few minutes to think about how Maslow's Hierarchy of Needs applies to you. What motivates you right now? What would it take to motivate you to complete high school, earn a college degree, or graduate from a health care educational program? How would you sustain that motivation over time? Is it having a job that leads to a nice home in a safe neighborhood? Is it having a career that brings meaning to your life? Is it knowing that you've achieved something that others have not, and earning their respect because of it?

Knowing and understanding what motivates you is an important step in beginning your journey. When the going gets rough and you become tired or frustrated, knowing what motivates you can help keep you on track and moving forward in your career plan.

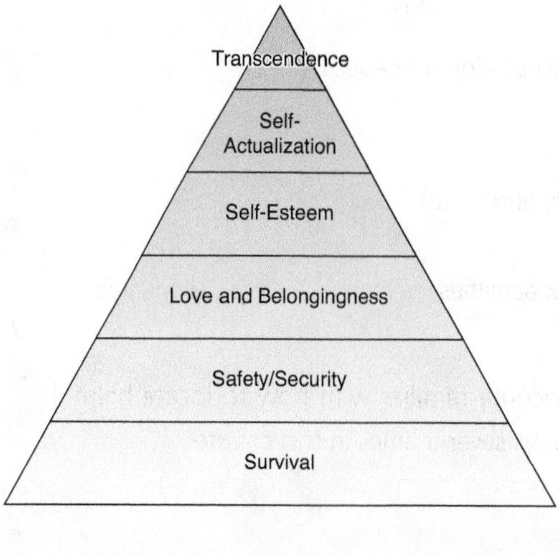

FIGURE 5.3
Maslow's Hierarchy of Needs

Identifying Your Values

An important step in self-discovery is identifying your values. Values are important elements in your life, and they guide you to act in certain ways. Your personal values represent needs that become clearer as you mature. Eventually, your values shape your behavior and help you set your goals. Values arise from the environment in which you grew up, and are influenced by your family, friends, school, and religious affiliations. Your values are also influenced by media (such as television, newspapers, and blogs) and by life experiences.

As you go through life, you view your experiences through the lens of your values and what your values mean to you. Choosing a career that allows you to *live out* your values will go a long way towards carving out a rewarding and fulfilling life. Values generally don't change much throughout a person's lifetime, so it's important to take your values into account when deciding on a career.

Here are some examples of personal values:

- ***Achievement.*** Doing work that yields results or a sense of accomplishment.
- ***Advancement.*** Increasing your level of responsibility through job promotions.
- ***Aesthetic.*** Creating beautiful things that make the world more attractive.
- ***Challenge.*** Performing difficult tasks.
- ***Collaboration.*** Working with other people.
- ***Competition.*** Pitting your abilities against other people with a win or lose outcome.
- ***Compensation.*** Receiving high pay.
- ***Creativity.*** Using your own ideas.
- ***Helping Others.*** Providing assistance to individuals or groups.
- ***Helping Society.*** Doing something to improve the world.
- ***Independence.*** Making your own decisions.
- ***Influence.*** Having the ability to affect people's opinions and ideas.
- ***Knowledge.*** Learning and understanding new information.
- ***Leadership.*** Leading others.
- ***Leisure.*** Enjoying time *away* from work.
- ***Location.*** Working in a place near your home, with a short commute.
- ***Personal Growth.*** Engaging in activities that offer opportunities to grow as a person.
- ***Power and Authority.*** Controlling the work activities of other people.
- ***Prestige.*** Having status and high standing.
- ***Recognition.*** Receiving credit for achievements, including money.
- ***Stability and Security.*** Having steady and predictable work with the likelihood that you will keep your job.
- ***Variety.*** Doing something different every day.
- ***Working Alone.*** Conducting work by oneself without other people.
- ***Working with Others.*** Working in close relationships with other people.
- ***Working Conditions.*** Working in a pleasant, clean, comfortable setting.

Learning About Your Personality Type

Discovering more about your personality preferences is an important part of career planning. You want to make sure that the occupation you choose is a good match for your personality type.

C. G. Jung developed a personality theory that describes how people differ on four *dimensions*. Each dimension contains a pair of opposite *preferences* or different ways that people respond to the same situation. There are sixteen potential *personality types*

work values
(WERK VAL-yews) Global aspects of work that are important to a person's satisfaction

recognition
(reh-kig-NIH-shen) Receiving credit for achievement

prestigious
(preh-STIH-jes) Admired and respected, of high esteem

THE MORE YOU KNOW

Work Values and Careers

Work values are global aspects of work that are important to a person's satisfaction. *Work values* are different from *personal values* because they relate specifically to your work life rather than your personal life. When you're aware of your work values, you're better prepared to choose a career that matches your values.

O*Net OnLine offers the ability to search careers by work values. The definitions of the work values used within O*Net are as follows:

- ***Achievement:*** Occupations that satisfy this work value are results-oriented. They allow people to use their strongest abilities, giving them a feeling of accomplishment.
- ***Independence:*** Occupations that satisfy this work value allow employees to work on their own and make decisions. People who value independence in their work want to try out their own ideas, make their own decisions, and plan their work with little supervision.
- ***Recognition:*** Occupations that satisfy this work value offer advancement and potential for leadership; these occupations are often considered **prestigious**.
- ***Relationships:*** Occupations that satisfy this work value allow employees to provide service to others and interact with coworkers in a friendly non-competitive environment.
- ***Support:*** Occupations that satisfy this work value offer supportive management that stands behind employees. People who value support want to be treated fairly by the company, and have supervisors who back them up and train their workers well.
- ***Working Conditions:*** Occupations that satisfy this work value offer job security and good working conditions.

Which one or two of these work values is most important to you? Search O*Net Online and explore careers that match these work values. Can you find some careers that sound interesting?

(4 dimensions × 4 preferences = 16 types). ALL of these types are valuable, and everyone exhibits each of the types at least some of the time. However, everyone has tendencies to use one preference over its opposite.

Over the years, people have developed assessments based on Jung's theory that can help you identify your personality type and careers where people with that type are naturally drawn.

The Myer's Briggs Type Indicator

introverts
(IN-tro-verts) People who focus on their inner world

extroverts
(ECK-stre-verts) People who focus on the outer world

The Myer's Briggs Type Indicator (MBTI) focuses on how people differ in perception and judgment. Perception is how people become aware of things and take in new information. Judgment is how people arrive at conclusions based on what they have perceived. The MBTI focuses on eight sets of preferences and identifies sixteen different personality types based on those preferences. For example, some people are **introverts** (prefer to focus on their inner world), while others are **extroverts** (prefer to

TABLE 5.1 C.G. Jung's Theory of Personality

Dimension	Preference on Scale				
Ways of Gaining Energy	E	Extroversion	You focus on your outside world and get energy through interacting with people and doing things.	Social Outspoken Action-oriented	Speaks well External focus
	I	Introversion	You focus on your inner world and get energy through reflecting on information, ideas, and concepts.	Thoughtful Detached Internal focus	Interest in ideas Works alone
Ways of Taking in Information	S	Sensing	You notice and trust facts, details, and present realities.	Realistic Practical Observant	Fun-loving Good at facts
	N	Intuition	You tend to and trust interrelationships, theories, and future possibilities.	Sees possibilities Imaginative Problem solver	Likes new ideas Sees relationship between things
Ways of Making Decisions	T	Thinking	You make decisions using logical, objective analysis.	Logical Objective Consistent	Analytical Looks at facts
	F	Feeling	You make decisions to create harmony by applying person-centered values.	Sympathetic Appreciative Tactful	Looks at values Skillful with people
Ways of Living in the World	J	Judging	You prefer to be organized and orderly and to make decisions quickly.	Planful Decisive Orderly	Stable Responsible
	P	Perceiving	You prefer to be flexible and adaptable and to keep your options open.	Imaginative Open to new ideas	Flexible Spontaneous Curious

focus on the outer world). Some people want to make decisions and bring closure to their work while others prefer to remain open to more options and new approaches.

Keirsey Temperament Sorter-II

The Keirsey Temperament Sorter-II (KTS-II) is another widely used personality assessment. Based on Dr. David Keirsey's theory, it proposes that behavior can be described in one of four *temperament groups*, with each group subdivided into four *character types*. The temperament groups and character types align with the sixteen different MBTI personality types.

According to Dr. Keirsey, temperament is based on a combination of personality traits, behavioral patterns, values, and so forth. Each temperament has its own characteristics. For example, some people talk about reality and everyday life—facts, figures, news, and so forth. Other people talk about the abstract world of ideas, dreams, and beliefs. Some people behave in a practical manner that is focused on getting results. Other people behave in a cooperative manner that is focused on social interactions more so than outcomes.

Golden Personality Type Profiler

Also based on Jung's theory, the Golden Personality Type Profiler is a personality assessment that provides information to help explain why an individual behaves in a certain way in both work and leisure situations. It helps people understand the basis for their decision making and the way they relate to other people. One of its five *global dimensions*, tense versus calm, helps explain differences in how people respond to stress at work.

Taking one or more of these assessments can help you learn more about your personality type and the health careers which most closely match your individual preferences.

Identifying Your Interests

Identifying your interests can help you discover your likes and dislikes. Interests are the activities and tasks that draw you in and cause you to be excited or curious. Knowing your interests can help you select a career because your interests are powerful predictors of career satisfaction. When you select a career that matches your interests, it increases the chances that you will be satisfied and fulfilled in your work. You may find a career that matches your motivations and values, but if it doesn't interest you, eventually you may experience frustration and dissatisfaction with your choice. If you're interested in a particular career, you may still choose to pursue that career even when faced with significant obstacles.

obstacles
(OB-sti-kuls) Things that stand in the way or oppose progress

John Holland's Interest Theory

John Holland explored interests and how they relate to career choice. Through his studies, he developed the RAISEC model that connects personal interests to careers. His theory suggests that people fall into one of six different personality types largely reflected by their interests; these include: Realistic, Investigative, Artistic, Social, Enterprising, and Conventional. Work environments reflect these same types, so people who choose to work in an environment similar to their personality type are more likely to be successful and satisfied.

A six-sided figure (called a hexagon) is used to show the similarities and differences among the six types. Types that are next to one another on the hexagon are most similar. For example, Realistic and Investigative types tend to have similar interests, whereas Realistic and Social types tend to be most different.

FIGURE 5.4
Holland's Six Kinds of Occupations

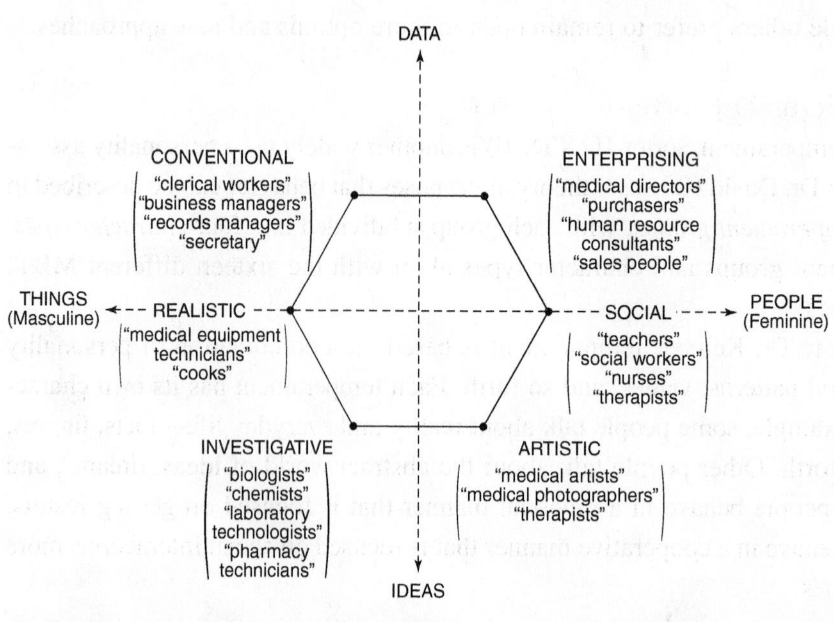

TABLE 5.2 John Holland's Interest Theory

Type	Description	Typical Characteristics	Examples of Health Careers
Realistic	People who have athletic or mechanical ability, prefer to work with objects, machines, tools, plants or animals, or to be outdoors.	Persistent Modest Natural Thrifty	Medical equipment technicians, Cooks
Investigative	People who like to observe, learn, investigate, analyze, evaluate or solve problems. Usually have math or science abilities and like to work alone and solve problems.	Analytical Complex Critical Methodical	Laboratory Technologists, Pharmacy Technicians, Chemists
Artistic	People who have artistic, innovating or intuitional abilities and like to work in unstructured situations using their imagination and creativity.	Expressive Imaginative Impulsive Intuitive	Therapists, Medical Artists, Medical Photographers
Social	People who like to work with other people to enlighten, inform, help, train, or cure them; or are skilled with words.	Understanding Generous Helpful Sympathetic	Nurses, Therapists, Social Workers
Enterprising	People who like to work with other people, influencing, persuading, performing, leading or managing for organizational goals or economic gain.	Acquisitive Domineering Energetic Self-confident	Medical Directors, Purchasers, Human Resource Consultants, Sales People
Conventional	People who like to work with data, have clerical or numerical abilities, carry out tasks in detail, or follow through on others' instructions.	Conscientious Obedient Persistent Practical	Business Managers, Records Managers, Clerical Workers

Self-Directed Search

The Self-Directed Search (SDS) is the most widely used interest assessment in the world. Developed by Holland, the assessment can be easily accessed online for a small fee and will help you identify your interests as well as your skills. The report will identify your 3-letter *Holland code* that you can then match to careers using O*Net Online.

Strong Interest Inventory

The Strong Interest Inventory is another assessment based off the RAISEC model. It is designed to identify your *likes* and *dislikes* and match your profile with the interests of people from a wide range of occupational groups. This assessment helps individuals select careers best suited to their personal interests. The Strong Interest Inventory is offered online or through many career centers.

If you've had a variety of life experiences, you may find the process of identifying your interests much simpler than someone who lacks varied experiences. The six personality types identified by Holland will aid with this process and may help you decide on your interests. As a student, one of the best ways to confirm your interests is to take a variety of courses. Another way is to look at the tasks of an occupation. If you discover that many of the tasks are not interesting to you, reconsider your choice and research careers that are more in line with your interests. Use O*Net's advanced search to learn more about which careers match your interests.

Identifying Your Knowledge, Skills, and Abilities

What have you learned over the years, and what are your unique talents and gifts? Talents and gifts are the skills and abilities that you're naturally *good at*. You may be a great athlete with physical strength and agility, an excellent student in math, or someone who's really good at leading a group and convincing others to follow you. These are all examples of your skills and abilities. It's important to evaluate your abilities and skills during self discovery. Identifying and tapping into both your abilities and your skills will make you marketable in the workplace.

Skills and abilities are the qualifications used to define what a person needs in order to perform in a job successfully. Skills are capabilities that can be acquired and developed through a learning process, practice, and repetition. Abilities are the underlying and enduring traits that are useful in performing the task. It is much more pleasant to work in an occupation that uses both your skills and abilities. If you choose an occupation that is below your skill and ability level, you may become bored. If you choose one above your skill and ability level, you may become frustrated and feel like giving up.

RECENT DEVELOPMENTS

Framework for 21st Century Learning

Skills and abilities are so important that a national organization, Partnership for 21st Century Skills (www.p21.org) has developed a list of skills that every student will need in order to be successful in a global economy. The framework includes the basic core skills that employers are seeking, as well as skills necessary for lifelong learning and innovation, the use of technology, and life and career skills.

Employers are looking for basic skills in mathematics, reading, and writing. In addition, they want employees who have the ability to learn, reason, think creatively, solve problems, and make decisions. These skills demonstrate a person's ability to apply what is learned to their work. Most organizations find these qualities very difficult to teach and therefore look for employees who already possess these talents. Learning these skills takes time and education but applicants who demonstrate these abilities are among the first hired.

As you think about your knowledge, skills, and abilities, you may immediately see some areas where you consistently meet requirements. On the other hand, you may notice some areas where you have low-level skills or an absence of skills altogether. Don't worry. You can acquire many skills and abilities through school and life experiences. For example, if your basic core skills are weak, you can take some extra coursework. To expand your life experiences, you can travel to other parts of the country and interact with people from different cultures.

For career planning purposes, you can start by identifying what you've learned in the past and what your talents are *now*. Make a list of your current skills and abilities. When researching health occupations, you can match your skills and abilities to the job description for each occupation of interest.

FIGURE 5.5

Framework for 21st Century Learning

Core Subjects and 21st Century Themes

Mastery of core subjects and 21st century themes is essential to student success. Core subjects include English, language arts, world languages, arts, mathematics, economics, science, geography, history, government and civics.

In addition, students must understand content at much higher levels by weaving 21st century themes into core subjects:

- Global Awareness
- Financial, Economic, Business and Entrepreneurial Literacy
- Civic Literacy
- Health Literacy
- Environmental Literacy

Learning and Innovation Skills

Learning and innovation skills are what separate students who are prepared for increasingly complex life and work environments in today's world and those who are not. They include:

- Creativity and Innovation
- Critical Thinking and Problem Solving
- Communication and Collaboration

Information, Media and Technology Skills

Today, we live in a technology and media-driven environment, marked by access to an abundance of information, rapid changes in technology tools and the ability to collaborate and make individual contributions on an unprecedented scale. Effective citizens and workers must be able to exhibit a range of functional and critical thinking skills, such as:

- Information Literacy
- Media Literacy
- ICT (Information, Communications, and Technology) Literacy

Life and Career Skills

Today's life and work environments require far more than thinking skills and content knowledge. The ability to navigate the complex life and work environments in the globally competitive information age requires students to pay rigorous attention to developing adequate life and career skills, such as:

- Flexibility and Adaptability
- Initiative and Self-Direction
- Social and Cross-Cultural Skills
- Productivity and Accountability
- Leadership and Responsibility

BUILD YOUR SKILLS *O*NET Assessments*

O*NET Online (http://www.onetonline.org/) offers some free, online assessments that you can take.

The O*NET Interest Profiler helps people identify their interests and how they relate to work. This assessment and the information it provides can help you decide what kinds of careers to explore. Six types of occupational interests are measured: realistic, investigative, artistic, social, enterprising, and conventional. You answer sixty questions by rating each work activity as Strongly Dislike, Dislike, Unsure, Like, or Strongly Like. The Interest Profiler doesn't consider how much education or training is required or how much income you could expect. However, it helps you focus on your individual interests and the types of jobs you might find interesting and rewarding.

The O*NET Work Importance Profiler (WIP) helps people identify what's important to them in a job. This assessment can help you focus on occupations that you might find satisfying based on your work values. The six types of work values measured include: achievement, independence, recognition, relationships, support, and working conditions. You place in rank-order twenty-one different *need statements* according to how much you value each one. You then receive a profile of your work values, which can be matched to different occupations.

The O*NET Skills Profiler helps people identify their skills and match them to jobs. You select the skills you already have, or plan to acquire, from six skill groups: basic skills, complex problem-solving skills, resource management skills, social skills, systems skills, and technical skills. The Profiler then matches your skills to jobs which require those skills.

There are many other assessments you can take to help you narrow down the long list of health occupations to find those which appear to be a good match for you.

FIGURE 5.6

Reviewing assessment results

Source: Carmen Martin/Pearson Education

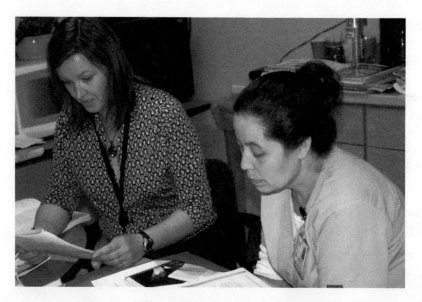

Pulling the Pieces Together

Once you have written your SMART goals and your vision statement, and completed some helpful assessments, you'll be ready to start pulling the pieces together into a career plan. The next step is to use the information you've gathered in exploring the health careers that sound most interesting to you.

REALITY CHECK

As you think about career planning, one thing should become clear—it's time to begin seizing control of your life and your future. What you *do for a living* will be extremely important as you mature and become self-dependent. Your network of family, friends, and advisors can help as you complete your secondary education and identify some occupations that match your motivations, values, personality type, interests, skills, and abilities. But it will be up to you to decide which career path to take and when to launch your plan.

As you finish your high school education or obtain your GED, enrolling in more courses or a training program might not sound very good. Getting a job and making some money might sound better. However, keep in mind that to *earn more* you must *learn more*. As mentioned previously, the first five years after you graduate from high school will fly by quickly. Wouldn't it be better to have a plan and get somewhere during those five years instead of wandering around, trying to figure out who you are and where you fit in the world? It's your future. Start planning now to make the most of it.

secondary
(SEH-ken-dair-ee) High school

Key Points

- Career planning starts with a dream and a vision of what you want to be in the future.
- Having a career plan is important even though it might change in the future.
- Developing SMART goals will help you stay on track and achieve your career plan.
- Self-discovery will help you learn more about yourself in order to choose a career that best matches your needs and personality.
- Assessments are tools to help you identify your motivations, values, personality type, interests, skills, and abilities.
- Knowing what motivates you can help keep you on track and moving forward in your career plan.
- Identifying your personal and work values can help you choose a career that leads to a rewarding and fulfilling life.
- Being aware of your personality type can help you find a career that matches your individual preferences.
- When your career matches your interests, you'll be more satisfied and fulfilled in your work.
- When researching career options, you can compare your knowledge, skills, and abilities to the job descriptions for occupations of interest to you.

Section Review Questions

Answer each of the following questions. Indicate which page in the textbook led you to your answer.

1. What role does dreaming play in career planning?
2. What is the purpose of a career plan?
3. What is a SMART goal?
4. List three ways to engage in self-discovery.
5. List three types of career assessments and explain their value.
6. Explain why you should identify your motivations, values, personality type, and interests when considering career options.
7. Identify four types of career information provided on O*Net Online.

Learn By Doing

Complete Worksheets 1–5 in Section 5.1 of your *Student Activity Guide*.

SECTION 5.2 Career Exploration and Preparation

Background

Exploring careers isn't the same thing as *finding a job*. Career exploration is a lengthy, in-depth process of decision making in which you identify an occupation, a school, an educational **program**, and a job, all of which are geared to aligning *who you are* with *what you do* for a living. Finding a job, on the other hand, is a shorter process of securing employment to meet your financial and career goals.

program
(PRO-gram) A planned set of courses and activities to prepare students for a particular career

Career exploration requires time and effort to research your occupations of interest and identify what it takes to prepare for a specific career. Career preparation includes identifying educational requirements, exploring options for schools and educational programs, and determining eligibility for funding and financial aid.

Objectives

After completing this section, you will be able to:

1. Define the key terms.
2. Identify three resources for career exploration.
3. Describe the value of role models and mentors.
4. List five key questions to ask when conducting occupational research.
5. Explain the role that labor trends and projections play in career exploration.
6. List four key questions to ask when choosing a school.
7. List four key questions to ask when choosing an educational program.
8. Describe the criteria that selection committees use to make admission decisions for schools.

9. Describe the criteria that selection committees use to make admission decisions for educational programs.
10. Name three types of funding and financial aid to help pay educational expenses.
11. List five things you should do in high school to prepare for your health career.

CAREER EXPLORATION

While completing your assessments, you've probably identified several occupations that interest you. Now it's time to explore those options in more detail. Your goal at this point in the process is to identify two or three occupations that might be a good match for you.

Perhaps you already have an idea of the occupation you want to pursue. Maybe you expect to *follow in the footsteps* of a family member ("My mom is a nurse," or "My brother is a respiratory therapist.") Or, you read a pamphlet, viewed a website, or watched a television program about a health career that looks appealing to you. Perhaps you were a patient or a visitor in a hospital, and spotted a job that looked interesting. Maybe your neighbor has made some suggestions, or you've heard that a certain type of worker is in high demand.

These are all good ways to become aware of career opportunities in health care. However, you can't always believe everything that you hear, read, or see. You need to *do your homework* first before making such an important decision. Continue to learn more about yourself, do lots of research, and give serious thought to selecting the best career for you.

Using Career Exploration Resources

A variety of resources and resource people are available to help you research careers. By conducting *occupational research*, you can learn about the **tasks** performed, the **job outlook**, the education required, the working environment, and many other things. Consider using your local library or career center. You can request career-related pamphlets, DVDs, and reference materials. Fortunately, there are also many free online resources available to you, including the following:

tasks
(TASKS) Pieces of work, or functions to be performed, as part of a job

job outlook
(JOB AUT-look) The demand of a career in a certain field

- O*NET Online. As mentioned previously, O*NET Online (http://www.onetonline.org/) is a major source of occupational information on hundreds of different jobs. It will take some work on your part to explore the entire website and learn how to find the detailed information you need, but your time and effort will be worth the investment.
- The *Dictionary of Occupational Titles* (http://www.occupationalinfo.org/) lists job titles, tasks, and duties for over 20,000 occupations.
- The *Occupational Outlook Handbook* (http://www.bls.gov/oco/) discusses the

FIGURE 5.7
Using library references for occupational research

Source: Carmen Martin/Pearson Education

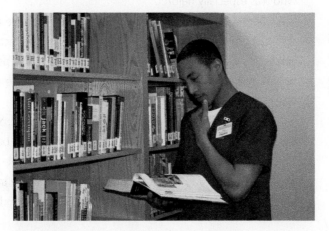

training
(TRANE-ing) Building skills

nature of the work, employment outlook, **training** and qualification requirements, earnings, and working conditions for a variety of occupations.

- CareerOneStop (http://www.careeronestop.org) provides tools for career exploration, including assessments and helpful information to create career goals, explore career options, gain skills, and find a job. You can also access assessments and view videos describing different occupational clusters.

Health care professional associations provide extensive information for people who are considering a career in that discipline. You can contact the professional association directly and ask that material be sent to you, or you can go online and view the organization's website. Many professional associations have state and local chapters that welcome students who wish to join the association and/or attend chapter meetings.

role model
(ROHL MA-dul) A person whom someone aspires to be like

mentor
(MEN-tawr) A wise, loyal adviser

A **role model** or **mentor** can be especially helpful in your career exploration and research. A role model is someone whom you aspire to be like. Role models have the education, work experience, and professional reputation that you want to achieve yourself. You can learn a lot from a role model because he or she has already traveled down the road on which you are starting. A mentor is a wise, loyal adviser who can be helpful as you work on career goals. Although mentors haven't necessarily achieved the same goals that you wish to achieve, they can help provide the insight, advice, and encouragement you need each step of the way. Consider who might make a good role model or

THE MORE YOU KNOW

Supporters and Non-Supporters

Everyone needs some help at some point in their lives, and this is especially true for young people who are planning and preparing for their futures. Whom can *you* turn to for help when you need it?

Identifying a *network of supporters* is a good strategy to ensure you'll have the help you need, when and where you need it. Parents, family members, and friends are a good place to start. Also consider teachers, counselors, school leaders, your friends' parents, and people you know from church, social clubs, and community and athletic organizations. Mentors and role models are part of your network of supporters, so put them on your list. If you've had a job, you might want to include your supervisor or a coworker who was especially helpful.

Choose people who know you well and who take an interest in your activities and well-being. Include people whom you admire and respect, and whose opinions and advice you value. Share your goals and career plan with each person and ask if he or she would be willing to provide some encouragement and advice along the way. If you've chosen wisely, most of them will *climb on board*.

The topic of non-supporters must also be addressed. You may find some people in your life who are not supportive of your efforts. They may be envious, overly competitive, or threatened by the thought of your success. Some people may question your goals or your abilities and claim you're *reaching too high*. Others may try to hold you back or even sabotage your efforts. Watch out for these negative forces and don't let them derail your plans.

mentor for you, and ask if he or she would be willing to serve. You might be surprised how quickly the person will say, "Yes!" Consider volunteering to serve as a role model or mentor for someone else. After all, everyone is on this road together.

Other opportunities for researching health careers include volunteering in a local hospital or nursing home, participating in summer health career camps, attending health career fairs, joining student organizations such as HOSA or a Medical Explorer post, and working a summer job in a health care facility. Participating in activities such as these will help you meet a variety of people who work in health care and who can help you explore and research career options.

HOSA
The student organization for health occupation students at the secondary, postsecondary, adult, and college level

Conducting Occupational Research

The goal of your exploration efforts is to find a career that provides satisfaction and an income. You'll be spending many hours *at work* during your career. So take time now to thoroughly investigate your options.

The following is a list of questions to be answered as you explore different careers:

1. ***What job tasks are required?*** Review the tasks involved in the job. Tasks are pieces of work, or functions to be performed, as part of a job. Are the job tasks things that you are interested in doing? Will performing these tasks satisfy your motivation and values? Are you physically, psychologically, and emotionally capable of performing these tasks? If you have physical, psychological, or emotional limitations, you should give them serious consideration when reviewing job task requirements.
2. ***What knowledge, skills, and abilities are required?*** Review the knowledge, skills, and abilities required for the job. Do they sound like things you could learn and do every day? Do they match your personality and preferences? For example, if you like to work alone in a quiet environment, would a job that requires a high level of customer service and social interaction be a good fit for you? If you want a job with a daily routine and predictable workload, would working as a paramedic on an emergency transport helicopter fit your preferences?
3. ***What are the education and training requirements?*** Education is acquiring knowledge and information. Training is building skills. Becoming a health care professional requires both education and training. For example, to become a competent radiographer, you need *education* to learn anatomy, physiology, pathology, and how ionizing radiation is used to study internal parts of the human body. You need *training* to learn the skills required to position patients and safely operate high tech diagnostic imaging equipment. Oftentimes, these terms are used interchangeably, such as referring to *an educational program* or *a training program.* In this chapter, the term *educational program* refers to *a planned set of courses and activities to prepare students for a particular career.* Educational programs for health careers include skills training as well.

   Review the educational requirements for the job. Consider your own situation and the resources you have to support your education. Should your first step after high school be on-the-job training, or do you have the resources to attend college or another postsecondary educational program before starting work? Decide which option might be best for you. Things may change as time goes by, but at least you'll have a general plan to get started.

education
(eh-jeh-KAY-shen) Acquiring knowledge and information

Several health careers have more than one level. For example, some of the options in the rehabilitation profession include occupational therapy aide, certified occupational therapy assistant, and occupational therapist. As you move from one level to the next, you will need more education and training. After considering your interests and resources, you may decide to pursue an associate's degree to become a certified occupational therapy assistant knowing that you may be able to return to school later on to become an occupational therapist.

4. ***What are the licensing, certification and/or registration requirements?*** Many occupations in health care require licensing, certification, registration, or a combination of these. What licensing, certification, or registration requirements must be met for the occupations you are considering? It's important to be aware of these, because you won't be eligible for employment in your discipline until you have complied with these requirements.
5. ***How much does the job pay?*** Compensation for jobs varies according to the region of the country where you work. Investigate the *average pay range* ($37,440 to $62,400 per year, for example) for the occupations of interest to you, based on where you plan to live and work. Compensation is either an hourly rate (such as $18.00/hour) or an annual rate (such as $37,440/year). A full-time employee with a 40-hour/week schedule will work about 2,080 hours per year. In addition to your *base pay*, you may be eligible to work *overtime* and receive a higher rate of pay for those hours. Employees who work holidays or the evening or night shift may also be paid at a higher rate for those hours.

   As a new employee, you will likely start at the bottom of the pay range. As time passes and you gain more experience and earn some pay raises, your compensation will move towards the mid-point of your pay range. If you remain employed with the organization for a significant period of time and earn outstanding performance evaluations, your rate of pay will move towards the top end of your pay range. If you secure a job promotion, your responsibilities will increase along with your hourly or annual pay rate.

   Be sure to investigate the *average cost-of-living* for the area of the country where you plan to live and work. If the cost-of-living is especially high, you'll need an occupation with higher pay than if you lived in a region where the cost-of-living is low. Pay rates are often higher in large cities than in rural areas. Employers base their compensation rates on *market factors* which often take the average cost-of-living for their area into consideration.
6. ***What are the continuing education requirements?*** Many licensing, certification, and registration bodies require **continuing education** in order to maintain your status. Continuing education is additional instruction for adults who have completed their **formal** education. This requires you to invest in your learning each year in order to keep your professional status. What are the continuing education requirements for the occupations of interest to you? Where can you obtain continuing education and how much will it cost? These are important details to identify as you choose an occupation.
7. ***What are the opportunities for career advancement and professional development?*** As you move from a **novice** to an expert, or as you mature and your needs change, you will probably want to seek opportunities for advancement and professional

continuing education
(con-TIN-you-ing eh-jeh-KAY-shen) Additional instruction for adults who have completed their formal education

formal
(FOR-mul) Structured, in accordance with accepted forms and regulations

novice
(NAH-ves) Someone new in a field or activity, a beginner

growth. This may require returning to school and/or earning more certifications. You may need to take on a new role with added responsibility within your field. Or, you may become cross-trained to function in a multiskilled role. By knowing what opportunities are available in advance, you can include them in your career plan and be well prepared when the time comes. Sometimes, opportunities for advancement and professional development can be difficult to identify, so you might need to speak with someone who works in the field to get the information you need.

8. ***What are the labor trends and projections for this occupation?*** It's important to learn about the labor trends and projections for your occupations of interest. Labor trends are forces that impact employers, workers, and job seekers. For example, in nursing the trend among hospital employers is a preference for hiring nurses with bachelor's degrees over nurses with associate's degrees. If you're interested in a nursing career, you need to know this. If you stop your nursing education at the associate's degree level, you may be limited in where you can work.

projections
(preh-JEK-shuns) Estimates of the number of positions needed in the future

labor trends
(LAY-bor TRENDS) Forces that impact employers, workers, and those seeking work

Labor trends are affected by workforce *supply and demand*. When there's a shortage of registered nurses, for example, employers may be more open to hiring nurses with associate's degrees because there aren't enough nurses with bachelor's degrees to fill their positions. However when there's a surplus of registered nurses, or fewer open nursing jobs, employers will likely hire candidates with bachelor's degrees. Labor trends vary from discipline to discipline, so it's important to research the trends for the specific occupations of interest to you.

Labor projections are estimates of the number of positions that will need to be filled in the future. When exploring health careers, you want to choose an occupation with ample employment opportunities, both when you enter the job market and in the future. If you choose an occupation that is shrinking, your employment options will be limited. Occupations referred to as *hot jobs* are typically those with the best employment opportunities.

labor projections
(LAY-bor pre-JEK-shun) Estimates of the number of positions needed in the future based on labor trends

Labor projections are presented as percentages and as actual numbers. It's best to look at the labor projections that are presented as actual numbers because projections presented as *the percentage of growth* can be misleading. For example, if the number of workers in an occupation is relatively small, such as 13,000 audiologists in the U.S., this means that even a high percent of growth, or 37%, will create a relatively small number of new jobs, such as 4,810 additional jobs for audiologists. However, if the number of workers in an occupation is higher, such as 108,800 respiratory therapists, then even a modest percent of growth of 19% will create many more new jobs, such as 20,672 additional jobs for respiratory therapists.

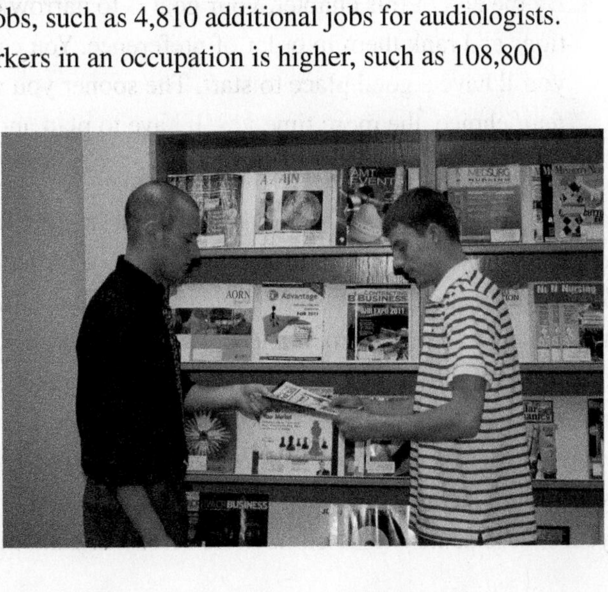

FIGURE 5.8

Researching careers by reviewing medical journals and speaking with a health care professional

Source: Carmen Martin/Pearson Education

Labor projections vary from state to state, so it's important to find projections for the state in which you want to work. State-specific information can be found at www.careerinfonet.org. When you look at the average number of openings for audiologists in Indiana, for example, between 2008 and 2011, it's only eleven.

As you can see, understanding how to use labor projections is a key element in career exploration. If your interests, values, motivations, and personality preferences point you to a career with just a modest projected growth rate, that's okay. You might still decide to pursue that career with the knowledge that finding a job could be more of a challenge.

Making Career Decisions

cognitive (COG-neh-tiv) Based on facts and logical conclusions

intuitive (in-TOO-eh-tiv) Based on instinct and feeling

Having completed your occupational research, you should have the information and resources you need to explore the careers of interest to you and begin making some decisions. People make decisions in different ways. People with a **cognitive** style of decision making prefer to consider all the information they have researched and documented, while others with an **intuitive** style of decision making like to go with their instinct based on how they feel at the time. Regardless of your decision making style, research shows that even people with an intuitive style make better decisions when they combine their decision making with factual information.

The process of decision making described in this chapter focuses on a cognitive style. If you use an intuitive style, consider how you might combine both styles to make your career decision more thoughtful. The following is a list of next steps:

1. Complete the assignments and activities in both sections of this chapter, including the assessments. Learn as much as you can about yourself and the careers that appeal to you, and use that information in your decision making.
2. Review the health occupation descriptions presented in this textbook. Consider the information you learned from your assessments and from your chapter assignments and activities. Identify the five occupations that sound like the best match for you.
3. Research your five careers of interest using the Career Exploration Resources discussed earlier. Answer the questions listed in Conducting Occupational Research for each career. Document the information you find. Based on what you learn, start eliminating some of the options which are no longer in consideration. Speak with your network of supporters to get their input and advice.
4. By the end of this chapter, your goal is to narrow down your list to three occupations and rank them in order of preference. You can change your mind later, but you'll have a good place to start. The sooner you narrow down your options to one *final* choice, the more time you'll have to plan and prepare.

Once you've obtained as much information as possible, you need to start thinking about a decision. One of three things might happen. You might review all of the information you've gathered and use it to make a logical choice. You might instinctively know which career is *the right choice* for you and start heading in that direction. Or you might feel so overwhelmed and pressured that you'll need to take more time to think and figure out things. How soon you need to make a decision will depend upon your age and other personal factors.

You may find yourself somewhat hesitant to make a decision. If so, that's okay. If you're missing a key piece of information that might make your decision easier, review your assessments and do some more research. Take time to think about what feels right

BUILD YOUR SKILLS *Job Shadowing and Informational Interviewing*

One of the best ways to learn more about a job is to meet with someone who works in that occupation. Job shadowing involves spending time with a health care professional in his or her work environment to observe job tasks and to see what a typical day is like.

Another option is informational interviewing. *Informational interviews* are different from *job interviews.* The purpose of an informational interview is to learn more about a particular occupation or job by speaking with someone in the field and asking for their advice. This could be a role model or a current or a recently-retired health care professional.

Teachers, counselors, or parents can help arrange a job shadow or an informational interview. Because you are asking for someone's time and attention, you should observe the following etiquette:

- Research the occupation and prepare for the discussion ahead of time.
- Arrange a time and meeting place convenient for the professional.
- Dress appropriately (business casual clothes, such as slacks and a nice shirt for males, and a pantsuit, skirt and blouse, or dress for females).
- Arrive on time, and don't stay longer than scheduled.
- Ask well-prepared questions and take notes.
- Don't ask questions in front of patients and or interrupt the work flow when meeting in a work environment.

The following are some questions you might want to ask:

- What attracted you to this career?
- What is your typical day like?
- What do you like the best and least about your work?
- What level of education do you need to work in this field?
- What types of continuing education are required?
- How should I prepare myself to enter this occupation?
- Where are the best job opportunities?
- Where do you see this occupation going in the next five years?
- What types of career advancement and professional growth opportunities are available?
- Is there someone else you would recommend I speak with? If so, would you help me get in touch with this person?
- Do you have any other advice to offer?

Be prepared to talk about why you are interested in this career. The person you speak with may have some insight and advice based on your interest.

Within two days of the job shadowing experience or the informational interview send the person a hand-written Thank You note to express your appreciation for the time he or she spent with you. You never know, you may want to touch base with this person again when you start seeking employment after graduation.

job shadowing
(JOB SHA-doe-ing) Spending time observing a professional in his or her work environment to see what a typical day is like

for you. If you still aren't sure which career to pursue, consider **job shadowing** and/or scheduling an informational interview to gather more information and advice.

If you're still hesitant, you may lack the confidence you need to become *who you really want to be*. If this is the case, now is the time to connect with your network of supporters to get the encouragement and advice you need to take that first step.

It takes courage, strength, and determination to step into the future, but you can do it. You're off to a good start on your journey, and right where you need to be at this stage of your life and your career.

CAREER PREPARATION

Once you've identified the occupation you want to pursue, you need to consider what it's going to take to make your dream a reality. You already have a lot of the information you need to write your SMART goals and begin preparing for your career. The most important step in career preparation is meeting the educational requirements.

Meeting Educational Requirements

Many occupations have multiple entry points to consider; these include:

- On-the-job training.
- Completion of a postsecondary certificate educational program.
- Completion of a college degree educational program.

Most health occupations require completion of either a postsecondary certificate educational program or a college degree educational program. Therefore, only a few occupations allow for on-the-job training. If you enter health care through on-the-job training, at some point you'll need to complete more formal education to qualify for job advancement.

Based on the research you've conducted, the educational requirements for your chosen career should be fairly clear. If you have the choice of either a certificate program or a college degree program, review your Vision Statement, consider your personal situation, and think about the resources available to support your education. Speak with your parents, teachers, and counselors to get their input. Once you've decided on an approach, include it in your career plan.

Meeting career-related educational requirements starts while you're still in high school. Regardless of the occupation you choose, you'll need to obtain your high school diploma or a GED. Very few jobs in health care don't require a high school education or a GED. If you plan to apply for admission to a postsecondary certificate program or a college degree program, you'll need to complete your high school education or obtain your GED first.

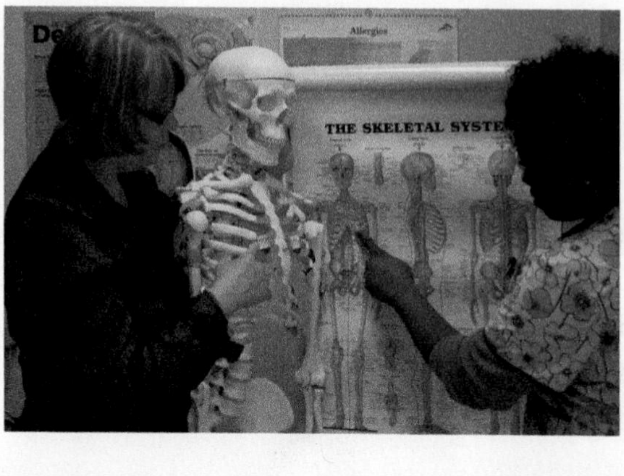

FIGURE 5.9

Studying human anatomy to learn about the skeletal system

Source: Carmen Martin/Pearson Education

Think about the courses you should take during your remaining time in high school. Which courses would provide the best academic foundation for your postsecondary education? Consider advanced courses in math and science, including pre-calculus or calculus, biology, chemistry, and physics. Also consider the humanities and social sciences, such as literature, history, writing, public speaking, and philosophy, to strengthen your reading, writing, oral communication, and critical thinking skills. Strengthen your computer skills and become proficient in several software applications, such as Microsoft Word, Excel, Outlook, Access, and PowerPoint. Learning to speak a foreign language is a good idea; bilingual skills can be highly valuable when applying for jobs in health care.

There's a major difference between high school courses and postsecondary courses. Once you're enrolled in college or a certificate program, your coursework will become more difficult, and your instructors will expect more from you in terms of grades and performance. You'll need good time management, stress management, and personal financial management skills. Effective study skills will be key to your success, along with motivation and the ability to *hang in there* when things get tough. Take a variety of courses in high school, especially those which challenge you and lead to **advanced placement** (AP) credit; they will help prepare you for the **rigors** of higher education.

advanced placement
(ad-VANS-d pleys-muhn) High school courses that qualify for college credit

rigors
(RI-gers) Things that are hard or severe

Consider This *Anticipating Delays, Obstacles, and Barriers*

Regardless of which health occupation you choose, chances are you'll encounter some bumps along the way. Delays might include getting married, becoming a parent, moving to a new town, or suffering the death of a loved one. Obstacles might include a lack of motivation, too much stress, poor study habits, or not gaining admission to the school or program of your choice. **Barriers** might include a cut in your financial aid, the loss of support from family or friends, or the inability to find a part-time job to help pay expenses.

A study from the Bill and Melinda Gates Foundation summed it up best when it found that the main barrier to staying in school was a conflict between school, work, and family commitments. By anticipating potential delays, obstacles, and barriers, you can plan ahead and have some strategies in mind to get your career plan back on track.

barriers
(BER-ee-ers) Things that obstruct or impede

Choosing a School and an Educational Program

To prepare for your health career, you'll need to choose a school and an educational program and gain admission.

Postsecondary schools are *institutions of higher learning* that offer several different educational programs. Most likely, the school you will choose will be a public, private, or for-profit college or university. However, several *teaching hospitals* also offer educational programs for people who wish to become health care professionals. Some of these hospitals operate as colleges; they *award college credit* and *grant college degrees*. Other hospitals don't award college credit or grant college degrees, but they do award *Certificates of Completion* for students who meet graduation requirements. All of these colleges, universities, and teaching hospitals must meet strict requirements to maintain their accreditation.

You will also need to choose an educational program. Educational programs provide discipline-specific courses to prepare for your health career. As you think about choosing an educational program, consider your own **learning style**. How do you learn best—through large or small classes, hands-on labs, online courses, self-study courses, or a combination of these? Many educational programs and courses are now offered online. Online courses are popular because they allow you to access the information and complete assignments at times most convenient for you. On the other hand, online courses lack the face-to-face instruction and interactions with other students that might be advantageous to your learning.

learning style
(LERN-ing STILE) The method in which a student learns best

Identifying and Researching Prospective Schools

Depending on where you live and want to attend school, you may have several schools from which to choose. The first step is to identify those schools which offer the type of educational program you need to prepare for your health career. Some schools, for example, offer educational programs in nursing, medical assisting, pharmacy technician, and health information technology, while other schools conduct programs in physical therapy, occupational therapy, radiography, and nuclear medicine technology. Take advantage of reference materials, online websites, and assistance from your teachers, counselors, mentors, and role models to help identify schools from which you may choose.

The following is a list of questions to answer as you explore different schools:

1. ***What is the school's accreditation status?*** The school's accreditation status, referred to as **institutional accreditation**, is extremely important. Accreditation is a quality assurance process that a school must undergo to verify that it is meeting necessary educational standards. If a school is not accredited, it might not offer the level of quality of education you need to become competent in your field. Schools are accredited by a variety of national and state agencies and must undergo periodic site-visits by teams of surveyors to maintain their *active accreditation status.* Accredited schools provide high quality education and opportunities for financial aid, and they give students the ability to transfer college credits from one accredited school to another.

   Be sure to investigate the accreditation status of the schools that you are considering. Also investigate the agency which accredits the school because some accrediting bodies have stricter requirements for quality than others. If the school is relatively new and not yet accredited, the benefits of accreditation might be withheld until the school's active status is awarded. If the school has lost its accreditation and is seeking reaccreditation, the benefits of accreditation may be withheld until the school's active status has been regained. To avoid problems that result from accreditation issues, it's best to choose a school which is currently accredited by an agency that requires high standards for quality education.

institutional accreditation
(in-steh-TOO-shen-al a-KREH-deh-tay-shun) A quality assurance process to ensure that a school meets high quality standards

2. ***What is the school's reputation?*** Is the school well regarded in both the community and the state in which it is located? Do past and present students speak highly of the school? Would they recommend the school to others? Does the school attract and retain well qualified instructors? Are the school's courses filled, or almost filled, to capacity? Do area employers hire the school's graduates? How is the school's reputation presented in the media?

If the school appears to have a poor reputation and difficulty recruiting and retaining top instructors, filling its classes, and placing its graduates in jobs, then you would probably be wise in choosing a different school.

3. ***Does the school grant college degrees or certificates of completion?*** If your career plan calls for earning a college degree, the school you choose will need to be either a college or university.

   - *Community colleges,* also known as *two-year schools,* award associate's degrees. They also award certificates of completion for certain educational programs that do not lead to a college degree.
   - *Colleges*, sometimes referred to as *four-year schools*, award associate's and bachelor's degrees. Some colleges also award certificates of completion for certain educational programs that do not lead to a college degree.
   - *Universities* award associate's and bachelor's degrees as well as *postgraduate* courses leading to master's and doctoral degrees.

   If your health career requires an associate's degree, you could attend a community college, a college, or a university.

   If your career requires a bachelor's degree, you could attend a community college for the first portion of your education and then transfer to a college or a university to complete your education. Community colleges tend to be less expensive than four-year schools, and they admit students who need **remedial** coursework or a stronger academic foundation before enrolling in a four-year school.

   If your health career requires a master's or doctoral degree, the school you choose will need to be a university.

   Depending on the occupation you've chosen, you may have the opportunity to consider a teaching hospital as your school. Acquiring your education in a medical setting offers several benefits, including a direct route to employment at graduation.

remedial
(ri-ME-dee-al) Correcting a deficiency

4. ***What does the school require for admission?*** Admission requirements are the minimum standards that an applicant must meet to be considered for admission to the school. Some schools have *open admission*, which means they accept applicants regardless of their academic background. Other schools have specific academic requirements, which must be met prior to admission. Admission requirements typically include a minimum score or higher on the ACT or SAT test (exams that measure your academic readiness for college) plus a minimum grade point average (**GPA**) for your high school courses. GPA is calculated by dividing the total amount of grade points earned by the total amount of credit hours attempted.

GPA
A measure of a student's academic achievement in school

5. ***How diverse is the school's student population?*** You might want to consider the diversity of the student population for each of the schools you're considering. Are you looking for a school that's populated with students like you, or would you prefer a school where you can meet and interact with students from a variety of different cultures and backgrounds? In which environment would you be most comfortable? Your assessment results should give you some clues.
6. ***What is the average class size?*** Some schools have very large classes, with as many as 300 students attending a lecture at one time. Other schools feature smaller classes and personal interaction with instructors. Do you learn best in a small class, or would larger classes meet your needs?

7. ***What is the travel distance to the school?*** Can you drive to the school or take public transportation, or will you need to move to another location to be closer to the school? If you move, will you be able to come back home frequently or during school breaks? Travel distance will affect your expenses, so this is an important factor to consider when choosing a school.
8. ***Does the schedule of classes offer flexibility?*** Are the courses that you need to take offered at times convenient for you? Are classes offered during the daytime or evening hours or on weekends? Are online courses available? If you plan to work a part-time or full-time job while you're in school, or if you have family and personal obligations to meet, the flexibility of class times could be an important factor to take into consideration.
9. ***How much does the school cost, and does it offer financial aid?*** Schools vary greatly in terms of what they charge for tuition, books, fees, room and board, and other costs. It's important to estimate these expenses and have a plan in place to cover them before you finalize your choice of school. Does the school appear to offer a *good value* for what they charge? How do the schools that you're considering compare with one another in terms of costs? What sources of financial aid are available through the school? On average, how much financial aid does the school award per student? Resources to support your education must be taken into consideration when choosing a school.

Based on these questions and others that are important to you, you should be able to gather enough information to decide which school would best meet your needs. You may want to apply to more than one school to increase you chances for selection and to give you more choices when the time comes to make a final decision.

Identifying and Researching Prospective Educational Programs

Choosing the right educational program to meet your needs is just as important as choosing the right school. The school you choose will provide general *core courses* to lay the foundation for your health care courses. Core courses include subjects such as English Composition, Psychology, Sociology, Mathematics, Chemistry, Biology, and Human Anatomy and Physiology. The educational program you choose will provide discipline-specific courses and training you need to prepare you for employment in health career.

FIGURE 5.10

Researching schools and educational programs online

Source: Carmen Martin/Pearson Education

Some of the same factors which are involved in choosing a school also apply in choosing an educational program. The following is a list of questions to answer as you explore different educational programs:

programmatic accreditation (PRO-gra-ma-tik a-KREH-deh-tay-shun) A quality assurance process to ensure that an educational program meets high quality standards

1. ***What is the educational program's accreditation status?*** The accreditation status of an educational program, referred to as **programmatic accreditation**, is an

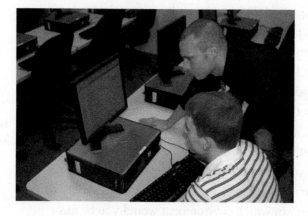

extremely important factor to consider when choosing a health care educational program. Programmatic accreditation ensures that the educational program, and the school that sponsors the program, have met high standards for quality education.

Many health careers require satisfactory completion of an accredited educational program before you can sit for your licensure, certification, or registration exam to obtain your professional credentials. If you enroll in an educational program that isn't appropriately accredited, you'll be investing your time and resources in an approach that ends with significant barriers to credentialing and employment.

Be sure to investigate the accreditation status of the educational programs you're considering. As is the case with schools, if the program is relatively new and not yet accredited, the benefits of accreditation might be withheld until the program's active status is awarded. (In other words, you might not be eligible to sit for credentialing exams and secure employment.) If the program has lost its accreditation, it might be best to consider another program.

2. ***What is the educational program's reputation?*** Is the program well regarded in the community? Do past and present students speak highly of the program? Would they recommend the program to others? Does the program attract and retain well qualified instructors? Are the program's classes filled, or almost filled, to capacity or does the program struggle to recruit students? Do area health care employers hire the graduates of the program, or do employers prefer to hire graduates from other programs? Find out which programs the employers prefer, and put those at the top of your list.
3. ***Does completion of the educational program lead to a college degree or a certificate of completion?*** Based on the health career you've chosen, make sure the educational program leads to the outcome required for credentialing and employment. If the career requires an associate's or bachelor's degree, then graduating from an educational program that awards a certificate of completion won't prepare you for credentialing or employment in your field.
4. ***What does the educational program require for admission?*** Like schools, educational programs have minimum standards that an applicant must meet to be considered for admission. Some educational programs in health care have open admission, but most are highly competitive. This means there will be more applicants vying for admission than *seats* to be filled. Admission requirements for health care educational programs typically include a minimum score on the ACT or SAT test plus a minimum grade point average for your high school courses.

   Knowing program admission requirements in advance can help you stay on track in high school, or get back on track if necessary. Many health care educational programs expect applicants to have at least a 3.0 GPA (out of 4.0) for high school courses.
5. ***How diverse is the educational program's student population?*** Once you complete your general education and begin your discipline-specific courses, you'll likely form close relationships with other students in your program. As in choosing a school, you might want to consider the diversity of the student population for each of the educational programs you're considering. Would you be more

comfortable in classes with students like you, or would you prefer a program with a more diverse array of classmates? Refer to your assessment results for some insight.

6. ***What is the average class size?*** Educational programs in health care have a *limited capacity*. This means there's a limit to how many students can be enrolled in an educational program at any given time. Some programs have a relatively large number of students while others have very small classes. Which type of environment would best meet your needs?
7. ***How does the program handle clinical experience?*** Most health care educational programs require *clinical experience* prior to graduation. Sometimes referred to as *internships, externships, practicum*, or *hands-on experience*, clinical experience gives students the opportunity to apply, practice, and improve their skills in an actual health care setting before they graduate from school and begin employment. As you might image, where and how you do your *clinicals* is a very important part of your health care education.

   Most high-quality educational programs *place* their students in pre-arranged *clinical sites* and *rotate* students within the site, or among different sites, to provide a variety of experience. But some educational programs expect students to find their own clinical sites and make the arrangements themselves. This situation can create major problems. Most health care facilities that are willing to provide clinical experience won't make arrangements directly with students. Instead, they sign a clinical affiliation agreement with the program and accommodate students when the program places the students in their site. If students contact the facility directly, they are usually referred back to their program for guidance. It's best to choose a program that has pre-arranged clinical sites. If it's a quality program, you shouldn't have to make your own arrangements. The following are some questions to ask to investigate the program's clinical experience:

   a. How much clinical experience do the students receive (the number of hours, weeks, or months over a certain period of time)?
   b. How much variety do the students experience through clinical rotations (the types of patients and kinds of procedures to which students are exposed)?
   c. Where exactly do the students do their clinical experience (the names and locations of specific hospitals, physician practices, clinics, and so on)?

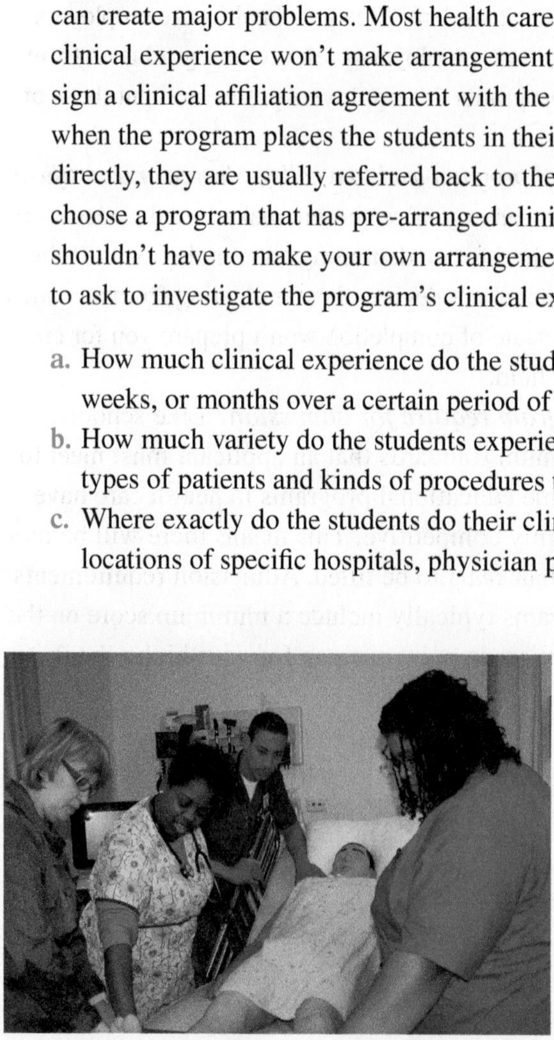

FIGURE 5.11

Learning clinical skills in a simulated environment before working with actual patients

Source: Carmen Martin/Pearson Education

Next to programmatic accreditation status, how and where a program provides clinical experience is probably the most important factor in choosing a health care educational program. You want to do your clinicals in a state-of-the-art facility that welcomes students and has a structured plan in place to help students build their skills. If your clinical experience falls short, you'll lack the competence and confidence you need to succeed on-the-job.

8. ***How long is the program and what is the graduation rate?*** How long is the program, and how long does it take the average student to complete program requirements? Does the program run on an academic calendar or is attendance required year round? Do you have a preference on program length or schedule? You'll want to choose an educational program where the majority of students can complete requirements and graduate within a reasonable amount of time. How many students are accepted into the program, and how many actually graduate? If the dropout or termination rate is high, it might signal poor admissions procedures or other quality-related problems.
9. ***What is the pass rate on board exams for program graduates?*** Depending on the health career you choose, you may have to pass a state or national exam to become licensed, certified or registered. So it's important to choose an educational program with a good track record in preparing its graduates to pass the exam. If the program's pass rate is high, you can rest assured that it offers quality education. If the program's pass rate is low, it's best to find another program.
10. ***What is the job placement and job retention rate for program graduates?*** Your primary reason for enrolling in an educational program is to eventually get, and keep, a good job in your discipline. So you need to identify the extent to which past and present graduates are getting jobs (job placement), and keeping their jobs (job retention).

    Of those students who graduate, how many have a job in their chosen field within one to three months of graduation? The job placement rate is helpful information for two reasons—it indicates the reputation of the program among area employers, and it reflects employment trends in that field and that area of the country. The job retention rate among program graduates is also important. If graduates get jobs but can't keep them, perhaps the educational program they attended was lacking in quality.

Applying for Admission to a School and an Educational Program

Once you've chosen the school and the educational program that best meet your needs, you must complete a two-step process before beginning your discipline-specific education. First, you have to apply to the school, get accepted, and complete your prerequisites. Second, you have to apply to the educational program and get accepted.

prerequisites (pre-REH-kwe-zets) Required or necessary as a prior condition

School Applications

You'll need to fill out and submit an Application for Admission to your school of choice. You may need to complete a lot of paperwork, so find a way to stay organized. Some applications are on paper while others are online.

Schools are looking for applicants who can perform well and meet requirements for graduation. School *selection committees* typically require and review the following application materials:

- ***Transcript.*** The selection committee will review the rigor of the courses you've taken in the five core subject areas (English, Math, Science, Foreign Language, and Social Studies) and the grades you've earned. Your GPA will be very important.

- ***ACT, SAT, or AP exam scores*** (if required). Many schools consider test scores as part of admissions. Consider taking a practice exam first, such as the PSAT. Prepare for these exams and do your best. If your score is too low and you have the opportunity, consider taking the test again.
- ***Essay*** (if required). Some schools require an application essay. The essay is an example of your communication skills and your ability to follow instructions. Give thought to what you want to say because selection committees may pay a lot of attention to applicants' essays. Be sure to answer the essay question and grab the reader's attention with a strong opening paragraph. Double-check your spelling and grammar, and make sure the essay is your own work. Never have someone else write your essay for you.
- ***Résumé of Activities or Career Portfolio*** (if required). The selection committee wants to know *who you are* and *what you would bring* to their school and campus. Highlight your accomplishments, interests, extracurricular activities, career plan, and any leadership experiences you've had.
- ***Letters of Recommendation*** (if required). Part of the process of communicating *who you are* comes from the recommendations provided by people who know you well. Choose people who are familiar with your academic history, strengths, interests, and goals to provide your letters of recommendation. Ask them in advance if they would be willing to recommend you for admission. Give them copies of your transcript and review your portfolio with them to help them describe you in a more holistic way.
- ***Personal Interview*** (if required). Some schools require a personal interview. If you must undergo an interview, make sure you present a professional image. Review the information in this textbook to help you prepare.

Once you've been accepted into the school, it's time to work with a counselor to arrange your schedule of courses. Depending on the school you've chosen and the health career you're pursing, your list of required courses should be fairly clear. Most of your courses will be designated as *required* while a few will be *electives*. You must complete certain prerequisite courses and earn good grades before applying to your educational program.

You'll need to manage your time well and set priorities for yourself in order to keep your GPA high. A general *rule of thumb* is three hours of study time for every hour of class time. If you fall behind in your assignments or earn less than satisfactory grades, it's going to be hard to catch up. Work with a tutor, participate in a study group, ask for extra help from your instructors, or reach out to your network of supporters if the going gets rough.

FIGURE 5.12

Student studying to prepare for class

Source: Carmen Martin/Pearson Education

Educational Program Applications

Once you've completed the necessary prerequisites, you'll be ready to submit your Application for Admission to the educational program. Some of the information from your school application will be considered as part of your program application.

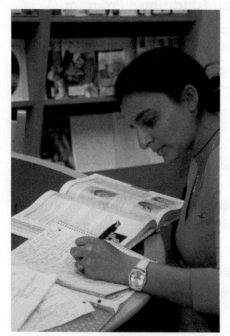

Program *selection committees* typically require and review the following application materials:

- ***Transcripts.*** The program selection committee may wish to review your high school transcript as well as the grades you've earned so far in your postsecondary courses. The grades you earn in your prerequisite courses will be very important since they are the best predictors of success in your discipline-specific courses.
- ***Standardized Entrance Exam Scores*** (such as the TEAS V, HOBET, or NET). These exams are used to assess your overall academic achievement. Sometimes, additional components to these assessments (such as critical thinking) are of interest to selection committees. Before taking an assessment, find out which parts of the assessment are reviewed and hold the most weight in the selection process. Make sure you study and prepare in advance. You can find review and preparation books in a library, or you can purchase them inexpensively from a used book store.
- ***Personal Health Assessment.*** Educational programs have health requirements you must meet to participate in the program. Your personal health assessment will likely include vaccination requirements and possibly a **drug screen**. If a personal health assessment and drug screen aren't required for acceptance into the program, they probably will be when you start your clinical experience. When you apply for a job after graduation, the employer will reassess your personal health and conduct another drug screen.
- ***Criminal History Background Check.*** This process is conducted to make sure that students are suitable for participation in the program and clinicals. Finger printing and a local, state, and national criminal history check may be conducted. Certain types of criminal offenses may not prevent you from acceptance into the program, whereas other types of offenses will.

  If a **criminal history background check** isn't required for acceptance into the program, it probably will be prior to starting your clinical experience. Health care facilities are very selective in whom they accept for clinicals. If your background includes a **felony** or a **misdemeanor**, you may be excluded from clinical sites depending on the specific offense and the circumstances surrounding the conviction. When you apply for a job after graduation, the employer will conduct another background check.
- ***Personal Interview*** (if required). You may have to undergo a personal interview with members of the program selection committee or with others who are involved in the program. You'll be asked why you chose this profession and how you know it's a good match for you. Having read this chapter and completed your assignments, you'll be well prepared to answer these questions. Review the information in this textbook and remember what it takes to make a positive and professional first impression.
- ***Career Portfolio*** (if required). By now you're familiar with the purpose of a career portfolio and you have started compiling one. Your portfolio documents your progress, achievements, and efforts throughout your academic and work career. It provides samples of your work and evidence of your growth and accomplishments

drug screen
(druhg skreen) Lab test to detect illegal substances in a job applicant

criminal history background check
(krim-uh-nl his-tuh-ree bak-ground chek) A review of legal records to search for misdemeanors and felonies

felony
(fel-uh-nee) A major offense with extensive jail time as a penalty

misdemeanor
(mis-di-mee-ner) A minor offense with a fine and/or short jail sentence as a penalty

over time. Some of this information may come in handy as you apply for admission to an educational program.

Gaining admission to your educational program of choice is a significant accomplishment. Now it's time to focus on how to cover your educational expenses.

Securing Funding and Financial Aid

Several sources of funding and financial aid are available to help students pay for their education. These include federal student aid, scholarships and grants, work study, and student loans. In order to receive financial aid, you must fill out applications and meet eligibility requirements.

To determine which sources of aid you might qualify for, start by completing the Free Application for Federal Student Aid (FAFSA), which collects information about you and your family's financial situation. Complete the FAFSA as soon as possible after January 1 and before early March of the year in which you are requesting aid. The FAFSA can be accessed at www.fafsa.ed.gov.

Based on the results of your FAFSA, you may be eligible for one or more of the following types of funding:

- ***State or federal grants*** such as Pell Grants and Academic Competitiveness Grants are considered *gift aid* and generally do not have to be repaid.
- ***Work-study programs*** provide jobs for *undergraduate* students with financial need. They allow you to earn money for expenses while gaining valuable work experience.
- ***Student loans*** have to be repaid, so consider this a last resort. The two basic types of student loans are private and federal. *Private loans* are through lending institutions such as banks, and they generally have higher interest rates. *Federal loans*, either subsidized or unsubsidized, are through the federal government and made available to both students and their parents. *Subsidized loans* are awarded based on financial need, and the government pays the interest until loan repayment begins. *Unsubsidized loans* are not based on family income, and the recipient must pay the interest. The amount of an unsubsidized loan is based on factors such as the student's year in school, his or her other financial aid awards, and the estimated cost of attending school. When certain criteria are met, students may be awarded both subsidized and unsubsidized loans.

  If you decide to borrow money for your education, learn more about how much you can afford, loan cancellation, and the consequences of default.
- ***Scholarships*** are sponsored by public or private organizations and are often awarded based on academics, athletics, field of study, ethnic background, religious affiliation, or special interest. While the FAFSA may qualify you for some scholarships, you can also look for, and apply for, other scholarships on your own. Scholarships are also gift aid and do not have to be repaid. Check with your school counselor to see if he or she has any suggestions regarding scholarships that you might apply for and how to locate additional scholarship opportunities.

Financial aid is one of the tools that makes higher education possible for many students who otherwise would not be able to afford it. Take time to consider all your options and plan wisely. For more information, check websites such as www.scholarships.com and speak with a career counselor.

RECENT DEVELOPMENTS

The Student Loan Debt Crisis

Student loan debt is growing at an unprecedented rate, raising concerns about the potential impact on the overall U.S. economy. In 2012, student loan debt will reach one trillion dollars, surpassing all credit card debt combined. Some predict that the student debt crisis will create the next *financial bubble*, similar to the subprime housing bubble that severely weakened the U.S. economy in 2008.

The rising cost of a college education is a big part of the problem. Tuition expenses at public colleges and universities where most students receive their education has increased steadily in recent years while government funding for schools has declined. The average tuition cost among public schools increased 8.3% in 2010.

Another contributing factor to rising student loan debt is the drop in family income due to pay cuts, job losses, and unemployment. Dwindling financial support from their families have lead students to take out additional loans in order to remain in school. The average student borrower currently has $25,250 in school debt.

Loan delinquency and default rates are rising, and student loan debt cannot be discharged or refinanced through bankruptcy. Efforts are underway to alleviate the situation, but for the time being people must seriously consider how much debt they can afford. Before taking out a loan, students and parents are cautioned to identify the earning power of a college degree and estimate how long it might take a graduate to repay his or her school loans. As a general rule of thumb, school debt should be no more than 10% of projected income after graduation. Students and parents are also encouraged to consider public colleges and universities rather than more expensive private and for-profit schools.

Ensuring Success

Once you've identified the best health career for you, chosen your school and educational program, figured out how to cover the costs, and finalized your career plan, your future will be off to a great start. Now it's time to do *everything in your power* to launch your career plan and achieve your SMART goals.

When the going gets rough, ask your network of supporters for assistance. They want you to be successful, so keep them informed and let them know how they can help. Hang in there and remember this—nothing of value comes easily.

Manage your time well. Don't fall behind in your studies. Devote three hours of study for every one hour of class time. If you're having difficulty, seek the assistance of a tutor. Many schools offer free tutoring services. If you can afford it, you may choose to pay a private tutor to help you learn the course material. Learn everything you need to know to get good grades and graduate. And learn it well—don't just memorize and regurgitate the information for a test and then forget it. You may have to demonstrate what you've learned on an entrance exam for your program application. You will have to demonstrate what you know when you take your certification, licensure, or board exam.

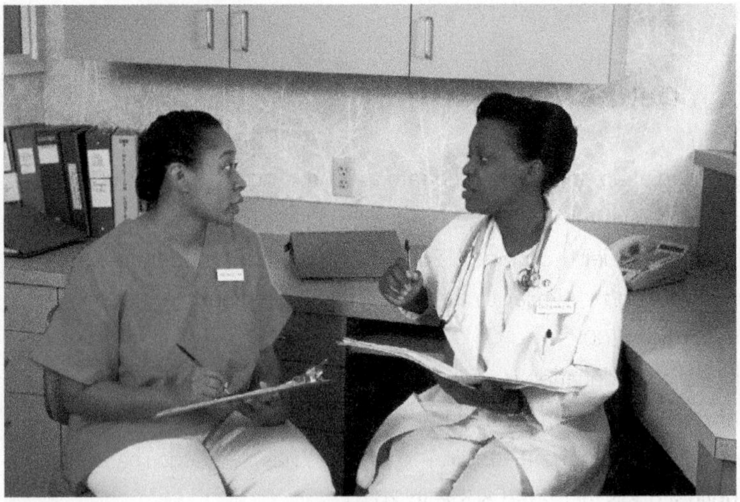

FIGURE 5.13

Meeting with a role model to adjust a career goal

Source: Michal Heron/Pearson Education

Once you're on the job, everything you've learned must come together to make you the very best health care professional you can possibly be.

If you find that your career goals aren't realistic, you can revise them. You may have to adjust a small piece of a SMART goal to make it work for you. You may decide that the occupation you were pursuing isn't a good fit after all. If that happens, you can always repeat the process that you learned in this chapter, research other career options, and pick something that fits you better. You may realize that your timeline needs to be adjusted to give you more time to achieve a long- or a short-term goal. Or you might need to change goals in order to fulfill your Vision Statement.

Keep reading. You'll learn most of what you need to know to succeed in your educational program, secure the job you want, and be recognized by others as a health care professional.

REALITY CHECK

Are you worn out and overwhelmed by all of this, or are you energized and ready to go? You may need to pause for awhile, reflect on what you've learned, and figure out how all of this information applies to you.

This chapter covers a lot of information and calls for some serious thinking on your part. If you're used to having parents or other adults make decisions on your behalf, at some point relatively soon it will be time to start making decisions yourself. If you've completed the activities in this chapter and spent time researching health careers, schools, educational programs, and financial aid, you should be ready to write your SMART goals, complete your career plan, and start making your dream a reality. The time and effort you devote at this stage of your life to career exploration and preparation will become an important investment in your future.

Key Points

- Career exploration is a process of decision making geared to aligning *who you are* with *what you do* for a living.
- Take advantage of resources and resource people to help you research career options.
- A role model or mentor can be especially helpful in career exploration. Participating in HOSA or a summer health care job can help you meet health care workers and research career options.
- Conduct occupational research and ask a series of key questions as you explore different careers.
- Identify labor trends and projections for occupations of interest.
- Consider job shadowing and/or scheduling an informational interview to gather more information and advice.
- Identify the educational requirements for the careers that interest you, and the schools and educational programs which offer the education.
- Decide which courses you should take while still in high school to prepare for your postsecondary education.
- Identify your learning style and use that information when making school and program decisions.
- Ask key questions as you explore different schools and educational programs.
- Selection committees review Applications for Admission and several types of supporting information when making school and program admission decisions.
- Complete the FAFSA to identify your eligibility for various types of funding and financial aid.
- Revise your career goals when necessary, and continue learning what it takes to achieve success.
- When the going gets rough, ask your network of supporters for assistance.

Section Review Questions

Answer each of the following questions. Indicate which page in the textbook led you to your answer.

1. Name three resources for career exploration.
2. What are role models and mentors?
3. What role do labor trends and projections play in career exploration?
4. List five key questions to ask when conducting occupational research.
5. Name three criteria that selection committees use to make admission decisions for schools.
6. Name three criteria that selection committees use to make admission decisions for educational programs.
7. Describe five things you should do in high school to prepare for your health career.

Learn By Doing

Complete Worksheets 1–5 in Section 5.2 of your *Student Activity Guide*.

CHAPTER 5 Review

Chapter Review Questions

Answer each of the following questions. Indicate which page in the textbook led you to your answer.

1. What role does a vision statement play in career planning?
2. Why should a career plan include SMART goals?
3. What is self-discovery and how is it helpful?
4. Name three skills included in the Framework for 21st Century Learning.
5. Why is it important to identify your knowledge, skills, and abilities when considering career options?
6. List four key questions to ask when choosing a school.
7. List four key questions to ask when choosing an educational program.
8. What are three types of funding and financial aid that can help pay educational expenses?

Chapter Review Activities

1. Make a list of your top five strengths and weaknesses. Next, ask four people who know you well to do the same. Compare your list with theirs and discuss any similarities and differences.
2. Review Maslow's Hierarchy of Needs, starting at the bottom of the pyramid with survival needs. Determine to what extent your needs are being met at each level in the hierarchy.
3. Go to www.bls.gov/ooh/healthcare. Identify labor projections for each of the following health occupations: dental hygienist, surgical technologist, registered nurse, cardiovascular technologist, and medical assistant. Identify the *number of jobs*, the *job outlook* from 2010 to 2020, and the *employment change* from 2010 to 2020. Using the *job outlook* percentages, rank the occupations from the highest percentage of job growth to the lowest. Which occupation appears to have the best job growth opportunities? Using the *employment change* actual numbers, rank the occupations from the highest number of new jobs to the lowest. Which occupation appears to have the best job growth opportunities? Explain why the occupation with the highest job growth ranked by percentage appears third on the list when ranked by actual numbers. Why is it important to examine actual numbers rather than percentages when researching labor projections for the occupations of interest to you?
4. Make a list of potential delays, obstacles, and barriers that you might encounter as you prepare for your health career and launch your career plan. List some steps you could take to get back on track if any of these things happen to you.

What If? Scenarios

What would you do in each of the following situations? Record your answer, explain it, and indicate which page in the textbook led you to your decision.

1. You're interested in pursuing a career as a pharmacy technician, but you think you lack the necessary math skills.
2. After reading an online article about careers in biotechnology research and development you're considering becoming a cell biologist, but you aren't sure if this occupation would be a good match for you.
3. Your teacher has encouraged you to develop a career plan, but you expect to get married and move out of town after graduation.
4. You're pretty sure you would like to become a medical coder, but your brother says he doesn't think you are capable of doing that job.

5. A career in sports medicine and athletic training sounds appealing, but you aren't sure what the job market might be after you complete your education.
6. You've narrowed your list of career choices to two, and your sister says you should *go with your gut* pick the one that *feels right* to you, but you aren't sure this is a good way to make such an important decision.
7. Your best friend has chosen the same health career as you, and she's just been accepted to an educational program that lost its accreditation last year. She's pressuring you to apply to the same program.
8. You're planning a career in physical therapy, but you don't have enough funding to enroll in the master's degree program at the private university in your town.

Media Connection

Use the companion website for additional interactive learning activities.

Portfolio Connection

As you research occupations, employment trends and projections, and potential schools and educational programs, document the information you find and file it in your career portfolio. Keep copies of your transcript, applications and application materials, and letters and other correspondence with schools and programs in your portfolio. Also keep names and contact information for your mentors, role models, and other members of your network of supporters. Keep records of job shadowing and informational interviews, and copies of your Thank You letters, in case you want to follow-up with people later on. Keep your portfolio well organized so you can find information quickly when you need it.

CHAPTER 6

Working with Patients

Source: Alexander Raths/Shutterstock

SECTIONS

6.1 **Meeting Patient Needs**

6.2 **Customer Service and Patient Satisfaction**

"How far you go in life depends on your being tender with the young, compassionate with the aged, sympathetic with the striving and tolerant of the weak and strong. Because, someday in life, you will have been all of these."

GEORGE WASHINGTON CARVER, AGRICULTURAL CHEMIST, 1861–1943

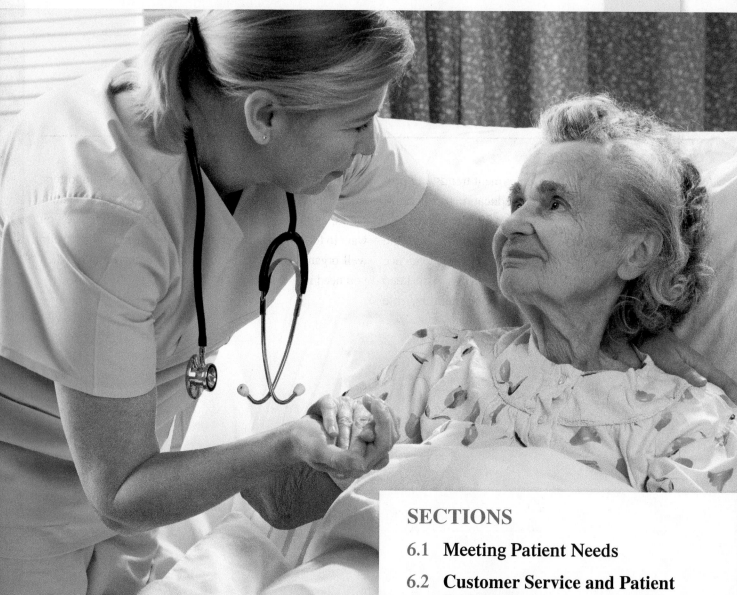

GETTING STARTED

As you will learn in this chapter, humans have a number of basic needs. They include shelter, food and water, work that is fulfilling, safety, family relationships, and access to health care. The level of access to these needs has a direct effect on a healthy lifestyle and quality of life.

Spend one school day experiencing a *disabling condition.* Select from the following: being wheelchair bound, walking with a cane, wearing cotton or another covering to restrict hearing capability, covering eyeglasses with petroleum jelly to impair vision, binding one arm to your side, or other limitations you might consider. Discuss your plan with your teacher ahead of time.

At the conclusion of your day, answer these questions: Was it difficult to perform normal daily activities with this condition? If so, give some examples. How would your lifestyle change if you actually had this condition? What would you need to do to adapt? How could public places (such as shopping malls, restaurants, and movie theatres) improve access and support for people with this condition?

Meeting Patient Needs

SECTION 6.1

Background

A physical **disability** or **mental illness** can strike anyone, at any age. When this happens, people have several different kinds of needs which must be met. Their ability to function may be limited, and they may become frustrated or depressed. Their basic human physiological and psychological needs must be addressed. Patients and families facing end-of-life decisions also have a unique and special set of needs which must be met.

As a health care worker, it's important to understand what your patients are experiencing and what it takes to provide the care and the support they need. Protecting the patients' safety and avoiding a preventable **mistake** or **error** is critical. When you focus on patient safety and comply with safety policies and procedures, you can avoid causing serious injury.

disability
(dis-eh-BIH-le-tee) Something a person is unable to do well due to a mental or physical impairment

mental illness
(MEN-tal ILL-ness) Health condition that changes a person's thoughts, emotions, and behavior and affects that person's ability to undertake daily functions

mistake
(meh-STAKE) To understand, interpret, or estimate incorrectly

error
(AIR-er) Something done incorrectly through ignorance or carelessness

Objectives

After completing this section, you will be able to:

1. Define the key terms.
2. List the three causes of physical disabilities.
3. List three categories of mental illness.
4. Describe one risk factor for mental illness.
5. Name four psychological needs that must be met, and give one example of each need.
6. Name four physiological needs that must be met, and give one example of each need.
7. Describe the five psychological stages that terminally ill patients experience.
8. List three ways to meet the needs of terminally ill patients.
9. Identify two mistakes or errors that jeopardize patient safety.
10. List three ways to protect patient safety.

UNDERSTANDING PATIENT NEEDS

The World Health Organization (WHO) defines *health* as "a state of complete physical, mental, and social well-being and not merely the absence of disease or infirmity." Health care workers strive to help patients overcome physical and mental disabilities, maintain their independence, and lead full and rewarding lives.

Daily Living and Independence

When people are ill or injured, they often have limitations. These usually affect their *activities of daily living*, such as eating, hygiene, dressing, toileting, and mobility. These limitations can also affect what's known as *Instrumental Activities of Daily Living*, which include shopping, cooking, laundry, managing finances, transportation, and telephone use. Some patients can do these activities with little or no help. Others need a lot of help to develop their adaptive skills. The goal is to allow each person to be as independent as he or she possibly can.

Health care workers should encourage their patients to try activities. For example, the patient may be able to put toothpaste on the brush but needs your help to brush the teeth. You can encourage the person by being positive and by letting him or her make choices. This helps the patient feel more independent and increases feelings of well-being and self-respect. Many assistive and adaptive devices are available. Occupational therapists specialize in assisting patients with adaptive devices for accomplishing activities of daily living and instrumental activities of daily living.

Physical Disabilities

When people become disabled, they are no longer capable of leading a normal life. Their disability may be temporary or permanent. In either case, they may need the assistance of health care professionals to adapt to their medical condition. A physical disability may be caused by a **congenital** condition, a **debilitating** illness, or an injury. Understanding disabilities helps you provide better care to your patients.

congenital
(con-jeh-neh-tul) Existing at, or before, birth

debilitating
(dih-BIH-le-tate-ing) Causing weakness or impairment

heredity
(he-REH-de-tee) Passed from parent to child

Congenital conditions usually occur through **heredity**. Examples include autism, cerebral palsy, cleft lip and/or palate, cystic fibrosis, Down syndrome, epilepsy, hydrocephaly, sickle-cell anemia, and spinal bifida.

Debilitating illness may occur at any age. Depending on the severity of the disease, physical changes may be minimal or very extensive. Elderly patients are more affected by a debilitating illness as they may not have sufficient physical, mental, or financial resources to accommodate recovery. An elderly person experiencing a fall or a hospitalization may undergo a spiraling downward effect in their health status. Common debilitating illnesses include Alzheimer's disease, cancer, cardiovascular disease, diabetes, emphysema, and leukemia, multiple sclerosis (MS), AIDS, and Parkinson's disease.

Injuries may occur at any age and may cause many different disabilities. Some of the most common are:

paralysis
(peh-RAH-leh-ses) Loss of sensation and muscle function

- Spinal cord injuries, which may cause **paralysis**
- Stroke, which may cause paralysis, brain dysfunction, speech impairments, and/or loss of memory

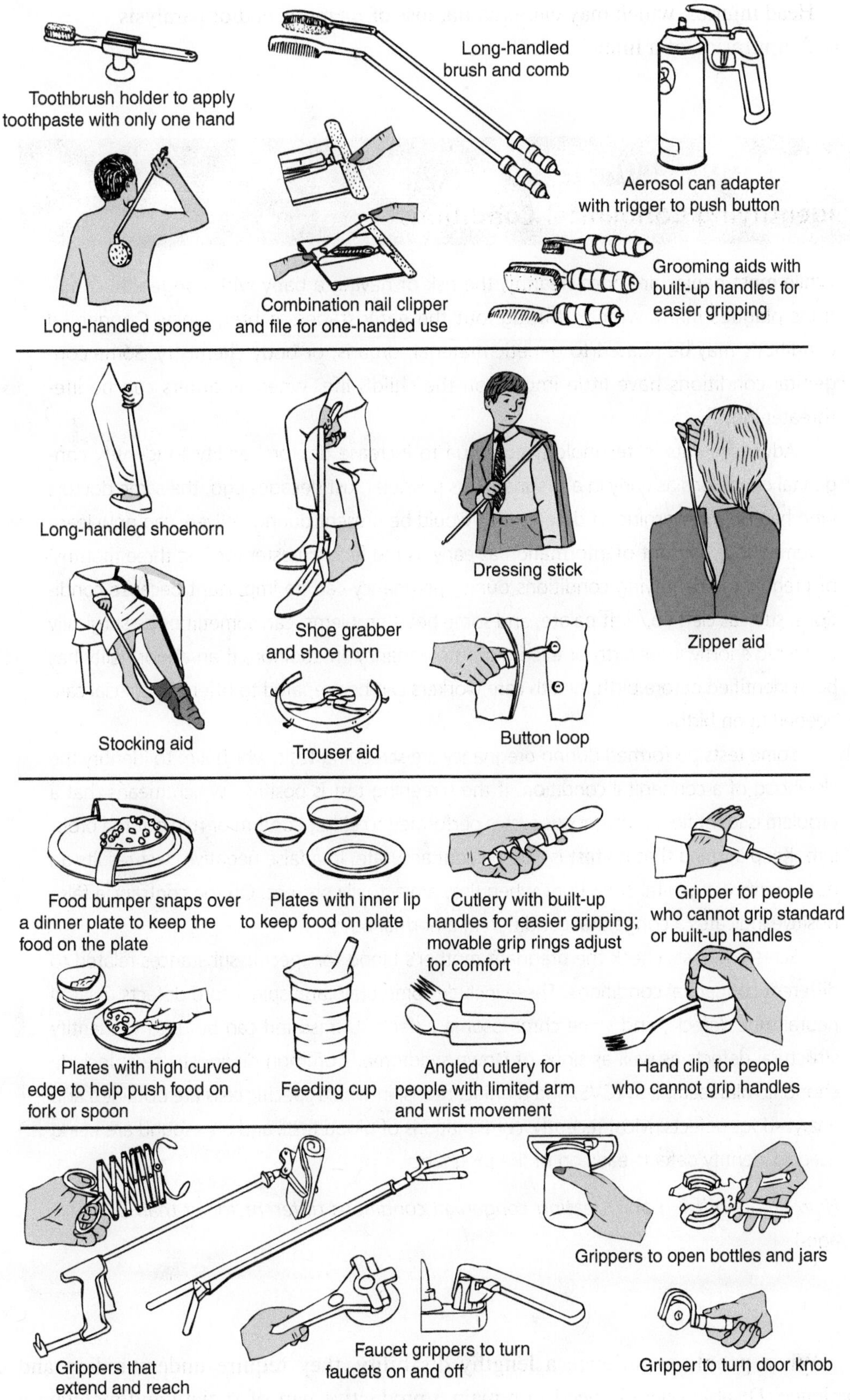
Toothbrush holder to apply toothpaste with only one hand
Long-handled brush and comb
Aerosol can adapter with trigger to push button
Long-handled sponge
Combination nail clipper and file for one-handed use
Grooming aids with built-up handles for easier gripping
Long-handled shoehorn
Dressing stick
Zipper aid
Shoe grabber and shoe horn
Stocking aid
Trouser aid
Button loop
Food bumper snaps over a dinner plate to keep the food on the plate
Plates with inner lip to keep food on plate
Cutlery with built-up handles for easier gripping; movable grip rings adjust for comfort
Gripper for people who cannot grip standard or built-up handles
Plates with high curved edge to help push food on fork or spoon
Feeding cup
Angled cutlery for people with limited arm and wrist movement
Hand clip for people who cannot grip handles
Grippers to open bottles and jars
Grippers that extend and reach
Faucet grippers to turn faucets on and off
Gripper to turn door knob

FIGURE 6.1

Assistive and adaptive devices to help overcome physical disabilities

coma
(COE-ma) Deep sleep, unconscious state for a period of time

amputation
(AM-pew-tay-shun) Removal of a body part

- Head injuries, which may cause **coma**, loss of memory, and/or paralysis
- **Amputation** of a limb

RECENT DEVELOPMENTS

Identifying Congenital Conditions

While most babies are born healthy, the risk of having a baby with congenital conditions plagues many women throughout the early stages of pregnancy. Congenital conditions may be related to genetic material, organs, or body chemistry. Some congenital conditions have little impact on the child's life, whereas others can be life-threatening.

Advancements in technology continue to increase doctors' ability to identify congenital conditions as early in a pregnancy as possible. Just decades ago, the same doctors who had no forewarning of defects that would be present during delivery can now learn a tremendous amount of information as early as the first trimester (or first three months) of pregnancy. Identifying conditions during pregnancy can be important because conditions, such as cleft lip, cleft palate, and some heart problems, can sometimes be surgically corrected shortly after birth or even during pregnancy. In addition, if an abnormality has been identified before birth, health care workers can be prepared to offer any special care needed upon birth.

Some tests performed during pregnancy are screening tests which aim to identify the likelihood of a congenital condition. If the screening test is positive, which means that a problem is identified, a diagnostic test is performed to either confirm or rule out the problem. Keep in mind that no test is 100 percent accurate. In a false negative, test results do not identify congenital conditions when they are actually present. On the contrary, a false positive indicates a congenital condition in a normal baby.

Screening tests check the pregnant mother's blood for specific substances related to different congenital conditions. These include some brain and spinal cord defects, related neural tube defects, and some chromosome defects. Ultrasound can be used to identify structural defects as well as signs of Down syndrome. Common diagnostic tests include chorionic villus sampling (CVS) and amniocentesis, in which specific cells are obtained and analyzed for defects. Most recently, combinations of blood tests and ultrasound are being used to identify defects early on in the pregnancy.

How are identifying and treating congenital conditions different today than 50 years ago?

When people experience a lengthy disability, they require understanding and patience. Disabled people need to remain a productive part of society and maintain a sense of well-being. The health care worker can be a positive influence on patients during the period of adjustment and rehabilitation.

People who lose a body part, or a part of their body functions, experience the same stages of loss as do people with a terminal illness. Many people who suddenly find

Language Arts Link — Debilitating Illnesses

Identify a physical disability that is caused by a debilitating illness. Research your topic. What causes the illness, what are its signs and symptoms, and how is it diagnosed? What limitations might patients with this illness face? What basic human needs would caregivers need to meet for such patients? What treatments are available for patients with this disease? Which health care professionals would be involved in the patients' diagnosis, treatment, and rehabilitation?

Prepare an oral report to present to your classmates and teacher to share what you have learned. Include a statement that describes the purpose of your report. Create an outline that organizes the material to be covered in a logical sequence. Ask another person to review your outline and offer some feedback before giving your presentation. Use printed materials or other visual aids to help explain your topic.

themselves disabled are dependent on others for many of their daily needs. Being dependent often leads to feelings of not being in control. Physical losses can cause various body functions to be impaired. Loss of body function often means that changes may occur in the following:

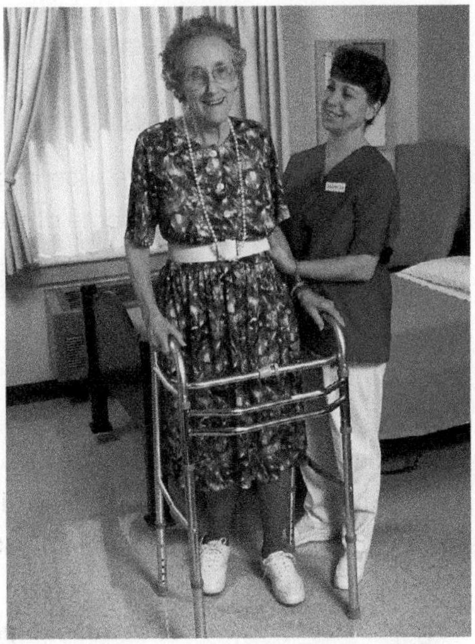

FIGURE 6.2

Learning to use a walker to regain stability and independence

Source: Michal Heron/Pearson Education

- Communication skills
- Sensory awareness
- Ability to think and comprehend
- Ability to move
- Elimination of waste products
- Ability to eat
- Ability to engage in sexual activity

Loss of physical functions may cause changes in a person's emotional stability. The areas of emotional insecurity usually focus around the following:

- Self-esteem
- Self-confidence
- Self-image

Physical impairments that lead to emotional changes may also create a sense of loss concerning the ability to:

- Develop relationships with others
- Earn a living
- Be a useful member of society

The health care worker helps patients reach their goals by being understanding and knowledgeable about the process involved in acceptance of a disability and rehabilitation. When physical changes occur, the goal of rehabilitation is to help the patient return to the highest level of functioning possible. Rehabilitation promotes a healthy return to a productive lifestyle. Many rehabilitation areas are involved in this process; the most common are as follows:

- Physical therapy restores the body to normal functioning when possible.
- Occupational therapy restores the ability to be involved in purposeful activity.
- Speech therapy restores the ability to communicate effectively.
- Psychotherapy changes inappropriate behavior patterns, improves interpersonal relationships, and resolves inner conflicts.

Several groups are available to aid the patient and family during the recovery and rehabilitation period. These groups, called *support groups,* are organized to help patients and family members cope with changes during this period. You can locate support groups in your area by contacting the social services department at hospitals, community centers, and organizations oriented to health care.

APPLY IT SUPPORT GROUPS

Research a local health care support group to find out more information. Who sponsors the group? What is the purpose of the group? Whom does the group serve? What kinds of activities or support do they provide? How is the support group funded?

Mental Illness

Emotions and thoughts can be overwhelming. Sometimes, people have a hard time dealing with their emotions and the world around them. When this happens frequently, a person may be diagnosed with a mental illness. According to the National Institutes of Mental Health, as many as 26 percent of Americans suffer from a mental illness or they know someone who does. A smaller percentage of Americans—about 6 percent—suffer from a serious mental illness.

Mental illnesses can be classified into the following categories:

- Anxiety disorders, including panic attacks, phobias, obsessive-compulsive disorder (OCD), and post-traumatic stress disorder (PTSD)
- Mood disorders, including bipolar disorder and depression
- Personality disorders, including schizophrenia
- Attention disorders, including attention deficit hyperactivity disorder (ADHD)
- Eating disorders, including anorexia nervosa and bulimia nervosa
- Drug abuse, including alcoholism and the abuse of drugs such as amphetamines, heroin, cocaine, and barbiturates.
- Alzheimer's disease, the most common form of dementia, is a progressive and fatal disease.

Mental illness affects people of all ages, regardless of gender. Some diseases are more common in certain groups. For example, Alzheimer's disease usually affects older adults. Attention disorders are more common in children and young adults. Scientists do not completely understand the causes of mental illness. Several risk factors can play a role in whether people develop mental illnesses. These risk factors include the following:

- ***Biological factors.*** Mental illnesses occur more often in some families than in others. This may be the result of genetics.
- ***Environmental factors.*** Head injuries, poor nutrition, and exposure to harmful or addictive chemicals can increase the risk of developing a mental illness.
- ***Social factors.*** Emotional trauma, abuse, exposure to violence, and other stressful events may affect whether someone develops a mental illness.

genetics
(jeh-NEH-tik) Traits passed from parent to child through heredity

BUILD YOUR SKILLS *Dealing with Depression*

Everyone feels sad or blue once in a while when situations go wrong or disappointments arise. For some people, however, sadness is a constant emotion—even when no obvious reason for it exists. This disorder, known as depression, is not a passing mood or a sign of weakness. People who suffer from depression cannot simply *get over it* or assume it will go away. The symptoms of depression go beyond mere sadness. People who suffer from depression may also experience any or all of the following symptoms:

- A change in sleeping patterns
- A change in eating habits
- An increase in fatigue
- Unexplained aches and pains
- A loss of interest in activities and friends
- Difficulty concentrating
- Feelings of hopelessness, helplessness, and worthlessness

The causes of depression vary from one person to another. Low self-esteem, pessimism, and anxiety are major contributing factors in some types of depression. Physical changes, such as a stroke, heart attack, or hormone disorders, can also lead to depression. Stresses at home or school, life and relationship changes, and family history are also important causative factors.

If you display any symptoms of depression, you can take several steps to start the healing process. Begin by identifying any problems that might be causing the symptoms. For example, consider living conditions, relationships, diet, physical fitness, and spiritual beliefs. Regain control of your life by looking for ways to fix problems and

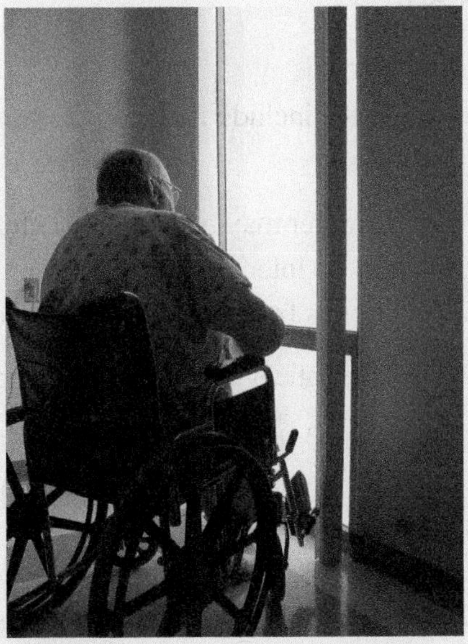

FIGURE 6.3

Patient experiencing depression and hopelessness

Source: Amanda Haddox/Shutterstock

eliminate sources of sorrow. Develop a healthier diet, get regular exercise and sleep, and establish a support system of friends and family. Set realistic goals each day, and determine priorities in your life. If symptoms persist, seek a professional counselor who can help you work through issues and refer you to a physician if medication is required.

Health care workers should be aware of the signs and symptoms of depression. Basic tools used to screen the patient for depression should be available for use in the health care setting. Mental health resources for referral should be made available to the patient. This is a part of providing the patient with comprehensive care. Treatment for depression can last for months or years, but a combination of psychotherapy and medication can often reduce or even eliminate symptoms of depression.

How might an increase in exercise help defeat mild depression?

BASIC HUMAN NEEDS

For many years, psychologists have studied people to better determine what makes each of us act the way we do. People act and behave differently but, as mentioned previously, Abraham Maslow identified some common characteristics over sixty years ago. He explained them in Maslow's Hierarchy, which focuses on five levels of basic needs. Health care workers should be aware of these basic human needs and the patient care techniques designed to meet each one. Let's take a closer look at how Maslow's work relates to patient care.

Physiological Needs

Physiological needs are divided into four categories: Biological, Safety, Sensory, and Motor Activity.

Biological Needs

elimination (ih-loh-meh-NAY-shun) Process of expelling or removing, especially waste products from the human body

holistic (hoe-LIS-tik) Pertaining to the whole; considering all factors

Biological needs include food, water, sleep, and **elimination**. When a person is threatened by illness:

- Food and water may be withheld before various procedures or surgery is performed.
- Sleep may be interrupted because of the environment, noises, or anxiety.
- Elimination is frequently affected by changes in routine, foods, or medication.

To meet the patient's biological needs, apply the following communication techniques:

- Be committed to reflecting the value of dignity.
- Use effective communication skills that demonstrate **holistic** care.
- Be alert to the biological needs and communicate how they will be met during patient care.
- Explain, or ensure that patients understand, the physician's orders concerning activity, food, use of the bathroom, and any expected special procedures; mealtimes; and how to request assistance or ask questions.
- Ask patients if they have any special requests or questions.
- If the patient's sleep must be interrupted, be sure to inform him or her prior to going to sleep.

- Use words that the patient can understand. If necessary, ask a translator to ensure that words and thoughts are fully communicated.
- Allow decisions concerning food and sleep to be made by the patient when possible.
- Tell patients what to expect.
- Reassure children and their parents of times they can be together.
- Address people by their proper names and titles, especially older people.
- Ask **coherent** patients if they have any specific fears. Address their fears honestly and with sensitivity, always treating people with dignity. Ask for assistance when necessary.
- Do not use comments like, "Don't worry" because they are rarely helpful.

coherent
(coe-HEER-ent) Capable of understanding

Keep cultural issues in mind. For example, many cultures of the world:

- Believe that illness is caused by a supernatural power.
- Use various herbs to treat illness and may request a specific diet.
- Consider the color white to be bad luck. Medical personnel in white may cause an increase in fear.
- Believe that hot and cold air currents negatively affect health. Be alert to drafts.

Safety Needs

Safety needs include the need to feel secure and to avoid bodily harm and injury. When threatened by illness, patients needing medical procedures and treatments may feel insecure. They may be facing hospitalization for the first time and are afraid they will be hurt or die. They may be entering a long-term care facility where they will live for the rest of their lives. They may wonder: What will happen to me? How will I be treated? Will I be safe? Patients may also be worried about pain or accidents that could occur during procedures.

To meet the patient's safety needs, apply the following communication techniques:

- Be sure that the patient fully understands what you are saying. Use pictures, culturally appropriate gestures, writing, and possibly a translator to ensure a patient's understanding.
- Tell patients what they can expect from you and your team. Introduce yourself and your team. Your reassuring presence and warm touch may be enough to help a patient feel safe.

FIGURE 6.4
Meeting safety needs through reassurance and a warm touch
Source: Yuri Arcurs/Shutterstock

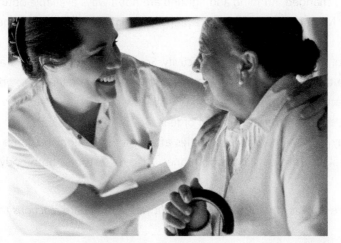

- Tell new hospital patients how to request assistance or contact you. Explain the call system and intercom.
- Show your commitment to service and treating others with dignity by always doing what you say you're going to do. This helps create trust and builds a sense of security for patients and their families.
- Think of the patient's age and ability to understand before speaking.
- Use the patient's words as much as possible. Speak at his or her level.
- Ask the family of pediatric patients if special words or objects communicate special things. For example, a child may call a special toy or blanket a "binki."
- Allow family or significant others to be present, when possible, if the patient requests their presence.
- Be alert to body language and other forms of communication that may provide clues to the patient's state of mind.

Science Link Fight or Flight Response

You can probably recall a situation in which you felt threatened or scared, a time when your basic human need for safety was called into question. Perhaps your teacher surprised you with an unexpected test or you had an argument with a classmate. In situations like these, your heart pounds, your muscles tighten, and your mind races. You are experiencing a fight-or-flight response.

The fight-or-flight response, also known as the *acute stress response*, was first described by the American physiologist Walter Cannon in 1927. He described it as an inborn response that prepares the body to either deal with, or flee from, a perceived threat to survival. In response to the threat, changes occur in the nerve cells of the body, and hormones such as adrenaline and cortisol are released into the blood stream.

The combination of nerve cell and chemical activities cause the respiration rate to increase. Blood is shunted away from the digestive tract and directed into muscles and limbs, which require extra energy and fuel for running or fighting. The pupils of the eyes dilate as the person's awareness of the surroundings intensifies. At the same time, the perception of pain decreases. Essentially, the fight-or-flight response bypasses your thinking mind and puts your body into an attack mode.

Long ago, the fight or flight response often saved people from physical threats, such as saber-toothed tigers and opposing warriors. Today, the threats are different. They might be found on the soccer field, in the classroom, or at work. The response has also changed. Running and fighting are not always available options—for example, in the case of an unexpected pop quiz. Nonetheless, the response prepares your body to deal with the situation in order to protect yourself.

The natural conclusion of fight-or-flight is physical activity. Some researchers suggest that without the physical conclusion, people can suffer from the buildup of stress hormones. Some people experience symptoms such as muscle tension, headache, upset stomach, racing heartbeat, deep sighing, or shallow breathing. Others may experience anxiety, poor concentration, depression, hopelessness, frustration, anger, or fear.

Perhaps the easiest way to slow the body's activities after a fight-or-flight response is through physical exercise. Exercise helps the body break down excess stress hormones, thereby restoring both body and mind to a calmer, more relaxed state.

What are some modern-day examples of when "fight" or "flight" are appropriate reactions to danger?

Sensory Needs

Sensory needs **stimulate** the five senses (hearing, seeing, feeling, smelling, tasting) as well as **intellectual stimulation**. When the senses are not stimulated, they diminish. For example, when a patient is not able to eat, intravenous fluids may be used. Because the smell and taste sensors are not stimulated, when the patient begins to eat again it will take time for taste and smell to return to normal.

stimulate
(stim-YOU-late) To cause an activity or heightened action

intellectual stimulation
(in-teh-LEK-shu-wul stim-you-LAY-shun) Causing deep thought

The senses are less responsive to stimulation as we age. Geriatric patients may have lost one or more of their senses. They may have difficulty hearing or seeing, which may increase their fear and cause anxiety. Communicating with people experiencing a sensory loss takes patience and imagination. Try some of the following techniques to stimulate their senses:

- Allow people with hearing loss to touch a speaker while it plays music. This may help them experience music because they can feel rhythm vibrate through the speaker.
- Touch the faces or arms of touch-impaired patients with the things that they want to feel, such as a warm towel, when reasonable. Such patients usually lose feeling in their hands and feet.
- Describe colors, smells, or flavors in the environment to sight-, smell-, and taste-impaired patients. For example, you might say, "Remember the smell of fresh bread baking? That's what it smells like today." They may appreciate your descriptions.

The loss of senses during the aging process also adds to the loss of well-being. As a health care worker you can help restore a sense of well-being by being aware and using techniques that help people experience or remember the feelings of their five senses. When you are aware of sensory loss, talk to the person and ask what helps him or her experience the lost sense. Try various techniques that will help stimulate the senses, always explaining what you are doing.

When working with people, show your commitment to excellence by being sensitive and remembering to use techniques that help people experience their senses. The various cultures of the world relate differently to touch, gestures, and personal space. As a health care worker, it is important that you are mindful of the various cultures and the potential barriers relative to the body senses.

atrophy
(AA-tre-fee) To shrink and become weak

Motor Activity Needs

Motor activity involves movement or exercise of the body. When muscles are not stimulated, they **atrophy** and eventually weaken and can even become frozen. The results of a lack of muscle stimulation may or may not be reversible depending on the length of time the muscle was not stimulated. For example, when a cast is removed from an arm or a leg after a long period, the arm or leg is usually much smaller than the one which was not in a cast. The casted limb was not able to stimulate the muscles so they shrank and became weak. Weakened muscles can prevent free and easy movement.

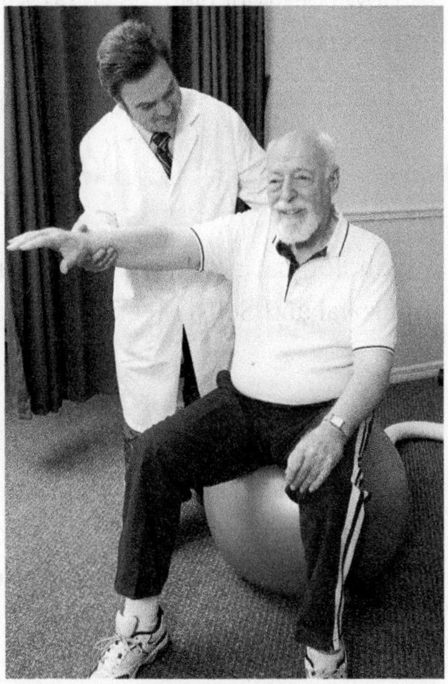

FIGURE 6.5

Exercising to prevent muscle atrophy

Source: Lisa F. Young/Shutterstock

To meet the patient's motor activity needs, apply the following communication techniques:

- Be sure that the patient fully understands what you are saying. Use pictures, culturally appropriate gestures, writing, and possibly a translator to ensure understanding.
- Inform people who experience difficulty moving around about how to reach you and others at all times.
- Inform the person that you are aware of his or her condition and will take precautions to protect any special needs.
- Explain the procedures that you will use to ensure the patient's safety as you help him or her move or as you do procedures.
- Remember to ask patients if they follow a certain procedure that best accommodates their limited or painful movement. Caution: Never do anything contradictory to your training or good judgment.
- Encourage people to do as much as possible on their own, as appropriate, to promote self-sufficiency.
- Be alert to your patient's customs concerning personal space. Always tell the patient what you are going to do before you start to move or touch him or her.
- Be aware of cultural taboos about touching the head and appropriate versus inappropriate hand gestures.

Community Service Rehabilitative Services

Volunteer in a local rehabilitation center to find out what kinds of patients receive care, what services are provided, and what types of health care professionals work there. Without violating confidentiality, review the case history of one of the center's previous patients. Consider the patient's condition, and develop a rehab plan that will meet at least one of the patient's needs. Ask one of the center's supervisors to review your plan. How does your plan match up with the actual plan created for the patient by a licensed professional?

Psychological Needs

Psychological needs are divided into four categories: Adequacy and Security, Social Approval and Self-Esteem, Order and Meaning in Life, and Self-Growth.

Adequacy and Security Needs

Adequacy and security is the need to feel in control and capable of coping. When a condition occurs that requires medical treatment, it is easy to feel a loss of control. Medications and various procedures and disease processes can change the way the body feels and what a person is capable of doing. Loss of a sense of control affects physical and emotional well-being.

Discuss what must be done to promote good health and treat specific conditions. Encourage the patient to comment and make decisions as much as possible. Show your commitment to dignity and justice by providing opportunities for patients to be involved as much as possible in decision making. For example, provide opportunities for patients to make decisions such as what they will eat or wear, when possible. Be aware of cultural customs that show respect or disrespect. For example, making direct eye contact in some cultures is disrespectful. Adapt your behavior and language to show respect for each person's dignity.

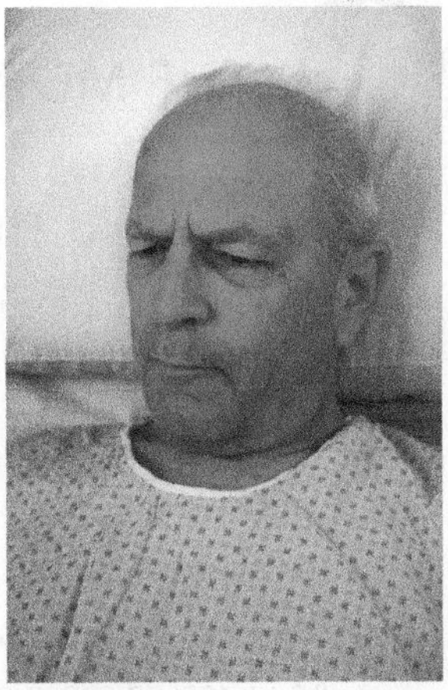

FIGURE 6.6

Hospitalized patient worries about his condition and his future

Source: George Dodson/Pearson Education

justice
(JUS-tess) Fairness; applying good rules equally to all people

Social Approval and Self-Esteem Needs

Social approval and self-esteem needs include recognition and acceptance by other people. When illness limits what a person is able to do at work, socially, or personally, depression can occur. This in turn can affect the success of treatment. The patient's ability to support his or her family may be taken away by an illness that causes job loss. This causes extreme stress.

It's important to spend time with patients who feel isolated. Patients in quarantine or who have visible body changes may feel different and isolated from their friends and family. Spending time with them and learning about their life can help them feel accepted. Consider the following:

isolated
(eye-seh-LAY-ted) Separated, lack of contact with others

quarantine
(kwor-en-TEEN) Isolating a person or animal to prevent the spread of disease

social services
(sew-SHAL SER-vis) Activities and resources to support well-being for individuals and families

- Encourage family and friends to include them in activities and events when possible.
- Show your commitment to dignity by practicing active listening skills.
- Show interest in the patient's concerns and past experiences.
- Inform the patient and family of available helpful resources such as social services.

Keep the following in mind:

- When caring for children, use terms they can understand.
- Be positive even when you want to say something negative.
- As a health care worker you can help restore a sense of well-being by staying alert to your patient's preferences and moods.
- Use resources within your facility to encourage and promote socialization with others who may be having similar experiences.
- Use age-appropriate vocabulary. Do not use childish gestures or language when speaking with an elderly person.
- Use culturally appropriate gestures and words to show respect. Honoring a person's culture is an effective way of reinforcing self-esteem and showing social approval.
- Be aware of dietary needs or restrictions.
- Encourage family and friends to display pictures and articles that may bring warm and comforting memories.
- Report any change in behavior such as withdrawal, passive behavior, wanting to give things away, refusing to see people, and so forth.

THE MORE YOU KNOW

Pet-Facilitated Therapy

Recent studies have focused on the value of the human-pet bond, showing that petting or stroking a pet has an immediate effect on the body. Most people studied showed:

- A slowing heartbeat.
- Deeper breaths.
- Fewer abnormal heartbeats.
- Lowered blood pressure.
- An increased sense of well-being.

Over 50 percent of American households have pets, primarily for the companionship that they provide. Research shows that even when people do not respond well to other people, they do respond to pets. They talk to their pets. They care for the needs of their pets. People who have a human–animal bond often find new meaning in life. They feel less lonely. They feel needed because their pets are totally dependent on them. They have a reason to get out of the house to buy food for their pets. The pet may be just the friend or responsibility they need to help feel better or to feel good about themselves. Research also shows that fish swimming gracefully in an aquarium with swaying plants creates a relaxing environment that reduces stress.

Hospitals, nursing homes, and long-term care facilities often allow specially-trained pets such as dogs and even miniature ponies to visit with patients and residents.

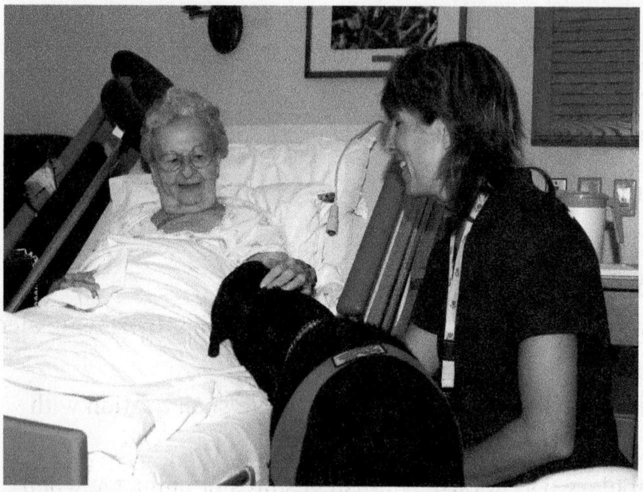

FIGURE 6.7

Pet therapy brightens the day for a hospice patient

Source: Dennis Sabo/Shutterstock

Order and Meaning in Life Needs

Order and meaning in life needs include having an understanding of what is going on in one's environment. When illness occurs, it is difficult to know what to expect or how to plan for the future. Meaning and purpose in life are in question if an illness changes the way we do things. Order that brings a sense of control is lost, leaving a feeling of being out of control and uncertain.

Tell patients what to expect before, during, and after procedures to help them psychologically prepare for the experience. Listen to the patient so you will have an understanding of his or her concerns. Respond with understanding. For example, "We will be starting your physical therapy today. I'm bringing you the schedule now so you will know when to expect the therapist."

Use words that the patient can understand. Ask for a translator when necessary to ensure that words and thoughts are fully communicated. Write information and schedules on a paper that the patient and family can use. Use pictures for children, like a clock with the hands pointing to a time you will return. Use culturally appropriate gestures and words to show respect. Be aware of routine cultural activities that bring meaning to the patient.

Self-Growth Needs

Self-growth is the need for fulfillment beyond basic needs. Illness often consumes our thoughts. Patients who experience a long illness or physical changes that limit their abilities may experience a loss of personal growth. Use active listening skills to identify patients' special interests. Allow them to share the details of these interests. When appropriate, discuss possible options with the care team that will allow the patient to experience learning. Your customer service and commitment to treating others with dignity are a reality when you take action in this way.

When caring for children, introduce activities at the child's level of understanding. Be sure to include enough time to teach and not frustrate the patient of any age. Seek culturally appropriate learning for the patient. Some cultures view games as childish. Being sensitive to cultural attitudes will help the patient accept new opportunities.

Meeting the Needs of Terminally Ill Patients

As a health care worker, you may come in contact with people who are nearing the end of their life. Patients who have an illness that cannot be cured are terminally ill. They are expected to die. When the patients learn of their illness, they usually pass through five different psychological stages. Elisabeth Kübler-Ross, MD (1926–2004) was a Swiss-born psychiatrist who first proposed the five stages of grief as a pattern of phases, most or all of which people tend to go through, in sequence, after being faced with the tragedy of their own upcoming death. The stages include the following:

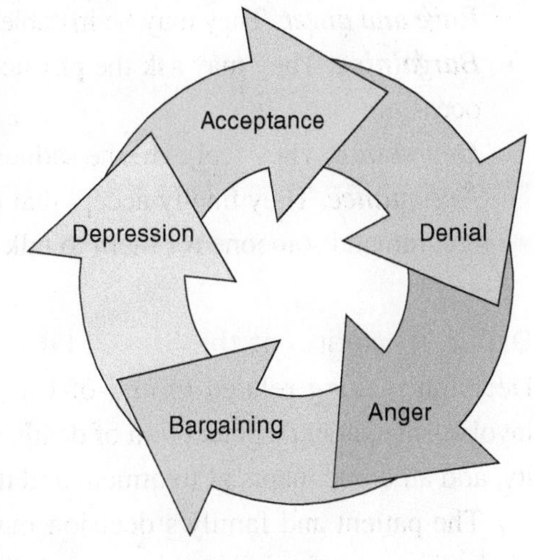

FIGURE 6.8
Stages of dying

- *Stage one: Shock and denial*. People find it very difficult to believe that they are really going to die. "No, not me!" is a

impending
(im-PEND-ing) About to happen

common reaction. During this stage, they feel very lonely and isolated. If they can discuss these feelings and talk about their impending death, they are able to move into the next stage. You may be the only health care worker available to listen to their feelings.

- ***Stage two: Rage and anger***. No matter how much kindness you have shown, your patient may become very insulting; there might be many complaints about everything you do. You may be tempted to leave them to their anger. If you realize it is not a personal attack, you will be able to listen and to understand that the anger is not directed at you. It is directed at the injustice of the situation. Be a good listener. When patients have exhausted their anger, they will move out of the anger stage.
- ***Stage three: Bargaining***. Although they now admit to themselves that they are dying, the patients try to prolong their life with bargaining. For example, they might say, "Just let me live until my children are independent." Listen and reflect what is said, express your understanding, and be aware of your voice tone and body language. Be aware of times when your presence in silence is helpful and when words are not helpful.
- ***Stage four: Depression***. Your patients may refuse to talk to you or even look at you. They are experiencing great sadness, for they are losing everyone and everything. Although they may not want to be bothered with friends or visitors, your touch is very important. Your understanding of their feelings of loss enables them to move into the last stage.
- ***Stage five: Acceptance***. At last your patients can accept their death. This is a time when your presence lets them know you will not desert them. They may want to discuss their death. Your willingness to be available will help your patients in a very difficult time.

Of course, a patient may skip stages. In addition, he or she may regress back to a stage after they have passed through it.

Friends and family often experience the same stages when someone they love and care about is terminally ill. As a health care worker, you need to be understanding. Family and friends may experience the following stages:

- ***Shock and denial.*** They may continue to make plans for the future that include the dying person.
- ***Rage and anger.*** They may be irritable and angry and say unkind things occasionally.
- ***Bargaining.*** They may ask the physician to keep the patient alive for a special occasion.
- ***Depression.*** They feel extreme sadness and even despair.
- ***Acceptance.*** They finally accept that death is going to occur. They may ask you to recommend someone for them to talk to.

Decision Making at the End of Life

Decision making related to end-of-life issues must consider all aspects of care. It involves the patient's perception of death, psychological aspects of culture and spirituality, and all components of treatment and its expected outcome.

The patient and family's decision making must be supported in an ethical framework of respect for independence and dignity. Without the support of an individual's right to decision making, there is the risk that the patient will be treated as an object rather than as a person. Health care decision making is built upon a relationship between patient and health care provider that requires mutual respect, trust, honesty, and confidentiality. Manipulation or intimidation must not hinder the resulting free exchange of information. Patients need to know and be informed of the following:

- Their condition
- The proposed treatment
- Expected results
- Alternative treatment options
- Potential risks, complications, and anticipated benefits

Consider This *Organ Procurement and Donation*

Organ donation is the removal of tissues of the human body from an individual who has recently died or from a living donor. Organ procurement is the obtaining of organs for transplantation. It includes the transporting of donor organs, after surgical removal, to the hospital for processing and transplant. The following organs can be procured: heart, intestines, kidneys, lungs, liver, pancreas, bones, and skin. In addition, the following tissues can be procured for donation: tendons, corneas, heart valves, bone marrow, and veins.

Everyone is a potential organ and tissue donor. Age and medical history are not the determining factors; instead, the critical factor is the condition of your organs and tissues at the time of death. If you are under age eighteen, a parent or guardian must give permission for you to become a donor. If you are eighteen or older, you can agree to be a donor by signing a donor card. It is also important to let your family know your wishes.

Pain Management

When the terminally ill patient decides jointly with health care providers and the family that prolonging life with therapy is no longer possible, then comfort and pain relief become the treatment goal. Most patients with a terminal illness fear physical pain much more than they fear death itself. Pain that is undertreated can have an extreme effect on the patient. It is important to work as a team with your coworkers to address the emotional, physical, spiritual, and psychological effects of pain and relieve discomfort as much as possible.

Relieving pain includes maintaining the patient's personal hygiene and body alignment, and speaking gently and clearly to the patient even if he or she is not able to respond to you. Reporting restlessness, excessive sweating, and rapid respirations to the charge nurse will provide information needed to determine if medication is appropriate. Scales of ten are commonly used in health care today for evaluating the level of discomfort. Teaching a patient to use a pain scale gives them a way of evaluating and communicating their pain to a caregiver.

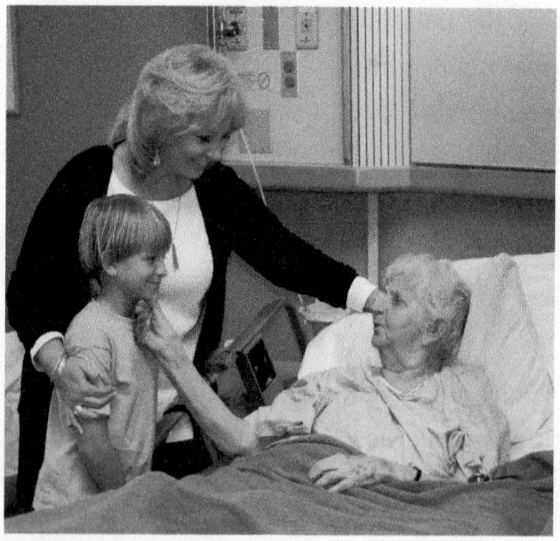

FIGURE 6.9
Hospice patient visits with family members
Source: James Steidl/Shutterstock

Hospice Care

In many communities, hospice care is available for terminally ill people. The goal of hospice care is to help patients nearing the end of life live each day to the fullest. This care is provided in the home or in a hospice facility. Patients are kept comfortable and free from pain. When the time for death comes, they are allowed to die peacefully. An important service of hospice is family involvement. Families are counseled and helped to accept the impending death of a loved one. Following the death, the family has continuing support for at least a year. This support helps make the grieving period more tolerable.

APPLY IT HOSPICE CARE

Investigate the availability of hospice services in your community. Where are the hospices located? Is home care hospice service available? At what point are patients eligible for hospice care? Make a list of things that hospice workers can do to help meet the needs of terminally ill patients and their family members. What information and community resources might they provide to help with making end-of-life decisions?

Euthanasia

Euthanasia, also referred to as a *mercy killing*, is the act of ending the life of an individual who is suffering from a terminal illness or an incurable condition. The word *euthanasia* originated from the Greek language: *eu* means *good* and *thanatos* means *death*; so, it actually means a *good death*.

However, if death is not intended, then it is not an act of euthanasia. Euthanasia is carried out by lethal injection or by suspending extraordinary medical treatment. The different types of euthanasia include:

- ***Voluntary euthanasia***. When a person killed requested to be killed.
- ***Non-voluntary euthanasia***. When the person killed gave no request or consent to be killed.
- ***Involuntary euthanasia.*** When the person killed made an expressed wish to not be euthanized.
- ***Assisted suicide***. When someone provides an individual with the information, guidance, and means to take his or her own life with the intention that they will be used for this purpose. When a doctor who helps an individual to kill themselves it is called "physician assisted suicide."

The issue of euthanasia is controversial. Some people argue that this is a case of freedom of choice—one that relieves an individual of extreme pain and suffering when his or her quality of life is low. Others believe that euthanasia devalues human life and can become a means of health care cost containment.

In April 2002, the Netherlands became the first country in the world to legalize euthanasia, soon followed by Belgium. Switzerland allows assisted suicide, under specific regulations, as does the state of Oregon. The U.S. government has tried to challenge this law, but has been unsuccessful so far.

PROTECTING PATIENT SAFETY

Health care is one of the most, if not THE most, complex industries on Earth. Due to recent advancements in medicine, health care providers now work with 13,600 different diagnoses, about 6,000 different drugs, and 4,000 different medical procedures. Hundreds of medical miracles occur every day as dedicated, hard-working health care professionals do their best to care for patients.

But the U.S. health care system is not perfect. Consider the following sober statistics:

- Death by a medical mistake is the third leading cause of death in the United States.
- Each year one million people are injured and 98,000 people die as a result of preventable medical errors. (This equals the number of deaths that would result from four jumbo jets crashing every week!)
- Of the thirty-seven million patients who are hospitalized each year, two million suffer hospital-acquired infections.

Awareness of the increasing need for patient safety started in 1999 with a report published by the Institute of Medicine entitled, "To Err is Human: Building a Safer Health System." The report highlighted several serious, yet preventable, problems and the need to focus on improvements. The Institute of Medicine set a goal of reducing medical errors by fifty percent over the next five years. However, based on follow-up studies, the risks associated with medical errors appear to be even higher than originally thought. Consider the following research findings:

- Hospital staff failed to report eighty-six percent of the harm done to Medicare patients. When errors aren't reported, they can't be tracked or corrected.
- One in seven Medicare patients suffered serious injuries or died as a result of hospital care. Forty-four percent of these outcomes were preventable.
- A review of patient records at three leading U.S. hospitals showed that one out of three admitted patients experienced some type of harm.

Examples of harm to a patient include:

- Performing surgery on the wrong patient or the wrong body part. This happens as often as forty times per week. Making mistakes in scheduling, marking the wrong site for surgery, and marking surgical sites with washable ink that comes off during the patient's prep lead to serious problems.
- Acquiring a new infection or disease while hospitalized. This happens when housekeepers don't adequately disinfect rooms, and when caregivers don't wash their hands properly. Despite training, continual reminders, and easy access to hand sanitizers, only half of hospital workers comply with hand-washing guidelines.

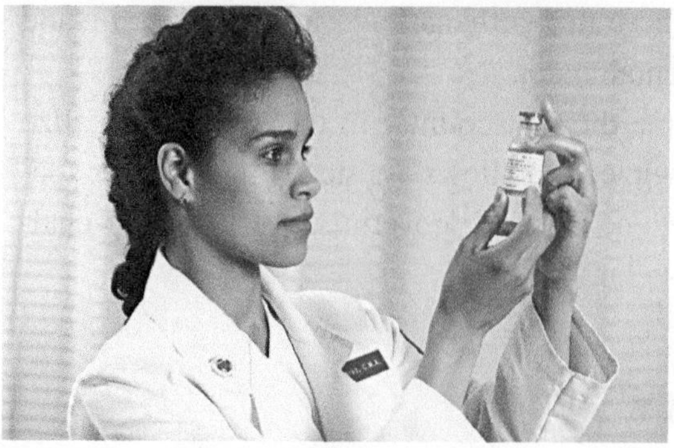

FIGURE 6.10

Checking a medication vial to make sure that it is what the doctor ordered

Source: Michal Heron/Pearson Education

- Receiving the wrong drug or the wrong dose of a drug. Drug containers may look alike even though the contents are very different. Errors result when nurses don't read the labels carefully.

Improving patient safety requires a heightened awareness of errors and mistakes and a culture that encourages health care workers to speak up when they see mistakes about to occur. Nurses and others who interact frequently with patients get to know their patients quite well. These caregivers must feel **empowered** to question things when they don't seem right. For example, a nurse might question the doctor's order to give the patient a certain drug if the nurse believes the drug might cause a complication with other drugs the patient is taking. Or a medical assistant might notice that a busy doctor forgot to properly wash his or her hands when moving from a patient with the flu to the next patient in for prenatal care.

empowered
(em-POW-er-ed) To give authority, to enable or permit

APPLY IT MEDICATION ERRORS

Find an article in a newspaper, magazine, medical journal, or web page that describes a situation where a patient was given the wrong **dose** of a drug. Who was responsible for the error, and under what circumstances was the error made? What drug was administered? What dose did the patient receive as compared with the appropriate dosage? Was the patient harmed and, if so, how? What steps have been taken to prevent this error from occurring again?

dose
(DOSE) The quantity of a medicine or a drug that is administered at one time

Speaking up when you spot something that doesn't seem right may require some courage on your part, especially if you are questioning someone with more authority. But it's absolutely essential in protecting the patient's safety. Ask yourself this—if you were about to make a mistake that could potentially harm a patient would you want someone to speak up, even if it might cause you some embarrassment? Health care professionals always put what is best for their patients ahead of what is best for them. Be on the lookout for potential mistakes and errors and never hesitate to speak up.

A primary goal of patient safety is preventing a **sentinel event**—an unexpected occurrence involving death or serious physical or psychological injury, or the risk thereof with *serious injuries* including the loss of a limb or function. Each accredited hospital or health care organization is required to define a sentinel event for their purposes and to have a plan in place to identify, report, and manage these kinds of events. Once the event has been reported, the circumstances can be studied and processes can be put into place to prevent the occurrence from happening again.

sentinel event
(SENT-nel EE-vent) An unexpected occurrence involving death or serious physical or psychological injury, or the risk thereof

Each year, National Patient Safety Goals provide a series of specific actions that accredited organizations are expected to implement to prevent medical errors. Here are a few examples:

- Identify patients correctly; use at least two ways to identify patients (such as the patient's name and date of birth) to make sure that each patient gets the medicine, treatment, and blood type meant for them.
- Use medicines safely; label all medicines that are not already labeled (such as medicine in syringes, cups, and basins); take extra care with patients who take blood thinners.
- Prevent infection; use hand cleaning guidelines to prevent difficult-to-treat infections; use proven guidelines to prevent infection of the blood from central lines (tubes inserted into a patient's vein to administer medications or fluids) and use safe practices to treat the part of the body where surgery was done.
- Improve staff communication; quickly get important test results to the right staff person.

Many efforts are underway to improve patient safety and reduce medical mistakes and errors. One example is the use of checklists to ensure that safety precautions are followed. About 30,000 patients die per year from infections they've acquired due to the improper handling of heart catheters. In the past, these deaths were thought to be unpreventable. However in a program launched in 2004 in intensive care units in 100 Michigan hospitals, the use of a short check list to ensure proper handling decreased the infection rate by two thirds. This seemingly simple intervention, plus a heightened focus on patient safety among hospital employees, saved 1,500 lives over an 18-month period. Since then, other hospitals have begun using the same techniques.

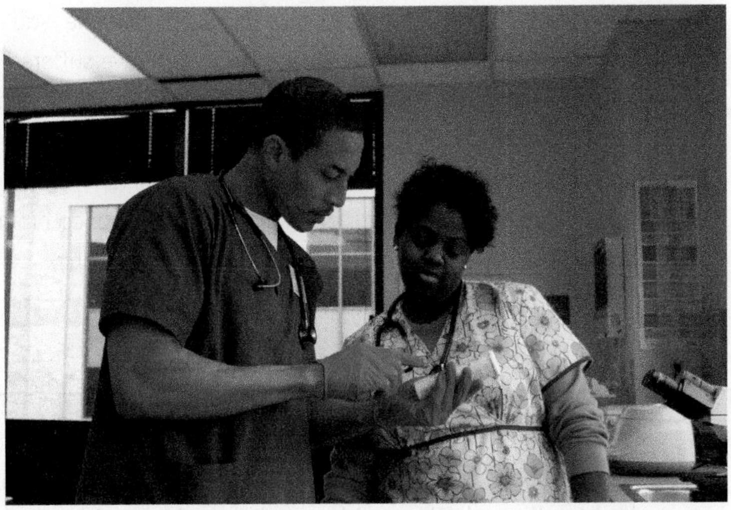

FIGURE 6.11

Double-checking labeling to ensure accuracy

Source: Carmen Martin/Pearson Education

Another strategy to improve patient safety is the public reporting of hospital performance. Twenty-nine states require hospitals to report their infection rates and information about medical errors. But exactly what to report to the public is still under debate. Reporting hospital infection rates is becoming more common because the Centers for Disease Control and Prevention have developed a standardized system that all hospitals can use. The government is adding financial incentives to improve patient safety. Starting in 2008, hospitals receive less reimbursement for treating Medicare patients when hospital-acquired conditions occur. In 2012, hospitals that earn high scores on quality and patient safety standards can receive extra income.

staffing level
(STAFF-ing LEH-vel) The number of people with certain qualifications who are assigned to work at a given time

Maintaining a safe **staffing level**, especially with registered nurses, is crucial to ensuring patient safety and quality care. Research has shown that having an adequate supply of RNs on patient care units is directly related to the quality of care those patients receive. When health care providers cut back on staff, there's a greater likelihood that safety and quality will suffer. So it's important for health care organizations to maintain sufficient staffing levels while monitoring their labor costs. Staffing models that give bedside nurses and other caregivers more responsibility for quality and safety lead to better patient outcomes.

REALITY CHECK

The information in this chapter will help you decide whether you want to work in direct patient care or in a role that supports patient care from behind the scenes. If your goal is to become a caregiver, you'll need to acquire the knowledge and skills it takes to be aware of your patients' needs and how to meet them. Depending on the occupation you choose, you may work with a variety of patients who are suffering from different kinds of illnesses and injuries.

After completing your general courses (also known as a *core curriculum*) and your initial educational program, you may wish to focus your future studies and professional work on a specific type of patient or disability. For example, you might want to specialize in pediatric physical therapy to help children who have suffered a serious injury learn to walk again. You might want to learn more about diagnosing and treating cancer and work in a radiation therapy department. Or, you might study mental illness and specialize in counseling Alzheimer's patients and family members.

Regardless of the health career that you choose, your commitment to meeting patient needs and protecting patient safety should be a high priority.

Key Points

- When people are ill or injured, their ability to perform normal daily activities may become limited. The goal is to help people remain as independent as possible.
- Physical disabilities are caused by a congenital condition, a debilitating illness, or an injury.
- Patients who lose a body part or a bodily function may experience the same stages of loss as do people with a terminal illness.
- The goal of rehabilitation is to promote a healthy return to a productive lifestyle.
- People who have a hard time dealing with their emotions, thoughts, and the world around them may suffer from a mental illness.

- Over sixty years ago, Abraham Maslow identified five levels of basic human needs. These include physiological needs; safety needs; the need for love, affection, and belonging; the need for esteem; and the need for self-actualization.
- Caregivers must understand what their patients are going through in order to meet their needs.
- In patient care, physiological needs are divided into four categories: Biological, Safety, Sensory, and Motor Activity.
- Psychological needs are divided into four categories: Adequacy and Security, Social Approval and Self-Esteem, Order and Meaning in Life, and Self-Growth.
- Terminally ill patients and their families go through five stages of grief; they have end-of-life decisions to make and special needs which must be met.
- Euthanasia, which is a highly controversial practice, is the act of ending the life of an individual suffering from a terminal illness or an incurable condition.
- Health care is an extremely complex and imperfect industry.
- Each year, about one million people are injured and almost 100,000 die as a result of preventable medical errors.
- Research conducted by the Institute of Medicine, plus follow-up studies, indicate the need for major improvements in patient safety.
- National Patient Safety Goals provide specific actions that providers must take to prevent sentinel events and reduce medical errors.
- Using standardized checklists, reporting medical outcomes to the public, and ensuring adequate staffing levels are some of the ways that health care providers are improving patient safety.

Section Review Questions

Answer each of the following questions. Indicate which page in the textbook led you to your answer.

1. Discuss the relationship between *activities of daily living* and the patient's independence.
2. List three causes of physical disabilities.
3. Describe two things than can happen when a person becomes disabled.
4. List three categories of mental illness, and describe one of the risk factors.
5. Name two types of therapy which are helpful in rehabilitation.
6. Explain how a caregiver can help the needs of a patient with sensory loss.
7. List three ways to meet the needs of terminally ill patients.
8. Give two examples of how medical errors can cause death.
9. Describe one National Patient Safety Goal.
10. Explain the relationship between staffing levels and patient safety.

Learn By Doing

Complete Worksheets 1–5 in Section 6.1 of your *Student Activity Guide*.

SECTION 6.2 Customer Service and Patient Satisfaction

Background

Health care workers interact with several different types of customers, including coworkers, doctors, visitors, guests, and vendors. However, the most important group of customers is the patients, of course. Patient and customer satisfaction is an essential element in providing effective health care. When health care professionals demonstrate the values of service and excellence, this helps patients, their families, and their friends feel satisfied with their care. Satisfaction does not always mean that people get what they want. However, it does mean that patients receive the very best care available, and that the care is given with respect and kindness. It also means that each patient is fully informed about the service being provided.

When a patient's expectations are not met, there are consequences. The patient may change doctors or refuse treatment from a particular provider or facility. Changing caregivers can compromise a patient's care. In addition, the loss of a patient, or customer, is detrimental to a health care facility's business. All health care workers need to develop and apply good customer service skills in order to meet, or better yet—exceed, their customers' expectations.

Objectives

After completing this section, you will be able to:

1. Define the key terms.
2. List three types of health care customers.
3. Discuss the purpose of patient centered care and list three benefits for patients.
4. Explain the difference between *empathy* and *sympathy*.
5. Describe how hospitals are measuring patient satisfaction.
6. Discuss the purpose of the HCAHPS survey and explain how it is administered.
7. List three concerns that patients may have when they become hospitalized.
8. Explain four ways to provide good customer service for patients.
9. List three ways to provide good customer service for the patient's family members.
10. Describe two ways to provide good customer service for visitors in your facility.

PATIENT CENTERED CARE

In *patient centered care*, the goal is to provide the right care, for the right person, every time. This requires meeting the needs of each patient in a manner that conveys respect and dignity for the individual.

In patient centered care, the patient is an active part of the decision making team. Physicians, who typically play an authority role, function more as partners with their patients. This partnership:

- Strengthens the patient-provider relationship.
- Encourages communication about things that matter to the individual patient.
- Helps patients understand more about their health and medical conditions.
- Gets patients more involved in their own care.

The goal is to treat the whole patient and to do what's best for the patient based on his or her needs. The focus on individual needs leads to *good outcomes*, which are defined as valuable and meaningful for the patient.

Health care providers are focusing on ways to help patients become more engaged in their health care. Patients who work *with* their doctors get better results, are more satisfied with their care, and are better prepared to manage their medical conditions. To increase their engagement, patients should:

engaged
(in-GAJED) Involved

- Share information about their symptoms and express expectations about their personal health in an open, honest manner.
- Jot down their symptoms and bring the lists with them to their appointments. They should include when the symptoms first appeared, how long they have lasted, and what actions have been taken thus far to treat the symptoms.
- Keep their appointments and arrive on time. If an appointment must be rescheduled, give the provider adequate advance notice.
- Bring lists of their current medications with them to their appointments. This should include the names of the drugs, dosages, and who prescribed the medications. Also include any over-the-counter drugs such as aspirin and vitamins.
- Bring a list of questions with them to their appointment. Patients should ask their questions, make sure they understand the answers, and write down any information they need to remember after the appointment.
- Make follow-up appointments and comply with post-appointment instructions.

over-the-counter drugs
(OH-ver the-COUN-ter DRUGS) Medications and supplements that don't require a prescription

To increase patient engagement, physicians and other health care providers should:

- Use language and terms that patients can understand, and explain things clearly.
- Ask about their patients' individual preferences and expectations regarding their health.
- Provide complete and accurate information about what patients should expect from their diagnostic tests and treatment plans.
- Communicate test results in a timely manner, and provide details for those patients who want detailed information.
- Demonstrate cultural competence when working with diverse groups of patients.
- Coordinate the care provided by different providers to ensure continuity of care for each patient.
- Display a genuine and sincere concern for the well-being of their patients.
- Protect the patients' confidentiality, and treat them with respect and dignity.

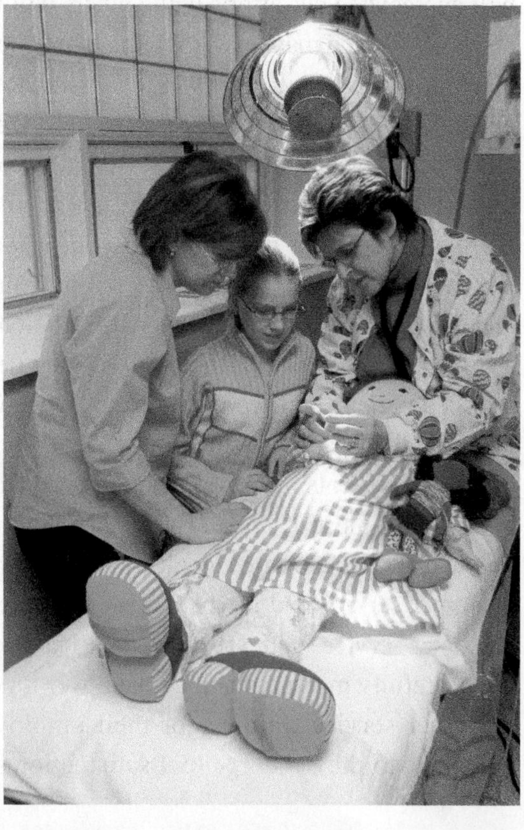

FIGURE 6.12

Demonstrating a procedure on a doll to show a young patient what to expect

Source: Corbis Cusp/Alamy

empathy
(EM-peh-thee) Understanding and relating to another person's emotions or situation

sympathy
(SIM-peh-thee) Feeling sorrow or pity for another person

In order to deliver patient centered care, health care workers must be able to understand and relate to what their patients are experiencing. **Empathy** is the ability to be sensitive to or understand the feelings of another person, and identify with what he or she is experiencing without necessarily experiencing the same thing yourself. When you empathize with patients, you put yourself in their place and feel what they are feeling. In other words, you *walk in their shoes* and experience things from their points of view. Empathy is different from **sympathy**. When you sympathize with patients, you feel sorry for them but you don't experience what they are experiencing yourself. Instead of *walking in their shoes*, you remain distant and express sorrow or pity for the patients and their situations.

APPLY IT PATIENTS, CLIENTS, OR RESIDENTS?

Do some research to find out the differences among the terms *patients*, *clients*, and *residents* with respect to the health care industry. When should a person be referred to as a *client* instead of a *patient*? Who would be considered as *residents*? Why is it important for health care workers to be aware of these differences?

CUSTOMER SERVICE

Some people cringe at the thought of referring to patients as *customers*. But health care is a business, and patients are the customers. It's important that health care customers are pleased and satisfied with the services they receive.

Similar to your coworkers, your patients are a highly diverse group of people. They represent all personality types and a wide variety of differences. Some will be easy to get along with; others will be more difficult; and some will be downright nasty. Some patients will appreciate your efforts while others will not. But they all deserve to be treated with respect and good manners. Applying what you've learned so far in your interactions with patients is *where the rubber meets the road*. Remember the difference between hard skills and soft skills? Everyone expects you to be competent (hard skills), that's just a given. What will set you apart as a professional is how you behave (soft skills.)

Working in direct patient care is a privilege. It's an honor to have another person entrust their health and safety to you. It's also an awesome responsibility. Today's patients have high expectations about how they will be treated by health care workers, and they have choices about where to obtain health care services. Patients won't hesitate to go someplace else for their care if they believe they haven't been treated well. Dissatisfied patients will complain to their doctors and before long, the doctors will start referring their patients elsewhere.

When patients have a decision to make about where to go for their health care, they assume that most, if not all, of the hospitals and doctors in town provide quality care. What differentiates one health care provider from another often comes down to customer service and the patient's experience. As a result of this increasing focus on customer service, *patient satisfaction* has become a top priority. Patient satisfaction is now carefully measured and tracked over time. Many health care organizations provide customer service training for their employees and are starting *service excellence* programs to raise their patient satisfaction scores.

APPLY IT EVIDENCE-BASED PRACTICE

Evidence-based practice (EBP) combines clinical expertise, the patient's values, and findings from the best medical research to make decisions about patient care. Clinical expertise is based on the physician's education, experience, and skills. The patient contributes his or her individual preferences, concerns, and expectations. Medical research that has been conducted following strict guidelines to ensure accurate outcomes provides valuable information.

Select a disease or another medical condition that's of interest to you. Investigate how EBP is helping to make the best decisions for the care of patients with this condition.

PATIENT SATISFACTION

Many hospitals have been collecting patient satisfaction data for their own internal use. However, until the H-CAPS survey was recently introduced, no standard approach existed for all hospitals to use in collecting this data and sharing it with the public. Also known as HCAHPS (Hospital Consumer Assessment of Healthcare Providers and Systems), the survey asks twenty-seven questions to collect data about the patient's perception of the quality of his or her hospital experience. The survey is given to a random sampling of adult patients with a variety of medical conditions between two days and six weeks after they've been discharged from the hospital. The survey can be conducted by mail, telephone, or combination of the two. Questions solicit feedback regarding communication with the nurses and doctors, pain management, cleanliness, noise levels, details about medications, and so forth. Patients are also asked to rate the hospital overall and whether or not they would recommend the hospital to other patients. Interestingly, patients who are admitted into the hospital via the emergency department (ED) tend to give lower scores on satisfaction surveys. Since the percentage of patient admissions via the ED is somewhat high in many hospitals, extra efforts should be taken to meet or exceed the expectations of these types of patients.

H-CAPS/HCAHPS
Hospital Consumer Assessment of Healthcare Providers and Systems

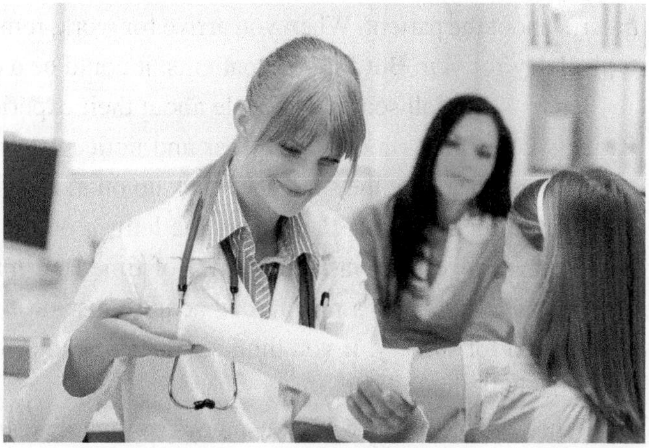

FIGURE 6.13

Patient satisfaction starts with customer service and caring

Source: CandyBox Images/Shutterstock

HCAHPS focuses on creating a culture of *always*—always delivering quality care to every patient during every encounter. Since data collection methods are standardized and hospitals post their results on a public website (www.hospitalcompare.hhs.gov), patients and other stakeholders have access to meaningful comparative data. Public reporting of survey results provides incentives for hospitals to improve the patient experience and increases transparency by sharing their outcomes.

Patient satisfaction data is expected to play a major role in health care reform because hospitals that fail to receive high marks for patient satisfaction will receive less financial reimbursement for services provided to Medicare patients. The federal government is gearing up to implement *pay for performance* or *value-based purchasing* as a way to encourage more high quality, patient centered care.

RECENT DEVELOPMENTS

Healing Environments

Green initiatives, which focus on protecting the environment, are leading to more healing environments in hospitals and other health care settings, offering beneficial effects for both patients and workers. Research has shown that the quality of the environment can improve the healing of patients and the morale and efficiency of staff. Calming spaces designed with carefully chosen colors, lighting, and building materials can lift the spirits of seriously-ill patients and reduce the stress of busy health care workers.

Green initiatives, which help save energy and reduce waste, are well-timed because many health care organizations are gearing up to build new hospitals, clinics, and nursing homes to replace out-dated facilities and respond to the increasing demands of the baby boomer population. Developers are designing energy-efficient utility plants, improving waste management and recycling efforts, and incorporating recycled materials, natural sources of light, and live plants and trees.

healing environments (HEEL-ing in-VIE-ren-ment) Physical spaces designed to reduce stress, ensure safety, and uplift the spirits of patients, visitors, and staff

BEING THERE FOR PATIENTS

When you work in direct patient care, you should make the patient the focus of everything you do. It's not about you, your department, or your schedule for the day. It's *always* about the patient. When you arrive for work, remember this. Today is just another typical day for you. But for your patients, it could be a day that they will never forget.

Patients will tell scores of people about their experience and how they were treated. Patients don't miss much—they hear and notice everything going on around them. If there's tension among the staff, they pick up on it. If a piece of equipment doesn't work, the restroom hasn't been cleaned, or the lettuce on the cafeteria salad bar is less-than-fresh, they notice. Patients spend a lot of time (too much time) waiting. It's amazing how much information a patient can acquire just sitting in a waiting room or lying on cart headed for surgery. If you think the patient can't overhear your phone conversation down the hall, think again.

When people become patients, they're vulnerable and at their worst. They're in pain and anxious, worried, confused, and overwhelmed with the medical experience. Many patients feel helpless, having to turn themselves over to strangers who will make decisions about their care. They're concerned about what might happen to them, how their lives will be affected, how their children and spouses will fare in their absence, and a whole host of other issues. Patients need reassurance and confidence that they're in good hands. How you look, communicate, and behave can have a tremendous impact on their feeling of security.

Everything that you say and do has an impact on patients. Your small act of kindness may be huge to a patient. Patients tend to pick their favorite caregivers. Upon returning, they may ask to have the same person take care of them again. Some caregivers *go the extra mile* and those are the people that your patients will remember.

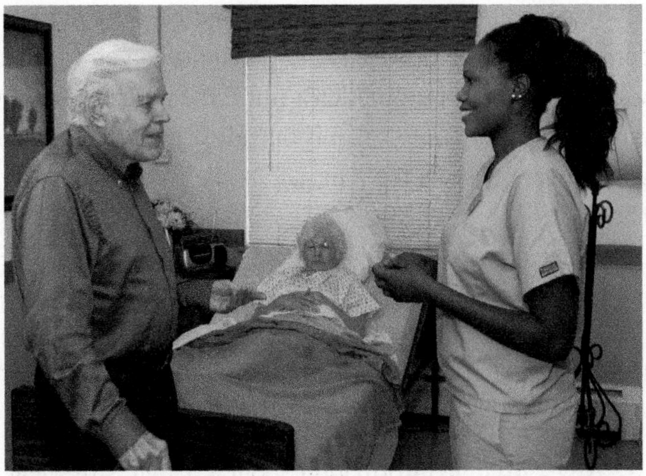

FIGURE 6.14
Providing reassurance and confidence that the patient is in good hands

Source: Patrick Watson/Pearson Education

Think back to the discussion about *being present in the moment*. This requires the ability to filter out everything else going on around you and concentrate on *being there* at that precise moment for that patient. The connections that professionals make with their patients are not the result of just acting or performing a duty. The ability to connect with patients is a reflection of the caregiver's personal values and professional priorities—an indication that caring for others comes straight from the heart. Isn't this the kind of person that you would want caring for you and your loved ones?

remarkable
(rih-MAR-keh-bul) Unusual, uncommon, and extraordinary

amenities
(ah-MEH-nih-tees) Pleasant and attractive features or benefits

Language Arts Link A Remarkable Experience

If you were a patient in the hospital for three days, what would it take to make your stay a **remarkable** experience? Would you want a private room with large windows and lots of sunlight? How about a flat screen TV and a bedside computer with Internet access for your personal use? Would you like to watch some DVDs to help you learn about your medical condition and how to regain your health? How about the option of ordering food and beverages from a room service menu any time of the day or night? Some hospitals already offer these **amenities** for the comfort and convenience of their patients.

Write a paper that describes the kind of hospital environment that you would prefer if you were the patient. Explain your reasoning, and discuss what it would take to make your ideal hospital stay a reality. Proofread your paper, correct any spelling or grammar errors, and share your report with your classmates and teacher.

Apply what you've learned about valuing differences and diversity in your interactions with patients and other customers. Remember the following:

- Do not be **judgmental**. It doesn't matter if your patient is wealthy, poor, homeless, elderly, a celebrity, or a criminal. Each patient deserves the same level of respect, quality of care, and customer service.
- Protect your patients' dignity, self-respect, and personal possessions.
- Refer to patients as *Mr.* or *Ms.* instead of *honey*, *sweetie*, or *dear*. You may think calling someone *honey* is a sign of caring, but keep in mind that many patients (and other customers) object to these kinds of terms.
- Be compassionate and empathetic. Try to see things from your patient's point of view.

judgmental
(jej-MEN-tul) Having or expressing a critical point of view

Anticipate your patients' needs and be prepared to meet them. No request or concern is too trivial. However, if a patient asks you for a drink, food, medication, or help walking to the rest room, don't fulfill the request unless your job includes these duties. Always refer any matter that is outside of your scope of practice to the patient's nurse or another caregiver on the unit, and make sure the appropriate person follows through to handle it.

When communicating with patients, use terms they can understand. If they ask you a question you aren't capable of answering or aren't authorized to answer, refer the question to the appropriate person. Be mindful of the need for patient **confidentiality**. Here are some things to remember:

confidentiality (con-fe-DENT-she-al0ih-tee) Maintaining the privacy of certain matters

divulge (de-VULJ) To make known

- Never read a patient's medical record unless it's part of your job.
- Never **divulge** information about a patient's medical status to the patient's family members, clergy, or other visitors without the patient's permission.
- Confine the exchange of confidential information to a *need to know* basis when discussing patients with other health care professionals.
- Protect the privacy of patients who are celebrities, leaders in your organization, or coworkers. Give them every consideration you would give other patients.
- Never ask questions or make comments in a public area that might embarrass a patient or violate their privacy. For example, a medical assistant should never raise his or her voice to ask Mr. Jones, who is sitting in the public waiting area, whether he remembered to bring his stool sample!
- Avoid the temptation to give your own personal opinion when a patient asks, "Which doctor in this group is the best?" or "Which doctor would you take your child to?"
- Don't discuss your own medical history, or the medical histories of your family members, with patients.
- Always stop and think—if *you* were the patient, how would you want to be treated?

PATIENT VISITORS

No discussion of customer service would be complete without mentioning the patient's visitors—their family members and close friends. A patient's family is his or her *lifeline* to normal life. When the patient invites other people to be a part of his or her medical experience, these people become part of the *patient's team*. Remember that *family* may mean something very different to the patient than to you. Accept who the patient identifies as family, and assist these individuals as they provide support for your patient.

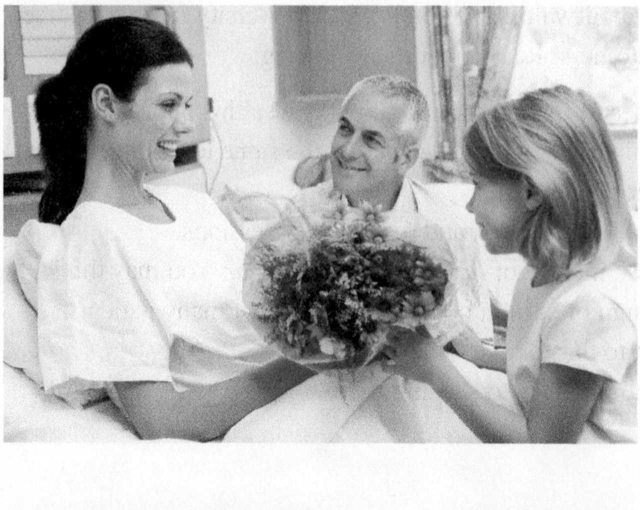

FIGURE 6.15

Family members are part of the patient's health care team

Source: Monkey Business Images/ Shutterstock

Patients need families and friends to help them through difficult situations.

Having clergy or other spiritual leaders present may help. Sadly, not all patients have a support system. Some patients will complete their entire hospital stay with no family or visitors present. These patients need some special compassion and attention from their caregivers. Other patients have large families and lots of friends, and sometimes this can cause problems. Policies regarding hospital visiting hours have always been controversial. Some hospitals strictly enforce limited visitation while others have abandoned visitation limitations altogether. The problem is that visitors don't always use common sense. If a person is sufficiently sick or injured to require hospitalization, then he or she needs rest and shouldn't be overtaxed with too many visitors. On the other hand, maintaining connections with family and friends is an important part of the healing process. Sometimes it's up to the caregiver to enforce limitations on visitors to carry out the wishes of the patient and what's best for his or her recovery.

clergy
(CLER-gee) People who perform religious functions

Consider This *Camping Out at the Hospital*

Families of seriously ill patients may literally *camp out* at the hospital. They want to be as close to their loved ones as possible, and for as much time as possible, even though it might be uncomfortable. Spouses may spend the night in their loved ones' rooms. Parents may hover nearby to watch over their babies and children. Family members may stay in the patient's room all day and refuse to leave for fear of *missing the doctor* during rounds. Families may bring things from home to comfort the patient, such as favorite foods, flowers, and personal items. They may bring their own clothes and toiletries because they are *living there* for the time being. The patient's room could become cluttered with people and things. Try to avoid viewing this as an inconvenience to you and remember—this is the patient's and his or her family's *home away from home* for the time being. Providing family support is an important part of customer service and patient care.

As mentioned earlier, patients notice everything. When a patient is hospitalized for several days, the patient and his or her family spend hours and hours, and days and days, waiting. Their lives are on hold until their medical situation is resolved and they can resume their normal lives. With so much time on their hands, they notice when the free coffee down the hall isn't strong enough, the upholstery on the chairs is threadbare, and the elevator doors close too quickly. When it's finally time to eat, they notice that there's never an extra wheelchair available to take grandma down to the cafeteria. The patient's room is too hot or too cold. The meal tray was supposed to be delivered twenty minutes ago and when it finally arrived, the milk was white instead of chocolate. The TV remote control doesn't work properly. Patients and families may become irritated when they don't get medical information about the patient's condition and treatment plans quickly enough. They may pressure you for information that you don't have and ask for answers that you can't give. Sometimes it's enough to make a sane health care worker crazy! When this happens, take a deep breath and remember why you went into health care. Give your patients and families some slack and rejoice that *you*, unlike your hospitalized patients, get to go home in a few hours.

Patients who receive health care in outpatient settings are also on a quest for information. After seeing their doctor in his or her office and undergoing diagnostic tests, patients want to hear the results of those tests as quickly as possible. They also have questions about the results and next steps. All too often, patients receive a postcard in the mail or a brief phone call from the doctor's nurse or medical assistant directing the patient to pick up a prescription at the pharmacy. Patients may not have the opportunity to get all of their questions answered until returning for a follow-up doctor's visit several weeks later. If part of your job is calling patients to inform them of test results, have sufficient information at hand to answer their questions.

THE MORE YOU KNOW

Smoking and Role Models

One of the best ways to protect your health and prevent disease is not to smoke. According to the Centers for Disease Control and Prevention, smoking causes harm to almost every organ in the body. One out of every five deaths in the U.S. each year is related to smoking. You might know that smoking causes lung cancer, emphysema, and other respiratory diseases. You might not know that smoking can also cause many other cancers, including cancers of the mouth, larynx, pharynx, esophagus, bladder, kidney, pancreas, cervix, and stomach. Smoking also puts people at a higher risk for coronary heart disease and stroke. Women who smoke when they are pregnant can damage the health of their fetus. Older women who smoke are more at risk for osteoporosis.

If you don't smoke, you should never start. Cigarettes are highly addictive, so it is difficult to quit smoking. If you smoke now, you should quit. Many health insurance companies have programs that can help smokers quit. Many resources on the Internet are also available to help smokers become nonsmokers.

Here's another good reason to avoid smoking—research shows that patients who smoke are less likely to stop smoking if their caregivers smoke themselves. Although doctors, nurses, and respiratory therapists encourage their patients to refrain from smoking, their efforts are less successful when they don't practice what they preach themselves. Patients view their caregivers as educators and trusted role models. When their caregivers continue to smoke despite the overwhelming evidence that smoking is hazardous to their health, patients are less likely to follow the advice given by their caregivers. One of the strategies, therefore, to reduce smoking among the general public is to reduce smoking among health care professionals.

What are some other good reasons to avoid smoking?

Today's health care consumers are often well informed. They don't just want to hear, "Your results were slightly elevated." They want details and actual numbers so they can go online and learn more about their conditions and potential treatment

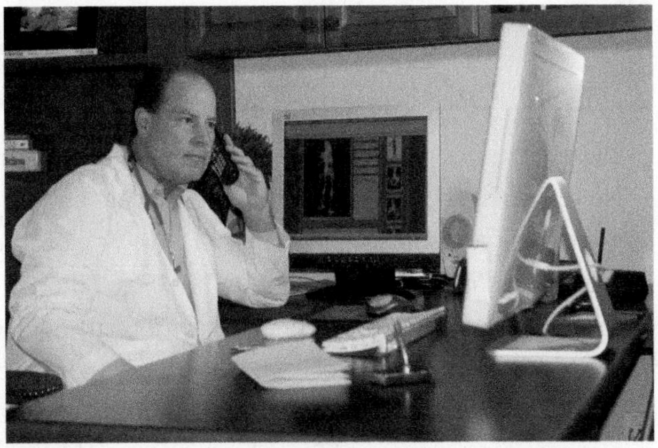

FIGURE 6.16
Physician speaking with his patient
Source: william casey/Shutterstock

options. In situations where you can't provide all of the information requested, don't be surprised if the patient asks to speak with the doctor. Some doctors willingly take phone calls while others may do so begrudgingly or not at all. Depending on your job, you may be in an assistant role to the physician, serving as a liaison between the patient and his or her doctor. Do your best to meet the patients' needs while still working within your scope of practice.

Try to give your patients and their family members the benefit of the doubt and remember that their lives are in limbo. They're temporarily living in suspended animation, in a surreal world, and usually not by choice. They're uncertain about what's going to happen next, and no one has all of the answers.

Avoid the temptation to give your patients personal advice or to express your own religious beliefs, even if the patient asks you for it. When appropriate, generate some humor and laughter. Be positive whenever you can. Even tiny improvements in the patient's condition mean a great deal to the patient and his or her family members. Here's where your optimistic *the glass is half full* attitude can be helpful. Consider the following:

- Perhaps the patient's blood pressure and heart rate haven't settled down during the past hour. But they haven't worsened either.
- Maybe the patient isn't well enough to be transported to radiology for a chest x-ray. But he can sit up in bed and have a portable radiograph taken in his room.
- Maybe the patient's IV supply can't be completely disconnected. But the dosage has been reduced.

Look for things to be happy about and express them. Optimism and a positive outlook on the part of caregivers are important to patients. A positive frame of mind can lead to improvements in a patient's condition. When undergoing high-risk procedures, patients who are optimistic and more relaxed may have better outcomes. If a patient thinks his or her medical team has given up, he or she may give up, too. But don't give patients **false hope** or *get their hopes up* inappropriately. Some of your patients won't get better. Some won't leave the hospital alive.

false hope
(FOLS HOPE) Looking forward to something that probably won't happen

You may be called upon to help prepare someone for death. The patient and his or her family will have difficult decisions to make. They will need privacy and time to talk, cry, and express their love and other emotions. These are the moments that your patients and family members will remember forever, and you are a part of it. Just as you may help usher in a new life in labor and delivery, you may also be present when someone passes. Both are humbling experiences that you cannot begin to imagine until you go through them yourself.

BUILD YOUR SKILLS *Protecting Yourself Against Health Risks*

Depending on your job, you may have a lot of contact with patients or very little. Nonetheless, anyone working in a health care environment is at some risk of infection. Therefore, you should consider your own risk of infection, and what can you do to reduce your risk.

Hepatitis B virus (HBV) is one of the most serious infections. It is typically spread through sexual contact, by sharing needles among drug users, and by accidental needle sticks, which represent the greatest risk to health care workers. HBV cannot be contracted by casual contact with infected patients. Some health care employers provide inoculation against HBV at no cost to the employee.

inoculation
(ih-nah-cue-LAY-shen) To introduce an antibody or antigen to prevent a disease

Human immunodeficiency virus (HIV) is primarily transmitted by sexual contact and intravenous drug use. It is not transmitted by casual contact, through contaminated food or water, or through the air.

Influenza, or the flu, is a common illness that often brings patients to a medical facility. To protect yourself from infection and avoid spreading the flu to other patients, you should consider getting an annual flu vaccination. Some health care employers provide free flu shots for their employees, and an increasing number now require flu shots.

Workers may be exposed to other microorganisms that can be spread through casual contact in the medical facility. The best precaution against infection is to wash your hands regularly and frequently. Keep your hands away from your mouth. If you develop any signs or symptoms of illness, report them immediately.

How does your health affect the health of patients? How can you protect patients from catching something from you?

WORKING WITH DOCTORS, GUESTS, AND VENDORS

In some health care settings such as hospitals, doctors are often considered customers, along with guests, vendors, and other people who come into your facility. As with other customers, you'll encounter doctors from various cultures, with different personality types and communication styles. You'll work with doctors whom you really like and respect, and others whom you would avoid if you could. Some will take an interest in you, answer your questions, and explain procedures as they are performed. They'll *go the extra mile* for their patients, and they'll express appreciation for the efforts of their staff. Other doctors may appear smug, dispassionate, or downright rude. To save time, they may dictate in front of a patient during an office visit rather than converse directly with the patient. (Yes, unfortunately this really happens.) As a worker, you may feel they treat you as if you're invisible or unimportant. One day a

dictate
(DIK-tate) Record patient information for medical records

doctor will be friendly, and the next day he or she will be grumpy. A doctor may appear angry when speaking with you, yet his or her anger may actually have nothing to do with you at all.

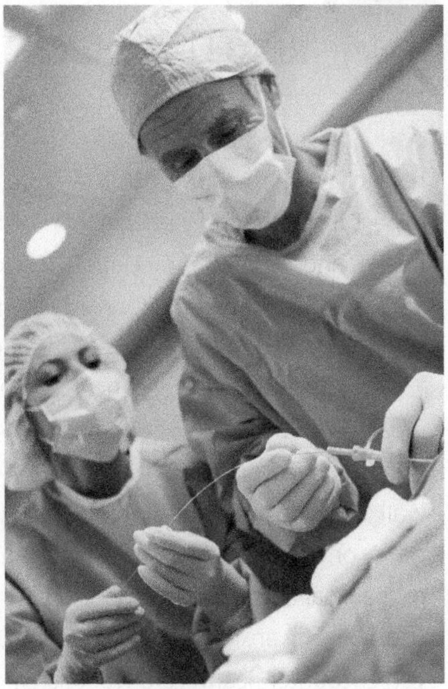

FIGURE 6.17

Working as a team to save a patient's life

Source: Monkey Business Images/ Shutterstock

Although some doctors will be demanding and intimidating, try to remember that doctors are just people, too. They have hopes and dreams, feelings and fears, frailties and flaws just like everyone else. Much of the time they're in a hurry and under a great deal of stress. Some of them literally hold life and death in their hands on a daily basis. Practicing medicine is an enormous responsibility, and it takes its toll. Until you have walked in a doctor's shoes, you have no idea what his or her job is like.

Occasionally a doctor may ask you to do something that's outside of your scope of practice. He or she may mistake you for a different type of worker or may not be familiar with your training and job duties. If this happens, speak up! Don't just go ahead and do something you aren't qualified to do because a doctor asked you or told you to do so. Say politely, "That's not within my scope of practice, but I'll go get someone who can help you." If you are competent and apply your best communication and customer service skills, you'll likely get along just fine with the doctors.

Guests in your facility are also customers and they, too, are a diverse group of people. Some may be lost or stressed out, running late for an important meeting or a job interview. Others may be in the building to attend a conference or keep an appointment with someone in management. The most frequent request that you'll get from guests is help with directions. Keep these suggestions in mind:

- If you work in a large building, make sure you know your way around so you can give good directions to other people.
- If you have the time or are headed in that direction anyway, offer to walk with the person to make sure he or she gets to their destination.
- If someone is waiting to see your supervisor or someone else in your area and you have access to coffee or a soft drink, offer the person a beverage.
- If you know someone is going to have to wait for awhile, let the person know and explain why.

Do whatever you can to make guests comfortable. Your customers will appreciate even a small gesture of kindness.

The last group of customers is vendors. Vendors might be salespeople from a patient supply company, insurance agents, drug company representatives, or people who work for advertising agencies or temporary services. Just like other customers, they, too, should be treated with respect, manners, and good customer service.

REALITY CHECK

As a customer yourself, you know the importance of being treated with kindness and respect. When you walk into a store, a restaurant, or another place of business, you expect to find friendly people who will welcome you, answer your questions, meet your needs, and express appreciation for your business. Of course, your expectations aren't always met, and you may leave feeling disappointed or angry. If you didn't receive good service, you'll probably take your business elsewhere the next time.

It's one thing to experience poor customer service in a store, a restaurant, or an auto repair shop. But experiencing poor service when your health is on the line is another matter. If you are ignored in a store, or served unappetizing food in a restaurant, you can just walk out and vow never to return. But if you're in your doctor's office, an outpatient clinic, or a hospital for medical tests or treatments, you have much more to lose. You're probably already nervous about what's going to happen to you before you even arrive. If you're overly anxious and stressed out, it won't take much to *push you over the edge* if you encounter health care workers who are insensitive, **indifferent**, or rude.

indifferent
(in-DIH-fer-ent) Showing no interest or concern

People who work in retail sales often say that dealing with customers is the most difficult part of their jobs. Health care workers, on the other hand, chose their occupations specifically because they *want* to work with customers (patients) and hopefully make a positive difference in their lives.

Are you cut-out to provide good customer service? Can you put the needs of your customers ahead of your own? Can you remain calm and reassuring when your customers are scared and stressed out? Can you make eye contact, smile, and convey a warm and friendly personality? Can you make everyone you encounter feel welcome and appreciated? If so, you're well on your way to supporting good customer service and a high level of patient satisfaction.

Key Points

- Health care is a business and its customers include doctors, visitors, guests, vendors, and most importantly—patients.
- Health care workers must apply good customer service skills in order to meet or, better yet, exceed customer expectations.
- Providing the right care, for the right person, every time is the goal of patient centered care.
- In patient centered care, doctors and patients work in partnership to seek medical outcomes which are of value and meaningful to the individual patient.
- Health care workers who are empathetic can put themselves in the place of their patients and relate to what they are feeling.
- Hospitals now use HCAHPS surveys to measure and improve patient satisfaction. Financial incentives penalize or reward providers based on their patient satisfaction scores.

- Health care workers must *be there* for their patients and deliver excellent customer service. They should express optimism and a positive outlook without giving patients false hope.
- Workers should also provide support for the patient's family and close friends who serve as members of the *patient's team*.
- Doctors, guests, vendors, and other people who come into the facility should also be treated as customers with kindness and respect.

Section Review Questions

Answer each of the following questions. Indicate which page in the textbook led you to your answer.

1. What is patient centered care and how does it benefit patients?
2. What is the purpose of the HCAHPS survey and how is it administered?
3. List four ways to provide good customer service for patients and their family members.
4. Explain two things that might happen if a patient experiences poor customer service.
5. Name two things that workers should do when they call patients to inform them of their test results.
6. What is the best precaution that health care workers can take to prevent getting an infection at work?

Learn By Doing

Complete Worksheets 1–5 in Section 6.2 of your *Student Activity Guide*.

CHAPTER 6 Review

Chapter Review Questions

Answer each of the following questions. Indicate which page in the textbook led you to your answer.

1. List three examples of Instrumental Activities of Daily Living.
2. Why are elderly patients more affected by a debilitating illness than younger patients?
3. Name four psychological needs that must be met, and give one example of each need.
4. Name four physiological needs that must be met, and give one example of each need.
5. List three types of health care customers.
6. Explain the difference between *empathy* and *sympathy*.
7. List three concerns that patients may have when they become hospitalized.

Chapter Review Activities

1. Investigate the availability of free, or low-cost, health screenings where you live. These might include screenings for high blood pressure, high cholesterol, and diabetes. What is the purpose of the health screenings, how are the procedures done, and how are the results reported? Who should have each type of screening, and when? What roles do age, gender, family history, and genetic risk factors play in determining if someone should undergo health screening?
2. How would you train a new health care employee to provide excellent customer service for his or her patients? Make a bulleted list of the topics and techniques that you would cover.
3. What advice would you give a close friend who appears to be suffering from depression? He's having trouble concentrating and sleeping; he's lost interest in his hobbies and friends; and he's expressing feelings of despair and hopelessness.

What If? Scenarios

What would you do in each of the following situations? Record your answer, explain it, and indicate which page in the textbook led you to your decision.

1. A new doctor in your department mistakes you for a registered nurse and tells you to administer a medication to one of his patients.
2. An elderly patient shows up for her appointment the day before she's scheduled to see a specialist. She's confused and says her son took a day off from work to drive her to the clinic. She lives two hours away and there's no specialist in the town where she lives.
3. It's 8:00 p.m. and you notice that one of your patients who just had surgery the day before has five visitors in his room. When you check on him, you notice that he looks tired and the group appears to be staying for awhile.
4. The husband of one of your critically ill patients wants to spend the night in his wife's room but there's no bed for him to sleep in.
5. One of your patients was just diagnosed with cancer. No one in his family has ever had cancer before, and he doesn't know where to turn for information, counseling, and support.
6. You are trying to meet the biological needs of an ill patient who must be awakened several times during the night to receive her medications.

Media Connection

Use the companion website for additional interactive learning activities.

Portfolio Connection

Working with people who are ill causes unfamiliar feelings and experiences. Your ability to identify your feelings and understand how you react to those feelings helps you carry on and continue to care for others.

Select a disability described in this chapter. Imagine that you are diagnosed with this disability. Identify your fears, feelings, and expectations. Explain what each day would be like, what type of care you would need, how others would respond to you, and how you would respond to others. Your explanation must clearly identify your self-evaluation and new insights about disabilities and behaviors, and show how you would approach others with disabilities.

This assignment helps you investigate your feelings and identify possible behaviors of patients who live with disabilities. Including this assignment in your portfolio gives you easy access to it for review during your education. Comparing assignments throughout your education shows how your experiences have brought about changes in your thinking.

CHAPTER 7

Your Legal and Ethical Responsibilities

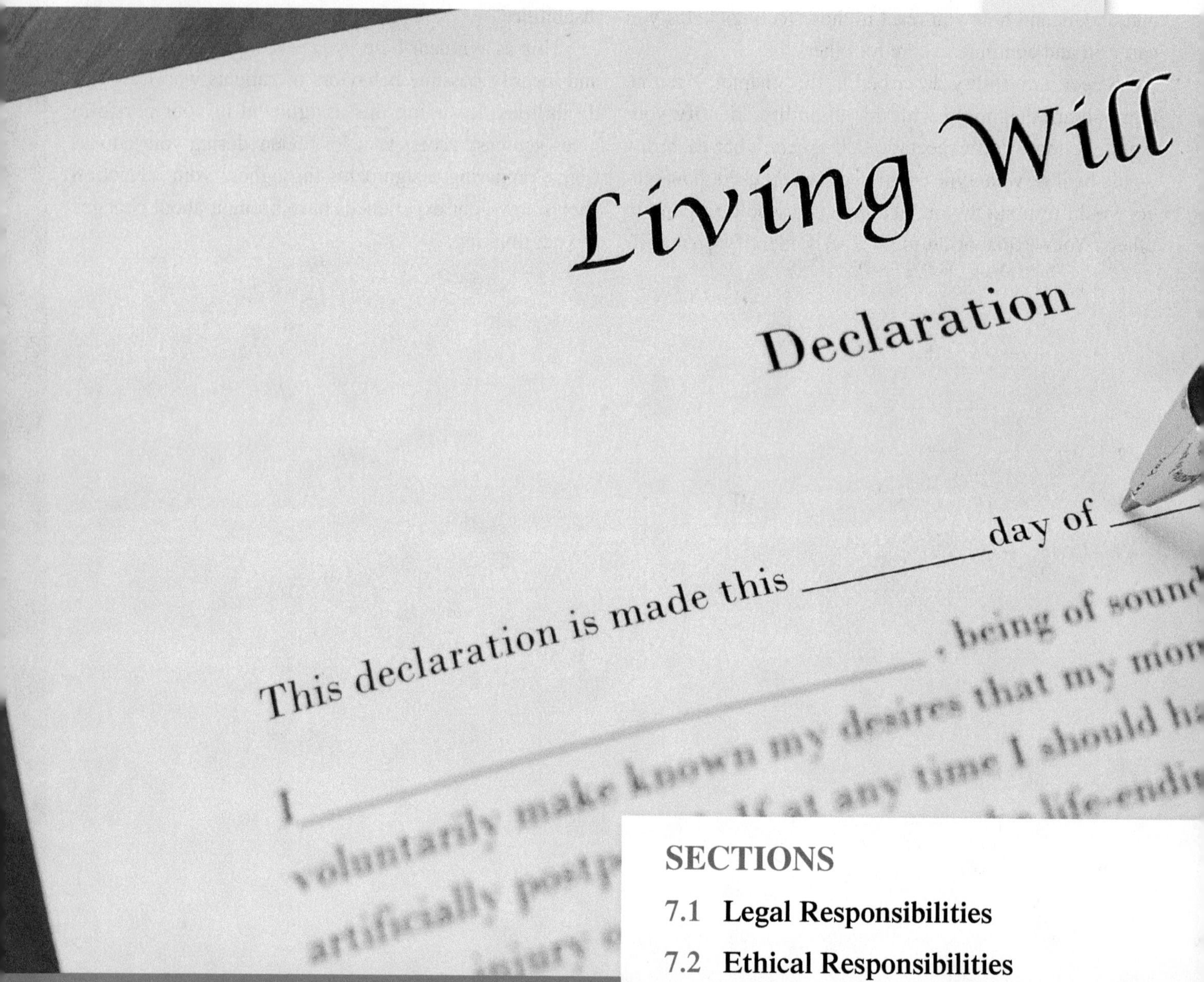

Living Will
Declaration
This declaration is made this ________ day of

Source: zimmytws/Shutterstock

SECTIONS

"The ultimate measure of a man is not where he stands in moments of comfort and convenience, but where he stands at times of challenge and controversy."

MARTIN LUTHER KING, JR., CIVIL RIGHTS LEADER, 1929–1968

GETTING STARTED

As you will learn in this chapter, ensuring the patient's right to privacy regarding health care practices and procedures, as well as a patient's condition, is a legal responsibility of the entire health care workforce. The Health Information Portability and Accountability Act (HIPAA) was signed into law in 1996, and on April 14, 2003, new regulations strengthening the Act went into effect. This law creates a national standard for medical privacy and gives patients greater control over their personal health information. If someone knowingly violates this law, they can be fined from $50,000 to $250,000 along with imprisonment, depending on the severity and intent of the offense. If you have been to your doctor or dentist, or received care in any other health care setting within the last ten years, you will have been asked to sign a form declaring you have been made aware of HIPAA. This is a requirement in the law.

As you learn more about the legal requirements relating to confidentiality, you become more aware of conversations taking place in various health care settings. Imagine that you are in a small medical office and can hear the staff discussing a patient, along with all the others who are awaiting their appointments. It is a small community and several people in the waiting area know the patient who is being discussed.

What would you do? Write down how you believe this situation should be handled. Be prepared to share your response with the rest of the class.

Legal Responsibilities

SECTION 7.1

Background

Health care workers have a legal responsibility to provide excellent care. Understanding legal responsibilities ensures a safe work environment, prevents lawsuits, and protects patients, workers, and health care facilities. Policies are in place to ensure that everyone practices and monitors sound legal behavior.

A failure to provide the best care to patients can result in lawsuits. Lawsuits are determined by the legal system based on the facts of the case. Avoiding illegal and unethical behavior promotes good patient care and helps avoid legal trouble.

Objectives

After completing this section, you will be able to:

1. Define the key terms.
2. Describe the rights to which a patient is entitled.
3. List the patient's responsibilities in the health care process.
4. Explain what might happen if health care workers fail to meet their legal responsibilities.
5. Define *licensure, certification,* and *registration,* and explain the role they play.
6. Summarize the importance of patient confidentiality.

7. Explain the purposes of HIPAA and the HITECH Act.
8. Describe the elements of a contract.
9. List the types of advance directives and explain their purpose.
10. Identify the difference between civil law and criminal law.
11. List six common categories of medical malpractice.

PATIENT RIGHTS AND RESPONSIBILITIES

Effective health care requires collaboration among patients and physicians and other health care professionals. Policies and procedures are established in health care settings to facilitate this type of collaboration. Open and honest communication, respect for personal and professional values, and sensitivity to differences are integral to optimal patient care.

As the setting for the provision of health services, hospitals must provide a foundation for understanding and respecting the rights and responsibilities of patients, their families, physicians, and other caregivers. Hospitals must ensure a health care ethic that respects the role of patients in decision making about treatment choices and other aspects of their care. Hospitals must be sensitive to cultural, racial, linguistic, religious, age, gender, and other differences as well as the needs of persons with disabilities.

"A Patient's Bill of Rights" was first adopted by the American Hospital Association in 1973. A revision was approved by the AHA Board of Trustees on October 21, 1992. The AHA presented "A Patient's Bill of Rights" with the expectation that it would contribute to more effective patient care and be supported by the hospital on behalf of the institution, its medical staff, employees, and patients. The AHA encouraged health care institutions to tailor this bill of rights to their patient community by translating and/or simplifying the language of the bill of rights as may be necessary to ensure that patients and their families understand their rights and responsibilities. In 2003, the AHA replaced its "A Patient's Bill of Rights" with "Patient Care Partnership: Understanding Expectations, Rights and Responsibilities" to make the information easier to understand and to emphasize the importance of collaborative effort between the patient and his or her health care providers.

APPLY IT PATIENT RIGHTS

A bill of rights is a document that sets limitations in order to guarantee rights. With your classmates, hold a round table discussion about the situations in which patients find themselves in hospitals and other health care settings. Discuss the ways in which cultural, social, and ethical issues affect people's needs and rights when they are patients. Explain the benefits of documents such as "Patient Care Partnership: Understanding Expectations, Rights and Responsibilities" for health care workers and patients.

A designated surrogate or proxy decision maker may exercise the patient's rights on behalf of the patient in situations where the patient is legally incompetent, a minor, or lacks decision-making capacity. To the extent permitted by law and by hospital policy, hospitals are expected to honor a patient's advance directive (such as a living will, health care proxy, or durable power of attorney for health care) and other directives regarding his or her treatment and care.

The following information is provided in the AHA's brochure, "The Patient Care Partnership: Understanding Expectations, Rights and Responsibilities." This information is given to patients upon admission to the hospital to help explain their rights and how to exercise their rights. (Reprinted from "The Patient Care Partnership: Understanding Expectations, Rights and Responsibilities" by permission, Copyright 2003, American Hospital Association.)

What to expect during your hospital stay:

- High quality hospital care.
- A clean and safe environment.
- Involvement in your care.
- Protection of your privacy.
- Help when leaving the hospital.
- Help with your billing claims.

When you need hospital care, your doctor and the nurses and other professionals at our hospital are committed to working with you and your family to meet your health care needs. Our dedicated doctors and staff serve the community in all its ethnic, religious and economic diversity. Our goal is for you and your family to have the same care and attention we would want for our families and ourselves.

The sections explain some of the basics about how you can expect to be treated during your hospital stay. They also cover what we will need from you to care for you better. If you have questions at any time, please ask them. Unasked or unanswered questions can add to the stress of being in the hospital. Your comfort and confidence in your care are very important to us.

High quality hospital care. Our first priority is to provide you the care you need, when you need it, with skill, compassion and respect. Tell your caregivers if you have concerns about your care or if you have pain. You have the right to know the identity of doctors, nurses and others involved in your care, and you have the right to know when they are students, residents or other trainees.

A clean and safe environment. Our hospital works hard to keep you safe. We use special policies and procedures to avoid mistakes in your care and keep you free from abuse or neglect. If anything unexpected and significant happens during your hospital stay, you will be told what happened, and any resulting changes in your care will be discussed with you.

Involvement in your care. You and your doctor often make decisions about your care before you go to the hospital. Other times, especially in emergencies, those decisions are made during your hospital stay. When decision-making takes place, it should include:

- Discussing your medical condition and information about medically appropriate treatment choices.
- Discussing your treatment plan.

surrogate
(SER-e-get) Substitute

proxy decision maker
(PRAK-see di-SIH-zhun MAY-ker) The advocate for a patient who isn't competent to make decisions about his or her own medical care

minor
(MY-ner) Under the legal age of full responsibility

law
(LAW) A rule of conduct or procedure recognized by a community as binding or enforceable by authority

advance directive
(ad-VANCE deh-REK-tiv) A written instruction such as a living will or a durable power of attorney recognized under state law relating to the provision of health care when the individual is incapacitated

living will
(LIV-ing WILL) A will in which the signer requests not to be kept alive by medical life-support systems in the event of a terminal illness

durable power of attorney
(DUR-eh-bul POW-er of eh-TER-nee) A type of advance medical directive in which legal documents provide the power of attorney, or the authorization to act on someone else's behalf in a legal or business matter, to another person in the case of an incapacitating medical condition

directive
(deh-REK-tiv) Something that serves to guide or impel towards an action or goal

- Getting information from you.
- Understanding your health care goals and values.
- Understanding who should make decisions when you cannot.

Discussing your medical condition and information about medically appropriate treatment choices. To make informed decisions with your doctor, you need to understand:

- The benefits and risks of each treatment.
- Whether your treatment is experimental or part of a research study.
- What you can reasonably expect from your treatment and any long-term effects it might have on your quality of life.
- What you and your family will need to do after you leave the hospital.
- The financial consequences of using uncovered services or out-of-network providers.

Please tell your caregivers if you need more information about treatment choices.

Discussing your treatment plan. When you enter the hospital, you sign a general consent to treatment. In some cases, such as surgery or experimental treatment, you may be asked to confirm in writing that you understand what is planned and agree to it. This process protects your right to consent to or refuse a treatment. Your doctor will explain the medical consequences of refusing recommended treatment. It also protects your right to decide if you want to participate in a research study.

Getting information from you. Your caregivers need complete and correct information about your health and coverage so that they can make good decisions about your care. That includes:

- Past illnesses, surgeries or hospital stays.
- Past allergic reactions.
- Any medicines or dietary supplements (such as vitamins and herbs) that you are taking.
- Any network or admission requirements under your health plan.

Understanding your health care goals and values. You may have health care goals and values or spiritual beliefs that are important to your well-being. They will be taken into account as much as possible throughout your hospital stay. Make sure your doctor, your family and your care team know your wishes.

Understanding who should make decisions when you cannot. If you have signed a health care power of attorney stating who should speak for you if you become unable to make health care decisions for yourself, or a "living will" or "advance directive" that states your wishes about end-of-life care; give copies to your doctor, your family and your care team. If you or your family need help making difficult decisions, counselors, chaplains and others are available to help.

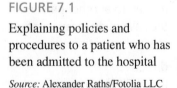

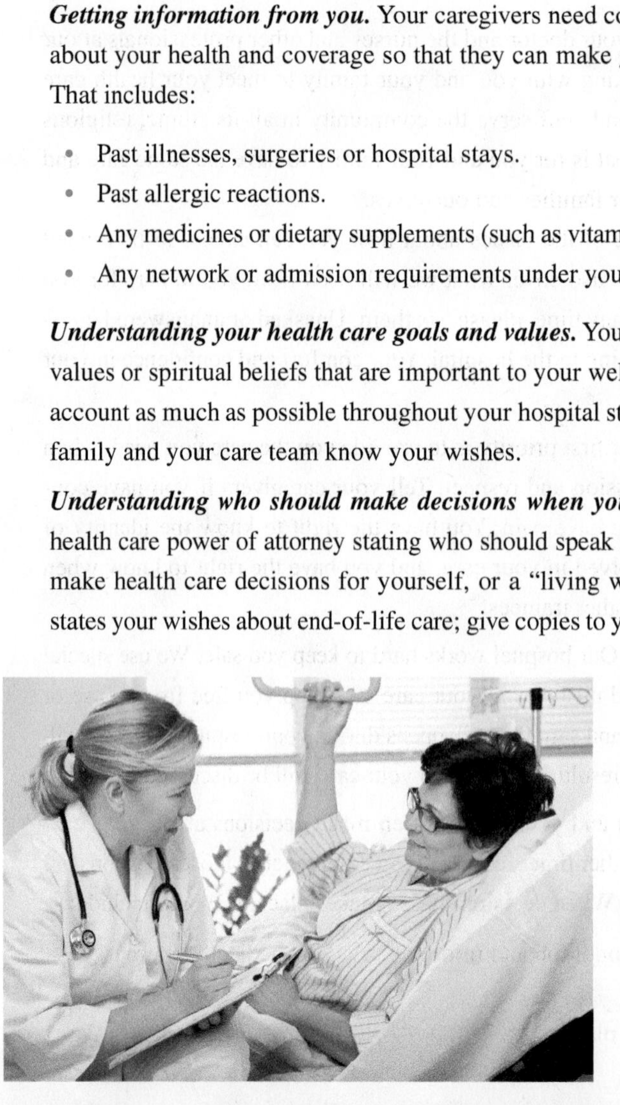

FIGURE 7.1

Explaining policies and procedures to a patient who has been admitted to the hospital

Source: Alexander Raths/Fotolia LLC

Protection of your privacy. We respect the confidentiality of your relationship with your doctor and other caregivers, and the sensitive information about your health and health care that are part of that relationship.

State and federal laws and hospital operating policies protect the privacy of your medical information. You will receive a Notice of Privacy Practices that describes the ways that we use, disclose and safeguard patient information and that explains how you can obtain a copy of information from our records about your care.

Preparing you and your family for when you leave the hospital. Your doctor works with hospital staff and professionals in your community. You and your family also play an important role in your care. The success of your treatment often depends on your efforts to follow medication, diet and therapy plans. Your family may need to help care for you at home. You can expect us to help you identify sources of follow-up care and to let you know if our hospital has a financial interest in any referrals. As long as you agree that we can share information about your care with them, we will coordinate our activities with your caregivers outside the hospital. You can also expect to receive information and, where possible, training about the self-care you will need when you go home.

Consider This *Residents' Rights in Nursing Homes*

The Omnibus Budget Reconciliation Act (OBRA) was passed in 1987 to implement certain basic patient rights and guidelines for nursing home care facilities. Patients who live in nursing homes are called *residents*. This Nursing Home Reform Act states that:

1. Each resident be fully evaluated upon admission and each year after in regards to health, memory, hobbies, habits, and so forth.
2. A plan must be created to maintain and possibly improve the resident's condition.
3. Patients have rights to a doctor. If they can't find one on their own, the medical director of the nursing home will help them find one.
4. Patients have a right to be informed about treatment, and to refuse if desired.
5. Patients have a right to privacy and a right to complain without fear of reprisal.

OBRA also contains the Resident's Bill of Rights, which is similar to the Patient's Bill of Rights. The Resident's Bill of Rights specifically addresses:

- Free choice of doctor, treatment, care, and participation in research.
- Freedom from abuse and chemical or physical restraints.
- Privacy and confidentiality of medical records.
- Accommodation of needs and choice regarding activities, schedules, and health care.
- The ability to voice grievances without fear.
- Organization and participation in family/resident groups and in social, religious, and community activities.
- Ability to manage their personal funds and use personal possessions.
- Unlimited access to immediate family, and can share room with spouse if both are residents.
- Access to information about medical benefits, medical records, deficiencies in the facility, and sources of **advocates** for the residents.
- The ability to stay in the facility and not be transferred or discharged except for medical reasons, failure to pay, or if the facility cannot meet the patient's needs.

advocates
(AD-veh-kets) People or groups who speak or write in support of something or someone

Help with your bill and filing insurance claims. Our staff will file claims for you with health care insurers or other programs such as Medicare and Medicaid. They also will help your doctor with needed documentation. Hospital bills and insurance coverage are often confusing. If you have questions about your bill, contact our business office. If you need help understanding your insurance coverage or health plan, start with your insurance company or health benefits manager. If you do not have health coverage, we will try to help you and your family find financial help or make other arrangements. We need your help with collecting needed information and other requirements to obtain coverage or assistance.

UNDERSTANDING YOUR LEGAL RESPONSIBILITIES

It is important for health care workers to remember that patients have rights that represent not only moral and ethical issues, but also rights legislated by both federal and state governments. A list of patient rights is meaningless unless the person working with the patient understands and follows them. All health care workers must commit to giving the best possible care—which means complying with the professional standards of care for their particular professions.

> *Community Service* **Patient Rights**
>
> Prepare a flier, brochure, or poster on patient rights and present the information to parents, teachers, and students at an upcoming school event. Include websites and other resources that people could use to locate more information.

Resources for Ensuring Legal Compliance

Policies, offices, and agencies exist to ensure that everyone working in a hospital practices and monitors legal behavior. An **ombudsman** is a social worker, nurse, or trained volunteer who makes certain that the patient is not abused and that the person's rights are secure. Most institutions have a designated office, officer, and phone number posted for an employee to use when reporting identified problems with patients rights or institutional practice.

ombudsman
(AHM-budz-men) A social worker, nurse, or trained volunteer who ensures that patients/residents are properly cared for and respected

registration
(re-je-STRAY-shen) A list of individuals on an official record who meet the qualifications for an occupation

Other systems help ensure that health care workers are properly trained and regulated. Licensure, certification, and **registration** indicate what a health care worker may or may not do. They determine the scope of practice for the health care worker. Controls help to improve the quality of care. Although not all health occupations require licensure, certification, or registration, it is important to be aware of these controls.

- *Licensure* is a credential from a state agency awarding legal permission to practice. Licensed individuals must meet pre-established qualifications.
- *Certification* is a credential from a state agency or a professional association awarding permission to use a special professional title. Certified individuals must meet pre-established competency standards. When specific guidelines are met, the certification equals licensure.

APPLY IT PROFESSIONAL CREDENTIALS

Form groups of four students. Each group member should choose a different health care profession. Research and list the licenses, certifications, or registrations necessary for your chosen occupation. Find out if there are additional educational or training requirements needed to move ahead in your chosen field. Discuss how these credentialing processes help ensure that health care workers are properly trained and regulated. How do professional credentials support quality care?

- *Registration* is a list of individuals on an official record who meet the qualifications for an occupation (such as a registered nurse or a registered radiographer). Registered nurses are registered with the state in which they practice.

Confidentiality

One of the most important aspects of patient care is confidentiality. Patient information is confidential. *Confidential* means *secret.* Only people who are authorized to use the information should have access to it. Health care workers are obligated to protect and keep all patient information confidential.

A good rule is to discuss a patient only when the discussion affects his or her care in some way. Here are some examples:

- When you find candy with the belongings of a diabetic.
- When you find alcohol or medications with the belongings of a patient.
- When patients discuss areas of stress in their personal lives, such as financial problems or relationship problems.

Even when a patient discusses information that does not pertain to his or her care, it is still subject to confidentiality. For example, if a patient mentions that her sister is married to a local public official and has information about an upcoming ordinance that will affect property tax rates, this information is also *privileged communication* and should be kept in confidence. Privileged communication covers any personal or private information given by a patient to medical personnel that is relevant to his or her care. For example, a health care worker should consider all information in the patient's chart as privileged communication. A medical facility, a physician, or a health care worker can be fined, sued, or fired for sharing *any* information about patients with others, including family members. You must report any violation of patient confidentiality.

Patients must provide written **consent** for the release of medical information pertaining to their care. Patients must also give consent for procedures affecting their care. This includes patient approval, usually in writing, for surgery, experimental treatment, and so forth after having been informed of the potential medical risks. It also includes any *legal document*, signed by the patient, or his or her designee, stating that the patient understands any potential medical risks in surgery, experimental treatment, and so forth.

consent
(con-SENT) Approve, agree

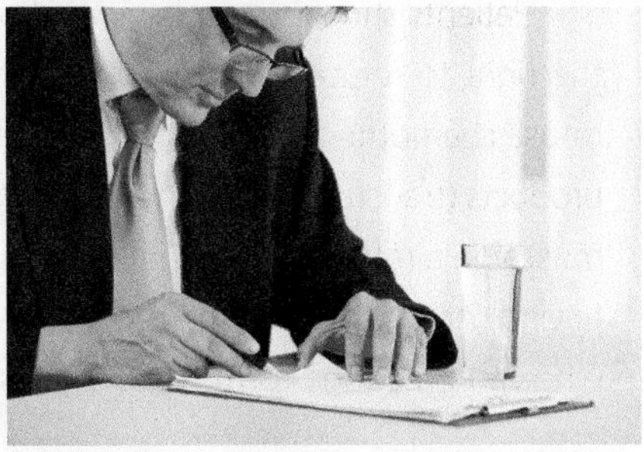

FIGURE 7.2

Reviewing and signing a consent form prior to treatment

Source: Lucky Business/Shutterstock

THE MORE YOU KNOW

Patient Consent

expressed consent (ik-SPRESS-ed con-SENT) Giving approval verbally or in writing

implied consent (im-PLIED con-SENT) Giving approval through an action

Before patients can be examined and treated they must give their consent. **Expressed consent** is when patients either sign a consent form or verbally agree to the care. **Implied consent** is when patients give approval through an action only, such as removing their clothing and putting on a patient gown. An invasive procedure, such as surgery, requires a signed consent. The signed consent form is evidence that the patient agreed to the care after having been informed of the risks involved.

Consent forms must be written in a language that the patient understands. Based on the Doctrine of Informed Consent, the following information must be included:

- The procedure to be performed
- The physician who will perform the procedure
- The person administering the anesthesia, when applicable
- Potential risks to the patient from having, or not having, the procedure
- Potential alternative treatments and their risks
- Verification that the patient has had his or her questions answered
- Exceptions or exclusions requested by the patient

Patients must be made aware of their diagnosis, if known, and the purpose, advantages, and risks of the procedure. Specialized consent forms are used for procedures such as blood transfusions, invasive procedures such as biopsies and lumbar punctures, chemotherapy, and cardiac or pulmonary stress testing.

incapacitated (in-keh-PAH-seh-tated) Permanently or temporarily impaired due to a mental and/or physical condition

emancipated (ih-MAN-she-pated) Legally considered an adult

Consent forms must be signed and dated by the patient or his or her representative. Patients must be mentally competent and at least eighteen years of age to sign their consent forms. If the patient is less than eighteen years old, a parent or guardian must sign for the patient. If the patient is mentally incompetent or temporarily **incapacitated** (unconscious, for example), the form will be signed by the patient's representative. Minors under the age of eighteen who are **emancipated** may sign their consent forms. Emancipated minors are married or otherwise responsible for paying their own bills, and have a court order stating they are emancipated. Minors who are in the armed services or undergoing care for a sexually transmitted disease or a pregnancy, or are being seen for birth control, abortion, or drug or alcohol abuse can sign their own consent forms.

Consent must be *informed*, meaning the patient must be told about the risks and benefits of the procedure plus any alternative treatments to be considered. Patients must be told about how much pain and discomfort to expect, and what their recovery or follow-up care will involve.

Patients should never be forced or threatened to sign a consent form, and they have the right to refuse the procedure. Patients near death due to cancer, for example, may refuse chemotherapy treatments because of the side effects, or patients may refuse blood products (transfusions) due to their religious beliefs. When patients refuse treatment, they must sign a refusal-of-consent form stating they were given information about the risks of having, or not having, the procedure. Patients who don't understand the procedure, or who can't read the form, should not sign a consent form.

Patients must give consent before their medical information can be released to other parties, such as physician specialists, insurance companies, and the patients' family members. Once the patient reaches eighteen years of age, the patient's medical information cannot be shared with anyone, including his or her spouse, parents, or guardian without the consent of the patient.

The Health Insurance Portability and Accountability Act (HIPAA)

The confidentiality of a patient's medical information is protected by the Health Insurance Portability and Accountability Act (HIPAA). This law regulates the sharing of medical information. Regulations in the act help ensure that a patient's medical information is kept secure and confidential. All employees of a health care system must be taught the HIPAA regulations that apply to their jobs. Here are a few examples of the kinds of information protected by HIPAA:

- Information in medical records
- Conversations between health care providers about patient care or treatment
- Health insurance information
- Patient billing information
- Most other information about a patient's health

The Health Information Technology for Economic and Clinical Health (HITECH) Act was signed into law in February 2009 as part of the American Recovery and Reinvestment Act (ARRA) of 2009. Portions of the HITECH Act address the confidentiality of health information transmitted electronically and strengthen the enforcement and penalties associated with HIPAA rules.

Confidential communications are protected under law against any disclosure (forced or voluntary) over the objection of the patient. The rationale behind the rule is that a level of trust must exist between a physician and the patient so that the physician can properly treat the patient. If the patient were fearful of telling the truth to the physician because he or she believed the physician would report such behavior to others, then the treatment process could be far more difficult. However, certain information may be considered **exempt** information, such as:

exempt
(ig-ZEMPT) To be free or released from some liability or requirement to which others are subject

- Suspected fraud
- Births and deaths
- Injuries caused by violence, including child abuse
- Drug abuse
- Communicable diseases
- Sexually transmitted infections

As the relationship between patients and health care professionals grows more complex, the definition of *privileged* or *confidential* information may be called into question.

FIGURE 7.3
Communication between a patient and her caregiver is confidential

Source: AISPIX by Image Source/Shutterstock

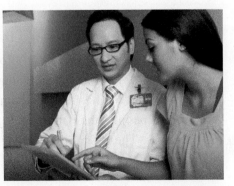

FIGURE 7.4
Reviewing the terms of a contract before signing
Source: Lucky Business/Shutterstock

Understanding Elements of a Contract

As an informed health care worker, it is important to understand the elements of a **contract**. Contracts are legal documents that are often used to define the terms of patient care. It is key to remember that these contracts are geared to the needs of the patient—he or she is the **principal** concern. Examples of contracts include the document patients sign declaring that they have been made aware of the terms of HIPAA regulation, as well as advance directive documents declaring their preferences in accepting or refusing medical care under certain circumstances.

Contracts are enforceable by law, and are composed of three main elements: offer, acceptance, and consideration. For a contract to be valid, one part must make an offer that the other party accepts. In many legal systems, consideration is also held to be a required component for a valid contract. Consideration means both parties bring something to the bargain specified in the agreement. Contracts can be either implied or expressed.

- **Implied contracts** occur when some of the terms of the agreement are not expressed in words. An example in health care is when a patient goes to a hospital for treatment and agrees that he will pay a fair price for the service. If he later refuses to pay for the treatment, he has breached the implied contract.
- **Expressed contracts** spell out the terms of the agreement in written form.

Contracts are typically made up of several parts, including **boilerplate language** and contract terms such as *provisions* or *warranties*, describing what is agreed to in the contract. Parties to a contract may only take legal action when the contract, or a part of it, is not fulfilled. Contracts are legally binding and breaching a contract can result in legal action, such as a lawsuit.

contract
(CON-trakt) A legally binding exchange of promises or an agreement between parties that the law will enforce

principal
(PRIN-se-pel) First, or among the first, in importance or rank

implied contracts
(im-PLIED CON-trakts) Contracts in which some terms are not specifically stated, but are understood by the parties based on the nature of the transaction

expressed contracts
(ik-SPRESS-ed CON-trakt s) Contracts in which terms are written out in the document

boilerplate language
(BOY-ler-playt LANG-gwidge) Standard language used repeatedly without change

Natural Death Guidelines and Declarations

For many years people were not allowed to make decisions about death with dignity. Today, new laws allow individuals to have a say in how they want to live their last days. Each state has adopted natural death guidelines and declarations that give direction to people about how to legally tell others their desire concerning end-of-life issues. These documents ensure the individual the right to accept or refuse medical care.

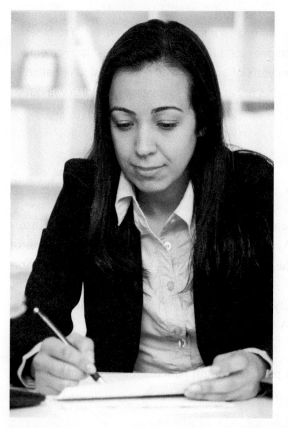

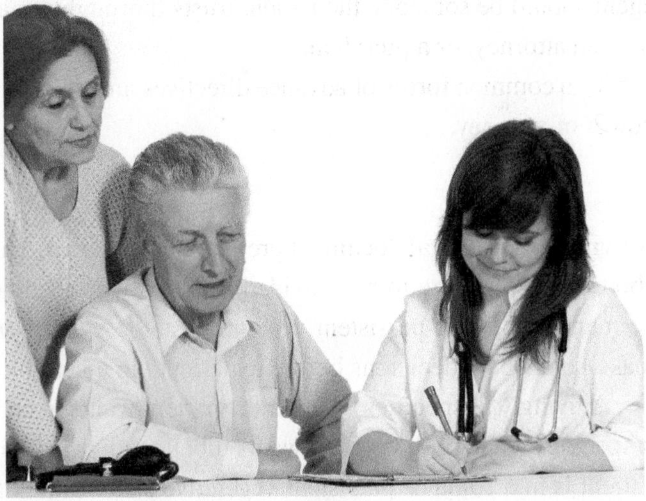

FIGURE 7.5

Discussing the terms of an advanced directive

Source: Aletia/Shutterstock

In the United States, every person is encouraged to prepare a document called an advance directive. Advance directives help ensure the person's right to accept or refuse medical care. Each state has slightly different laws that govern the interpretation of these documents. The advance directive is a written form providing a way for people to express how they want medical decisions made if they are unable to make decisions for themselves.

The advance directive contract is designed to help patients communicate their wishes about medical treatment at a time in which illness or injury might make them unable to make their wishes known. A formal contract will identify the **agent** (or health care surrogate) who makes the decisions once the patient cannot do so. Then, the contract will specify the directive, which states the patient's wishes in terms of a terminal illness or irreversible condition. There may be additional specific requests, such as whether or not the patient wishes to be kept on life support, fed through a tube, or treated with antibiotics. The contract is then signed, witnessed by two competent adults who cannot benefit from the patient's will, and **notarized**.

agent
(AY-jent) A person or business authorized to act on another's behalf

notarized
(NO-ta-rized) Certified as to the validity of a signature

The advance directive takes effect when the patient is no longer able to make personal decisions about medical treatment, or if they are legally disabled. A person is considered to be under a **legal disability** if they are a minor, mentally incompetent, under the influence of drugs or alcohol, semi-conscious, or unconscious.

legal disability
(LEE-gal dis-eh-BIH-le-tee) A person has a disability for legal purposes if he or she has a physical or mental impairment which has a substantial and long-term adverse effect on his or her ability to carry out normal day-to-day activities

As discussed previously, in the case of a minor, a legal mechanism exists that allows the minor to become *emancipated*. This means he or she is free from any authority from his or her parents or other legal guardians. In other words, the minor can make his or her own decisions. Minors can be emancipated in a variety of ways—through marriage, pregnancy, economic self sufficiency, educational degree/diploma, and military service, for example.

If a patient lacks decision-making capacity and/or is unable to communicate his or her wishes, decisions regarding the patient's health care will need to be made by someone else—his or her agent. The agent, appointed by the patient, will have the authority to see that the patient's wishes are enforced. Since this person will be acting on the patient's behalf if the patient is unconscious or unable to make health care decisions, the agent should be someone the patient trusts thoroughly—a spouse, an adult child, a relative, an attorney, or a guardian.

Two common forms of advance directives are a living will and a health care (durable) power of attorney.

Living Wills

A living will is a legal document prepared by a patient. This document gives instructions about the health care to be provided if the patient becomes terminally ill or falls into a permanent coma or persistent vegetative state. A living will is a way for the patient to make health care decisions before experiencing a health care emergency.

A living will specifies whether the patient wants to be kept on life-support machines. It specifies whether the patient wants tube feedings or artificial (IV) hydration when the patient is in a coma or persistent vegetative state. It may also contain other instructions related to health care. For example, the living will may contain a Do Not Resuscitate (DNR) order. This order instructs any health care worker not to use cardiopulmonary resuscitation (CPR) if the comatose or terminally ill patient experiences a life threatening event, such as a heart attack or stroke.

A living will should be on file with the patient's general health care provider. This information will be provided to any facility that is treating the patient. The physician providing treatment should add instructions from the living will to the patient's chart. Health care professionals must follow these instructions or risk legal action.

Health Care (Durable) Power of Attorney

Some patients may choose to legally appoint a health care power of attorney, or proxy. A health care proxy is a family member or close friend who is trusted to make health care decisions on behalf of the patient. A health care proxy may also be a doctor. However, a doctor who is a patient's proxy may not provide treatment and make health care decisions for the patient at the same time.

FIGURE 7.6

Deciding who to appoint as a health care proxy

Source: StockLite/Shutterstock

The health care proxy is asked to make decisions only when the patient can no longer think clearly or communicate. Therefore, it is important that the patient and health care proxy discuss potential medical situations and the patient's wishes for treatment before the patient becomes too ill. The patient may also choose to write down instructions for treatment in a living will. In the event that the patient needs life support, the health care proxy works with physicians and other health care workers to carry out the patient's wishes or living will instructions.

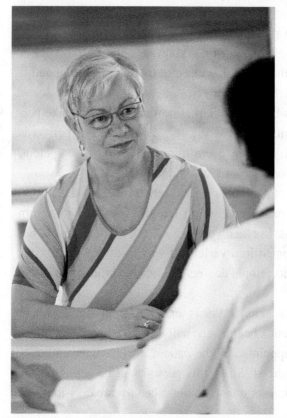

LIVING WILL DECLARATION

Declaration made this __________ day of ____________________, 20______ . I, ______________________________ being at least eighteen (18) years of age and of sound mind, willfully and voluntarily make known my desires that my dying shall not be artificially prolonged under the circumstances set forth below, and I declare:

If at any time my attending physician certifies in writing that: (1) I have an incurable injury, disease, or illness; (2) my death will occur within a short time; and (3) the use of life prolonging procedures would serve only to artificially prolong the dying process, I direct that such procedures be withheld or withdrawn, and that I be permitted to die naturally with only the performance or provision of any medical procedure or medication necessary to provide me with comfort care or to alleviate pain, and, if I have so indicated below, the provision of artificially supplied nutrition and hydration. (Indicate your choice by initialing or making your mark before signing this declaration):

_____ I wish to receive artificially supplied nutrition and hydration, even if the effort to sustain life is futile or excessively burdensome to me.

_____ I do not wish to receive artificially supplied nutrition and hydration, if the effort to sustain life is futile or excessively burdensome to me.

_____ I intentionally make no decision concerning artificially supplied nutrition and hydration, leaving the decision to my health care representative appointed under IC 16-36-1-7 or my attorney in fact with health care powers under IC 30-5-5.

In the absence of my ability to give directions regarding the use of life prolonging procedures, it is my intention that this declaration be honored by my family and physician as the final expression of my legal right to refuse medical or surgical treatment and accept the consequences of the refusal.

I understand the full import of this declaration.

I am a resident of

The declarant has been personally known to me, and I believe him or her to be of sound mind, I did not sign the declarant's signature above for or at the direction of the declarant. I am not a parent, spouse, or child of the declarant. I am not entitled to any part of the declarant's estate or directly financially responsible for the declarant's medical care. I am competent and at least eighteen (18) years of age.

______________________________ ______________________________
Witness Signature City and State of Residence

______________________________ Date ______________________
Printed Name

______________________________ ______________________________
Witness Signature City and State of Residence

______________________________ Date ______________________
Printed Name

FIGURE 7.7

Sample living will declaration

A health care proxy becomes the patient's legal representative when the patient can no longer make decisions. In this situation, physicians and other health care workers must follow the instructions provided by the health care proxy. Other family members and friends do not have the legal right to override the decisions of the proxy. If a patient recovers and is able to communicate, the patient then regains the right to make health

POWER OF ATTORNEY FOR HEALTH CARE

(1) **DESIGNATION OF AGENT:** I designate the following individual as my agent to make health care decisions for me: ______________________

(Name of individual you choose as agent)

(address) (city) (state) (zip code)

(home phone) (work phone)

OPTIONAL: If I revoke my agent's authority or if my agent is not willing, able, or reasonably available to make a health-care decision for me, I designate as my first alternate agent:

(Name of individual you choose as first alternate agent)

(address) (city) (state) (zip code)

(home phone) (work phone)

OPTIONAL: If I revoke the authority of my agent and first alternate agent or if neither is willing, able, or'reasonably available to make a health care decision for me, I designate as my second alternate agent:

(Name of individual you choose as second alternate agent)

(address) (city) (state) (zip code)

(home phone) (work phone)

(2) **AGENT'S AUTHORITY:** My agent is authorized to make all health care decisions for me, including decisions to provide, withhold, or withdraw artificial nutrition and hydration, and all other forms of health care to keep me alive, **except** as I state here:

(3) **WHEN AGENT'S AUTHORITY BECOMES EFFECTIVE:** My agent's authority becomes effective when my primary physician determines that I am unable to make my own health care decisions unless I mark the following box. If I mark this box [ ], my agent's authority to make health care decisions for me takes effect immediately.

(4) **AGENT'S OBLIGATION:** My agent shall make health care decisions for me in accordance with this power of attorney for health care, any instructions I give below, and my other wishes to the extent known to my agent. To the extent my wishes are unknown, my agent shall make health care decisions for me in accordance with what my agent determines to be in my best interest. In determining my best interest, my agent shall consider my personal values to the extent known to my agent.

(5) **AGENT'S POSTDEATH AUTHORITY:** My agent is authorized to make anatomical gifts, authorize an autopsy, and direct disposition of my remains, except as I state here or elsewhere in this form:

INSTRUCTIONS FOR HEALTH CARE
Strike any wording you do not want.

(6) **END-OF-LIFE DECISIONS:** I direct that my health care providers and others involved in my care provide, withhold, or withdraw treatment in accordance with the choice I have marked below: **(Initial only one box)**
[ ] (a) **Choice NOT To Prolong Life**
I do not want my life to be prolonged if (1) I have an incurable and irreversible condition that will result in my death within a relatively short time, (2) I become unconscious and, to a reasonable degree of medical certainty, I will not regain consciousness, or (3) the likely risks and burdens of treatment would outweigh the expected benefits, **OR**
[ ] (b) **Choice To Prolong Life**
I want my life to be prolonged as long as possible within the limits of generally accepted health care standards.

(7) **RELIEF FROM PAIN:** Except as I state in the following space, I direct that treatment for alleviation of pain or discomfort should be provided at all times even if it hastens my death:

DONATION OF ORGANS AT DEATH
(8) Upon my death: (mark applicable box)
[ ] (a) I give any needed organs, tissues, or parts,
OR
[ ] (b) I give the following organs, tissues, or parts only: ______________________
[ ] (c) My gift is for the following purposes:
(strike any of the following you do not want)
(1) Transplant
(2) Therapy
(3) Research
(4) Education

(9) **EFFECT OF COPY:** A copy of this form has the same effect as the original.

(10) **SIGNATURE:** Sign and date the form here:

(date)	(sign your name)
(address)	(print your name)
(city)	(state)

(11) **WITNESSES:** This advance health care directive will not be valid for making health care decisions unless it is either: (1) signed by two (2) qualified adult witnesses who are personally known to you and who are present when you sign or acknowledge your signature; or (2) acknowledged before a notary public.

FIGURE 7.8

Sample of power of attorney for health care

care decisions. Health care workers must respect decisions made by the patient. The health care proxy cannot override these decisions.

Patient Self-Determination Act

The Patient Self-Determination Act (PSDA) was passed by Congress in November 1990 as an amendment to the Omnibus Budget Reconciliation Act of 1990. The law requires that most health care institutions (not individual doctors) inform a patient, at the time of admission or enrollment, about their rights under state laws regarding advance directives including:

- The right to participate in and direct their own health care decisions.
- The right to accept or refuse medical or surgical treatment.
- The right to prepare an advance directive.
- Information on the provider's policies with respect to recognizing advance directives.
- Information regarding the prohibition of discrimination against a patient who does not have an advance directive.

It is important to remember that even without a written change, a patient's wishes stated directly to the doctor generally carry more weight than a living will, health care power of attorney, or durable power of attorney, as long as the patient can decide and communicate his or her wishes.

Life-Prolonging Procedures Declaration

Declaration made this ________________________ day of ____________ (month, year). I, ________________________, being at least eighteen (18) years of age and of sound mind, willfully and voluntarily make known my desire that if, at any time I have an incurable injury, disease or illness determined to be a terminal condition, I request the use of life-prolonging procedures that would extend my life. This includes appropriate nutrition and hydration, the administration of medication and the performance of all other medical procedures necessary to extend my life, to provide comfort care or to alleviate pain.

In the absence of my ability to give directions regarding the use of life-prolonging procedures, it is my intention that this declaration be honored by my family and physician as the final expression of my legal right to request medical or surgical treatment and accept the consequences of the request.

I understand the full import of this declaration.

Signed ________________________
City, Country, and State of Residence ________________________
____

The declarant has been personally known to me, and I believe (him/her) to be of sound mind. I am competent and at least eighteen (18) years of age.

Witness ________________________ Date ________
Witness ________________________ Date ________

FIGURE 7.9

Sample of life-prolonging procedures declaration

criminal law
(KRI-meh-nul LAW) The body of law that defines criminal offenses, deals with the apprehension, charging, and trial of suspected persons, and fixes penalties applicable to convicted offenders

civil law
(SI-vel LAW) The body of law governing certain relationships between people, such as marriage, contracts, and torts

torts
(TORTS) Under civil law, wrongs committed by one person against another

MEDICAL LIABILITY

Health care workers must perform to the best of their abilities or risk legal repercussions. These repercussions can fall under criminal or civil law. **Criminal law** is the type of law involved in punishing people for committing crimes against the state. Crimes against the state include many types of infractions of the law, such as stealing controlled substances from the hospital or stealing a patient's belongings. **Civil law**, on the other hand, covers **torts**—wrongful acts that result in physical injury, property damages, or damages to a person's reputation for which the injured person is entitled to compensation. Tort law usually provides people with rights to compensation for the damages done. Torts may be categorized in two ways: intentional torts and unintentional (negligent) torts.

Health care workers need to understand the law as it applies to clinical (medical) **negligence**.

Medical malpractice, one type of tort, can result from any mistake in medical treatment. An example of malpractice would be when a health care worker mislabels a tissue sample, and the patient has a mastectomy based on a misdiagnosis of breast cancer.

Language Arts Link Tort Law

A tort is a wrongful act that results in physical injury, property damage, or damage to a person's reputation. Tort law usually provides people with rights to compensation for the damages done. Torts may be categorized in two ways: intentional torts and unintentional torts. Intentional torts are wrongful acts committed on purpose. Unintentional torts are wrongful acts that result from negligence.

Using the Internet or a library, find one example of an intentional tort and one example of an unintentional tort that involve patient care. Write a report describing these two situations and what happened as a result. Create a new document on the computer, or use a blank sheet of paper. Include a title for your report and a thesis statement (a sentence stating your main ideas) in the opening paragraph. Check the spelling and grammar and correct any errors. Be sure to cite any sources that you use in the format required by your teacher. Exchange reports with a classmate. Provide feedback and corrections as necessary, and then exchange back. Read your classmate's comments and revise your report as necessary.

negligence
(NE-gli-jents) Failure to perform in a reasonably prudent manner

prudent
(PRUE-dent) Careful or cautious

Professional Standards of Care and Scope of Practice

A *professional standard of care* is established on the basis of the standard that would be used by a reasonably **prudent** professional in that line of work. Professional standards of care are specific to professions. For example, a medical assistant is not held to the same standard of care as a physician. Health care workers must always remember, however, that their actions have legal consequences. To that end, laws exist that authorize the scope of practice—or scope of care—under which health care workers operate, or function. For example, certain tasks are within the scope of practice for a registered nurse, such as administering medications, and certain tasks are *not* within the registered nurse's scope of practice, such as prescribing medications.

In any health care setting, a worker must limit the methods and procedures he or she uses to the appropriate legal scope of practice for his or her health occupation. A health care facility's policies and procedures manual provides further guidelines as

BUILD YOUR SKILLS *Using Policies and Procedures Manuals*

A policy is a principle, or rule, that guides decisions and actions in order to achieve as consistent an outcome as possible. A procedure is a series of steps also intended to achieve as consistent an outcome as possible, but for a specific task. A health care facility develops and enacts policies and procedures to ensure patient safety and to make sure the facility is in compliance with legal requirements. Federal and state laws regarding health care are continually updated and revised, so health care workers must stay up-to-date with legislation that affects their occupations.

Information about legislation that specifically applies to health care facilities is presented in *policies and procedures manuals*. Policies and procedures manuals also provide guidance and information for workers. This includes descriptions of how to carry out all tasks, so workers have information to do their jobs properly.

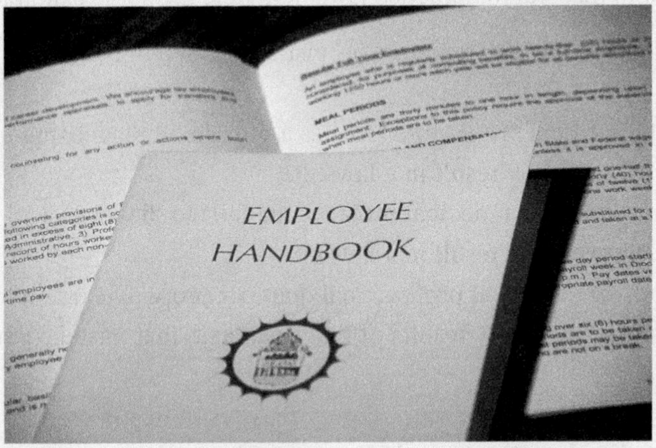

FIGURE 7.10

Employee handbooks and policies and procedures manuals provide detailed information to ensure employee compliance with rules and regulations

Source: Tony Freeman/ PhotoEdit

To fulfill your legal responsibilities, you should be familiar with the content of your facility's policies and procedures manual and know how to find information quickly when you need it. Pay attention to e-mails, memos, and other correspondence about updates and changes. If you violate a policy, claiming that you weren't aware of it is not an acceptable excuse.

to the authority and responsibilities of each type of health care worker employed in that facility.

Emergency Care

In emergency situations, medical professionals have legal responsibilities. The first responsibility of a medical worker is a duty to act within the scope of care for his or her profession. In an emergency, health care workers are accountable to themselves, their employers, and the public for actions that are in keeping with their medical training. The second responsibility is to stay constantly ready for emergencies by understanding policies of the place of employment, and staying current with procedures and equipment. A responsibility shared by everyone who works in a health care setting is to do all that is possible to prevent emergencies.

Understanding Medical Liabilities

Health care workers are obliged to do everything they can to offer high-quality care to their patients and take steps to reduce errors. If a health care worker does anything less than provide the best quality care, that professional may have committed medical malpractice. Malpractice means *bad practice*—care that leads to faulty practice or neglect. Malpractice is a commonly heard term, but actually refers to one type of unintentional tort. For example, suppose a patient falls on a nail, and the doctor does not order a tetanus shot or check to see when the patient last had one. The patient then develops tetanus or lockjaw. The failure to order a tetanus shot, or to check when the patient last had one, would be considered malpractice. The doctor could be held legally responsible, or **liable**, for his or her actions.

liable
(LIE-eh-bel) Legally responsible

Although these are medical issues, medical malpractice is a legal term. The legal system examines the facts of each case and determines whether or not the health care professional is guilty of malpractice. The specific facts are very important. Two very similar cases can be decided differently because of one small, but significant, difference.

What kinds of errors lead to medical malpractice lawsuits? Here are some examples:

- ***Medical errors and mistakes***. Any serious error or mistake by a caregiver may result in a lawsuit.
- ***Inaccurate diagnosis***. If a medical professional makes a mistake in diagnosing a patient's condition, that mistake may result in a lawsuit.
- ***Failure to diagnose a condition***. If a medical professional fails to diagnose a patient's condition, that mistake may result in a lawsuit.
- ***Lack of informed consent***. If a medical professional does not properly explain to a patient his or her treatment or the likely results of that treatment, that mistake may result in a lawsuit.
- ***Mistakes during surgery***. Any mistake during surgery may result in a lawsuit.
- ***Medical instruments left inside patients during surgery***. If any instruments or equipment used in surgery remain inside a patient after the surgery is completed, that mistake may result in a lawsuit.

Just because a mistake was made and a lawsuit was filed, the professional who made the mistake has not necessarily committed medical malpractice. All the facts are presented to the legal system, and the decision is made there. Avoiding these mistakes in the first place, of course, ensures good care and helps avoid legal problems.

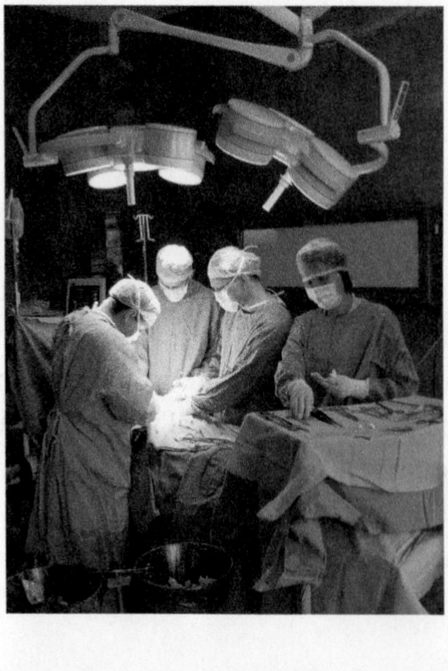

FIGURE 7.11
Leaving an instrument or a sponge in a patient after surgery may result in a lawsuit
Source: Brasiliao/Shutterstock

Other Legal Issues

Medical malpractice is just one of many legal problems that health care workers may face. Health care workers need to be aware of the whole range of possible medical-legal problems that can affect them. Read the following terms. They explain some of the other ways in which a health care worker can have a legal problem under criminal or civil law.

RECENT DEVELOPMENTS

Medical Lawsuits and Malpractice Insurance Rates

According to a recent survey by the American Medical Association (AMA), more than 60% of doctors age fifty-five or older have been sued at least once, and most physicians will be sued for malpractice at least one time during their careers. About five percent of all doctors are sued each year, with 65% of the lawsuits dropped, dismissed, or found in favor of the physician. Consider the following:

- Surgeons and OB/GYN doctors get sued five times more often than pediatricians and psychiatrists. Ninety percent of all surgeons age fifty-five and older have been sued at least once.
- Male doctors are twice as likely to be sued as female doctors. This is due in part because male doctors tend to specialize in areas with higher lawsuit rates, plus most male doctors have been in practice longer than most females.
- Doctors who own their practices are sued more often than those who work for hospitals or multi-specialty physician groups. OB/GYN doctors are the exception because they're usually sued for childbirth—a procedure which occurs in hospitals.
- Rates for medical malpractice insurance vary greatly from state to state. In California, for example, general surgeons pay $20,000 to $32,000 per year, while coverage in Minnesota costs $10,000 per year.
- OB/GYN doctors pay the highest rates, ranging from $85,000 to as much as $200,000 per year for medical malpractice insurance. Malpractice insurance for internal medicine doctors costs about $20,000 per year.

When states pass laws to increase the caps on medical liability, doctors are charged less for medical malpractice insurance. Before Florida enacted its new limits, OB/GYN doctors were paying more than $200,000 per year for insurance. California's liability cap reduced the price of malpractice insurance to an average of $57,000. Because of these differences, doctors are relocating from states with higher premiums to states with lower premiums. This represents good news for the doctors, but bad news for states that might possibly be left with a shortage of physicians.

Criminal Law Terms:

- ***Assault*** is a threat or an attempt to injure another person. *Example*: A health care worker threatens to hit a patient or coworker.
- ***Battery*** is the unlawful touching of another person without his or her consent, with or without an injury. Assault and battery are often charged together because of the successful attempt to injure. Both assault and battery are violations of criminal law, but they may also be subject to a civil lawsuit filed by a patient to recoup damages. *Example*: A health care worker hits a patient or coworker, or a doctor operates on a patient without obtaining a signed consent form.
- ***Felony*** is a serious criminal offense that carries a penalty of imprisonment for more than one year and possibly the death penalty. *Example*: A health care worker

withholds treatment for a terminally ill patient, which causes the patient's premature death.

- ***Harassment*** is any verbal or physical abuse of a person because of race, religion, age, gender, or disability. Any conduct that creates significant anguish for another person is harassment. Both state and federal criminal laws apply to harassment, but a civil lawsuit for harassment may also be filed. *Example:* A health care worker makes a joke about the religion of a patient.

Civil Law Terms:

defamatory (de-feh-MAH-toor-ee) Statement that causes injury to another person's reputation

misrepresentations (mis-reh-prih-zen-TAY-shenz) Untruths, lies

obligation (AH-bleh-GAY-shen) Moral responsibility

- ***Libel*** is writing untrue matter that is **defamatory** about an individual or group to a third party. Libel is a violation that pertains to civil law. *Example*: A newspaper writes damaging information about a local health care institution. The information is false. The paper is charged with libel. What you write in a patient record could be libel if you make a statement such as, "Mr. M. is hoarding painkillers," when—in reality—Mr. M. is only requesting, and taking, the medication that has been prescribed.
- ***Slander*** is a spoken statement of false charges or **misrepresentations** that defame or damage another's reputation. Slander is also a violation pertaining to civil law. *Example*: A health care worker tells friends that a famous person was treated for a drug overdose when in fact he or she was treated for a serious medical problem.
- ***False imprisonment*** is a civil tort in which a person is held or retained against his or her will. *Example*: A physician or a health care worker refuses to allow a patient to leave the hospital.
- ***Invasion of privacy*** is a civil tort that unlawfully makes public knowledge of any private or personal information without the consent of the wronged person. *Example*: A health care worker gives personal information to a newspaper about a patient or coworker, or a health care worker leaves the door open while bathing a patient.
- ***Reportable conditions***, such as *abuse.* Abuse falls under the heading of intentional torts. There are three types of abuse: physical, verbal, and sexual. The health care worker is obligated to file a confidential report to the county health department when child or adult abuse is suspected. Reports are also required when certain diseases are diagnosed. It is important to check your facility's policies and procedures manual for a current listing of reportable diseases and the procedure for reporting abuse. *Example*: A child is at the doctor for a checkup, and the doctor sees bruises and burns and suspects child abuse. Or, a health care worker intentionally pinches an elderly person in a nursing home.
- ***Negligence*** is the failure to perform in a reasonably prudent manner. The legal definition of negligence can offer more clarification of this unintentional tort: Negligence occurs when a person "does not do what a reasonable and careful person would do, or does what a reasonable and careful person would not do." *Example*: A health care worker forgets to lock the brakes on a wheelchair, and the patient is injured.
- ***Reasonable care*** is the legal **obligation** of health care workers. They must perform according to the standards of practice expected in their community for comparable workers. *Example*: Drawing blood takes training and skill. If a laboratory aide draws blood from a patient after watching the procedure several times but without proper training in the procedure, then reasonable care was not exercised.

- *Sexual harassment* is defined by federal regulations as "unwelcome sexual advances, requests for sexual favors, and other verbal and physical contact of a sexual nature." Innocent remarks, inappropriate pictures, and written material can be perceived as sexual. You can guard against harassment accusations by not making personal remarks or sexual gestures and by not participating in sexually explicit discussions around coworkers. *Example:* A coworker gets really close and frequently touches another person when talking. The closeness and physical touch could be interpreted as sexual harassment, even if it is innocent.

These definitions and examples provide the knowledge you need to avoid medical-legal problems.

REALITY CHECK

When you violate a policy, regulation, or law, you put yourself and your employer in legal jeopardy. Health care employers have enormous expenses to cover, and they react very quickly when the illegal behavior of an employee results in extra legal fees, fines, or penalties. You can be one of the best-educated, most highly-skilled professionals in your organization, but if you fail to meet your legal responsibilities, you won't have a job for long.

Violating patient confidentiality, divulging private business information, or slandering a physician or coworker is a sure way to get fired. Stealing from a patient, assaulting a coworker, and performing a procedure outside your scope of practice are examples of **gross misconduct** typically leading to immediate termination. Your employer may be sued and banned from participating in certain programs, and you may end up in jail.

Then there are the patients, the people who put their trust in you and your facility during some of the most vulnerable times in their lives. They're counting on their caregivers to put the needs of their patients first. The last thing a patient needs is a health care worker who makes mistakes and errors, abuses other people, or fails to live up to their legal obligations.

Policies, regulations, and laws are put into place to protect patients, employees, and health care employers. Every health care worker, regardless of job title or specific occupation, has the responsibility to comply with these rules.

gross misconduct (GROSE mis-KAHN-dekt) Unacceptable behavior of a serious nature, often leading to job dismissal

Key Points

- Health care policies and procedures help facilitate effective collaboration between patients and their caregivers.
- Health care providers must respect the patient's role in making decisions about his or her medical care.
- Hospitals must be sensitive to each patient's individual needs.
- The American Hospital Association adopted the first "A Patient's Bill of Rights" in 1973 and later updated the document in 1992. The document was replaced by "Patient Care Partnership" in 2003.

- Patient rights support effective patient care on behalf of the facility and its medical staff, employees, and patients.
- The patient must also fulfill certain responsibilities as an active participant in his or her care.
- The Omnibus Budget Reconciliation Act, passed in 1987, implements patient rights and guidelines for nursing homes.
- Policies, offices, and agencies ensure that workers practice and monitor legal behavior.
- Ombudsmen make certain that patients are not abused and their rights are secure.
- The licensure, certification, and registration of health care workers determine their scope of practice and help ensure quality health care.
- Patient information and patient communications must be kept confidential.
- The Health Information Portability and Accountability Act (HIPAA), signed into law in 1996 and strengthened in 2003, creates national standards for medical privacy and increases patients' control over their personal health information.
- The Health Information Technology for Economic and Clinical Health (HITECH) Act, signed into law in 2009, addresses the confidentiality of health information transmitted electronically and strengthens HIPAA rules.
- Contracts, implied and expressed, are legal documents often used to define the terms of patient care.
- Natural death guidelines and declarations state the patient's desires concerning end-of-life issues, and give patients the right to accept or refuse medical care.
- A living will helps patients make health care decisions before health care emergencies occur.
- A health care surrogate, agent, or proxy who has been identified by the patient can make care decisions when the patient is unable to do so for himself or herself.
- Health care workers must comply with all criminal and civil laws or face serious repercussions.
- Torts are wrongful acts that result in physical injury, property damages, or damages to a person's reputation for which the injured person is entitled to compensation.
- Medical malpractice, one type of tort, can result from negligence and any mistake in medical treatment.
- Health care workers must function within the *standard of care* and *scope of practice* established for their profession.
- Several types of errors can lead to charges of medical malpractice and lawsuits.

Section Review Questions

Answer each of the following questions. Indicate which page in the textbook led you to your answer.

1. Discuss the purpose of the AHA's "A Patient's Bill of Rights" and "Patient Care Partnership."
2. List three patient rights and three patient responsibilities.
3. Explain two things that might happen if health care workers don't fulfill their legal responsibilities.

4. Describe the purpose of licensure, certification, and registration.
5. Explain the purposes of HIPAA and the HITECH Act.
6. Identify the difference between civil law and criminal law.
7. List six common categories of medical malpractice.

Learn By Doing

Complete Worksheets 1–5 in Section 7.1 of your *Student Activity Guide*.

Ethical Responsibilities

SECTION 7.2

Background

Medical ethics has a long history dating back to guidelines for the practice of early physicians such as the Hippocratic Oath, widely believed to have been written by Hippocrates in the 4th century B.C. One of the earliest principles to come from this oath is to "First, do no harm." Western medical ethics has evolved to include values derived from the Muslim, Jewish, and Christian religions, including noted thinkers such as al-Razi, Maimonides, and Thomas Aquinas. In recent times, professional codes of medical ethics have incorporated legal principles to spell out more formally what conduct is expected of health care workers.

Members of the health care team must be aware of their ethical roles and responsibilities. This awareness protects them, the patients, their coworkers, and the facility where they work. Ethical issues differ from legal issues in health care settings. Legal issues protect patients and workers because they are based on laws, which, if not obeyed, will result in legal consequences. Ethical behavior is not based on laws, but ensures quality patient care, positive work relationships, and a well-managed workplace environment. One of a health care worker's main responsibilities is to recognize and report unsafe, illegal, or unethical behaviors occurring in their work environment.

Objectives

After completing this section, you will be able to:

1. Define the key terms.
2. Explain the difference between unethical and illegal behavior.
3. Identify two factors that influence a person's perspective on right versus wrong.
4. Summarize the code of ethics that every health care worker must follow.
5. List three questions to answer when making ethical decisions.
6. Explain the importance of reporting illegal and unethical conduct.
7. Give two examples of reportable incidences.
8. Identify three resources to help you report illegal or unethical behavior.
9. Identify four examples of complex, controversial bioethical issues.

VALUES AND ETHICAL CONDUCT

Recognition as a health care professional requires meeting your ethical responsibilities as well as your legal responsibilities. Ethics is a system of moral principles—the standard of *right* versus *wrong*. Knowing how to comply with laws is fairly straightforward. Laws appear in writing and, if you violate a law, you know what the penalties could involve. Living up to ethical responsibilities, on the other hand, is more challenging. Standards of moral **conduct** are subject to interpretation, and not everyone is held to the same penalties for unethical behavior.

conduct
(KAHN-dukt) Standard of behavior

A person's perspective on right versus wrong is influenced by his or her family, friends, teachers, coworkers, religion, and society in general. If you associate with people who lie and cheat, at some point you may decide there's nothing wrong with lying and cheating. If your supervisor gets personal gifts from a vendor in exchange for giving the vendor your organization's business, you may decide the practice is acceptable. If your mother uses someone else's membership card to qualify for a discount, you may think it is okay to be dishonest.

People are subjected to many different influences every day, from television and magazine advertisements, to political and religious perspectives. All of these messages can influence your morals and your sense of right and wrong. But when it comes down to behavior, ethical conduct is up to the individual. This is where professionalism plays such an important role.

Health care professionals meet high standards for ethical conduct. They reveal their character traits in everything that they say and do. They show their commitment to serving others by living certain values. These core values include:

- ***Dignity.*** You treat people with dignity when you are honest, truthful, trustworthy, sincere, and respectful of others. Always do what is needed to the best of your abilities and ask for assistance when tasks are beyond your understanding or ability. Dignity is communicated through listening actively, being positive, showing understanding, and being respectful of all people.
- ***Service.*** Service means responding to patients and coworkers with an understanding of their unique needs. You show kindness and patience, and make comments that are positive, courteous, and helpful.
- ***Excellence.*** Performance excellence is taking responsibility for yourself, your team's decisions, and the results. You adapt to changing needs by learning new skills, knowledge, and behaviors that encourage continuous improvement. Accepting and seeking feedback help you improve your performance excellence.
- ***Fairness and Justice.*** You treat all people with mutual respect and provide the same dignity, service, and performance excellence regardless of the patient's race, beliefs, ethnic background, or financial resources. You also use supplies and available resources effectively to provide **appropriate** care and a safe environment for everyone.

appropriate
(ah-PRO-pree-at) Suitable, correct

code of ethics
(CODE of EH-thiks) Principles of conduct for decision making and behavior

Each health care professional association has a written **code of ethics** for its members. These statements outline the *principles of conduct* for decision making and behavior which are considered ethical by the profession. Let's take a look at how to apply core values and codes of ethics in patient care.

APPLY IT PROFESSIONAL CODES OF ETHICS

Research various codes of ethics from different health care professions. Choose two ethical codes and compare them, citing differences and similarities. Identify any legal principles addressed by the codes. Prepare a brief speech for the class, explaining what you agree with in each code, and why.

Dignity

- ***Know your limitations.*** Know what you are trained to do and what you are capable of doing.
- ***Be sincere.*** Always be honest and trustworthy in the performance of your duties. Earn your pay. Do not solicit gifts or additional money.
- ***Be well groomed.*** Always clean your uniform, shoes, hair, nails, skin, teeth, and body to prevent the spread of disease-causing bacteria. Be sure your uniform is free of wrinkles, tears, and stains. All buttons must match. Shoes and laces must be clean and bright. Wear a name tag. This helps people you work with know you and your title. It is required in most states. Do not wear excessive jewelry. It harbors bacteria and can cause you or your patients injury. Wedding rings and watches are acceptable. Never wear perfume or aftershave lotion to work. They make some people who are ill feel even worse and may trigger an allergic reaction.
- ***Communicate effectively.*** Express ideas, information, and viewpoints clearly. Use active listening skills and seek to understand others. Create and maintain positive working relationships. Understand and respect differences in people. Be supportive of others' success when they do well.

Service

- ***Be a good citizen.*** Demonstrate concern and respond to the needs of others.
- ***Be caring.*** Try to understand the unique needs of others. Respond quickly and effectively to problems that arise while you are working.
- ***Have a good attitude.*** Be willing to help your coworkers. Be aware of your body language and facial expressions, and reflect a positive outlook. Be respectful by changing your behavior when it appears to irritate others. Work effectively under pressure.

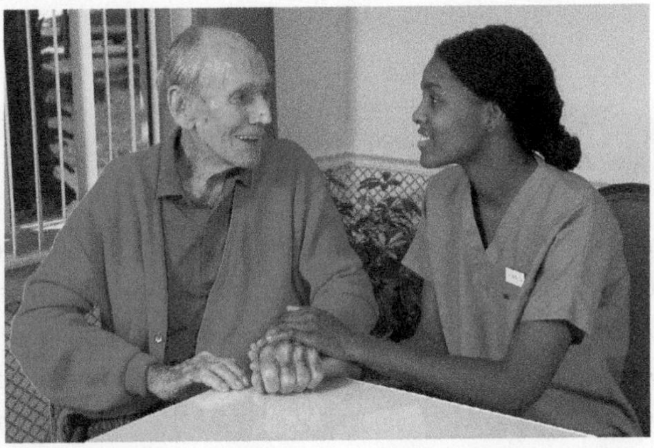

FIGURE 7.12

Demonstrating core values conveys kindness and respect

Source: Michal Heron/Pearson Education

APPLY IT PERSONAL AND PROFESSIONAL ETHICS

You are conducting an orientation session for new employees at your hospital. Your topic includes the core values that support ethical standards of behavior. In your presentation, explain each of the four core values. Give examples to illustrate how these values should be applied in caring for patients. Be clear about your organization's expectations for ethical conduct. Create this speech and present it to your class. Afterwards, answer questions from the audience.

Excellence

- ***Be accountable.*** Seek out and use feedback from others to learn how to improve. Take responsibility for yourself and for your team's actions, decisions, and results.
- ***Be informed.*** Learn from your experiences. Seek growth and development opportunities for yourself and others.
- ***Follow the rules and regulations.*** Read the policies and procedures manual. Ask for clarity if you aren't sure how these rules apply to you.
- ***Be dependable.*** Be on time. Report in when you arrive. Report to the person taking care of your assignment prior to leaving your area. Do your job to the best of your ability. Call your supervisor ahead of time on those few occasions when you are unable to be at work.

Fairness and Justice

project
(PRA-jekt) To show or reflect

- ***Be loyal.*** This applies to patients, coworkers, and your employer. Always **project** a positive attitude toward the institution where you are employed.
- ***Respect the privacy of others.*** Always keep privileged information about any personal or private matter confidential.
- ***Be honest.*** Never clock in or out for another person. Never take anything from the facility that is not yours. Never say that you have completed a task when you have not. Work with commitment and enthusiasm to improve the care that patients receive.

Language Arts Link Ethical and Professional Standards

Health care workers must comply with professional standards and codes of ethics that describe how to apply core values when caring for patients. These core values include dignity, service, excellence, and fairness/justice.

Create a scenario where a health care worker applies all four core values in caring for one patient. Then create a second scenario where a health care worker fails to apply any of these values in caring for one patient.

Create a document that describes your two scenarios. Discuss how the patient might be affected, and what he or she might do as a result. Proofread your work to see if you can improve it by making it more clear, concise, or interesting to read. Check the spelling and grammar and correct any errors. Exchange your document with another student. Provide feedback and then exchange back. Read your classmates' comments and revise your document as necessary.

ETHICS IN DECISION MAKING

During a typical day, health care workers must make many different kinds of decisions. Some decisions are easy ones—when to take a break, which procedure comes next, and so forth. But some decisions require more thought—which patient should I care for first, should the patient be charged for this expense, and so forth. This is where ethics enter the picture.

Ask yourself the following three questions when making ethical decisions:

1. ***Is it legal?*** When facing an ethical issue, if what you decide to do is illegal, then it's also unethical.
2. ***Is it fair?*** Ethical standards require that you treat everyone fairly. This doesn't mean that you must give everyone the same treatment, or that other people will be pleased with the decision that you make. But your decision should be made in an impartial and unbiased manner.

   A behavior that is legal may still be unethical. Here's an example. A cashier at a local store mistakenly gives you $20 back in change when he should have given you just $10. Keeping the extra $10 would not be illegal, but it would be unethical.
3. ***What would my conscience say?*** This is where your core values and character traits enter the picture. When most people behave inappropriately, they know it. They regret their behavior and feel badly about it, especially if someone else was harmed. Their conscience reminds them of the difference between right and wrong and helps guides them in the right direction. But when people have no conscience, or have learned to ignore their conscience, they may think that their behavior is acceptable when, in reality, it's not.

impartial
(im-PAR-shel) Not favoring one side or opinion over another

unbiased
(un-BIE-est) Free from prejudice and favoritism

A behavior can be legal and fair, but still unethical. Consider this example. You signed up a month ago to have next Monday off to spend the day relaxing. But a special session was just scheduled on Monday to train people to use some new technology. You are one of just five people in your department who will operate the new equipment. The session can only be offered once because an expert is coming in from another state to demonstrate the safe and proper use of the equipment. All four of your coworkers plan to attend.

Now you have some options to consider and a decision to make. When you return to work on Tuesday, you could ask a coworker to teach you what she had learned the day before. However, you know you would feel more competent and confident if you received training from the expert instead of by someone who just completed the training herself. It would be fair for you to go ahead and take the day off. You are eligible for the time off; you followed your employer's policy in requesting it, and you gave your supervisor plenty of advance notice.

Yet missing an important training session to spend the day relaxing just doesn't feel right to you. Expecting your coworker to teach you something that she just learned herself would put her under a lot of pressure.

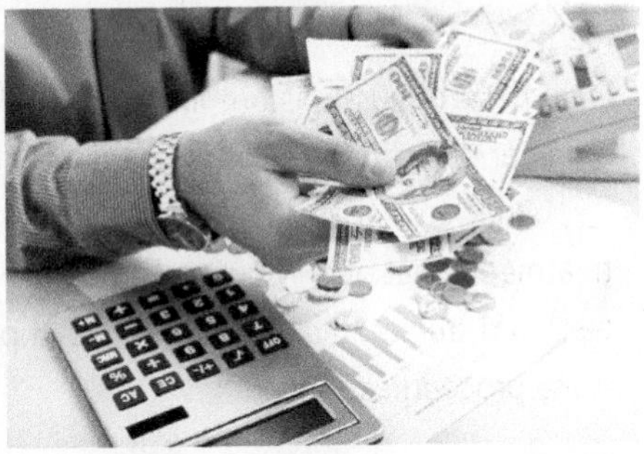

FIGURE 7.13
Ethical decision making requires honesty in fulfilling the standards of professional conduct

Source: docent/Shutterstock

You don't want to run the risk of damaging the equipment or hurting a patient because you don't have the skills you need to safely operate the equipment. Your supervisor says she regrets having to schedule the session on a day that you are planning to be off, but it's the only day that the expert is available to do the training. You know your supervisor would really appreciate it if you would change your plans and be there for the session.

Some people would say, "This isn't my problem. I've got the day off, and I'm taking it." A health care professional would say, "I need to be there. My supervisor, coworkers, and patients are counting on me to learn how to operate this equipment safely and properly. I'll change my plans and take a different day off. Besides, could I really relax and enjoy the day knowing what I was missing at work?"

This example not only points out the best ethical decision, but also illustrates several other core values and character traits. When you work in health care, you have to put the needs of other people ahead of your own. That's what professionals do.

BUILD YOUR SKILLS *Is This Procedure Really Necessary?*

Several groups of physicians are recommending ways to reduce wasteful spending without harming patients. This involves curtailing the use of certain medical tests and treatments that the physicians believe are overused, don't benefit patients, and are ordered largely to prevent possible lawsuits. If adopted, this approach would also help protect patients since some of the medical procedures involve risks and exposure to radiation. According to the doctors, reducing unnecessary expense would make more resources available for procedures that truly benefit patients. This movement aligns with current efforts to reform the health care industry and health insurance in order to cover more patients and provide better care. Instead of rewarding doctors for the volume of services they provide, the plan is to base payments on positive results and more highly coordinated care.

The doctors recommend no longer automatically ordering the following procedures:

- Repeat colonoscopies within ten years of the first test
- Early imaging for most back pain
- Brain scans for patients who fainted but didn't have seizures
- Cardiac stress tests for patients without coronary symptoms

They also suggest that cancer doctors stop treating tumors in end-stage patients who have not responded to multiple therapies and who are not eligible for experimental treatments.

These discussions are likely to continue as stakeholders search for ways to provide more, and better, care at an affordable cost.

What ethical and legal issues might arise if some doctors continue to order tests and treatments that other doctors believe are wasteful and unnecessary? Should doctors order tests and treatments primarily to avoid potential lawsuits? Should health insurance cover these procedures?

RECOGNIZING AND REPORTING ILLEGAL AND UNETHICAL BEHAVIOR

Health care workers are responsible for helping to protect everyone in the work environment. If you suspect that you or another employee has been responsible for an illegal behavior or unethical conduct, you must report that incident. How can you recognize reportable incidents? A **reportable incident** is any event that can have an **adverse** effect on the health, safety, or welfare of patients, coworkers, or other people in the facility.

reportable incident
(ri-PORT-abul in-SIH-dent) Any event that can have an adverse effect on the health, safety, or welfare of people in the facility

adverse
(ad-VERS) To oppose

harass
(heh-RAS) To behave in an offensively annoying or manipulative way

Someone's behavior can negatively affect people in countless ways. Here are a few examples:

- A nurse might administer the wrong medicine.
- A housekeeper might unplug important equipment.
- A doctor might **harass** another employee.
- A manager might misuse hospital funds.
- An employee might disclose a patient's condition to a reporter.

No set list of reportable behaviors exists. Rather, it is required and expected that every employee will:

- Obey the laws of the city, state, and federal government.
- Fulfill his or her job requirements to the best of his or her ability, including following a code of ethics and respecting others.
- Treat everyone in the environment with care, dignity, and respect.

If you or anyone fails to fulfill these obligations, that behavior must be reported. Reporting an illegal or unethical incident helps ensure the health, safety, and welfare of everyone in the hospital environment.

APPLY IT REPORTABLE ACTIVITY

Engage in a role playing activity. You will be an emergency room health care employee who has witnessed what you consider to be a reportable activity. Another student should act as your supervisor. Report the incident to your supervisor. Does he or she agree with your concerns? If not, what should you do? Once this situation is resolved, switch roles with your classmate.

To accuse someone of unethical or illegal behavior, you need to have facts and evidence. Write down important details such as when and where the incident occurred, who was involved, and what happened. If other people witnessed the incident or have facts to share, record their names, job titles, and contact information. Make copies of any related documents, e-mail messages, correspondence, or other pertinent information. If you suspect that an incident might be illegal or unethical but you aren't certain, go ahead and report it. The person who is responsible for following-up on incident reports will investigate the situation and decide if further investigation is warranted.

Follow your employer's policy regarding how to report illegal and unethical incidents. If the situation involves serious and extreme illegal behavior, you have a duty to report it to your local law enforcement agency. Examples include suspected child abuse and the abduction of a baby from the nursery.

Here are some resources to help you report unethical or illegal behavior:

- Your employee handbook should explain clearly how you should report illegal and unethical conduct.
- Your supervisor should be able to help you report illegal and unethical behavior in most cases.
- A confidential **hotline** may be available for reporting the incident in an **anonymous** manner.
- Your human resources department, a legal services representative, or your facility's security officer serves as a resource if you have any doubt about how to report an incident. They will either help you report it, or direct you to those who can.

hotline
(HOT-line) Direct and immediate telephone assistance

anonymous
(eh-NAH-ne-mus) Not named or identified

Keep in mind that both illegal and unethical behaviors have consequences. Both illegal and unethical behaviors may result in an employee being put on probation or fired. Illegal behavior can result in a criminal charge or a civil lawsuit. In some cases, an employee who has exhibited unethical behavior will be required to undergo training to better understand, and meet, his or her employer's expectations for ethical behavior.

In rare cases, the organization which employs you may be guilty of illegal or unethical business practices. If you suspect Medicare or Medicaid fraud or abuse, you can contact the Office of the Inspector General (OIG) of the U.S. Department of Health and Human Services (HHS) at www.StopMedicareFraud.gov or 1-800-447-8477. The OIG provides a hotline and investigates concerns about fraud, waste, abuse, and mismanagement by conducting audits, investigations, and evaluations.

Consider This *Reporting Illegal Behavior*

If you know someone is engaged in illegal behavior, it's your responsibility to report it. If you don't, you could get in trouble as well. In fact, even if you didn't know the illegal behavior was occurring, but you should have known, you can be liable for legal action.

For example, if you observe someone stealing from a patient, report it immediately. If you don't report it and your supervisor finds out that you knew what was going on, you could be disciplined as well as the thief. If your job involves maintaining an inventory of supplies and a coworker gets fired for stealing some of them, you could get in trouble for not noticing the items were missing.

Although you might be tempted to say, "It's none of my business," reporting the illegal behavior of a coworker actually *is* your business.

ETHICAL, MORAL, AND LEGAL ISSUES

People who work in the health care industry, as well as other stakeholders, face a multitude of complex ethical, moral, and legal issues that stretch well beyond how just one person thinks or behaves. Ethical decisions that pertain to *life issues* are called **bioethics**. Hospitals usually have an ethics committee to help patients and workers make ethical decisions about patient care.

bioethics
(BI-oh-eth-iks) Ethical decisions that are related to life issues

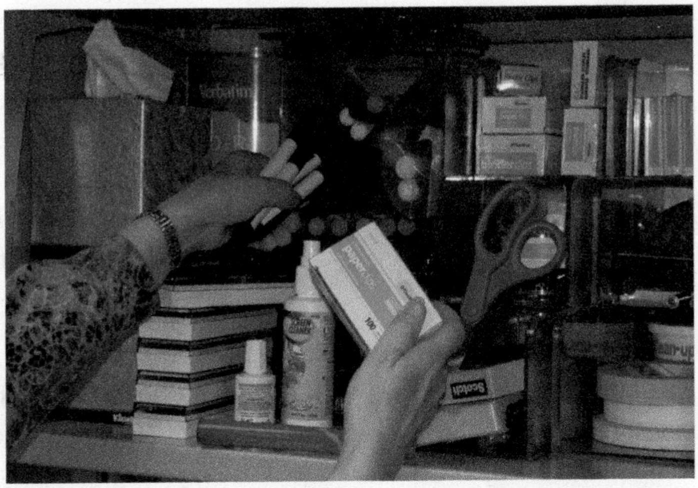

FIGURE 7.14

Taking office supplies from work for personal use at home is unethical and illegal

Source: Carmen Martin/Pearson Education

Physicians and scientists who are involved in medical research also deal with complex ethical issues. Years ago, patients were used for research studies without their knowledge or permission. Today, Institutional Review Boards (IRBs) composed of doctors, scientists, clergy, and consumers meet regularly to oversee clinical trials. IRBs establish policies and procedures to protect participants from unnecessary risks. They review details of the research plan to make sure the study is well defined and carried out in a way that safeguards patients to the extent possible.

clinical trials
(KLI-ni-kel TRY-als) Research to evaluate the effectiveness and safety of a medical procedure, device, or drug

Bioethical issues can be highly controversial. Depending on the occupation you choose, you may become directly involved in some of these issues yourself. Here are some examples:

- ***Abortion.*** Should abortion remain legal? Should an abortion to save the mother's life or in cases of rape be legal? Should late-term abortions be legal? Should tax dollars be used to pay for abortions?
- ***Genetic testing.*** Should insurance companies be permitted to cancel a patient's coverage based on the results of genetic testing? When prenatal genetic testing uncovers serious medical problems, is aborting the fetus acceptable?
- ***Embryonic stem cell research.*** Should embryonic stem cells be used for medical research when considering that the embryos must be destroyed as part of the process?
- ***Rationing.*** Should health care be rationed to reduce costs and reserve limited resources for those patients who would benefit from them the most?
- ***Cloning.*** Should scientists be permitted to clone human beings to produce organs for use in transplants and other medical procedures?
- ***Medical marijuana.*** Should patients who could benefit from using marijuana to reduce pain and increase appetite be permitted to buy and possess the drug even though federal laws, and some state laws, make medical marijuana illegal?
- ***End-of-life care.*** Should life-sustaining treatments such as feeding tubes or ventilators be withdrawn to facilitate the death of terminally ill patients?
- ***Euthanasia.*** Is assisting someone with suicide justifiable, and if so, under what conditions?

embryos
(EM-bree-oh) Living human beings during the first eight weeks of development in the uterus

rationed
(RA-shend) A fixed portion or amount

clone
(CLONE) A group of cells that is genetically identical to the unit from which it was derived

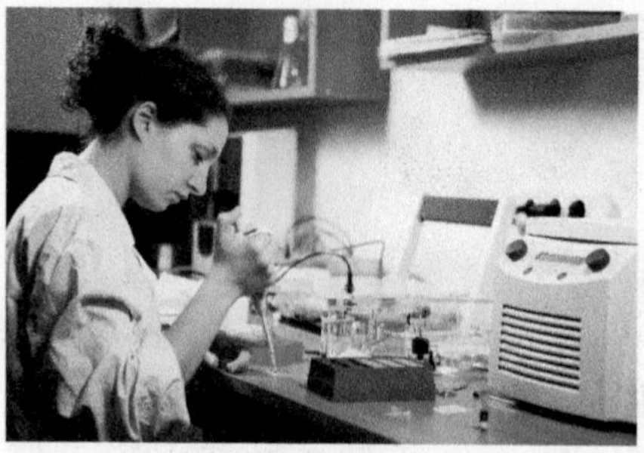

FIGURE 7.15

Performing sample preparation for a DNA laboratory procedure

Source: rimmer/Shutterstock

- ***Organ transplants.*** When several patients are awaiting an organ for transplantation, should age be a factor? Should an alcoholic patient about to die from liver disease be eligible for a liver transplant?
- ***Refusing treatment.*** Should parents be allowed to refuse treatment for a sick child based on their religious beliefs?

These are just a few of the complex ethical, moral, and legal issues under debate. There are no easy answers. Based on your personal values, morals, and ethics, how do you think each of these questions should be answered? How would you respond to someone whose opinions are different from yours? Is it possible to decide who is right and who is wrong?

As a health care worker, you may have strong personal opinions about some, or all, of these issues. You might be called upon to participate in patient procedures that you find to be **inconsistent** with your personal values, morals, and beliefs. When choosing the right health career for you, it's important to think about these issues ahead of time. If you don't want to participate in abortions or sex change operations, for example, no one will force you to compromise your principles. However, you need to make your **moral convictions** known in advance so that patient care won't be interrupted.

inconsistent
(in-ken-SIS-tent) Not satisfied by the same set of values

moral convictions
(MOOR-al ken-VIK-shens) Strong and absolute beliefs about what is right or wrong

THE MORE YOU KNOW

You Can't Always Trust Your Caregivers

Doctors are supposed to be open and honest in sharing information with patients about their medical conditions. Yet according to a recent survey, more than half of all doctors admitted to giving patients false hope. Ten percent of doctors reported telling their patients a lie within the past year. These findings emphasize why it's important for patients to make their wishes clearly known. If patients want the truth from their doctors, they need to speak up. Seriously ill patients who get accurate information can plan ahead and get their affairs in order. Yet many doctors are reluctant to convey bad news.

Almost 20% of the doctors surveyed failed to disclose mistakes they had made, based on the fear of being sued. Yet studies among patients indicate that when doctors admit up-front they've made a mistake and apologize for it, patients are less likely to sue them. One third of the doctors included in the survey don't agree that mistakes should be divulged.

In very rare situations, caregivers cause intentional harm to their patients. A nurse anesthetist in Minnesota addicted to pain medications took most of a surgery patient's painkillers herself. As the patient screamed in pain on the surgery table, she told him to "man up" because he couldn't be given any more medication. Prior to surgery, the patient had been told that his kidney stone removal wouldn't be painful because patients are typically heavily sedated or asleep during the procedure. As the man told doctors he was in terrible pain, he heard staff members discuss putting him in restraints. The patient's medical records revealed that he had only been given one-third of the drug he should have received. After the incident, officials found empty syringes in the nurse's pocket. She refused to take a drug test and resigned.

There have been several cases where health care workers have killed one or more patients for various reasons. Fortunately, incidences involving such extreme and heinous unethical, illegal, and immoral conduct are very rare.

REALITY CHECK

Let's come back to a statement made earlier in this section, "When it comes down to behavior, ethical conduct is up to the individual." This means *you*. This means it's up to you to understand how society in general defines the moral difference between right and wrong, and to live your life accordingly. If you want to succeed in health care, you must ignore the negative, unethical influences in life and focus on what really matters—displaying ethical and professional conduct in service to others.

Depending on the situation, it may be difficult to separate the different ethical, moral, and legal dilemmas from one another because there's so much overlap. The important thing to remember is that your patients and your employer are counting on you to fulfill the responsibilities of your job. This brings us back to ethical conduct. If you behave in a way that supports quality, safety, and service at work, and always put your patients first, you'll be well on your way to recognition as a health care professional.

dilemma
(deh-LEH-ma) A difficult situation or problem that requires making a choice

Key Points

- Fulfilling ethical responsibilities helps protect your patients, coworkers, and employer.
- Ethical issues and legal issues are different. Legal issues are based on laws with legal consequences for noncompliance; ethical issues are codes of moral behavior based on right versus wrong.
- An individual's morals may be influenced by his or her family, friends, teachers, coworkers, religion, and society in general.
- Health care professionals serve others by living the core values of dignity, service, excellence, and fairness/justice.
- Each professional association has a code of ethics for its members that outlines ethical standards for decision making and behavior.
- When making difficult ethical decisions, ask yourself three questions: Is it legal? Is it fair? What would my conscience say?
- Health care workers must report illegal and unethical behavior in order to protect everyone in the work environment.
- A reportable incident is any event that can have an adverse effect on the health, safety, or welfare of patients, coworkers, or other people in the facility.

- You should report serious and extreme illegal behavior to your local law enforcement agency. Use your employer's policy to report concerns about unethical or illegal behavior at work. Concerns about possible Medicare or Medicaid fraud or abuse should be reported to the Office of the Inspector General.
- Health care workers and other stakeholders face many complex ethical, moral, and legal issues. Ethical decisions that pertain to life issues are called bioethics.
- Scientists and physicians encounter complex ethical issues when conducting medical research. Institutional Review Boards oversee research studies to protect participants from unnecessary risks.
- Bioethical issues include abortion, genetic testing, and cloning, to name just a few.
- Health care workers who do not wish to participate in certain patient procedures, such as abortions or sex change operations, based on their moral convictions should discuss the matter with their supervisors.

Section Review Questions

Answer each of the following questions. Indicate which page in the textbook led you to your answer.

1. Explain the difference between unethical and illegal behavior.
2. Identify two factors that influence a person's perspective on right versus wrong.
3. Name three questions to answer when making ethical decisions.
4. List the four core values that lead to ethical conduct in patient care.
5. Discuss the relationship between fairness and ethical conduct.
6. What is a *reportable incident*, and why is reporting these incidents important?
7. Identify four examples of complex, controversial bioethical issues.
8. Explain the role of Institutional Review Boards.

Learn By Doing

Complete Worksheets 1–5 in Section 7.2 of your *Student Activity Guide*.

Chapter Review Questions

Answer each of the following questions. Indicate which page in the textbook led you to your answer.

1. Explain the difference between *libel* and *slander*.
2. What offense have you committed if you hit a patient?
3. What offense has a surgeon committed by leaving a surgical tool inside a patient?
4. Identify a law that helps ensure the confidentiality of medical information.
5. What is the purpose of an ombudsman?
6. Summarize the code of ethics that every health care worker must follow.
7. Give two examples of reportable incidences.
8. Explain the purpose of the Office of the Inspector General.

Chapter Review Activities

1. Create a scenario where a health care worker has a legal obligation to break the confidence of a conversation with a patient.
2. One of your patients tells you he cannot eat because he is worried about having no will. He has no money to pay for an attorney. How would you advise this patient? What resources are available in your community for such a person? Use this as a research opportunity. Check with the county court and your local bar association. Look for current articles about similar scenarios.
3. Investigate the practice of cloning. What is cloning? Why is cloning controversial? Who performed the first successful cloning procedure, and how was this accomplished? How is cloning used today? Who benefits from cloning? What does the future hold for cloning?
4. Conduct research to identify local government agencies, law enforcement agencies, advocacy groups, and hospital departments whose missions include protecting patients from unethical and illegal health care practices. Make a list of contact information and share it with people who might have a use for the information.

What If? Scenarios

What would you do in each of the following situations? Record your answer, explain it, and indicate which page in the textbook led you to your decision.

1. You witness a coworker taking money from the petty cash box in your department. She says she needs to borrow the money to get her car fixed, and she'll pay it back when she gets her next paycheck. She reminds you that she did you a big favor when you first started your job and asks that you not report her to the supervisor.
2. You have one more paper to turn in for a course you're taking that's required for your job. You keep the weekend open to write it, but a dear friend calls and says he'll be in town for the weekend and would like to spend it with you. You have a copy of a paper that someone else wrote for the course two years ago that earned a grade of "B." The instructor is new and would never know that you didn't write the paper yourself.
3. You overhear a coworker speaking on the telephone, sharing confidential information about a patient's diagnosis. The patient is a local celebrity. You have a feeling that your coworker was speaking with someone from the media.
4. When you open up your paycheck, you realize that you got paid for a day that you didn't work.

5. Your sons are returning to school tomorrow after summer break. You haven't had time to shop for school supplies and are short on cash. Your organization is overstocked with office supplies, and no one would miss a few pencils, pens, and tablets of paper.
6. Your best friend, who works in the same department you do, asks you to clock her out at 3:00 pm so that she can leave work at 2:00 pm to attend her daughter's dance recital.
7. After reviewing some financial records, you're beginning to wonder if your manager is billing Medicare for patient procedures that were never done.
8. A famous actress is in the hospital under an assumed name for elective surgery. The next day, a tabloid carries a story of her admission for a drug overdose, citing an "inside" hospital source. You know who is responsible.

Media Connection

Use the companion website for additional interactive learning activities.

Portfolio Connection

Patient advocacy defends and promotes issues that help ensure appropriate health care. With the many challenges that affect health care today, there is a greater awareness of the need to defend patient rights. Concerns about patient rights are frequently in the news and have been presented to the U.S. House of Representatives and the U.S. Senate on several occasions.

Search the newspapers, public library, and the Internet for the latest information on the struggle to protect patient rights. Identify three ways in which you can be an advocate for patient rights. Write a short report explaining the current status of patient rights and include your ideas on how you can be a patient advocate. Keep this in your portfolio for future reference.

CHAPTER 8

Your Clinical Internship

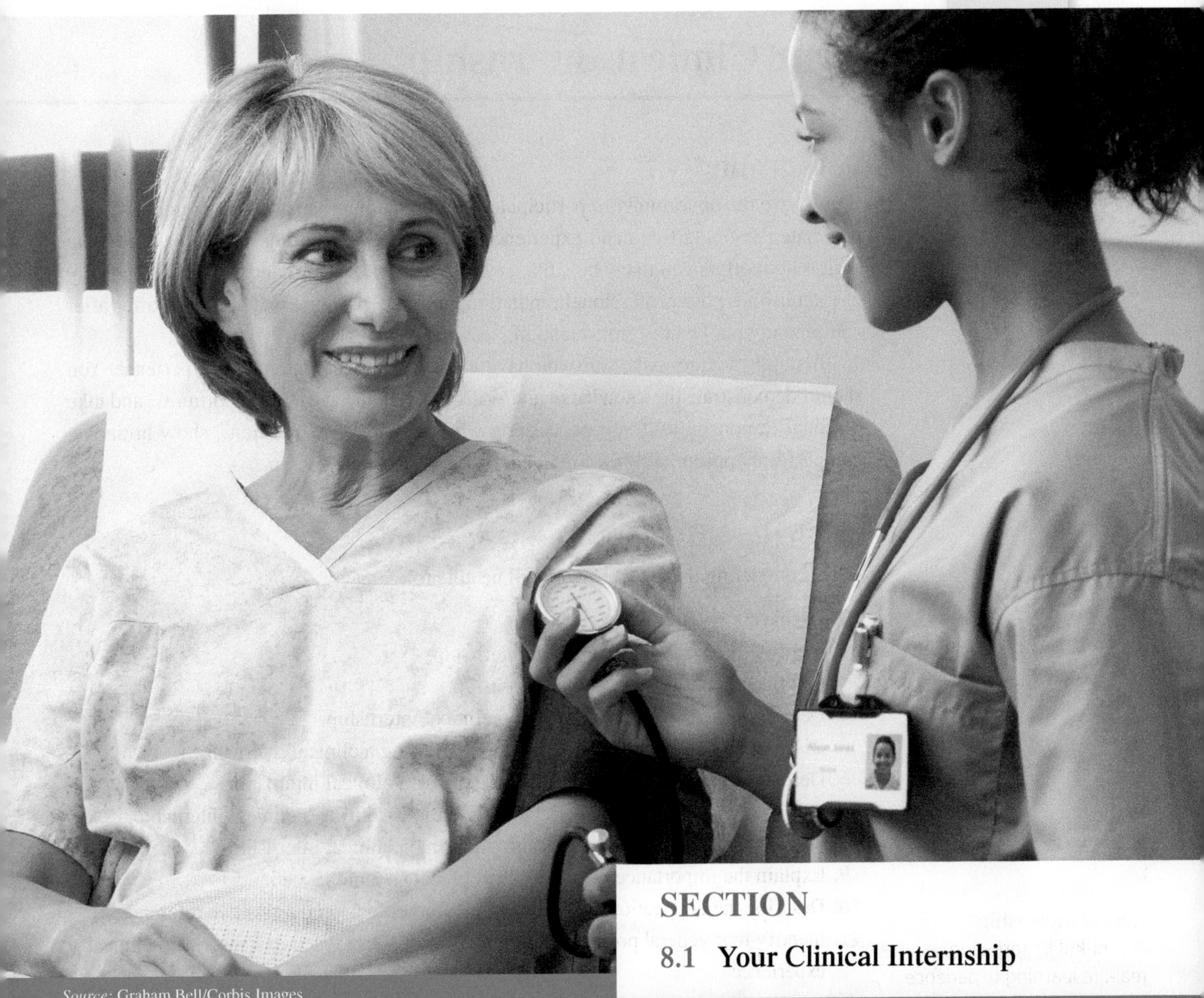

Source: Graham Bell/Corbis Images

SECTION

8.1 Your Clinical Internship

"My mother said to me, 'If you become a soldier, you'll be a general; if you become a monk, you'll end up as the Pope.' Instead, I became a painter and wound up as Picasso."

PABLO PICASSO, ARTIST, 1881–1973

GETTING STARTED

Why do you think your school includes clinical internships for its students? Make a list of the reasons. Why do you think health care employers offer internship experiences for high school students? Make a list of the reasons. Keep these lists handy as you read this chapter and prepare for your internship.

SECTION 8.1 Your Clinical Internship

Background

If you have the opportunity to participate in a clinical internship, consider yourself very fortunate. Having a first-hand experience in a health care setting before you complete high school offers you many benefits. Your attitude and performance will go a long way in establishing your professional reputation, and may pave the way for a job offer after completing your health care education.

It's up to you to make sure you have a positive clinical internship experience. You should demonstrate the knowledge and skills that you bring to this opportunity, and take personal responsibility for your learning while on-site. Ask questions, show initiative, and perform appropriately as a member of the clinical site's team.

Objectives

After completing this chapter, you will be able to:

1. Define the key terms.
2. Identify the purpose of a clinical internship.
3. List three benefits of a clinical internship.
4. Describe three ways to prepare for a clinical internship.
5. Discuss four examples of proper behavior during a clinical internship.
6. Describe three ways to ensure success during a clinical internship.
7. Explain the importance of patient confidentiality during a clinical internship.
8. Discuss the value of keeping a journal during a clinical internship.
9. Explain the importance of putting the clinical site and its patients first.
10. Describe the connection between a clinical internship and a positive reference.
11. Identify four general policies, procedures, and issues related to a successful clinical experience.

clinical internship
(KLI-ni-kul IN-tern-ship) A real-life learning experience obtained through working on-site in a health care facility or other setting while enrolled as a student

rotation
(row-TAY-shen) Movement from one place to another

GETTING READY FOR YOUR CLINICAL INTERNSHIP

A **clinical internship** is a real-life learning experience obtained through working on-site in a health care facility or other setting while enrolled as a student. Schools and educational programs use different terms for this activity, such as a practicum, clinicals, clinical **rotation**, externship, hands-on experience, and so forth.

Once you graduate from high school and begin your postsecondary education, you'll probably participate in another internship as part of your health care education. Some health care programs begin the clinical experience early in the curriculum, integrating classroom instruction with hands-on experience. Other programs complete classroom instruction first and schedule the clinical portion at the end of the program just prior to graduation.

The Purpose and Benefits of a Clinical Internship

You may be thinking, "Should I worry about my clinical internship? Isn't it just another assignment to complete before I can graduate?" In reality, your internship is much more than just another assignment. In fact, it could be one of the most important parts of your education.

Your internship is an opportunity to apply the knowledge and skills you've learned during the classroom portion of your curriculum. If you perform well, your internship could also result in a positive **reference** when you submit your application for admission into a health care educational program. You might even receive a job offer from the site after you complete your health care education and obtain your license or certification.

reference
(REH-fer-ens) A person who can provide information about a job applicant

Your clinical internship is an opportunity to make a positive first impression and successfully kick-off your new health career. Let's take a closer look at what you can expect, and what will be expected of you.

Student Versus Employee

Internship experiences vary in length, depending on your school and program. Some internships may be relatively short, lasting just a few days or weeks. Others may extend over several weeks or months. You won't be paid for the work you do during your internship. If you spend a lot of time at the site, you may feel like *free labor*. But keep one very important fact in mind—you are there as a *student* to learn and to hone your knowledge and skills. Even though the site supervisor will assign your work hours, break times, duties, and responsibilities, you are *not* there as an employee. There's a big difference between being in the site as a student and working there as an employee. You need to keep these differences in mind as you progress through the experience.

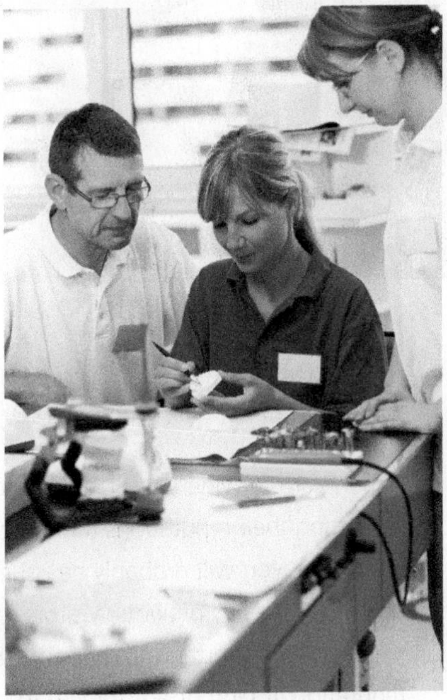

FIGURE 8.1
Participating in an internship experience in a dental lab
Source: Robert Kneschke/Shutterstock

Participating in a clinical internship is a privilege. Whether your internship is in a hospital, outpatient clinic, physician practice, or another setting, you are a guest in the facility. The site supervisor has the right to terminate your internship at any point in time if he or she believes that your appearance, attitude, or performance negatively impacts the site's patients, visitors, physicians, or employees. So you must *prove yourself* in the early stages of your internship to convince the site supervisor that you

mature
(mah-CHUR) Having reached adult development

are mature, prepared, and personally committed to performing well. It's time to apply everything you've learned thus far in establishing your reputation.

Identifying Your Preferences

A benefit of a clinical internship is the opportunity to decide what types of patients you'd like to work with in your new health career. It's not unusual to hear students say they want to work in pediatrics (*peds*). Working with pediatric patients can be highly rewarding, but it takes a certain type of person to do this type of work. Sometimes students have an unrealistic image of what it's like to work with children. They imagine themselves holding and cuddling newborns and small children. They don't always think about the children being sick and their parents being anxious and upset. Experience shows that about half of the students who say they want to work in peds change their minds after a pediatric internship. Students who think they want to work with cancer patients or scrub in on surgery cases may change their minds after some on-site clinical experience.

The same may be true when considering different employment settings. Students may think they want to work in a large, urban hospital or in a small, rural clinic. Yet after their internships, they may change their minds. There's nothing like *being there* to know for sure where you'd like to work and the types of patients and procedures with which you would like to be involved. Your internship can help you make those decisions before you apply for a health care educational program and a job after graduation.

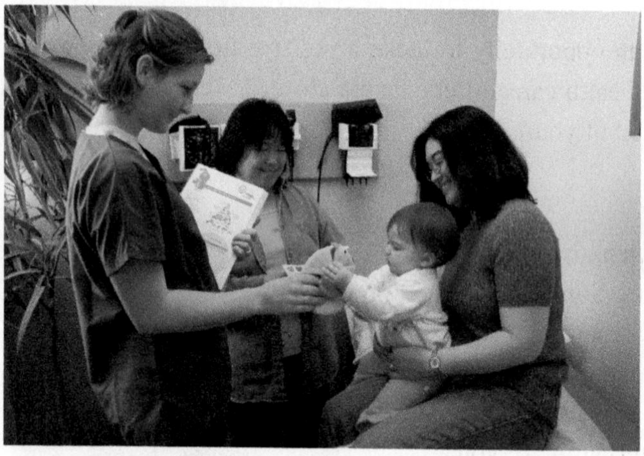

FIGURE 8.2
An intern gains first-hand experience working with a pediatric patient

Source: George Dodson/Pearson Education

Consider This *Site Orientation*

Health care providers are highly focused on customer service and patient satisfaction. Protecting their reputations for quality and service is a high priority. When you start your internship, you will probably be issued an identification (ID) badge to wear while you're on site. The site's patients, visitors, and guests may assume from your ID that you are part of the organization. Your appearance, attitude, and behavior will impact the site's reputation. It's important for you to be familiar with the site's mission, vision, and values and to support them while you're there.

Expect to participate in an orientation when you start your internship. Your orientation may be short, such as a conversation with your site supervisor. Or it might involve attending a half-day or a full-day orientation session with some of the site's new employees who are starting their jobs. Pay attention to the information you are given, and do your best to help the site maintain and enhance its reputation in the community.

Evaluating Your Performance

As you prepare for your clinical internship, you need to think about how your performance will be evaluated. Performance evaluations are typically based on criteria established by your school and program. You may receive a grade based on your attendance, attitude, appearance, and overall performance. Regardless of whether you will receive a grade or not, it's still very important to do your best.

The employees who work at the site will know that you're a student. They will expect you to be a little bit nervous at first, and they won't hold you accountable for knowing everything when you start. But if it's clear that you aren't well prepared or serious about why you are there, your deficiencies will soon become apparent. Feel free to ask questions and show an interest in what goes on at the site. But don't ask the same question over and over again. Keep a small notepad and pen in your pocket, and jot down information that you want to remember.

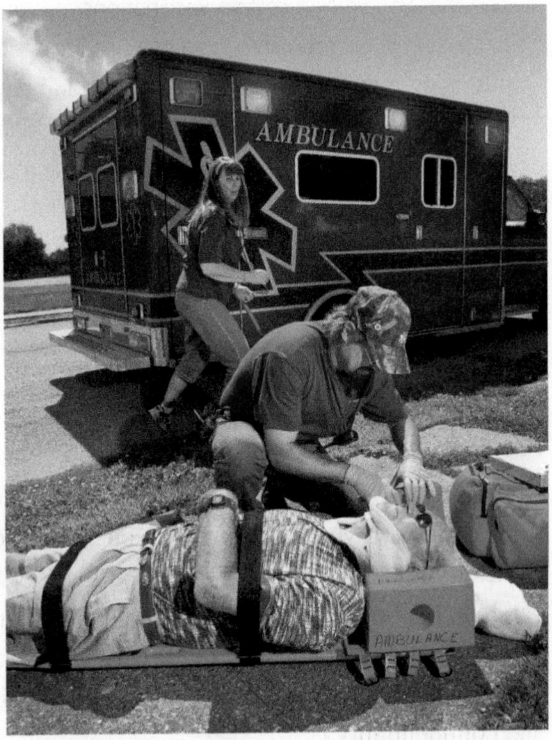

FIGURE 8.3

Observing how an emergency medical technician cares for a patient with a back injury

Source: Craig Stocks Arts/Shutterstock

Picture an internship site with two students present. One student is always visible, asking questions, and stepping in to help. He takes notes and pays attention. The other student is usually off someplace, socializing or taking a smoke break. She rarely asks questions, shows no initiative, and often asks to leave early. It should be obvious which student will earn the best evaluation. But what neither student knows is that the site supervisor prefers to fill his vacant positions by hiring graduates from the local community college's health education programs. One of the reasons he provides internships for high school students is having the opportunity to spot young people who show a lot of potential. In this situation, the students' clinical internship was not just another high school assignment; it was actually an early job interview.

RECENT DEVELOPMENTS

Gaining Clearance

Based on growing concerns about workplace theft, sexual harassment, and the breach of patient confidentiality, health care employers are becoming more selective about whom they accept for internships. As a result, the requirements that students must meet to gain clearance for an internship are becoming increasingly restrictive.

To be cleared for a clinical internship, you may have to undergo a criminal history background check, drug test, and physical exam. If you anticipate problems passing a background check or a drug screen, you should discuss the situation with your teacher as soon as possible. You may also need to prove that you'll be covered by personal health insurance during the internship period.

With respect to vaccinations, you'll have to submit documentation from your physician that you've had certain vaccinations, or you'll need to receive the vaccinations prior to starting your internship. Vaccinations include mumps, rubella, varicella, measles, tetanus, diphtheria, and pertussis. Many sites also require students to have an annual flu shot, a tuberculosis (TB) test, and a hepatitis B immunization.

If your internship site doesn't have these requirements for high school students, they probably will for postsecondary students doing internship experiences as part of their health care education. These clearances are also commonly included in the employment process prior to starting a new job.

Pre-Internship Preparation

Depending on your program, you may be assigned to an internship site or you may have some choices. If you have choices, you'll have some important things to consider before making your decision. Don't choose a site where you or your family members are patients. It's best to choose a location where you can be viewed solely as a student. It's also preferable to choose a site where you don't know the patients. Having personal relationships with patients at your internship site can create some issues with privacy and confidentiality.

Health care employers may have limitations on what you will be allowed to see and do during your internship experience. These limitations may be based on federal and state laws regarding age restrictions. If you are younger than 18 years of age when you start your internship, you might not be permitted to observe or work in certain areas. Hospitals and other health care employers may have their own policies and procedures regarding age restrictions. It's best to investigate these limitations before identifying your site.

FIGURE 8.4

Visiting the site and reviewing printed materials prior to starting an internship

Source: Lilyana Vynogradova/ Shutterstock

Some schools schedule a pre-internship observation for students to visit potential sites prior to selecting, or being assigned to, a location. If you have the option of doing one or more observations before starting your internship, take advantage of this opportunity. During an observation, you'll gain valuable information about the people who work there and the pace at which they work. Is it a friendly, service-oriented facility? How do the employees interact with their coworkers, patients, physicians, and

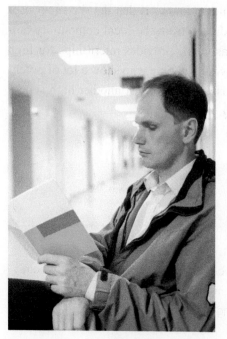

visitors? Is the environment fast-paced or slow-paced? Which type of environment would be most comfortable for you? Some students prefer a fast-paced environment, and they get restless when things move too slowly. Other students prefer a slower pace and feel rushed if things move too quickly.

Regardless of whether you're assigned to a site or have some choices, it's a good idea to do some research before you get there.

- Review the organization's website and printed materials. The more that you know about the site, the better prepared you will be and the more at ease you will feel on your first day.
- Ask your teacher for permission to contact the site ahead of time. Speak with the site supervisor and introduce yourself. Confirm your start date, the hours that you'll be there, and the site's dress code. Discuss any days you'll need to leave early for class or a prior commitment with your site supervisor before your start date.
- Obtain the uniform or professional clothing that's required for students at your site. Review the information in this textbook about how to display a professional image.
- Arrange your transportation and travel to the site a few days before your internship starts. Note the travel time. What time do you need to leave home or school in order to arrive at your site on time? How much traffic should you anticipate? What if the parking lot is full? What if your bus connection is running late? Imagine the *worst case scenario* and have contingency plans.
- On your first assigned day, allow sufficient travel time to arrive at the site at least fifteen minutes early so you'll feel more comfortable and less rushed. You don't want to arrive late or appear unprepared.

Remember, you never get a second chance to make a good first impression.

Language Arts Link Postsecondary Internships

Identify a postsecondary health care educational program offered in your community, such as nursing, medical assisting, surgical technology, medical laboratory technology, certified nursing assisting, or cardiovascular technology. Investigate the internship requirements for this program. The *internship* experience might be called externship, clinicals, practicum, and so forth.

What is the total length of the program, and how much of that time is spent on an internship? At what point during training does the internship occur? Where do the students do their internships? Do they rotate within the internship site, or among more than one internship site? If so, what is the purpose of the rotations? What types of clinical experience must they complete? How is their performance evaluated? Do the internship sites typically hire graduates from the program?

Write a report describing what you have learned from this research. How does this information apply to your own internship experience? Be sure to proofread your work to see if you can improve it by making it more clear, concise, or interesting to read. Check the spelling and grammar and correct any errors. When you've completed your report, exchange it with a classmate. Provide feedback on your classmate's report, and then exchange back. Read your classmate's comments and revise your report as necessary.

ENSURING A POSITIVE CLINICAL EXPERIENCE

As mentioned earlier, keep a small notepad with you and take notes. Write down questions that you may want to ask later on. When you think of a question, it may not be the appropriate time to ask it. For example, if you have a question about the way a physician performed a certain patient procedure, it would be inappropriate to ask in front of the patient. Asking in front of the patient could make both the patient and physician feel uncomfortable. You may have questions that you want to hold until you meet with your teacher again. During the course of a week, many things will happen and your notepad will really come in handy.

Keeping a Journal

journal
(JER-nal) A written record of a person's thoughts and experiences

Consider keeping a journal during your internship. Some programs require that you keep a journal and include certain types of information. Your school may be required to keep a copy of your journal in your student file. In such cases, it is best to record your personal thoughts and emotions in a separate document or notepad. To protect patient confidentiality, you should not mention patient names in your journal. Take a few minutes at the end of each day to record what happened, how you reacted, how you felt about it, and whether you could have handled it differently or better. Journaling can help you *re-group* your feelings, process your experiences, and reflect on what you've learned.

Write about both the good and not-so-good things that you see and experience. Record both the things you *do* and *do not* want to do again in the future. Sometimes you may hear an employee being impolite to a patient. Write down what you heard to remind yourself how others may perceive the things that you say.

You may see some things that surprise you. By recording these occurrences, you'll remember to bring them up when you meet with your teacher and classmates again. Expect to be nervous and busy at the same time. If you don't write things down, you may forget something important. If it's written in your journal, you'll have it as a reference whenever you need it.

APPLY IT KEEPING A JOURNAL

Make a list of the benefits of keeping a journal. Why do some educational programs recommend or require journals? What role does keeping a journal play? How might a journal help you during your internship? How might your internship journal help you later on, after you've graduated from high school and enrolled in a postsecondary educational program? How is a journal different from a diary? What information should, and should not, be included in your journal?

Following Protocol

protocol
(PRO-the-kol) Policies and procedures

Your site will have policies and procedures outlining what you may, and may not, do as a student. These policies and procedures are called protocol, and they will vary from site to site. Familiarize yourself with these at the beginning of your internship and comply with them. Find out how the site handles cell phone and computer use. Some sites won't allow students or staff to use personal cell phones during work hours. In some

Clinical Internship Journal

Print out and complete the following Journal worksheet while you are working as a clinical intern.

Name: **Date:**

Clinical Site: **Area:**

Summary of clinical experience: ____________________

Describe two things you learned today and explain how you will be able to use them in the future.

1. ____________________

2. ____________________

Describe one procedure or treatment you saw today and the patient's response: ____________________

List one new medical term you learned today and explain what it means:

1. ____________________

I performed these hands-on-skills today: ____________________

Name one positive and one negative experience you had in your clinical rotation today: ____________________

Feelings, Smells, Sounds:

I felt ____________________
I smelled ____________________
I heard ____________________

FIGURE 8.5

Sample clinical internship journal form

situations, cell phones may interfere with technical equipment. Avoid making personal telephone calls and texting during your internship hours. Keep in mind that the site's computers may be strictly limited to business use. It's always wise to ask before logging on to someone else's computer. Observe the site's policies regarding smoking, taking breaks, and wearing an ID badge. Don't leave an assigned area without telling the person who is supervising you.

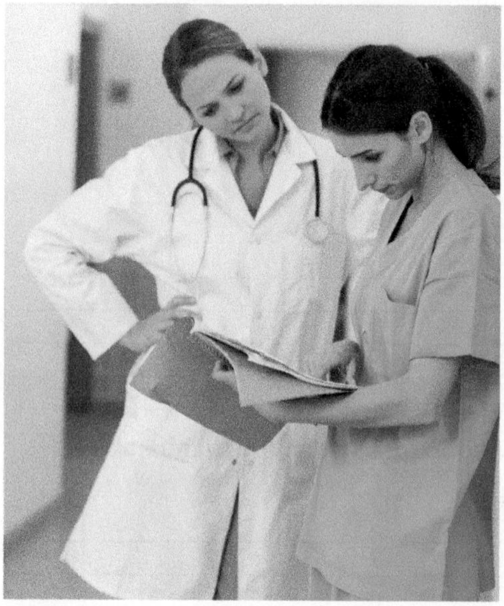

FIGURE 8.6
Reviewing internship policies, procedures, and protocol
Source: wavebreakmedia/Shutterstock

Depending on the site, the employees may need to get permission from patients before they allow you to observe or participate in procedures. Patients have rights, and some patients are more comfortable having a student present during their procedure than others. As a student, you have the right to observe and participate in procedures related to your educational experience. *But the patient's rights always come first.* If a female patient, for example, isn't comfortable with having a male student present during her procedure, the male student will need to comply with the patient's wishes. In most sites, a sufficient number of other patients are available who are comfortable with having students present to ensure that the students' educational goals can be met. Make sure you know how your site protects the rights of its patients and comply with protocol.

Confidentiality

Maintaining confidentiality and adhering to HIPAA and HITECH Act rules are top priorities. During your internship, you may have access to patient medical records and other private information. You may even know some of the patients. What you see, hear, or read at the site *must* stay at the site. Never read a patient's medical record unless you are instructed to do so.

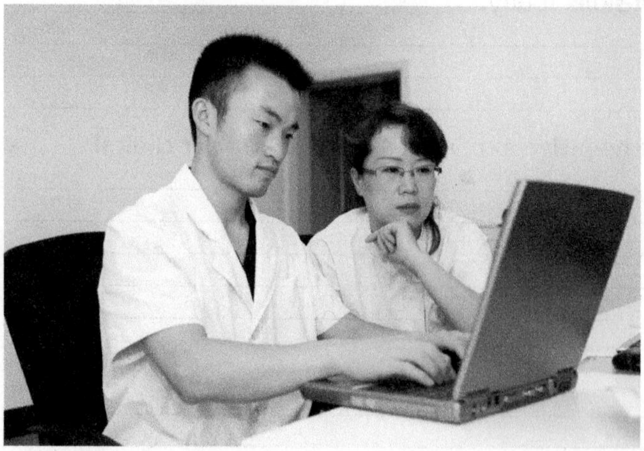

FIGURE 8.7
Protecting the confidentiality of financial and medical records during an internship
Source: bendao/Shutterstock

You will undoubtedly see and do things that you'll want to tell your family and friends about. It's natural to be excited and want to share your experiences. But you must remember to never use the patient's name or provide any other descriptive information that could reveal the patient's identity.

Here's an example of an unacceptable comment:

> You won't believe what I saw today. They removed a mole from Tom Smith's arm. I got to prepare the woman who lives next door for minor surgery and assist the doctor in removing her cyst.

Here's an example of an acceptable comment:

> You won't believe what I did today. They removed a mole from a patient's arm. I got to prepare a patient for minor surgery and assist the doctor with the procedure.

Describe what happened without breaking confidentiality. When you meet with your teacher and classmates to discuss what you've seen and done during the week, continue to protect the confidentiality of the site and its patients.

In addition to medical records, you may have access to other information, such as patient financial records or the site's patient charges or financial transactions. This is information that must remain within the site, and you should not talk about it with people outside the site. Private information is shared only on a *need to know* basis. This means the information is made available only to those people who need to know it to care for patients and conduct the site's business.

You may be rotating to different sites during your internship and working in organizations that compete with one another. Maintain the privacy of business-related information and use discretion when making comparisons among the different places you work. Remember—you are a guest at the site and the supervisor has the right to terminate your internship at any point should your performance pose a problem. Violation of confidentiality or the unauthorized sharing of sensitive information is a legitimate reason for immediate termination. If you are terminated from your internship site, you might find it difficult to gain access to another site, and your quest for recognition as a health care professional will suffer a major setback.

Free Samples

Many sites have what's called a **samples room**. This is a place (sometimes a closet) where they keep samples of drugs and medical supplies. You may be asked to go there to get samples of something for a patient. Just because the sales reps leave samples at the site at no charge, and the site gives samples to patients at no charge, you shouldn't assume that you can help yourself to anything that you want out of the samples room at no charge. Remember the internship student mentioned earlier who didn't get a good evaluation? One of the places she visited frequently was the samples room. Needless to say, this behavior didn't support a positive reputation.

samples room
(SAM-pels ROOM) A place where health care facilities keep samples of drugs and medical supplies

Office Politics

No discussion about proper behavior while on an internship would be complete without talking about **office politics** and how to avoid them. If you've had a job, you've probably already discovered that workplaces have office politics. Whether you're doing your internship in a physician practice, outpatient clinic, or a hospital nursing unit, you may encounter coworkers who don't get along well with one another.

office politics
(AW-fes PA-le-tiks) Clique-like relationships among groups of coworkers that involve scheming and plotting

One employee may tell you something negative about another employee or complain about something that someone else has done. This happens frequently with students and it's easy to get caught in the middle. Stay neutral and don't get involved. Remember, you are not employed by the site, and you probably don't have all of the facts. If you allow yourself to become involved in office politics, you could be labeled a troublemaker. The site supervisor may reconsider allowing you to remain there. You could be terminated from the site or lose your opportunity for a good reference or job offer later on. There's more to an internship than just practicing your hands-on skills. Practicing your *people skills* and your *professionalism skills* are equally important in ensuring success.

One of the reasons why sites accept students for internships is that having a student present helps keep the staff *on their toes*. Students tend to ask a lot of questions. They watch how coworkers interact with one another and with patients, visitors, and physicians. The employees at the site are all aware of this. They must be able to explain things, answer questions, and set a good example. This helps keep the employees focused on the correct way to do things and more cautious about their behavior.

More than One Right Way

There is often more than one right way to do things, and your way might not be the only *right way*. For example, when you clean a room, do you dust or vacuum first? It doesn't matter because both ways lead to the same result. If you observe a site employee doing something in a way that's different from the way you were taught, don't say, "That's wrong" or "You aren't doing that right" or "That's not the way we were taught." Instead, turn it into a learning opportunity. Ask the person to explain why and how he or she did it that way. You might learn a new technique that's easier and more efficient.

You will likely see different equipment in your internship site as compared with your classroom or lab at school. This is one of the benefits of doing an internship—you get to experience different technologies. You should approach this situation by saying, "This machine is different than the one I was taught on. Would you please show me how this one works?" This sounds much better than saying, "I don't know how to work this machine. We weren't shown this in school." With the first example, you're indicating that you know the correct procedure, but aren't familiar with the specific equipment. Medical equipment can be complicated to operate; mistakes can be expensive, and failure to use equipment properly can jeopardize patient care and patient safety. Make sure you know how to operate the equipment correctly or ask for help.

Showing Initiative

You are there to learn and to help, not to get in the way. Show initiative. One of the quickest ways to get labeled as unprofessional is to stand around doing nothing. Everyone from the receptionist to the physicians will be watching your every move. Avoid spending too much time chatting with the staff. Be productive and help keep the site moving smoothly.

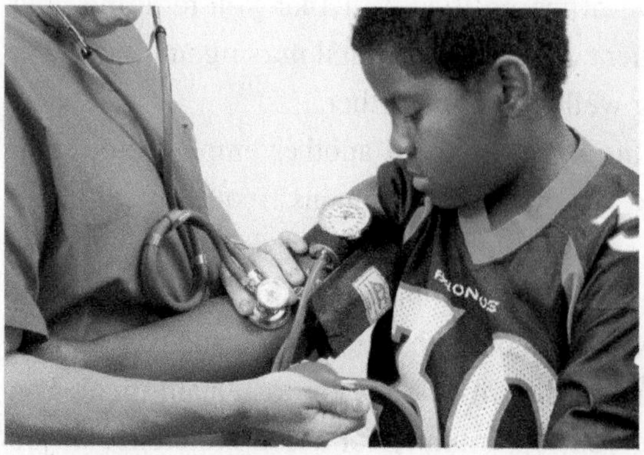

FIGURE 8.8

Showing initiative by taking a young patient's blood pressure

Source: Michal Heron Pearson Education

Once you've learned what is expected of you, and you feel comfortable with the equipment and procedures, it's important to begin functioning with less direct supervision. If you are uncertain about something, by all means ask! But if you've been given a responsibility, and it's *your job* to do it, then do it. If a patient has checked in, and it's your job to escort the patient to the exam room, do so without waiting to be told. Don't make patients wait. If you hear the phone ring, and you've been instructed how to answer it, you should answer it. The more you can do, the better.

Language

Here's a story that actually happened in a large medical office. A student reported to the site on the first day of her internship. When she arrived, she couldn't remember the name of her site supervisor. As she was talking to the person seated at the receptionist desk, she became frustrated and used some **profane** language. As it turned out, the *receptionist* was actually the office manager in charge of hiring for the practice. Needless to say, the student's clinical experience didn't get off to a very good start, and no reference was offered at the end of the internship.

profane
(pro-FANE) Improper and contemptible

BUILD YOUR SKILLS *Securing a Positive Reference*

When you apply for admission into a postsecondary health care educational program, you might be asked to provide one or more references. References are people who can provide information about you. They can verify your education and training, work experience, and attendance. They can provide insight to your work ethic, character, people skills, and ability to learn more and learn quickly.

Your internship site supervisor could serve as a valuable reference if he or she is impressed with you and your performance. Your supervisor's feedback is helpful to people who are considering whether you're a good match for an educational program or a job opening. Your supervisor has *seen you in action* in a real-life health care setting and can describe your level of interest, commitment, and motivation.

If you live in a small town, it's possible that your site supervisor knows the people who make selection decisions for local health care education programs. He or she probably knows the people in other health care organizations who do the hiring for those facilities. So it's very important to make a positive impression during your internship. Once you've begun developing your reputation, it will travel with you from place to place.

Unprofessional language should never be used in your internship site. That is not to say that you won't hear it yourself, because you will. However, hearing the employees using profane language is not an excuse to use it yourself. Put yourself in the patients' positions. If you were sitting in the waiting room and heard the staff using profanity, how would you feel? What impact would it have on your opinion of the organization? At each step of the way, put yourself in the patients' shoes. Although you are there as a student, the patients will consider you part of the staff. Your behavior not only affects your own reputation but also that of the site. Using profanity or any other type of unprofessional language will undermine both reputations.

Teamwork

Don't become part of a clique. Depending on how long you're at the site, you may start to feel comfortable with the staff and feel as if you *belong there*. Belonging is a good

FIGURE 8.9
Working as a team to make sure the ambulance is properly equipped for emergency care

Source: Monkey Business Images/ Shutterstock

feeling, but there's a difference between *fitting in* and being part of a clique. Fitting in simply means that you work well with the staff and you are viewed as cooperative. Your personality may blend well with the personalities of the employees. But being part of a clique can work against you. Cliques stick together and don't associate with the rest of the staff. They're exclusionary and impede teamwork. Employees in cliques are typically less productive because they spend too much time socializing and gossiping.

Supporting teamwork should be one of your goals. When everyone works well together, the site can function smoothly. During your internship, pay attention to which employees are good team players. Note the differences between team players and non-team players. You'll notice that non-team players have to work harder to get the work done, while team players pitch in and help each other out. Strive to be a team player and avoid cliques. This could become a major factor in getting a positive evaluation and a reference at the end of your internship.

You should consider several other things during your internship. Protect yourself and others from communicable diseases by applying everything you've learned about infection control and Standard Precautions. Use protective devices correctly. If you become ill during your internship, stay home and don't report for duty. Avoid spreading your germs to the patients and staff. Remember everything you've learned about safety in the workplace, and obey safety rules. You should report any accidents or incidents immediately.

Patient Preferences

You may come in contact with patients who are familiar with the staff and uncomfortable with anyone who is *new,* including students. Don't take this personally as it's very common. Some patients will refuse to tell the student (or a new employee) anything. If a student tries to assist with a procedure, for example, the patient may resist and ask for someone whom he or she knows. Patients can bond with members of their health care team and reject the involvement of people they don't know. If this happens to you, don't argue with the patient. Explain who you are and why you're there. If the patient still insists on interacting with someone they know, simply excuse yourself and go get one of the staff.

Personal Issues

When you walk through the door to your internship site, leave your personal problems outside. If you had a disagreement with someone that morning, don't discuss it with the people working at your site. If you're upset, distracted, and not thinking clearly, you're more likely to make a mistake.

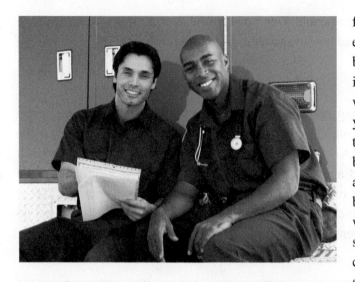

Never discuss your personal life or your own medical history with patients. You're there to focus on the patient's situation, not on your own. The medical profession is a relatively *small world*. People who work for one employer often know their counterparts at other employers. They participate in the same professional associations and attend the same continuing education conferences. When they get together, it's not uncommon for them to discuss personnel issues. Your performance and reputation as a student can easily spread from one place to the next without you ever knowing about it.

Achieving Success

Achieving success, especially during a lengthy internship, isn't easy. Working without pay can become frustrating and tiresome, especially when you're a student with bills to pay and family obligations to meet. If your internship occurs at the end of your school year, you're probably counting the days until it ends.

When you look at employment ads, you'll notice that employers prefer to hire applicants who have work experience. Once you've finished your internship, you can count that as experience even though you weren't a paid employee. You will know more about how the *real world* operates. You'll have first-hand knowledge and insights to share when you apply for admission into a health care educational program. You'll be more polished in your communication skills, and you'll present yourself in a professional manner. You didn't get paid for the hours you worked during your internship, but the experience you gained is priceless.

Be sure to list your internship experience on your résumé. Ask your site supervisor if you may use him or her as a reference. If you've had a positive experience, most supervisors will be happy to assist you in getting accepted into an educational program and finding a good job. If you arrived on time, avoided unnecessary absences, and did your best to fulfill the goals of your internship—all without pay, then your site supervisor will assume that you will work just as hard, or even harder, when you become an employee.

If you secure admission into a health care education program prior to completing your internship, don't make the mistake of slacking off just because you've already been accepted. Too many students have made this mistake. Once they get their acceptance letter, they start arriving a few minutes late, take longer breaks than they should, or fail to show as much initiative. This behavior indicates that they were making a good impression just to get into an education program.

As mentioned earlier, you may receive a grade for your internship. When you use your site supervisor as a reference, he or she will be contacted and asked a series of questions about you and your performance. The following criteria are the types of things that will be considered when assigning your grade and providing a reference:

1. *Were you dependable?*

   Did you show up on time, ready to work? How many times were you absent? When absent, did you follow procedures for calling in? No matter how competent you are, if you aren't there, you aren't doing your job. Employers would rather have a less experienced employee with a good attendance record than an experienced employee with a poor attendance record.

FIGURE 8.10
A clinical intern displays her friendly personality
Source: Rob Marmion/Shutterstock

2. *Was your appearance professional?*
   Were you dressed appropriately and neat and clean? Did your appearance reflect a positive image to your patients and the site's staff? Avoid trendy clothing and appearance. You may think that hair streaked in purple is fashionable, but it's not appropriate in a business setting. If you wear jewelry, make sure it's conducive to the work you're doing. Safety comes first when working with body fluids, equipment, and patients. Remember that some professions don't allow any jewelry to be worn for this reason.
3. *Did you display a friendly personality and good customer service?*
   Did you get along well with patients, physicians, and the site's staff? Were you cooperative with the staff and a team player?
4. *How well did you work under stress?*
   Did you maintain a calm demeanor and balance the priorities of your work appropriately? Did you adapt well to change?
5. *How well did you perform your duties with limited supervision?*
   Did you demonstrate initiative or wait to be told what to do? Did you accept responsibility and perform your duties competently?
6. *Did you display a positive attitude and a desire to learn?*
   Were you motivated? Did you ask good questions? Were you eager to learn new procedures and practice what you learned?
7. *Did you display a professional image?*
   Did you apply everything that's been discussed in this textbook to make the very best impression you could possibly make?

If you can answer "yes" to all of these questions, you are well on your way to achieving a good grade, a positive reference, and recognition as a health care professional.

After Your Internship

On the last day of your internship, thank everyone at your site. Let them know how much you appreciate the time they allowed you to be there and all of the encouragement and help they provided. Within a few days (no longer than a week) of leaving, send a handwritten thank you note. Sending a thank you note conveys appreciation and courtesy. Make sure you spell the person's name correctly and use good grammar and **penmanship**. Believe it or not, thank you notes can be the deciding factor in who gets a reference and who doesn't.

penmanship
(pen-MAN-ship) Handwriting

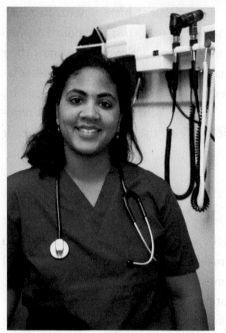

THE MORE YOU KNOW

Observations, Internships, and Job Offers

Some internship sites won't accept students unless they've done an observation there first. This pre-internship observation gives students a chance to check out the site before starting their clinical experience. But more importantly, it gives the site a chance to check out the students before accepting them into the facility. If students make a poor impression during the observation, there's a good chance they won't be invited back for an internship.

An increasing number of employers are now hiring primarily from the pool of graduates who did internships at the site. In some cases, new employees start with higher pay if they did their internship at the site. Think about it. If you did your internship at the site that hired you, you save them time and money. You're already oriented and ready to work. You're familiar with the staff, physicians, and patients. You know how the department or work unit functions, and you can operate the equipment, perform the procedures, and handle the paperwork. You can *hit the ground running* when compared with someone else who might need weeks or months of work experience to ramp-up to the level from which you started. This is just one more reason to impress the staff at your internship site and aim for a job there, after graduating from high school or from a postsecondary health care educational program.

Community Service Opening the Door for Future Interns

Depending on the size of the town where you attend school, it may offer a limited number of places where students can do internships. Some health care facilities won't accept students for clinical experiences. Their primary mission is patient care, and they don't have sufficient staff, time, space, or other resources to accommodate students. Facilities that do provide internships may only accept students from postsecondary educational programs. When employers fill their vacancies by hiring program graduates, they're more likely to be involved with those programs than with high school students. High school students require more direct supervision than postsecondary students. Postsecondary students have more health care education and a higher level of maturity when working in patient care areas. In other words, there's competition for internship slots, and health care facilities have to set their priorities.

One way you can serve your community is by performing exceptionally well during your internship. If you prove to be a serious, mature, well-informed intern who clearly appreciates being there and is willing to go above and beyond the minimum requirements, you may *open the door* for other high school students to follow. On the other hand, if you *slack off* and give the impression that you really don't want to be there, or if you giggle and act like a child, the site may decide to stop taking students altogether.

It comes back to the ripple effect. Your attitude, appearance, and behavior during your internship could make a far-reaching impact well beyond your ability to see it—for better, or worse.

REALITY CHECK

If you haven't taken your studies seriously up to this point, your internship experience could be somewhat disappointing. Your site supervisor is expecting you to be mature and well prepared. If you show up unprepared or behave in an immature manner, your opportunity may be cut short. You could be sent back to school to try to line up a different site. If your attitude is poor and your performance is weak, it's possible that no site may be willing to take you. Do you really want to get to this stage in your education only to be excluded from your internship because you didn't take your studies seriously enough?

Health care providers that offer internship experiences don't exist to serve students, they exist to serve patients. Having students on site provides some benefit to the organization, but many employers refuse to offer student experiences for a variety of reasons. Supervising students, answering their questions, and showing them how to operate equipment takes time and results in an expense to the facility. Students who perform poorly may damage equipment, waste supplies, and have a negative impact on the organization's reputation and its patient satisfaction scores.

So when a provider offers you an internship experience, don't just take it for granted. The people who work at the site are taking a chance on you. If you perform poorly, you may close the door for future students who want to do their internship there. On the other hand, if you perform well, you may actually open the door for future students.

Key Points

- Research the site in advance and visit there before your first day.
- Follow the site's protocol.
- Keep a journal and use a notepad to jot down things that you want to remember.
- Arrive on time and avoid unnecessary absences.
- Show initiative, ask questions, and remember the answers.
- Dress appropriately and display a positive attitude.
- Show respect, and put the site and its patients first.
- Remember that you are a student at the site, not an employee.
- Follow HIPAA and HITECH rules, protect confidentiality, and don't share private information.
- Don't use profane language.
- Avoid discussing your personal life with the site's patients and staff.
- Don't participate in office politics or become part of a clique.
- Send a thank you note shortly after your internship ends.

Learn By Doing

Complete Worksheets 1–5 in Chapter 8 of your *Student Activity Guide*.

Chapter Review Questions

Answer each of the following questions. Indicate which page in the textbook led you to your answer.

1. List three benefits of an internship experience.
2. How should you prepare for your internship?
3. List four examples of proper behavior while on an internship.
4. Name two things that must be kept confidential during your internship.
5. Why should you keep a journal during your internship?
6. What does it mean to *put your site first*?
7. Describe the connection between an internship and a positive reference.
8. What is *protocol* and why must students follow it?

Chapter Review Activities

1. Write a paragraph describing the attitudes and behaviors that could result in the termination of a student's internship experience by his or her site supervisor. Explain what the student should have done to prevent this situation from happening.
2. Write two scenarios where a student on internship is faced with *office politics*. Describe the situations. In the first scenario, discuss what happens when the student decides not to become involved in office politics. Why did the student make this decision, and what happened as a result? In the second scenario, discuss what happens when the student does decide to become involved in office politics. Why did the student make this decision, what did he or she do in terms of involvement, and what happened as a result?

What If? Scenarios

What would you do in each of the following situations? Record your answer, explain it, and indicate which page in the textbook led you to your decision.

1. While escorting a patient to the exam room, she asks you if her husband's tests results are back yet. You know that the results are back, but you don't have permission to give the results to anyone except the patient himself.
2. You notice the constant ringing of telephones in the office. You notice that the receptionist is talking on the telephone. But several times during the day, she's involved in personal calls. In the meantime, the ringing telephones are ignored.
3. One of your patients is a friend of your mother. She's at the doctor's office to find out if she's pregnant. After she leaves, her pregnancy test comes back as negative. You've been unable to reach her by telephone to give her the results. The next day you see her at the shopping mall with her family.
4. You realize that your neighbor is a patient at your internship site. You see her medical record and are wondering why she always looks so tired all of the time. Her records are right there and no one is watching.
5. During your internship, a patient mentions that he would prefer that no one other than his physician be in the room during his medical procedure. It's a procedure you've never seen before and you would like to observe. The patient will be under the influence of medication and probably won't remember what happened during the procedure.

6. You're short on money and need some antibiotics for your child. Her prescription has run out, but there is a large supply of the same drug in your site's sample room. You notice that samples are given to patients free of charge.

7. During your internship, you notice that an employee has left work thirty minutes early every day for the past week. Two other employees, who suspect this behavior but haven't witnessed it themselves, ask you to report it to the site supervisor.

Media Connection

Use the companion website for additional interactive learning activities.

Portfolio Connection

Keep a copy of your internship journal and your final internship evaluation in your portfolio. These items not only document your experience in a real-life health care setting, they also demonstrate your commitment and your ability to perform appropriately *on-the-job*. If your site supervisor offers to provide you with a reference, take advantage of his or her offer. Even if you aren't ready to apply for a postsecondary education program or a job yet, your reference will come in handy at some point in the future. Keep your supervisor's contact information in your portfolio. If he or she is willing to give you a reference letter, keep the original letter plus a few copies in your portfolio for future use.

CHAPTER 9

Health, Wellness, and Safety

Source: Tyler Olson/Shutterstock

SECTIONS

"He who has health has hope, and he who has hope has everything."

ARABIC PROVERB

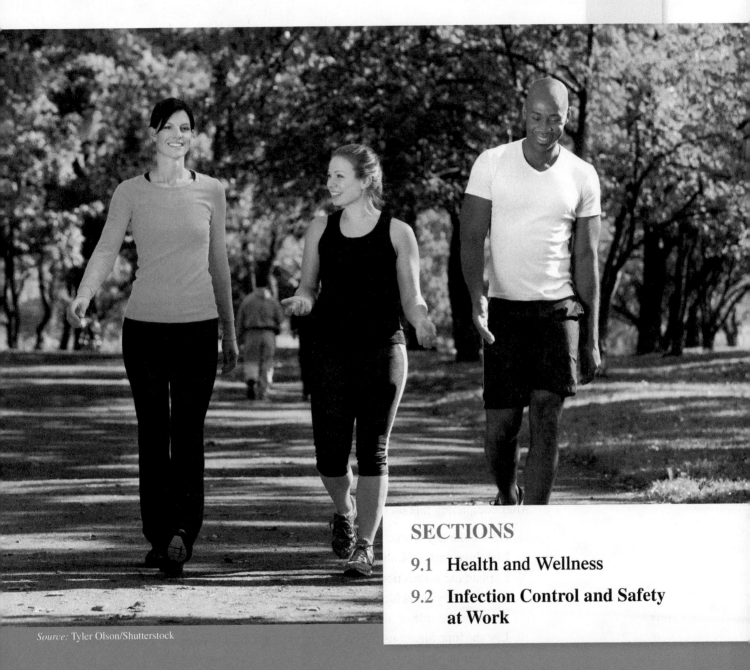

GETTING STARTED

Health care workers must be healthy workers. It is well documented that those with good health habits miss fewer work days, are able to meet the required work schedule more efficiently, and maintain a more rigorous work ethic. Eating right is a major factor in reaching and maintaining good health.

Keep a journal for one week of everything you eat and drink. Analyze the strengths and weaknesses of your dietary habits, including potential diseases/disorders that might result from your eating habits.

SECTION 9.1 Health and Wellness

Background

Responsible health care promotes lifestyles that encourage wellness. It is important for the health care worker to understand that mind, body, spirit, and social involvement must be balanced. Understanding wellness promotes good health in the health care worker and in the patient.

The holistic approach to health is important because it includes all aspects of a person's well-being. When a person is in balance physically, mentally, and spiritually, that person can experience life in a positive way and enjoy a greater sense of well-being. The trend in health care is toward wellness and preventive care. The health care worker has a responsibility to help the patient understand different care choices and the role that each of these therapies may play in seeking a goal of optimal wellness.

vitality
(vye-TA-leh-tee) The ability of an organism to go on living

When you eat the proper foods, you have the energy and vitality to function effectively. Patients need a healthy diet to maintain or restore good health. Knowledge of nutrition and the benefits of therapeutic diets help you understand how to maintain good health for yourself and your patients.

Objectives

After completing this section, you will be able to:

1. Define the key terms.
2. List three parts of holistic health.
3. Explain the connection between wellness and preventive care.
4. List five ways to achieve physical fitness.
5. Describe the role of alternative health care.
6. List the four functions of food when the right combination of nutrients work together in the body.
7. List five basic nutrients and explain how they maintain body function.
8. Describe the USDA's MyPlate and explain its purpose.
9. Identify the characteristics of three common eating disorders.
10. List four commonly abused substances and their negative impact on the human body.

11. Give three examples of therapeutic diets.
12. Discuss why health care employers are focusing on the health and wellness of their workers.

WELLNESS AND PREVENTIVE HEALTH CARE

The World Health Organization's definition of health, "Health is a state of complete physical, mental, and social well-being and not merely the absence of disease or infirmity" (http://www.who.int/about/definition/en/print.html), has been expanded with the recent growth and emphasis on holistic health. Today we think in terms of the body working as a unit (mental, physical, spiritual) to maintain and promote optimum wellness through daily actions. *Holistic* refers to the well-being of the whole person. It is important to meet physical needs and also mental and spiritual needs when giving care. Holistic health care is a part of the wellness approach, which encourages good health and a positive self-image. Understanding these needs helps you care for yourself and for your patients.

infirmity
(in-FER-meh-tee) Unsound or unhealthy state of being

self-image
(CELF-ih-MIJ) The mental picture that a person has of himself or herself

Wellness and preventive health care emphasize keeping patients well, not waiting until they are ill to provide treatment. Screenings are tests or examinations that are done to find a disease or condition before symptoms appear. Conditions that are commonly screened for before symptoms occur include: breast cancer in women, colorectal cancer, diabetes, high blood pressure, glaucoma, high cholesterol, osteoporosis, and prostate cancer in men. Age, gender, family history, and genetic risk factors are indications for whether a person should have particular screenings. This type of preventive care makes it easier to treat most diseases and conditions early, when treatment is often more successful.

screenings
(SKREEN-ings) Tests or examinations that are done to find a disease or condition before symptoms appear

Health education is vital to helping people maintain good health. A holistic approach includes physical fitness, mental fitness, and spiritual fitness.

Physical Fitness

Physical fitness keeps us alert and energetic in activities of daily living. It gives us enough energy to enjoy leisure time and to respond when emergencies arise. It can be achieved through:

- Routine physicals.
- Aerobic exercise.
- Adequate rest.
- Immunizations.
- Good nutrition.
- Well-baby checks.
- Good posture.
- Weight control.
- Elimination of body wastes.
- Avoiding substance abuse, including alcohol, tobacco, and excessive food intake.

aerobic
(air-OH-bik) Requiring oxygen

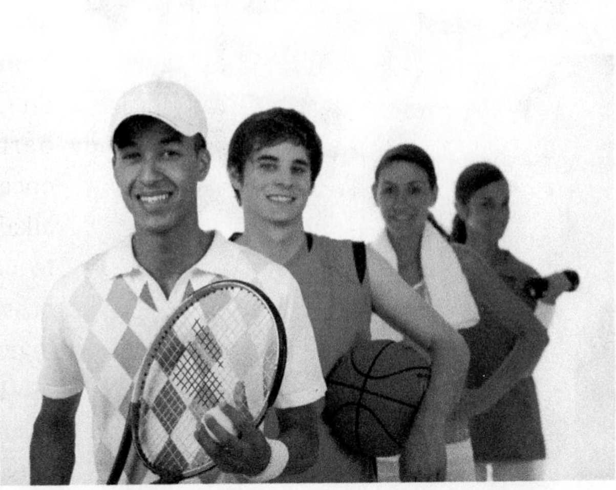

FIGURE 9.1
Regular exercise supports good physical fitness
Source: auremar/Shutterstock

Physical fitness is good bodily health and is the result of regular exercise, proper diet and nutrition, and proper rest for physical recovery. *Physical exercise* is bodily activity that develops and maintains physical fitness and overall health. This helps to strengthen muscles and the cardiovascular system, and to boost the immune system. Exercise helps prevent heart disease, cardiovascular disease, diabetes, and obesity. It also improves mental health and helps prevent depression.

cosmetic
(kahz-MEH-tik) Something done for the sake of appearance

taboos
(ta-BOOS) Banned from social custom

Besides exercise, correct posture is a simple but very important way to keep the back and spine healthy. It is more than cosmetic—good posture and back support are critical to reducing the incidence and levels of back and neck pain.

A diet is all of the food consumed by a person. Dietary habits are the decisions an individual or culture makes when choosing what foods to eat. Each culture holds some food preferences and some food taboos. Individual dietary choices may be more or less healthy, but proper nutrition requires the appropriate intake and absorption of vitamins, minerals, and fuel in the form of carbohydrates, proteins, and fats. Dietary habits and choices play a significant role in health and mortality, since deficiencies, excesses, and imbalances in diet can produce negative impacts on health, which may lead to diseases and conditions such as cardiovascular disease, diabetes, scurvy, obesity, or osteoporosis.

The impact of substance abuse, including tobacco, alcohol, and drugs, crosses all societal boundaries and can harm everyone. Smoking tobacco particularly damages the respiratory and the circulatory systems. Regular use results in diseases that cause death or severe disability. During pregnancy, chemicals from the tobacco smoke pass through the mother's blood to the baby through the placenta, reducing the oxygen and blood.

Excessive alcohol use increases the risk of many harmful health conditions, such as unintentional injuries, including traffic injuries, or falls. It is associated with violence, child neglect, and risky sexual behavior. In addition, alcohol poisoning can occur, a medical emergency that results from high blood alcohol levels which suppress the central nervous system and cause loss of consciousness, low blood pressure and body temperature, coma, respiratory depression, and death. Long-term alcohol problems include chronic disease and neurological impairments. Drinking alcohol during pregnancy can result in miscarriage, stillbirth, and a combination of physical and mental birth defects that last throughout the baby's life.

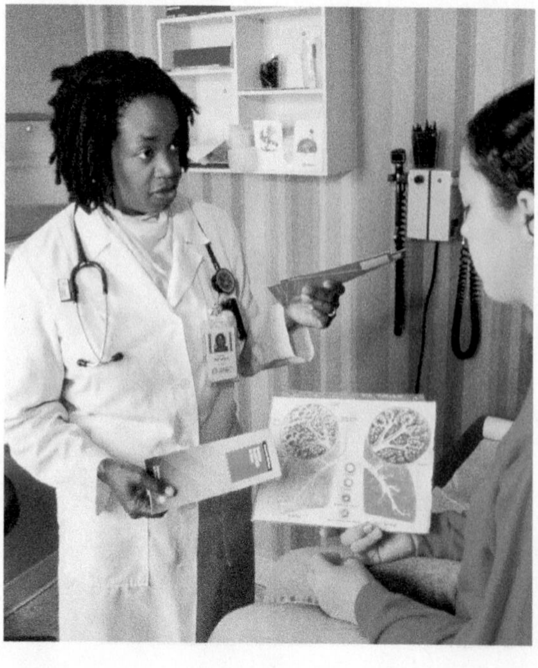

FIGURE 9.2
Explaining the dangers of smoking to a young patient
Source: Michael Newman/PhotoEdit

Drug abuse has a wide range of definitions related to taking a *prescription drug, psychoactive drug,* or *performance enhancing drug* for a non-therapeutic or non-medical effect. Some of the most commonly abused drugs include alcohol, amphetamines, barbiturates, benzodiazepines, cocaine, methaqualone, and opium alkaloids. Use of these drugs may lead to criminal penalties in addition to possible physical, social, and psychological harm.

Physical and mental activities require energy and create waste products. As our energy level goes down

THE MORE YOU KNOW

Substance Abuse, Alcohol, and Tobacco

Substance Abuse

Substance abuse refers to the use of legal or illegal substances that cause harm to a person's health or life. Abused substances usually produce some form of intoxication that alters judgment, perception, or physical control. Substance abuse in the United States is widespread. In 2009, about 8.7% of Americans over the age of twelve used illicit drugs and 17.6 million were heavy alcohol users. About one out of five Americans smokes cigarettes.

People use alcohol and other drugs because they like the way these substances make them feel. However, substance abuse may lead to **addiction**, a compulsion to continue using a substance despite its negative consequences. People can become addicted to illegal drugs, prescription drugs, or to things they may not think of as drugs, such as alcohol and the nicotine in cigarettes.

Many abused substances can produce a phenomenon known as *tolerance*. This means a person requires a larger amount of the drug to produce the same level of intoxication. Once a person is addicted to a drug, it becomes almost impossible to stop using it. Sometimes, when people stop using a drug, they experience withdrawal. Withdrawal can range from mild anxiety to seizures and hallucinations.

Alcohol

Despite the focus on illegal drugs, alcohol remains the main drug problem in the United States.

Alcohol lessens a person's inhibitions, slurs speech, and decreases coordination. Many people use alcohol without any negative consequences. However, approximately 15 million people in the country are addicted to alcohol; more than 4.5 million of them are women.

Alcohol is the most common cause of liver failure in the U.S. The drug can also cause heart enlargement and cancer of the pancreas, esophagus, and stomach. Alcohol abuse is associated with nearly half of all fatal motor vehicle accidents. Every year in the United States, alcohol abuse also causes 500,000 injuries, 600,000 assaults, and 70,000 sexual assaults.

Tobacco

Cigarettes kill more Americans than alcohol, car accidents, suicide, AIDS, homicide, and illegal drugs combined. Yet, amazingly, people continue to smoke. Cigarettes and other forms of tobacco contain nicotine, one of the most addictive of all drugs. Despite the rising cost of cigarettes, 19.3% of U.S. adults were smokers in 2010.

About half of all Americans who continue to smoke will die because of the habit. Each year about 440,000 people die in the United States from illnesses related to cigarette smoking, such as heart disease, lung cancer, emphysema, and stroke. Although 70 percent of smokers want to quit and 35 percent attempt to quit each year, fewer than 5 percent succeed. This is because smokers not only become physically addicted to nicotine, but they also become psychologically addicted to it. Nicotine withdrawal symptoms of smoking include anxiety, hunger, sleep disturbances, and depression. All these factors make it very difficult for a person to stop smoking once he or she starts.

addiction
(eh-DIK-shen) A compulsion to continue using a substance even though it has negative consequences

and wastes accumulate, we experience fatigue and a need to rest. During rest, energy is restored, and the waste buildup is diminished, allowing for recovery and growth. Rest and sleep are dependent upon our ability to relax. To get a good night's rest, try to sleep in a dark, quiet, cool room.

Mental Fitness

Mental fitness allows people to interact effectively with others and to feel balanced. Mental fitness manifests in a positive self-image. Mentally healthy people:

- Self-direct.
- Have a sense of belonging.
- Trust their own senses and feelings.
- Accept themselves.
- Have self-esteem.
- Practice stress management.

Stress is what you feel when you have to handle more than you are used to normally handling. Often, your body responds in the same way as it would if you were in danger—hormones speed up your heart, make you breathe faster, and give you a burst of energy. This is sometimes known as the fight-or-flight stress response. Some stress is normal and even useful; for example, it can help you win a race or finish an important job on time. However, if stress happens too often or lasts too long, it can have bad effects. You can experience headaches, an upset stomach, back pain, or trouble sleeping. Stress can weaken your immune system, making it harder to fight off disease. It can make you moody, tense, or depressed. Relationships may suffer, and you may not do well at work or school.

APPLY IT STRESS AT WORK

As a class, divide into teams of two or three. Each group should discuss potentially stressful situations in the workplace, such as having a heavy workload, or not getting along with a coworker. Then develop a list of strategies for dealing with stressful situations in the workplace. Share your lists as a class to compare and contrast strategies and gain insight about dealing with employment stress.

To identify stressors, you have to know:

- What event caused the stress.
- Why you feel stress.
- How much stress you are feeling.
- If you feel negatively or positively about the situation.

Before you can get stress under control, you need to find out what is causing it. Therefore, you should:

- Gather information or data.
- Identify the problem.
- List possible solutions.
- Make a plan.

- Act on your solution.
- Evaluate the results.
- Change the solution if the plan doesn't work the first time.

In order to cope with stress, look for ways to reduce it, and learn healthy ways to relieve it. Some methods might include better time management, taking good care of your health, getting plenty of rest and regular exercise, not smoking, limiting alcohol intake, learning to say "no" if you are too busy, and asking for help. You can talk to family, friends, or a counselor. You can write down things that are bothering you, or find other ways to express your feelings. Finally, you can take some time to do something you enjoy or find a way to relax, such as through yoga, massage, aromatherapy, and so forth. Also, manage your physical reaction to stress by stopping, breathing deeply, reflecting on the cause of stress, and choosing another way to react.

BUILD YOUR SKILLS *Managing Time to Reduce Your Stress*

Good time management skills can help you personally and professionally. These skills help you use time effectively; they keep you in charge of what's happening. By keeping things in perspective, these skills can increase your productivity. That means you can get your work done efficiently, and have more time to relax and enjoy life.

Time management starts with setting goals. These can be short-term, such as the stages and timeframe for getting a report done, or a long-term strategy, such as a timeframe for running for class president. Setting effective goals means that you state them positively, define them clearly and precisely, prioritize them, write them down, and make sure each goal is appropriate.

For example, you would *not* say: "Oh, I have to write my term paper by April 15." Instead, you would create a time management plan to meet that deadline. You would analyze and prioritize your work. And, of course, take into account your habits and preferences.

You might say: "My term paper is due on April 15. It is now April 1, so I have two weeks to finish it. Researching the topic is always the hardest part for me." Then, you would schedule the tasks that you must complete, make a daily *To Do* list, and plan your work. Here's how it might look:

- On April 1, I will create an outline.
- On April 2, I will review my outline with my teacher.
- From April 3–April 8, I will research my topic and take notes.
  - On April 3, I will use the school library.
  - On April 4, I will go to the public library and search online.
  - On April 5, I will conduct my interview.
  - On April 6 and 7, I will organize my notes.
  - On April 8, I will review my outline and notes to make sure I have no gaps.
- From April 9–11, I will write the first draft.
- From April 12–14, I will review and revise.

If you avoid distractions and concentrate on following your schedule, your term paper will be done on time—and you'll be able to take credit for a job well done.

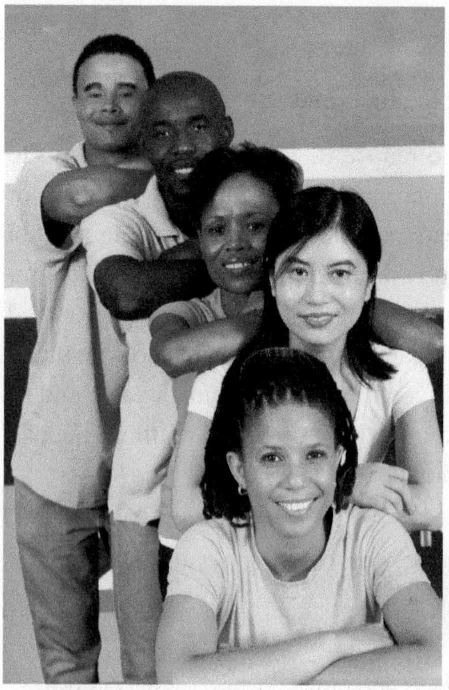

FIGURE 9.3

Enjoying friends and companionship supports good spiritual fitness

Source: michaeljung/Shutterstock

Spiritual Fitness

Spiritual fitness allows us to experience meaning and purpose in life. It provides a sense of comfort with others, creating greater acceptance of behaviors, attitudes, and beliefs. It includes:

- Enjoying companionship.
- Sharing ideas and thoughts.
- Having a sense of belonging.
- Showing enthusiasm for life.

Holistic health requires health care workers to promote physical, mental, and spiritual well-being. For example, a patient experiencing stomach pain may be referred to a psychologist if the physician suspects that the patient is under emotional stress. The psychologist may refer him to a biofeedback specialist for stress management. This process continues until the patient's needs are met in all areas.

THE MORE YOU KNOW

Illegal Drugs and Steroids

Illegal Drugs

Marijuana comes from the plant Cannabis sativa and is the most commonly used illegal drug in the United States. More than 83 million Americans have tried marijuana. However, dangers are associated with it. Like anything that is smoked, it can irritate a person's lungs. Smoking marijuana also impairs coordination and memory. Perhaps most importantly, possession of even small amounts of marijuana in the United States remains a crime. In 2010, 52% of all drug arrests were for marijuana.

Americans in large numbers use many other types of illegal drugs. Cocaine, derived from the coca plant of South America, is the most abused major stimulant in America. More than 2 million Americans use heroin despite the very real danger of death through overdose. Methamphetamines are a powerful stimulant that increases alertness and decreases appetite.

An assortment of so-called *club drugs* have also become popular in the last two decades, including Ecstasy, PCP, GHB, Rohypnol, ketamine, and LSD. Most of these drugs deliver a feeling of happiness, excitement, and energy. However, most of them are physically and/or psychologically addictive. Withdrawal symptoms can be particularly harrowing for some drugs such as heroin. In addition, prolonged use of any of them can lead to serious health problems including coronary problems, dangerously high blood pressure, and stroke.

Steroids

Anabolic steroids are artificial versions of the hormone testosterone. Testosterone brings out male sexual traits. Steroids are often used to treat delayed puberty and the wasting of the body caused by diseases. However, anabolic steroids also help the growth of skeletal muscle. For this reason, these compounds have been abused by bodybuilders, weightlifters, and athletes in many other sports.

By the 2000s, the use of steroids was becoming epidemic among college and high school athletes. In 2006, 1.6% of eighth graders and 2.7% of twelfth graders reported using steroids without a prescription at least once in their lifetimes.

Anabolic steroids can be injected, taken by mouth, or rubbed on the skin as gels or creams. Anabolic steroid abuse has been associated with a wide range of adverse side effects such as irritability, aggression, acne, breast development in men, liver cancer, and heart attacks. Most of the effects are reversible if the abuser stops taking the drug, but some can be permanent.

Alternative Health Care

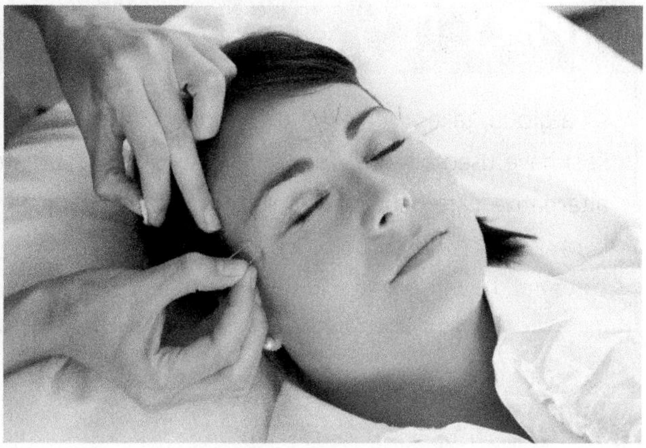

FIGURE 9.4

Undergoing an acupuncture treatment

Source: Tyler Olson/Shutterstock

The National Library of Medicine classifies alternative medicine as complementary therapy. These therapeutic practices are not currently considered an integral part of conventional medical practice. They do not follow generally accepted medical methods and may not have a scientific explanation for their effectiveness; they are unconventional. However, as researchers continue studying the effectiveness of many modalities, such as acupuncture, their use is becoming more widely accepted by the medical community. Other alternative therapies, such as humors or radium therapy, have become no more than historical footnotes. Therapies are considered *complementary* when used in addition to conventional treatments; they are considered *alternative* when used instead of conventional treatment.

Fundamental to alternative medical practice is a strong bond between patient and provider; they need to work as a team. These providers do not see themselves as the source of healing; patients must take active responsibility for their health and well-being. Initially, these therapies were used by individuals who had run out of other options—individuals with immune deficiencies, cancer, chronic back pain, arthritis, and other conditions. Today, more and more people are turning to alternative health care for wellness care. Some examples of alternative medicine include herbal medicine, acupuncture, yoga, massage therapy, and spiritual healing. For example, a woman with breast cancer chooses to treat her cancer by eating a special macrobiotic diet instead of having radiation and chemotherapy, which is the standard medical practice. Or, an elderly person with arthritis uses acupuncture to treat arthritis pain instead of taking medications.

The use of alternative medicine, of course, has its drawbacks. Many in the mainstream medical community believe that these alternative therapies, in conjunction with standard treatments, provide comfort for the patient. However, they argue that relying on these therapies alone and without doctor approval is dangerous and can even be fatal. The disease might be getting worse, even if the patient *feels better*, because it is not being adequately treated. Using herbs that are not FDA-approved may cause interactions with other medications or vitamins. It may be easier to overdose on a specific regimen that has not been adequately tested. Just because a product is *natural* does not mean it is safe. One example of this is the foxglove plant, an extract from which digitalis, a drug used to treat heart conditions, is produced. Foxglove, with unsupervised use, can also be a poison. Minimal, if any, regulations or federal guidelines are currently associated with alternative medicine. For example, over-the-counter herbs are not regulated, meaning the patient cannot be sure of any standard of preparation in their formulation. Finally, insurance companies may not cover alternative medical treatments unless they are used in conjunction with traditional therapies.

APPLY IT TAKING ADVANTAGE OF ALTERNATIVE HEALTH CARE

As a group, take a survey of the students in your class. How many of them (or their families) have used alternative medical treatments? Create a chart that shows the types of alternative care delivered—for example, chiropractic, acupuncture, aromatherapy, and hypnosis. List the purposes and benefits of each type of alternative care. Of the people surveyed, how many would be likely to try each alternative treatment again?

NUTRITION AND HEALTH

resistance
(ri-ZIS-tence) The ability of the body to protect itself from disease

malnutrition
(mal-new-TRISH-en) Poor nutrition caused by an insufficient or poorly balanced diet or by a medical condition

regulate
(RE-gyu-late) To control or adjust

Good nutrition promotes a healthier body and mind. It also aids in **resistance** to illness. When we eat a healthy diet, our energy and vitality are increased. The right foods speed the healing process and help a person feel better and sleep better. Good nutrition enhances your appearance and increases your stamina. It is important to plan meals and snacks that include all of the basic nutrients each day. Poor nutrition can lead to **malnutrition**.

Your patients are all from different cultural and religious backgrounds. Each culture and religion has dietary differences. Appetites, food budgets, cultural food preferences, and religious restrictions influence some of these differences. You and your patients need the same basic nutrients provided by a balanced, healthy diet. The health care worker must be knowledgeable about food choices and their effects on the body in order to assess his or her own diet and the patient's diet.

When food is taken into the body, it is used in many different ways. The right combination of nutrients work together in the body to:

- Provide heat.
- Repair tissue.
- Promote growth.
- **Regulate** body processes.

Essential Nutrients

Nutrients are chemical compounds found in food. When the food we eat enters the digestive tract, it is changed into a simple form and absorbed into the blood. The blood carries these nutrients to body cells, where they are used to maintain body functions. The body needs a certain amount of each nutrient to support good health. Too little of a nutrient causes a **deficiency**, and too much of a nutrient causes a **toxicity**. There is a range between the two that is optimal for most humans. Recommended Dietary Allowances (RDAs, also known as Recommended Daily Allowances) for each nutrient help you prevent diseases associated with getting too much or too little of a specific vitamin or nutrient.

Essential nutrients include **proteins**, **carbohydrates**, **fats**, **minerals**, **vitamins**, and water.

Proteins

- Build and renew body tissues.
- Provide heat energy.
- Help produce antibodies.
- Formed by organic compounds called **amino acids**.
- Made up of twenty-two amino acids; nine are essential, which means the body cannot produce them and they must be supplemented through the diet. They are found in almost all animal sources.
- Main sources of complete proteins: meat, fish, milk, cheese, and eggs.
- Incomplete proteins: cereal, soybeans, dry beans, peas, and peanuts.
- Complementary incomplete proteins can be combined to form complete proteins.
- Vegetarians combine foods to create complete proteins; for example, combining rice with red beans results in a complete protein.

Fats/Lipids

- Provide fatty acids for normal growth and development.
- Provide energy.
- Carry vitamins A and D to the cells.
- Help maintain body temperature by providing insulation; helps cushion organs and bones.
- Provide flavor to foods.
- Serve as an essential component of every cell membrane.
- Main sources: butter, margarine, oils, creams, fatty meats, cheeses, and egg yolk.
- Classified as saturated (solid at room temperature) or polyunsaturated (liquid at room temperature).

Minerals

- Regulate the activity of the heart, nerves, and muscles.
- Build and renew teeth, bones, and other tissues.
- Inorganic (non-living) elements found in all body tissue.
- More than 1/3 of the dietary nutrients needed each day are minerals.
- Major dietary minerals: calcium, chloride, magnesium, phosphorus, potassium, sodium, and sulfur.

nutrients
(NEW-tree-ents) Chemical compounds found in food

deficiency
(di-FIH-shen-see) A disease caused by lack of a nutrient

toxicity
(TAUK-sis-ih-tee) A disease caused by too much of a nutrient

essential
(i-SENT-shel) Necessary

proteins
(PRO-teen) Complex compounds found in plant and animal tissue, essential for heat, energy, and growth

carbohydrates
(CAR-bo-high-drates) Groups of organic compounds that include sugars, starches, celluloses, and gums that provide major sources of energy

fats
(FATS) Groups of organic compounds that, together with carbohydrates and proteins, constitute the primary structural material of living cells; also known as lipids

minerals
(MIN-rels) Inorganic elements that occur in nature; essential to every cell

vitamins
(VYE-the-mens) Groups of substances necessary for normal functioning and maintenance of health

amino acids
(eh-MEE-no AS-eds) Compounds found in living cells that contain carbon, oxygen, hydrogen, and nitrogen and join together to form proteins

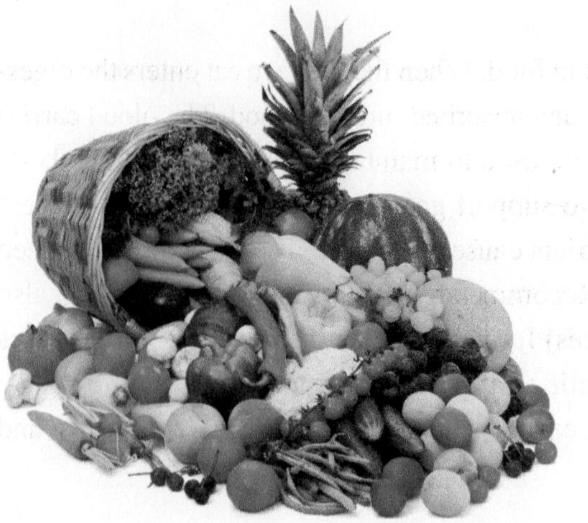

FIGURE 9.5

Fresh fruit and vegetables provide essential nutrients to support a healthy diet

Source: Tischenko Irina/Shutterstock

- Trace dietary minerals: chromium, copper, fluoride, iodine, iron, manganese, molybdenum, selenium, and zinc.

Vitamins

- Essential for normal metabolism, growth, and body development.
- Inorganic (non-living) elements found in all body tissues.
- Regulate the following body functions:
  - Help release energy from other nutrients (metabolism).
  - Play a vital role in almost every chemical reaction within the body.
  - Supply co-enzyme for normal health/growth (some behave like hormones).
- Only a small amount required; a well balanced diet provides required vitamins.
- Excess or deficiency can cause poor health.

Water

- Found in all body tissues; all cells in the body must be bathed in water.
- Makes up most of blood plasma; accounts for about 60% of an adult's body weight.
- Active in most chemical reactions; carries nutrients to the body cells and carries toxins and waste products away from the body cells.
- Lubricates the joints and helps regulate body temperature and body processes.
- Lost through evaporation, urination, and respiration so it must be replaced every day.
- Dehydration, or under-hydration, is when the body loses more water than it takes in; may occur during hot weather through profuse sweating or as a result of prolonged exertion; older people may not recognize dehydration because their bodies are not registering thirst, although thirst isn't the only sign.
- Over-hydration is when the body takes in more water than it loses; may occur in people whose kidneys do not excrete urine normally or in athletes who drink more water than they need when trying to avoid dehydration.
- The average person should drink 6–8 glasses of water daily.

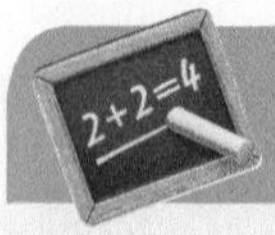

Math Link Liquid Conversions

Even after the United States became independent from England, its citizens continued to use the English system of measurement. This system had grown naturally for hundreds of years. People used familiar objects and parts of the body, such as *feet*, as measuring devices. They measured liquid volume with common household items such as teaspoons, cups, and pails (the word *gallon* comes from an old name for a pail). Although this system could be quite confusing, it is still used in the United States today.

The metric system was developed in France during the French Revolution in the 1790s. The metric system has several advantages over the English system. The metric system was based on a decimal system, which made it much easier to do calculations. The scientific community adopted the metric system almost from its inception. It came to be used by most other nations of the world.

The dual systems create problems for Americans. Liquid measurement seems to be an incomprehensible whirl of drams, milliliters, cups, and tablespoons. The situation is not helped by the fact that one cubic centimeter (cc) equals one milliliter (ml); they are the same. Here's a conversion chart to help you with trickier volume conversions:

- one teaspoon = 5 cc = 5 ml
- one tablespoon = three teaspoons
- one tablespoon = 15 cc = 15 ml
- one fluid ounce (U.S. liquid) = 30 cc = 30 ml
- 2 tablespoons = 6 teaspoons
- one cup = eight fluid ounces = 16 tablespoons
- one pint = 2 cups = 16 fluid ounces

Actually, one teaspoon equals 4.928921594 milliliters, but the chart has rounded it off to make things easier. Similarly, one fluid ounce (U.S.) equals 29.573529562 milliliters. Believe it or not, it actually makes a difference. At some point, *rounding off* errors would become serious. However, for the problems below, you can use the easier equivalents.

What is the volume in cc of 500 ml? The answer is 500 ml; they are equivalent amounts.

There are two bottles of electrolyte supplement on the shelf at the pharmacy. One contains 9.5 oz, and the other has 300 cc. Which has the larger volume?

1 fl. oz = 30

9.5 fl. oz = 285

The 300 cc bottle contains more liquid than the 9.5 oz. bottle.

Example 1

Billy must drink 2,250 cc of water each day. How many pints of water will he drink? Round to the nearest tenth of a pint.

1 pint = 16 oz.

1 oz = 30 cc

16 oz × 30 cc = 480 cc

2,250 cc divided 480 cc = 4.688 pints

4.7 pints

Example 2

Convert 55 tbsp into an equal volume of cups. Round to the nearest tenth of a cup.

1 cup = 6 tbsp

55 divided by 6 = 9.167 cups

9.2 cups

1. A dose of a specific medicine is 1 tbs. How many doses does an 8 oz bottle contain?
2. A bottle of juice contains 2 liters. If 1 liter equals 33.8 fl. oz, how many cc of juice are in the 2-liter bottle?
3. The humidifier for the nursing station holds 14 pints of water.
   a. How many ounces will completely fill the reservoir?
   b. How many 8-oz bottles will be needed to fill the reservoir?

U.S. fluid ounces and British fluid ounces are not the same volume. One British fluid ounce equals only 28.41 milliliters. *Why is this evidence that the metric system is easier to use than the English system of measurement?*

Fiber and Calories

cellulose
(SELL-you-lows) The primary component of plant cell walls, which provides the fiber and bulk necessary for optimal functioning of the digestive tract

Fiber adds bulk to the diet and helps prevent bowel and colon diseases. Cellulose is often referred to as dietary fiber or roughage. It is not digestible by humans and acts as a bulking agent by absorbing water; this helps to prevent constipation. The diet many people eat is high in protein, fats, and carbohydrates, but very low in fiber. To keep the bowel healthy, a person should eat several servings of fiber each day. Fiber is found in greens, kale, cabbage, celery, vegetable salads, raw and cooked fruits, whole-grain food, and cereals.

metabolize
(meh-TAB-oh-lize) To break down substances in cells to obtain energy

calorie
(KA-le-ree) Unit of measure of the fuel value of food

Food is the source of energy for our bodies. The body metabolizes food nutrients to create energy. As the body creates energy, it produces heat. Energy ensures that all of the body systems function. The amount of energy created by the food we eat is measured in calories. Calorie needs vary from person to person. A large, active person needs more calories than a smaller, inactive person does. Basal metabolic rate (BMR) is the amount of energy, or calories, your body uses when it is at rest in a neutral environment. BMR is usually calculated after twelve hours of fasting so that the body is not even using energy to digest food. Prior to calculating BMR, set the room temperature to a comfortable level to ensure that the environment is not hot or cold enough for the body to have to try and stay cool or warm.

The number of calories we eat and the amount of exercise we do balance our body weight. If we eat more calories than we burn, we gain weight. If we burn more calories than we eat, we lose weight. The FDA food labeling standard adopted the Recommended Dietary Allowances (RDAs) from the average USDA 2,000 calorie dietary guidelines. When a patient is inactive and feels ill, he or she may not want to eat. It is the health care worker's responsibility to encourage him or her to take in enough calories to produce the energy needed to heal the body.

Community Service Distributing Healthy Food

Volunteer at a local food distribution organization such as Meals on Wheels, the Salvation Army, or another group. Help the group plan and serve (or deliver) a well-balanced nutritious menu for one day. How does the organization make decisions about its menus? What factors are considered?

Digestion and Absorption

digestion
(dy-JES-chen) The process of making food absorbable by dissolving it and breaking it down into simpler chemical compounds that occur in the living body chiefly through the action of enzymes secreted into the alimentary canal

cholesterol
(keh-LES-the-ral) A type of lipid or fat found in the body; produced by the liver or eaten in food

Digestion is a complex process of turning the food we eat into the energy that we need to survive. Digestion begins before you even put food your mouth. When you smell, see, or think of food, saliva forms in your mouth. Saliva helps to break down the chemicals, specifically carbohydrates, in food. The tongue pushes food to the esophagus, which then carries the food to the stomach. The stomach acts as a mixer by grinding the food into smaller pieces and breaking down proteins which then go into the small intestine.

Cholesterol is often thought of only as a factor in heart disease. However, cholesterol is a component in digestion. It is a lipid made by the liver and, in addition to being involved in digestion, cholesterol is part of the transport process for nutrients. The job of the small intestine is to break the food down even more, so that the body can absorb all the vitamins, minerals, proteins, carbohydrates, and fats. This is the process of absorption. Although most nutrients are absorbed by the body, there is waste left. The waste travels through the colon where any excess water is absorbed, and the waste becomes solid. The solid waste, stool, then is excreted from the body.

The body gets the energy it needs from food through a process called metabolism. Metabolism is a constant process that occurs from the beginning of life to the end of life. The *Estimated Energy Requirement* (EER) is the average dietary energy intake that is predicted to maintain energy balance in a healthy adult. In other words, if the individual is currently a healthy weight, this amount of intake will cause him or her to maintain that healthy weight. EER deals with overall calorie intake; it does not specify which nutrients should comprise that total. The overall number of calories a person needs depends on his or her age, gender, weight, height, physical activity level, and health status. For many people, about 2,000 calories per day is the usual amount. However, in actual practice, this varies greatly from person to person.

absorption
(ab-SORP-shen) To take up liquid or other matter

excreted
(ik-SKRETED) When waste matter is discharged from the blood, tissues, or organs

metabolism
(meh-TAB-eh-lizm) Collection of chemical reactions that takes place in the body's cells to convert the fuel in food into energy

MyPlate

Good nutrition and a healthy diet help maintain good health. The U.S. Department of Agriculture (USDA) has provided MyPlate as a guideline. Using a *place setting* example, MyPlate illustrates the five food groups that your plate should contain. These dietary guidelines encourage people to eat more fruit and vegetables, whole grains, fat-free and low-fat dairy products, and seafood while reducing sodium, saturated and trans fats, refined grains, and added sugars. Reducing calories and increasing physical activity are also important aspects of the guidelines.

For more information about the USDA's new guidelines, go to www.choosemyplate.gov.

Follow these guidelines for yourself and your patients. The food choices of all cultures fit into these guidelines when you plan carefully.

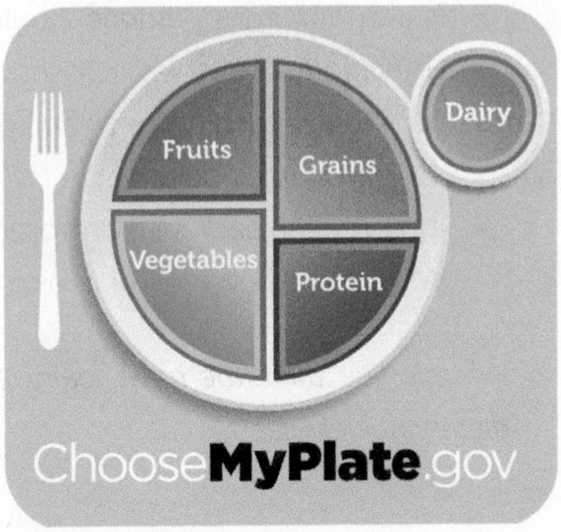

FIGURE 9.6

MyPlate from the U.S. Department of Agriculture

Consider This *The USDA's Dietary Guidelines*

The U.S. government has been issuing dietary recommendations for more than 100 years. In 1992, the USDA released a nutrition guide known as the American food pyramid. This illustration suggested how much of each food category a person should eat each day. Many nutritional experts, however, complained that the 1992 pyramid was not accurate based on the latest nutrition research. They believed it was heavy on beef and dairy and did not put enough emphasis on fruits and vegetables. For example, the food pyramid allowed some dietary choices that had been linked to heart disease, such as three cups of whole milk and an eight-ounce serving of hamburger every day. In addition, the pyramid lumped together all members of the protein-rich group ("Meat, Poultry, Fish, Dry Beans, Eggs, and Nuts") and made no distinction between whole grains and refined products. Many people complained that the USDA was influenced by corporate interests such as the dairy, meat, and sugar industries and had allowed lobbyists to change the wording of the guidelines.

As a result, in 2005, the USDA released a new nutritional guide known as MyPyramid. There were no foods pictured on the new MyPyramid image and no text. Instead, the new logo emphasized the importance of physical activity by showing a sort of stick figure climbing the stairs of the pyramid. MyPyramid was designed to be simple; colored vertical bands represented different food groups. Six bands of color ran from the top of MyPyramid to the base: orange for grains, green for vegetables, red for fruits, a tiny band of yellow for oils, blue for milk, and purple for meat and beans. Each stripe started out as the same size, but didn't end that way at the base. The widths suggested how much food a person should choose from each group.

In January 2011, the USDA released MyPlate as its latest effort to promote a healthy diet and to reduce obesity and the risk of chronic diseases. According to the USDA:

- Fruit and vegetables should cover half of your "plate," with grains and protein covering the other half.
- Half of the grains you consume should be whole grains.
- Eating seafood twice a week should provide your protein, along with beans, which are also a good source of fiber.
- Poultry and meat portions should be lean and small.
- Dairy products such as milk should be fat-free or low-fat (1%).
- Fatty foods, such as ice cream, pizza, hot dogs, and cookies, should be *treats* and not part of your daily diet.
- When eating packaged or frozen meals, choose low- or reduced-sodium options.
- Water is the beverage of choice as opposed to sugary drinks.

Why do you think the meat, dairy, and sugar industries would care about the USDA's dietary guidelines?

How Poor Nutrition Affects the Body

When we do not supply our bodies with the proper nutrients, many things can go wrong. We lose stamina and vitality. An unhealthy diet often results in illness and disease. Not having the proper nutrients for good health may come from either excessive or inadequate intake of essential nutrients. The following are a few of the problems that poor nutrition can cause:

hemoglobin
(HEE-meh-glow-ben)
Complex chemical in the blood; carries oxygen and carbon dioxide

- *Anemia,* a decreased number of red blood cells or a decreased amount of **hemoglobin**, results in:
  - Fatigue.
  - Headache.
  - Paleness.
  - Indigestion.
  - Rapid heartbeat.

- Insomnia (inability to sleep).
- Dyspnea (shortness of breath) on exertion.

- *Anorexia nervosa* occurs when a person refuses to eat or drastically reduces his or her intake of food. This disorder is related to an emotional disturbance about image (such as a person who is very underweight sees herself or himself as overweight). Anorexia nervosa is seen primarily in teenage girls. It results in:
  - Absence of menstrual periods.
  - Loss of teeth and hair.
  - Skeleton-like appearance.
  - Muscle spasms.
- *Bulimia* occurs when a person experiences intervals of food craving and **bingeing** and then **purging**. The side effects are the same as those of anorexia and result in depression.
- *Constipation* is infrequent, difficult defecation. It is commonly caused by lack of activity and by not eating enough vegetables, fruit, or water.
- *Dull hair and eyes* are symptoms of poor diet.
- *Mental slowdown* can occur when nutrition is poor.
- *Obesity* occurs when a person takes in more calories than the body uses. This results in increasing amounts of fatty tissue.
- *Osteoporosis* occurs when bones become porous, causing them to break easily. This is caused by inadequate calcium intake or absorption.
- *Rickets* is a softening of the bones in children, potentially leading to fractures and deformity. This occurs from a lack of vitamin D.
- *Dehydration* occurs when more water is lost than taken in. This can be caused by not drinking enough liquids, diarrhea, vomiting, excessive sweating, and some diseases such as diabetes.

bingeing
(BINJ-ing) Eating or drinking excessively

purging
(PERJ-ing) Causing oneself to vomit

Due to a variety of factors, malnutrition is prominent among the elderly population. As people age they experience sensory loss, especially in taste and smell, leading to decreased appetite. Dental problems may put the patient at risk because the patient will select foods high in carbohydrates and sugars, which are easier to chew. Another factor can be health issues that prevent the patient from obtaining food (grocery shopping) or preparing food (cooking). They may benefit from the home delivery of prepared meals or the purchase of pre-packaged meals which can be easily prepared in a microwave. The presence of disease in the elderly can also affect their dietary intake.

RECENT DEVELOPMENTS

Obesity in the United States

Americans, especially young people, are getting fatter. In the past 25 years, obesity has dramatically increased in the United States. In 1980, 25% of adults in the United States were overweight. By 1991, this figure had risen to 33%. In 2009, about two-thirds of the adult population, more than 120 million people, were classified as overweight.

In a way, the numbers are even bleaker for children. The number of overweight children between the ages of six and nineteen tripled between 1980 and 2004. An estimated 9 million children over the age of six (about 15%) are currently obese. About four out of every five of these obese children will remain overweight into adulthood.

What is so bad about being overweight? The answer is quite simple. Overweight and obese people have an increased risk for many diseases and health conditions such as the following:

- Hypertension (high blood pressure).
- Diabetes.
- Coronary heart disease.
- Stroke.
- Gallbladder disease.
- Sleep apnea and respiratory problems.
- Some cancers (endometrial, breast, and colon.)
- Osteoarthritis (a degeneration of cartilage and its underlying bone within a joint.)

The U.S. government estimates that the cost of obesity in the United States in 2011 was nearly $300 billion, considered one of the major health crises affecting the United States.

The solution to the problem is simple, but instituting it is not. People need to eat less, eat smarter, and exercise more. Fatty, sugary diets have contributed to growing waistlines. Fast food and junk food are not nutritionally sound. More than half of all Americans do not get the recommended amount of physical activity—thirty minutes daily for adults; sixty minutes daily for children. Children spend more time staring at television and computer screens than they do in physical play, devoting about 55 hours per week to watching television, texting, or playing video games. Both children and adults need to limit their time in front of the television or computer and follow the recommendations of the new dietary guidelines.

Eating Disorders

Eating disorders are not due to a failure of will. They are real and treatable medical illnesses. The three main types of eating disorders are anorexia nervosa, bulimia, and binge-eating. All three can affect a person's health including causing serious heart conditions, kidney failure, and electrolyte imbalance. The cause of eating disorders is not entirely clear. They seem to have a basis in biology but they are also affected by emotions, genes, and culture.

Eating is controlled by many factors, including a person's appetite; food availability; family, peer, and cultural practices; and attempts at voluntary control. An eating disorder involves a serious disturbance in eating behavior, such as extreme reduction of food intake, severe overeating, or intentional vomiting. Eating disorders frequently develop during adolescence or early adulthood and often occur in conjunction with other problems, such as depression, substance abuse, and anxiety disorders.

Women and girls are much more likely than men to develop an eating disorder. Women's magazines, fashion trends, and some activities and professions promote dieting

FIGURE 9.7

Depression may lead to an eating disorder

Source: Trish Gant/Dorling Kindersley Limited

to achieve the *perfect* lean body. This can lead to pressure on women to be thin. Eating disorders are sometimes triggered by the stress of being unable to reach an unattainable goal. Males make up only about 10% of people with anorexia or bulimia.

Anorexia Nervosa

People with *anorexia nervosa* see themselves as overweight and have an immense fear of becoming fat even though they are dangerously thin. People with anorexia may repeatedly check their body weight or exercise compulsively. People with anorexia are often perfectionists. They are driven to succeed, but cannot achieve the unattainable standards they set for themselves. When they fail to meet these standards, they often look for a part of their lives they can control such as food intake or weight. In addition, many athletes have eating disorders. For them, eating becomes an obsession. They develop unusual eating habits such as avoiding meals, eating only a few foods in small quantities, or carefully weighing food.

Bulimia Nervosa and Binge-Eating Disorder

Bingeing means eating an excessive amount of food within a short period of time. Bulimia sufferers have recurring episodes of binge eating. They usually feel unable to control their appetite during a bingeing episode. Afterwards, they try desperately to compensate in order to avoid gaining weight. A person with bulimia might engage in inappropriate behavior known as *purging*, brought on by self-induced vomiting, or misuse of laxatives, diuretics, or other medications. Because purging follows the binge-eating episodes, people with bulimia usually have a *normal* weight for their age and height. However, like people with anorexia, people with bulimia often feel extremely dissatisfied with their bodies. They might also feel disgusted and ashamed when they binge and perform both bingeing and purging behavior in secret.

Binge-eating disorder is similar to bulimia, but without the purging. Therefore, many people with the disorder are overweight for their age and height. The out-of-control eating may be associated with eating rapidly, eating until feeling uncomfortably full, or eating large amounts when not feeling hungry. Binge-eaters often feel embarrassed, depressed, or guilty after overeating. This can lead to overeating again, creating a cycle of binge eating.

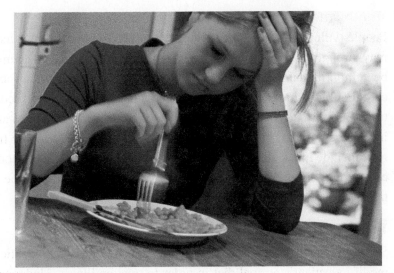

Treatment

People with eating disorders often do not recognize or admit that they are ill. They may strongly resist getting and staying in treatment. Family members or friends can be helpful in making sure that a person with an eating disorder receives the necessary care. Eating disorders can be treated and a healthy weight restored. The sooner a doctor diagnoses and treats these disorders, the better the outcomes are likely to be. Eating disorders often have multiple causes and require a complex treatment plan. This may include medical care, psychological treatment, nutritional counseling, and medication. Ongoing research by scientists continues to advance the understanding and treatment of eating disorders.

Therapeutic Diets

Some patients have illnesses that require special diets. Therapeutic diets are diets that modify a patient's normal diet in order to treat an illness. Understanding why the diet has been changed helps you to encourage patients to eat the food prepared for them. When you are knowledgeable about their diet, you are able to explain how important it is to their recovery.

Therapeutic diets are given to:

- Regulate the amount of food in metabolic disorders.
- Prevent or restrict edema (swelling) by restricting sodium intake.
- Assist body organs to regain and/or maintain normal function.
- Aid in digestion by avoiding foods that irritate the digestive tract.
- Increase or decrease body weight by adding or eliminating calories.

Examples of therapeutic diets include:

- ***Clear liquid.*** Replaces liquids lost from vomiting, diarrhea, or surgery.
- ***Full liquid.*** Provides nutrition for patients who have difficulty chewing or swallowing.
- ***Soft.*** Provides nutrition for patients who have trouble chewing after surgery.
- ***Bland.*** Soothes the gastrointestinal tract and avoids irritation in ulcers or other conditions.
- ***Restricted residue.*** Reduces the normal work of the intestines in cases of rectal diseases.
- ***Low carbohydrate.*** Matches food intake with insulin uptake and nutritional requirements for diabetics.
- ***Low fat.*** Provides nutrition for patients with gallbladder and liver disease, obesity, and heart conditions.
- ***Low cholesterol.*** Regulates the amount of cholesterol in the blood for patients with coronary disease and atherosclerosis (hardening of the arteries).
- ***Low calorie.*** Reduces the number of calories for overweight patients and for people with arthritis and cardiac conditions.
- ***High calorie.*** Increases caloric intake for patients who are 10% or more below desired weight.
- ***Low sodium.*** Reduces salt intake for patients with kidney disease, hypertension, and so on.
- ***High protein.*** Provides protein for children and adolescents who need additional protein for growth, and during pregnancy and **lactation**.

lactation
(lak-TAY-shen) The female body's process of producing milk to feed newborn babies

When a patient is put on a therapeutic diet, it's especially important to remember the factors that influence food habits: personal attitudes and preferences, nationality, race, and religious needs. A therapeutic diet is often very different from the foods the patient normally eats. Your understanding of the reason for the diet and your patients' special needs helps ease their concerns. In many situations, a dietitian will speak with the patient and try to adapt a therapeutic diet to meet his or her nutritional and personal needs.

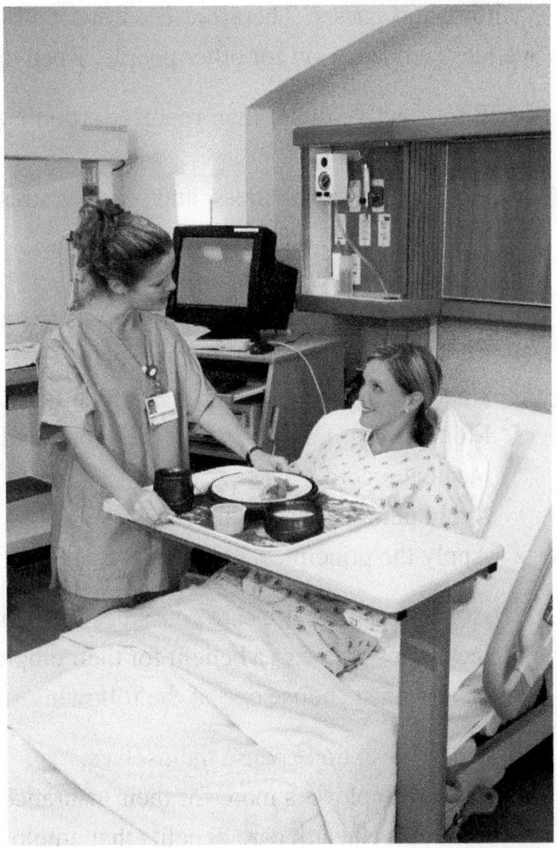

FIGURE 9.8

Explaining the therapeutic benefits of the patient's special diet

Source: Thinkstock/Corbis Images

An example of a special or personal need is religious restrictions. Many religions of the world follow specific dietary laws. These guidelines are very important to patients. When patients are on a therapeutic diet, the stress caused by breaking the dietary law may cause added worry. Always be respectful of dietary requests and report them to the appropriate person.

Language Arts Link Dietary Careers

Proper nutrition is vital for both health care workers and their patients. As many Americans fail to follow a healthy diet, the roles of dietary workers are becoming increasingly important to the population's health. Dietary professionals include registered dietitians, dietetic technicians, and food service workers.

Research a dietary career. Using the Internet or a library, investigate the education and skills required and identify different employment options. After you've completed your research, create a report to share what you have learned. Be sure to proofread your work to see if you can improve it by making it clearer, more concise, or more interesting to read. Check the spelling and grammar and correct any errors.

HEALTH AND WELLNESS FOR HEALTH CARE WORKERS

Health care is one of most physically demanding, emotionally draining, and stress-producing industries in which to work. Meeting the needs of patients, operating high tech equipment, dealing with lean staffing, adhering to tight schedules, and handling life and death situations can result in high levels of stress. Lifting patients and heavy objects can cause back injuries, and employees can catch infectious diseases from patients, visitors, and guests. Therefore it's important to pay attention to your own health and wellness while caring for other people. Keep the following in mind:

proactive
(pro-AK-tiv) Anticipating and acting in advance

reactive
(ree-AK-tiv) Responding to something that has happened

- Be proactive rather than reactive—don't wait to discuss any health concerns with your physician.
- Watch for signs of stress, and practice stress management techniques.
- Practice safe lifting techniques.
- Keep your vaccinations up-to-date.
- Comply with policies and procedures to guard against infectious disease.
- Maintain adequate health insurance.
- Undergo an annual physical exam and health screenings; follow-up on the results.
- Monitor your family's medical history, and make sure it's part of your personal medical record.
- Avoid taking unnecessary risks.
- Apply the principles of workplace safety.

As the cost of health care continues to rise in the United States, employers who provide health insurance as a benefit for their employees are experiencing financial distress. Employers must choose one of the following strategies:

- Cover the extra expense themselves.
- Charge employees more for their insurance coverage.
- Reduce the health care benefits that employees receive.

When you stop to think about it, health care organizations are employers, too. They must also figure out how to handle the rising cost of health insurance for their employees.

These financial pressures have resulted in a variety of programs to encourage employees to become healthier. In some health care organizations, employees get a discount on their health insurance when they meet certain health indicators. In other organizations, employees are charged higher rates for their health insurance if they fail to meet certain health indicators. Either way you look at it, these financial incentives are generating some visible improvements in the way health care workers manage their own health and wellness.

Health care organizations want their employees to set a good example for patients and the community when it comes to health and wellness. Many employers now offer *wellness tracks* that include free:

health risk assessments
(HELTH risk a-SES-ment) Questionnaires that identify which health issues a person needs to focus on based on his or her medical history and lifestyle

body mass index
(BAA-dee mass IN-dex) Measure of body fat based on height and weight for adult men and women

- Health risk assessments.
- Health screenings to measure body mass index (BMI), blood pressure, blood glucose, and cholesterol levels.
- Exercise, nutrition, weight loss, smoking cessation, and stress management classes.
- Coaching and support provided by wellness counselors.

Health care organizations are offering healthier food in their cafeterias and vending machines, setting aside bicycle and walking paths on their campuses, planting gardens to provide fresh produce, and offering employee discounts on memberships at local fitness clubs. Some health care employers provide an Employee Assistance Program (EAP) to help workers deal with personal problems such as alcohol and drug abuse, financial and legal issues, interpersonal difficulties, mental health concerns, and stress and burnout. EAP counselors can refer workers to community resources such as day care and elder care facilities, free or reduced-cost legal aid, and public assistance agencies. Even though EAP services are free to employees, people may resist taking advantage of them. Workers may fear being stigmatized as *needing help* or may deny that they suffer from an addiction.

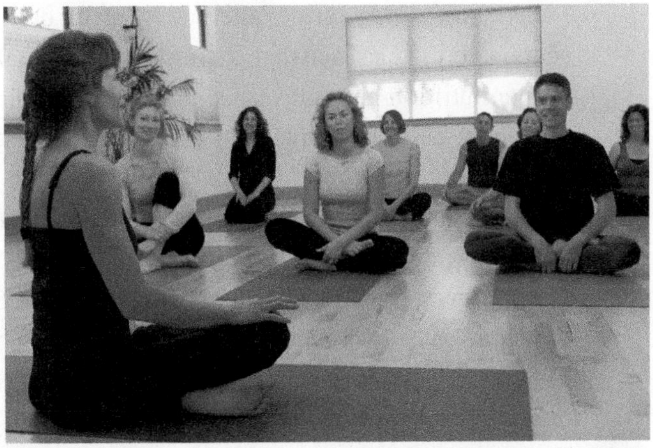

FIGURE 9.9

Participating in a yoga class as part of an employer-sponsored wellness track

Source: Pete Saloutos/Shutterstock

All of this attention on the health and wellness of employees is good news for health care workers who recognize the connection between a healthy personal life and a healthy professional life.

REALITY CHECK

Your health care education and training will provide the knowledge and skills you need to support the health and wellness of your patients. But it's up to you to protect, maintain, and improve your own health. How healthy are you? What lifestyle factors are affecting your health and wellness? Are you physically, mentally, and spiritually fit? Do you eat a healthy diet and avoid the dangers of smoking, alcohol, and drugs? Do you get a physical exam every year and undergo health screenings? Are you aware of your family's medical history and taking proactive steps to watch for similar signs and symptoms yourself? Or, are you taking unnecessary risks such as binge drinking, driving drunk, having unprotected sex, or texting while behind the wheel?

Many young people tend to think they are invincible, and that health problems and diseases are for *old people*. Nothing could be further from the truth. If you're serious about pursuing a career in health care, it's never too early to start focusing on your own health and wellness.

invincible
(in-VIN-she-bel) Incapable of being overcome

Key Points

- Health and wellness require a balance among mind, body, spirit, and social involvement.
- The holistic approach to health includes all aspects of a person's well-being.
- Health screenings offer a preventive approach to health and wellness.
- To be healthy, a person must have physical fitness, mental fitness, and spiritual fitness.
- Physical fitness results from regular exercise, a proper diet, and sufficient rest.

- Many patients now turn to alternative health care, including herbal medicine, acupuncture, yoga, massage therapy, and spiritual healing.
- Proper nutrition promotes a healthy body and mind and helps protect against illness; poor nutrition can lead to malnutrition and a variety of diseases and abnormalities.
- Good nutrition requires the proper amount of vitamins, minerals, carbohydrates, proteins, and fats.
- Water is an essential nutrient, accounting for about 60% of an adult's body weight.
- Watching calories and getting plenty of exercise help balance a person's weight.
- The USDA's MyPlate serves as a guideline for healthy eating.
- Elderly people are susceptible to malnutrition for a variety of reasons.
- Therapeutic diets help patients overcome nutrition-related diseases and health issues.
- Working in health care can be physically demanding, emotionally draining, and stressful.
- Like other types of employers, health care organizations are struggling with the rising cost of health care and health insurance.
- Health care employers are implementing wellness tracks and other types of programs and services to help improve the health and well-being of their workers.

Section Review Questions

Answer each of the following questions. Indicate which page in the textbook led you to your answer.

1. List three parts of holistic health.
2. What are five ways to achieve physical fitness?
3. What is body mass index and how is it measured?
4. Describe the role of alternative health care.
5. What three factors influence a person's food habits?
6. List five basic nutrients and explain how they maintain body function.
7. Give three examples of therapeutic diets.
8. Explain why health care employers are implementing programs to improve the health and wellness of their workers.

Learn By Doing

Complete Worksheets 1–5 in Section 9.1 of your *Student Activity Guide*.

SECTION 9.2 Infection Control and Safety at Work

Background

Health care workers are responsible for following infection control and safety precautions to protect themselves, coworkers, patients, and visitors from preventable infections and injuries. The health care environment contains larger numbers of microorganisms than most other environments. Workers must acquire the knowledge and skills required to restrict the spread of pathogenic microorganisms, practice good aseptic technique, and follow Standard Precautions.

Workers must follow Occupational Safety and Health Administration (OSHA) rules and their employer's policies and procedures for safe practices. If you or your employer fails to provide appropriate safety for all workers and patients, OSHA will penalize your employer with a large fine or lock the doors of the facility until the safety violation is corrected. If you are at fault for not providing safe conditions, you could lose your job.

Disasters can occur anywhere and at any moment, and workers must respond quickly according to their facility's disaster plan. A disaster is anything that causes damage and injury to a group of people, including floods, earthquakes, tornados, explosions, fires, and bioterrorism.

Health care workers lift, move, and carry many different objects and patients. It is important to use ergonomic practices and proper body mechanics when you are lifting or moving anything. Ergonomic practices prevent both fatigue and injury.

When employees apply infection control and safety procedures at work, everyone in the facility benefits.

pathogenic
(path-eh-JEH-nik)
Disease-causing

aseptic technique
(ay-SEP-tik tek-NEEK)
Method used to make the environment, the worker, and the patient as germ-free as possible

Standard Precautions
(STAN-derd pre-CAW-shens)
Guidelines designed to reduce the risk of transmission of microorganisms from recognized and unrecognized sources of infection in the hospital

ergonomic
(er-geh-NAW-miks) An object or practice designed to reduce injury

Objectives

After completing this section, you will be able to:

1. Define the key terms.
2. Differentiate between *pathogenic* and *nonpathogenic* microorganisms.
3. List five ways to prevent the spread of microorganisms and viruses.
4. Define *medical asepsis* and list five aseptic techniques.
5. List three ways by which bloodborne diseases are accidentally passed.
6. Describe the purpose of Universal Precautions.
7. Define *OSHA* and explain the agency's role in safety.
8. Explain the health care worker's role in maintaining a safe workplace.
9. Identify five general safety rules.
10. Identify what you are responsible for knowing and doing when a disaster occurs.
11. List the three elements required to start a fire, and four ways to prevent fires.
12. List six rules of correct body mechanics.
13. Demonstrate the correct techniques for lifting and moving objects.

CONTROLLING INFECTION

Controlling infection is a critical component of safety in the health care workplace. In order to prevent patients and workers from acquiring infections in hospitals and other health care facilities, workers must understand the nature of microorganisms, how they affect the body, how microorganisms and viruses spread, and how to protect people from infection.

The Nature of Microorganisms and Viruses

People are surrounded by tiny microorganisms and viruses. They are in the air you breathe, on your skin, in your food, and on everything you touch. You cannot see

viruses
(VIE-res-ez) Genetic material that is surrounded by a protective coat and that can only reproduce inside a host cell; can only be seen under a microscope

these organisms and viruses without a microscope because they are so small. Viruses are much smaller than microorganisms, so stronger microscopes are used to look at viruses.

Some microorganisms and viruses cause illness, infection, or disease and are called pathogenic. Some microorganisms help keep a balance in the environment and in the body. These microorganisms are called **nonpathogenic**. Viruses do not have all of the characteristics of living organisms. For example, viruses do not eat. They also cannot reproduce on their own. So, unlike microorganisms, viruses are not considered *living*. For microorganisms to live, they must have certain elements in their environment. Some organisms require oxygen in order to survive. These are called *aerobic*. Other microorganisms live in an environment without oxygen. These are called **anaerobic**.

nonpathogenic (non-path-eh-JEH-nik) Not disease-causing

anaerobic (a-ne-ROW-bik) Able to grow and function without oxygen

Most microorganisms that cause illness thrive in warm temperatures—about the same temperature as the human body. All organisms need moisture, and most microorganisms prefer a dark area in which to grow. Microorganisms also need food to survive. Some of these organisms live on dead matter or tissues and are called **saprophytes**. Other organisms that live on living matter or tissues are called **parasites**.

saprophytes (SAP-re-fites) Organisms that live on dead organic matter

parasites (PAIR-eh-sites) Organisms obtaining nourishment from other organisms they are living in or on

Nonpathogenic Microorganisms

Many microorganisms are not disease causing. These nonpathogenic microorganisms are *good* microorganisms that are used in different ways. For example, these microorganisms can be used to make buttermilk, ferment grain for alcoholic beverages, make bread rise, and so on. Many nonpathogenic organisms also **decompose** organic materials in nature.

decompose (dee-kom-POZE) To decay, to break down

In the body, nonpathogenic microorganisms work in the digestive system to break down the food elements that the body cannot use. This broken down food is eventually eliminated as a part of **feces**. Nonpathogenic microorganisms also help control the growth of pathogenic organisms.

feces (FEE-seez) Solid waste that is evacuated from the body through the anus; also known as stools

Pathogenic Microorganisms and Viruses

Health care workers must be aware of the different kinds of pathogens that cause disease. There are several kinds of disease-causing microorganisms: **bacteria**, protozoa, fungi, and **rickettsiae**. Viruses are also pathogens.

bacteria (bak-TIR-ee-a) A disease-causing microorganism

rickettsiae (ri-KET-see-eh) Parasitic microorganisms that live on another living organism and cause disease

- ***Bacteria.*** Bacteria are responsible for many diseases. For example, strep throat is caused by streptococci; staph infection is caused by staphylococci, and syphilis is caused by **spirochetes**. These are only a few of the diseases that bacteria cause.

spirochetes (SPY-reh-keets) Slender, coil-shaped organisms

Staphylococcus and streptococcus are organisms that are always present in health care environments. Staphylococcus (staph) infections can have a serious impact on patients, caregivers, and families. An uncontrolled or untreated staph infection in a newborn nursery, for example, can cause infants to die. People who have a stressed immune system have trouble fighting a staph infection and may die.

Hospital stays are prolonged because of staph infections. Staph is usually the cause of pimples or boils found on the skin. All drainage from a pimple or boil should be handled according to Standard Precautions to prevent the spread of infection. Patients who have staph infections are always treated with Standard Precautions.

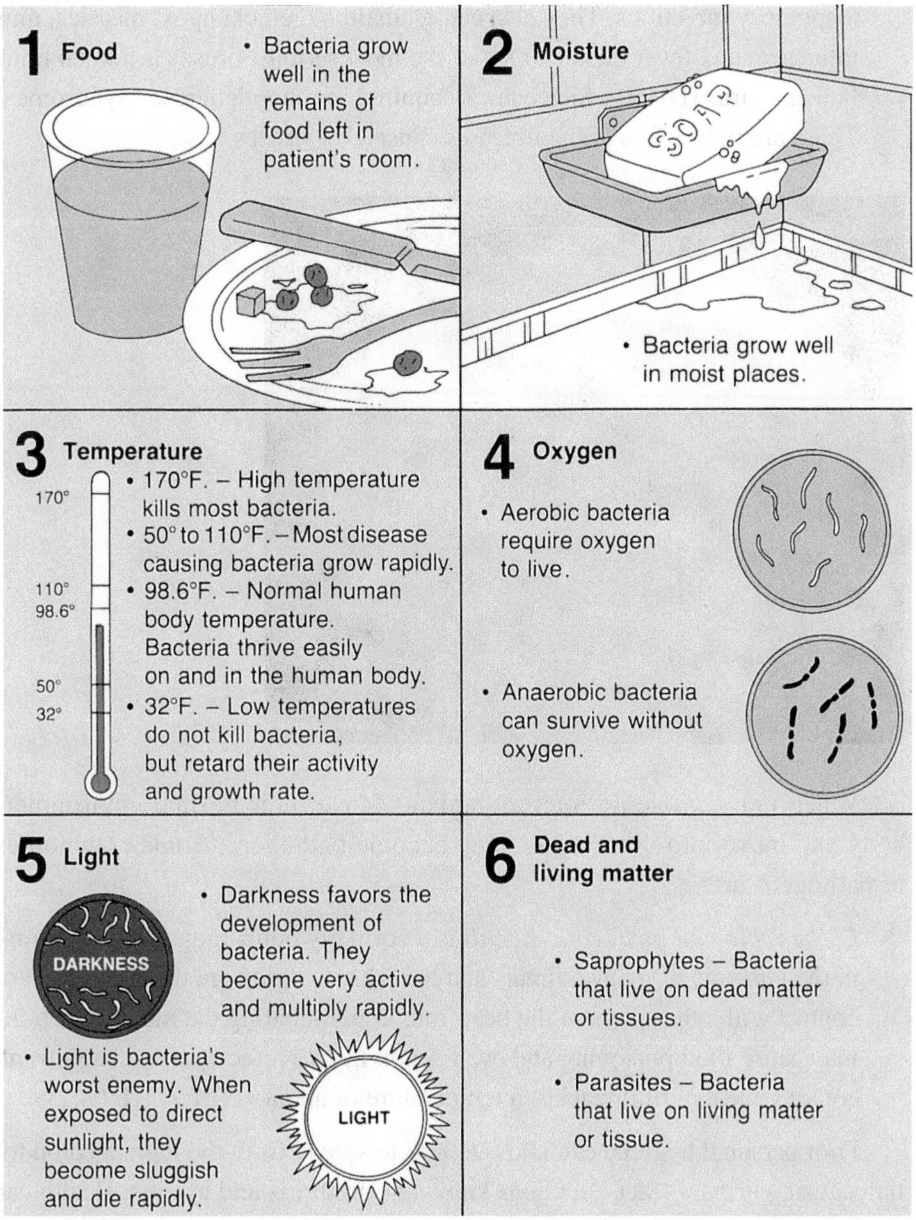

FIGURE 9.10

Conditions which affect the growth of bacteria

- ***Protozoa.*** Protozoa are larger than viruses but also grow within a host cell. They cause trichomoniasis, amebic dysentery, and malaria. Most protozoa are too small to be seen with the naked eye, but can easily be found under a microscope. Protozoa are found in water and soil environments and play an important role in their ecology.
- ***Fungi.*** Microscopic fungi include molds and yeasts. Some fungi can cause disease, such as athlete's foot, thrush, vaginitis, and serious lung diseases.
- ***Rickettsiae.*** Rickettsiae are parasites that live in lice, fleas, ticks, and mites. When one of these organisms is infected with rickettsiae, the disease is transferred to a person after he or she is bitten. Rickettsiae are responsible for many of the world's worst epidemics, including various types of typhus and spotted fever. Rodent and insect control helps prevent rickettsiae infection.
- ***Viruses.*** Viruses are much smaller than bacteria. They cannot reproduce until they have taken over a living cell. Viruses cause the common cold and many upper

host
(HOSTE) The organism from which a microorganism takes nourishment; the microorganism gives nothing in return and causes disease or illness

respiratory infections. They also cause smallpox, chickenpox, measles, mumps, influenza, and fever blisters. One of the most serious viruses is human immunodeficiency virus (HIV), which causes acquired immunodeficiency syndrome (AIDS). These are only a few of the illnesses caused by viruses.

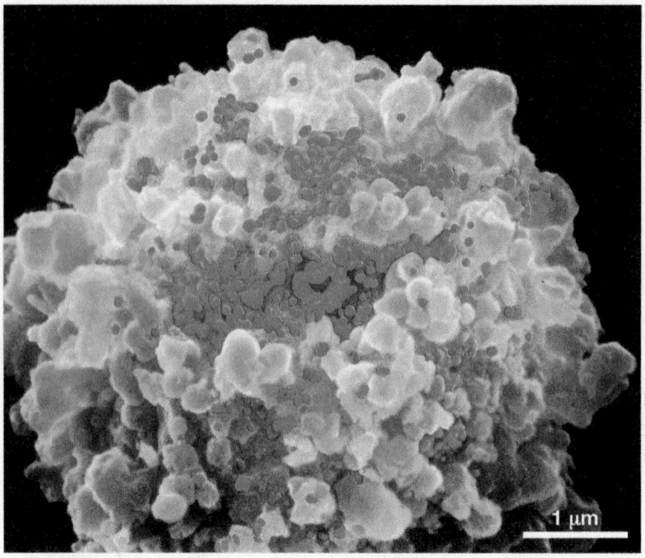

FIGURE 9.11

The human immunodeficiency virus (HIV)

Source: NIBSC/Science Photo Library/ Photo Researchers, Inc.

When nonpathogenic microorganisms leave their normal environment in the body and move into other areas, they become pathogens. Some common examples of pathogens are:

- *Escherichia coli* **or** *E. coli.* *E. coli* is a normally nonpathogenic bacterium found in the intestine of many animals and humans. *E. coli* from the colon can come in contact with other parts of the beef, thus contaminating the meat. *E. coli* infections may cause food poisoning and even death. *E. coli* infections can be prevented by cooking meat until it reaches a temperature of about 160°F (71.1°C).

Poor personal hygiene can allow *E. coli* to spread from the human colon to the urethra causing urinary tract infections known as urethritis and cystitis. Health care workers who have dirty hands—especially hands that are not washed after using the toilet—can spread *E. coli* to patients' food or onto equipment used to provide care.

salmonella
(sal-meh-NEL-a) A rod-shaped bacterium found in the intestine that can cause food poisoning, gastroenteritis, and typhoid fever

- **Salmonella.** Salmonella infections are caused by bacteria. Salmonella infections may cause food poisoning or death. Salmonella infections can be caused by eating chicken that is undercooked or from eating foods that contain raw eggs. Salmonella can also be spread to food when food service workers do not wash their hands. Salmonella is also spread when cooking utensils or surfaces are not cleaned properly after preparing raw meat, chicken, or egg dishes in particular.

Acute infections occur suddenly or last a short time. Chronic infections happen slowly over a long period of time and may last months, or even years. Infections are caused by pathogens and fall into two groups: *endogenous* and *exogenous*. An endogenous infection grows or develops from within an organism, tissue, or cell when an individual is in an already weakened state. An endogenous infection is caused by an infectious agent already present in the body, with the previous infection having been dormant or non-apparent.

An exogenous infection originates from outside the body. Examples of exogenous infections include salmonella poisoning after eating an uncooked egg or poultry, catching a cold after eating off of someone else's fork, or contracting rabies after getting bit by a dog.

An opportunistic infection occurs when there is weakness or compromise in the immune defenses of an individual. Opportunistic infections may be caused by bacteria, fungi, viruses, or parasites. These infections can be fought off by people with strong immune systems; however, they can be fatal for AIDS patients.

How Microorganisms Affect the Body

Pathogens cause disease in several different ways. Some microorganisms produce **toxins** that affect the body. For instance, staphylococcus produces an **enterotoxin** that is the cause of food poisoning. The toxin causes fatigue, diarrhea, and vomiting. The tetanus bacilli produce a toxin that enters the bloodstream and attacks the central nervous system, causing severe damage and frequently death.

Some microorganisms and all viruses invade living cells and destroy them; this is called *cell invasion*. For example, there is a **protist** that invades the red blood cells of the host. As the protists grow, the cells rupture and cause chills and fever. The presence of some microorganisms causes a violent *allergic reaction* in the body. A runny nose, watery eyes, and sneezing can be caused by the presence of a microorganism to which the host is allergic.

toxins
(TOK-sens) Poisonous substances

enterotoxin
(en-te-row-TOK-sen) Poisonous substance that is produced in, or originates in, the contents of the intestine

protist
(PRO-tist) An organism belonging to the kingdom that includes protozoans, bacteria, and single-celled algae and fungi

contaminated
(ken-TA-me-nate-ed) Soiled, unclean, not suitable for use

Science Link — Prions

Unlike bacteria, protists, and fungi, viruses are not living organisms. Another type of nonliving pathogen is called a *prion*. Prions are infectious protein molecules. Prions are a defective version of a protein found in normal brain cells. They cause several brain diseases, including Creutzfeld-Jakob disease and mad cow disease.

Unlike viruses and microorganisms, prions do not replicate themselves. So, how do they infect people and animals? According to one theory, the prion is taken into the body. In the case of mad cow disease, humans eat infected beef. The prions enter brain cells, and the cells begin producing the prion instead of the normal protein. This happens because the prion comes in contact with normal proteins. The normal proteins become prions, which in turn spread to other cells.

Prions cause the death of the brain cells that send signals to and from the body. Over time, the cell death keeps the body from sending signals to and from the brain. So, the body stops functioning properly, eventually leading to death.

Prion infections are rare. In the case of mad cow disease, they can be prevented by avoiding raw meat, especially meat that has been or may have been **contaminated** with the prion. Other prion diseases are transmitted by contaminated equipment used during medical procedures. Proper cleaning and sterilization of equipment prevents the spread of prions. Some prion diseases are inherited, so little action can be taken to prevent the disease.

Proteins are *denatured*, or inactivated, by heat. *How does this reaction to heat apply to the prevention of prion infection?*

How Microorganisms and Viruses Spread

Now that you have a basic knowledge of microorganisms and viruses, you need to know how they are spread and how they enter the body. This helps you protect yourself and your patients from infection.

susceptible
(se-SEP-the-bel) Capable of being affected or infected; the body can be attacked by microorganisms and become ill

chain of infection
(CHAYN of in-FEK-shen) A chain of events, all interconnected, is required for an infection to spread

For microorganisms or viruses to cause disease or infection, they must have a **susceptible** host. This host is unable to fight off infection because its resistance to the pathogen is low. Low resistance may be caused by poor diet, fatigue, inadequate rest, stress, or poor health. A model used to understand the infection process is the **chain of infection**. This model represents each component in the cycle. Each component must be present and in sequential order:

- Infectious agent
- Reservoir
- Portal of exit from the reservoir
- Mode of transmission
- Portal of entry into the susceptible host

Understanding the characteristics of each link provides the health care professional with methods to support vulnerable patients, prevent the spread of infection, and protect themselves.

There are five ways that microorganisms and viruses are spread:

- *Direct contact.* Occurs when organisms or viruses are transmitted directly from one person to another. Examples include:
  - Physical contact by touch on open or closed skin or a body opening.
  - Sexual contact.
  - Breathing in pathogens directly from an infected person.

  Prevention guidelines include:

  - Abstain from sex.
  - Do not drink or eat from dishes or utensils used by another person.
  - Stay an appropriate distance away from individuals who are coughing or sneezing.
  - Do not, without proper protection, touch objects used by someone who has an infection.
- *Indirect contact.* Occurs when organisms or viruses are transferred from one object to another. Examples include:
  - Contaminated substances and objects, such as food, air, soil, feces, clothing, and equipment.

  Prevention guidelines include:

  - Do not, without proper protection, touch objects used by someone who has an infection.
  - Hold contaminated linen, belongings, or other items, away from your uniform.
- *Airborne.* Some microorganisms and viruses are carried in the air. Coughing and sneezing project droplets into the air, and these droplets are carried on air currents until they find a place to land. The droplets cling to hair, uniforms, and medical equipment, or they fall on the floor. As you move from place to place, you may spread these pathogens. Examples include:
  - Influenza (the flu)
  - Chickenpox
  - Wound infections

Prevention guidelines include:

- Keep your hair short or tied back so that it does not swing around, spreading microorganisms.
- Cover your mouth and nose with your sleeve when you sneeze or cough, and then wash your hands.
- Change out of your uniform after working and before going anywhere other than home.
- Consider anything dropped on the floor as contaminated, and DO NOT USE IT.
- Stay home when you are sick with an acute respiratory infection.

- ***Oral Route.*** Microorganisms or viruses enter the body through the mouth by way of contaminated water and food, dirty hands, and from other contaminated objects. Examples include:
  - Food poisoning
  - Polio
  - Hepatitis
  - Salmonellosis
  - Typhoid fever

  Prevention guidelines include:
  - Wash your hands before eating or handling food, after using the toilet, and before and after helping patients.
  - Refrigerate food properly to prevent contamination and microorganism growth.
  - Dispose of wound drainage promptly and according to policy.

- ***Insects and Pests.*** Organisms or viruses are picked up by insects and other pests from contaminated areas and carried to water, food, and people. Examples include:
  - Bubonic plague
  - Malaria
  - Amebic dysentery

  Prevention guidelines include:
  - Keep all flies and insects out of the environment.
  - Report insects or pests immediately.

FIGURE 9.12

Surgical hand washing, also known as a sterile scrub, to reduce microorganisms and the possibility of cross-infection among staff and patients

Source: Tyler Olson/Shutterstock

Fallacies of Disease Transmission

In the nineteenth and twentieth centuries, developments such as the culture plate method of identifying disease-causing organisms, pasteurization, vaccines, antiseptics, and asepsis dramatically lowered the incidence of disease. A common fallacy, however, is to think that an infectious disease is

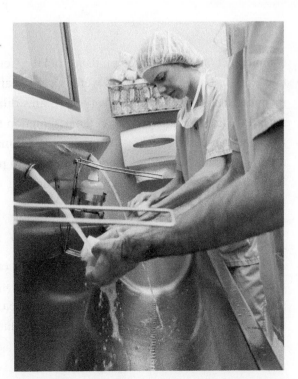

RECENT DEVELOPMENTS

Green Cleaning

Most traditional cleaning supplies, even the mildest of them, come with warnings. They may cause blindness, vomiting, or even death if swallowed. Although they are effective cleaners, they seem to be an odd choice to use around extremely sick people. At least that's the thinking that has inspired some institutions to search for green cleaning supplies and other eco-friendly products. These products, which are made from natural products, are often far safer for use around people and have a lower impact on the environment.

Green cleaning goes beyond just using natural products. It sometimes also means using less of the chemicals that have always been used. Frequently, people simply use more cleaners than they need for a particular job. For instance, new ways of cleaning using microfibers can reduce the need for chemicals. Microfiber mops require less water, and less chemical cleaners, than traditional cotton mops.

In the past, many facilities have stayed away from green products because they thought they would be more costly. Green products do not have to be more expensive, particularly when all costs are taken into account. Government agencies closely regulate many toxic chemicals. With green products, there are fewer toxic chemicals to track, which cuts regulatory costs and results in fewer injuries due to chemical accidents.

While green cleaning is not yet widespread, more and more institutions are beginning to see its advantages. Look for even more hospitals and environmental services departments to begin considering green cleaning in the future.

What additional benefits can you see in the use of eco-friendly products?

completely controlled. Based on data from the Centers for Disease Control and Prevention (CDC), U.S. measles cases were at a 15-year high in 2011 with over 200 cases, a reminder that effective immunization requires diligence. Another example of a fallacy related to disease transmission is the assumption that bats carry rabies. Bats are mammals and can contract rabies, but that does not make them specific carriers of the disease. Many fallacies and misunderstandings also persist concerning the transmission of **bloodborne** diseases, but standard precautions have been developed to effectively address realistic risks.

bloodborne
(BLUD-born) Carried in the blood

Signs and Symptoms of Infection

An infection may be **generalized**, or it may be **localized**. If the infection is generalized, it usually results in headache, fatigue, fever, and increased pulse and respiration. A person may also experience vomiting and/or diarrhea. If the infection is localized, you can see and feel one or more of the following: redness, swelling, heat, and/or drainage. There is usually pain at the site of the infection.

generalized
(JEN-reh-lized) Affecting all of the body

localized
(LOW-keh-lized) Affecting one area of the body

APPLY IT STATE BOARDS OF HEALTH

In addition to national agencies that deal with safety guidelines in regard to transmission of infectious agents, each state has a board of health. A state board of health licenses health care facilities and requires compliance with OSHA and CDC guidelines. Locate your state board of health online and learn what the expectations are for preventing the transmission of infectious agents. What other types of regulations do state boards of health impose on health care facilities?

ASEPSIS AND STANDARD PRECAUTIONS

Health care facilities are filled with people who are ill. Some of their illnesses are caused by body dysfunctions; other illnesses are caused by infections or injury. Thus, health care environments are constantly contaminated with the pathogens carried by patients, visitors, and employees.

Asepsis

This constant presence of pathogens requires the staff to wage an all-out battle against these microorganisms and viruses. This battle is waged by the continual use of medical **asepsis**, or the destruction of the environment that allows pathogens to live, breed, and spread. Medical asepsis is accomplished by using aseptic technique. Aseptic technique is very important when you are working with patients. The practice of aseptic technique helps to prevent:

- Cross infection, which is caused by infecting the patient with a new microorganism or virus from another patient or health care worker (**nosocomial infection**).
- Re-infection with the same microorganism or virus that caused the original illness.
- Self-inoculation by the patient's own organisms, such as *E. coli* from the intestines entering the urethra.
- Transmission of an illness from the patient to the health care worker, or from the health care worker to the patient.

Aseptic technique includes:

- Following proper hand washing technique.
- Ensuring employees are clean and neat.
- Handling all equipment properly.
- Using sterile procedure when necessary.
- Using proper cleaning solutions: **bacteriostatic** solutions, which slow or stop the growth of bacteria, or **bactericidal** solutions, which kill bacteria.
- Following Standard Precautions.

The health care team must strive toward achieving an aseptic environment to reduce the infection rate in the health care setting.

asepsis
(ay-SEP-ses) Sterile condition, free from all germs

nosocomial infection
(no-she-KOE-mee-al) An infection acquired while in a health care setting, such as a hospital

bacteriostatic
(bak-TIR-eh-oh-stat-ik) Slows or stops the growth of bacteria

bactericidal
(bak-TIR-eh-sigh-dell) Kills bacteria

Language Arts Link **Infection Control and Soiled Linen**

You are concerned that workers on your unit are not handling soiled linen properly. Write a letter to the manager in charge of infection control. Describe the types of patients who receive care on your unit. Include specific examples of your concerns along with suggestions for improvement.

Be sure to proofread your work to see if you can improve it by making it clearer, more concise, or more interesting to read. Check the spelling and grammar and correct any errors. When you've completed your letter, exchange it with a classmate. Provide feedback on your classmate's letter, and then exchange back. Read your classmate's comments and revise your letter as necessary.

Standard Precautions

Transmission of infectious agents requires three elements: 1) a source of infectious agents; 2) a susceptible host with a source of entry receptive to the agent; and 3) a mode of transmission for the agent. All blood, body fluids, secretions, excretions (except sweat), nonintact skin, and mucous membranes may contain contagious infectious agents.

transmitting (tranz-MIT-ing) Causing to go from one person to another person

Because of the risk of **transmitting** these infectious agents, a set of standard precautions was developed. In 1985, health care isolation practices in the United States changed to defend against the increased risk of exposure to hepatitis B virus (HBV) and human immunodeficiency virus (HIV). For the first time, all blood and body fluids were treated as infected substances.

The Occupational Safety and Health Administration (OSHA) of the U.S. Department of Labor established mandatory guidelines published in the *Occupational Exposure to Bloodborne Pathogens; Needlestick and Other Sharps Injuries; Final Rule.* These guidelines ensure that all employers provide personal protective equipment to employees at risk of exposure to body fluids. In 1992, OSHA increased its mandate to employers, insisting that training and immunization be provided to all employees within ten days of hire. This means that employees at risk for exposure to body fluids must:

- Be offered hepatitis B vaccine (HBV) at no charge.
- Be trained to use the appropriate protective equipment to prevent exposure to body fluids.
- Receive an annual update and review.

In 1996, the CDC expanded the bloodborne pathogen guidelines to assist in the prevention of nosocomial infections. These expanded guidelines are known as Standard Precautions. The CDC updated these Standard Precautions in 2007 to include a new section on Respiratory Hygiene/Cough Etiquette, primarily in response to the Severe Acute Respiratory Syndrome (SARS) virus outbreak in 2003.

Standard Precautions are appropriate for all patients receiving care or service in a health care environment regardless of their diagnosis. Standard Precautions provide protection from contact with blood, mucous membranes, nonintact skin, and all body fluids. Body fluids include the following:

- Blood.
- Vaginal secretions.
- Pericardial fluid (liquid that surrounds the heart).
- Body fluids containing visible blood.
- Amniotic fluid (liquid that surrounds the fetus during pregnancy).

- Peritoneal fluid (liquid in the peritoneal cavity).
- Tissue specimens.
- Cerebrospinal fluid (liquid that flows through and around brain and spinal tissue).
- Interstitial fluid (liquid that fills the space between most of the cells of the body).
- Semen (fluid from the testes, seminal vesicles, prostate gland, and bulbourethral glands).
- Pleural fluid (liquid that surrounds the lungs).

Infection with HBV and HIV occur through:

- Direct injection of infected blood or a contaminated needle that punctures the skin.
- Contact of infected body fluids with mucous membranes such as the eye or inside of the mouth.
- Sexual contact.
- Pregnancy; when the mother is infected, the infection is transferred to the newborn infant.

The risk of being infected in the health care setting is high. It is important for you to treat all patients as though they were infected. If you provide hands-on care to patients, you must follow all Standard Precaution guidelines to protect yourself and others. Make it a habit to follow each step in the Standard Precaution guidelines.

These include practices that apply to all health care providers, patients, visitors, and family members. Hand hygiene is the single-most effective way to prevent the spread of infections. Other safe practices may involve the use of gloves, goggles, face shield, and/or a gown when there is a risk of splashing or spray of blood or body fluids. Safe handling of soiled linens also reduces the risks of spreading infectious agents. Listed below are procedures to follow to minimize the risk of spreading infectious agents.

Surgical Asepsis

Medical asepsis includes all practices used to limit the number of microorganisms, their growth, and their transmission and to confine them to a specific area. Surgical asepsis, or sterile technique, includes all practices that keep an area completely free of microorganisms.

Controlling the Spread of Infection

Skin and hair cannot be sterilized because any solutions or procedures that kill microorganisms are harmful to skin. You use a bacteriostatic solution for cleaning skin. Bacteriocidal solutions are used on equipment. This method of controlling the spread of infection is called disinfection.

sterilized
(STER-eh-lized) Made free from all living organisms

disinfection
(dis-in-FEKT-shen) Process of freeing from microorganisms by physical or chemical means

A variety of methods are possible for disinfection. You can use boiling water to kill germs. You can add a 10% solution of household bleach to disinfect items that tolerate exposure to mild bleach solution. You can use stronger disinfection for cleaning inanimate items, such as floors, walls, tables, and patient care equipment. There are also ultrasonic cleaners, which offer a fast, consistent, and inexpensive way to remove contaminants from all kinds of surfaces. Ultrasonic cleaners are especially useful for precision cleaning of small parts that contain contamination in small hard-to-reach crevices. These machines mean you use less cleaning solution. (CAUTION: Never use bleach on any item that will be put into the body or with any other product such as cleansers or sprays.)

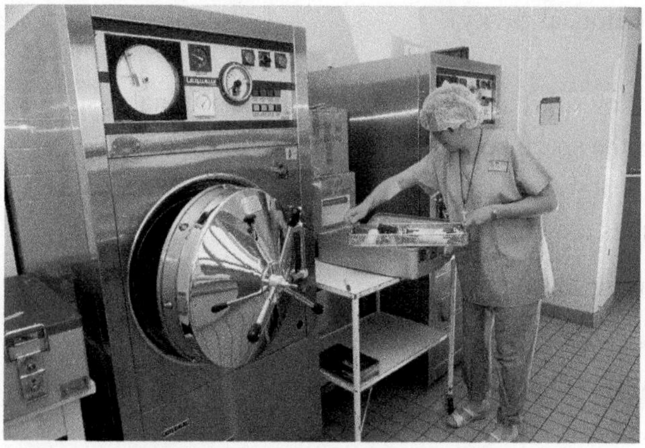

FIGURE 9.13

Sterilizing surgical instruments in an autoclave to kill microorganisms

Source: BSIP SA/Alamy

Sterilization is the process of killing all microorganisms, even spores, bacteria that have a protective shell around them. Spores are killed when they are exposed to steam under pressure at high temperatures. **Autoclaves** are used to produce steam. Gas autoclaves and chemical baths are used to sterilize equipment that would be damaged by steam, such as plastic and rubber devices and fiber optics. Items needing sterilization are those that are put into the body or around an open wound.

autoclaves
(AW-toe-klaves) Sterilizers that use steam under pressure to kill all forms of bacteria on objects that pathogens live on and can transfer infection

Consider This *Antibiotic-Resistant Bacteria*

Bacterial diseases are treated with drugs called antibiotics. Antibiotics can be highly effective in treating bacterial infections, but many bacteria have developed a resistance to antibiotics. As a result, these infections are more difficult to treat.

Why does antibiotic resistance occur? Some bacteria are naturally resistant to antibiotics or mutate to develop a resistance. Sometimes, these bacteria survive to produce more antibiotic resistant bacteria. Resistant bacteria arise when antibiotics are used incorrectly:

- A prescription for antibiotics is not completed. Some people stop taking their antibiotics after they feel better. Doing so increases the chance that resistant bacteria will survive. Often, these patients become ill again.
- Antibiotics are taken when a patient does not need them, such as a patient who has the flu. The antibiotics will not help the patient get over the flu because the flu is caused by a virus, which is not affected by antibiotics. As a result, resistant bacteria may arise. Doctors often avoid prescribing antibiotics in such a case.
- The widespread use of antibiotics in cleaning products has been linked to antibiotic resistance. Repeated exposure to an antibiotic can result in strains of bacteria that are resistant to the drug.

Several bacteria that were once easily controlled by antibiotics are now major health threats. Examples of these bacteria include:

- Tuberculosis: Tuberculosis (TB) is a contagious disease that affects the lungs. About one percent of tuberculosis cases involve a strain of bacteria that is resistant to multiple antibiotics. These cases need almost four times more recovery time than nonresistant strains of tuberculosis. Treatment of resistant strains is also more expensive and has more uncomfortable and dangerous side effects.
- Methicillin-resistant *Staphylococcus aureus* (MRSA): Resistant forms of *S. aureus* were first noted in the 1960s. Since, it has become one of the most common antibiotic resistant bacteria found in hospitals. Infection by *S. aureus* has been linked

to longer hospital stays and increased risk of death from secondary infections. In addition to the ongoing incidence of MRSA in hospitals, school-based outbreaks of the infection have also occurred. Although not considered a "superbug" by public health officials, MRSA is a threat that should be respected.

- Streptococcus: Various species of streptococci are resistant to antibiotics. These bacteria cause diseases such as pneumonia, meningitis, and arthritis.

While some antibiotics have little effect on bacteria, some substances, such as alcohol and bleach, are effective. Additionally, some equipment can be autoclaved to destroy bacteria. Regardless, careful monitoring of antibiotic use and proper equipment care are needed to prevent the development of resistance and the spread of resistant bacteria.

One of your patients is refusing to finish his antibiotic prescription. What would you tell him to make sure that he finishes his medicine?

Hand Washing

Hand washing is the process of removing microorganisms from contaminated hands. Proper hand washing is the most effective way to prevent infecting yourself or others.

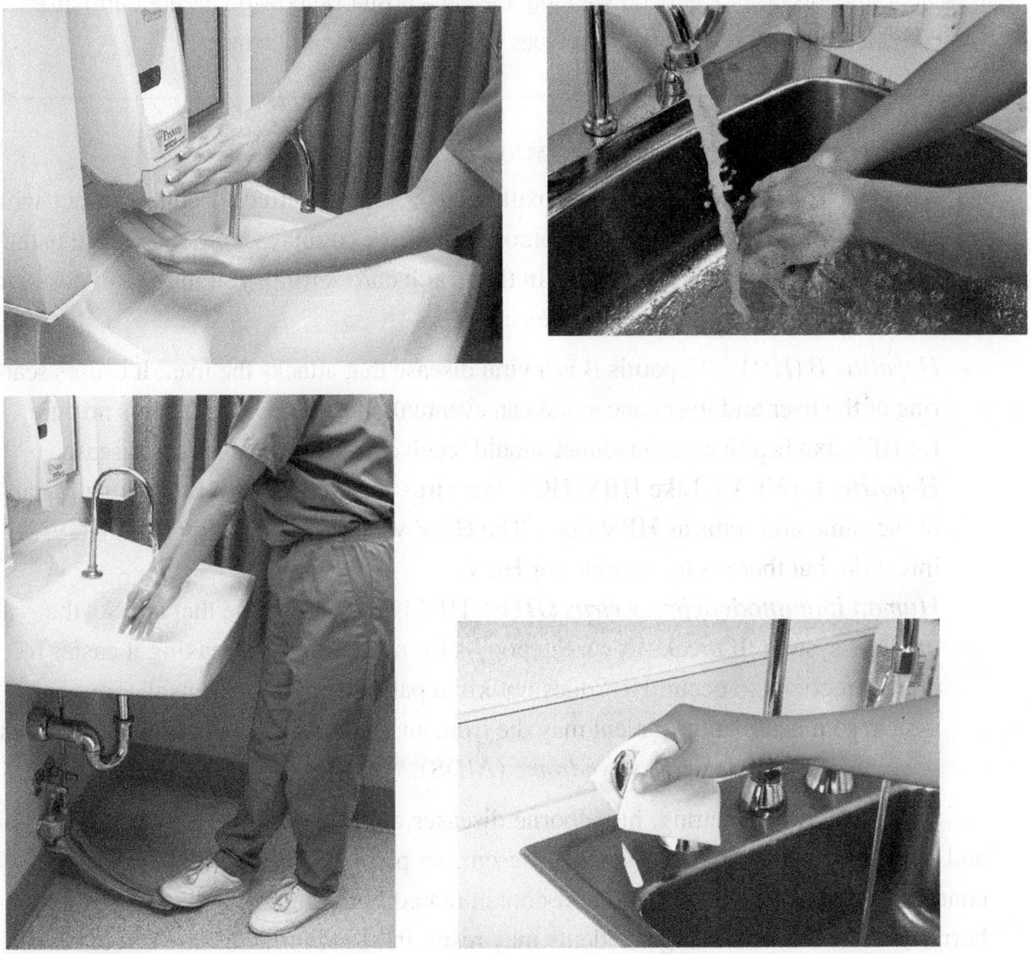

FIGURE 9.14

Hand hygiene

Source: Michal Heron/ Pearson Education

Hand Cleansing

If hands are not visibly soiled, a facility's procedures may allow the use of an alcohol-based hand rub for cleansing hands instead of washing them. According to CDC guidelines, situations where hand cleansing, instead of washing, may be appropriate include:

- Before having direct contact with patients.
- After contact with a patient's intact skin, for example after taking a pulse or blood pressure, or after lifting a patient.
- After removing gloves.
- After contact with inanimate objects, including medical equipment, when near a patient.

A facility-approved hand lotion should be used to prevent irritation and chapping from frequent hand washing or cleansing, because repeatedly using an alcohol-based hand-rub can irritate the skin. Irritated skin poses a risk of an individual becoming infected or infecting others.

Community Service Hand Washing Techniques

In a team of three or four students, prepare a presentation for elementary or middle school students on proper hand washing. Design a poster on how germs are transmitted and how proper hand washing techniques limit transmission of germs.

Bloodborne Diseases and Precautions

As previously mentioned, sometimes pathogens are transmitted through contact with blood, body fluids contaminated with blood, semen, or vaginal secretions. These pathogens are called bloodborne pathogens. In the health care setting, you may be exposed to the following three bloodborne pathogens:

- ***Hepatitis B (HBV):*** Hepatitis B is a viral disease that attacks the liver. It causes scarring of the liver and liver cancer and can eventually lead to death. There is no cure for HBV, but health care personnel should receive a vaccine against the disease.
- ***Hepatitis C (HCV):*** Like HBV, HCV is a virus that attacks the liver, causing many of the same problems as HBV does. The HBV vaccine may help prevent HCV infection, but there is no vaccine for HCV.
- ***Human immunodeficiency virus (HIV):*** HIV is a viral disease that attacks the immune system. It breaks down the body's immune defenses, making it easier for other infections to occur. HIV does not kill a patient, but it weakens the immune system so much that the patient may die from an opportunistic infection. HIV causes *acquired immunodeficiency syndrome* (AIDS).

In the health care setting, bloodborne diseases are rarely passed between caregiver and patient. However, the risk is still present, so precautions should be taken. Direct contact with infected blood and blood-contaminated body fluids can introduce a bloodborne disease. The following accidents may result in bloodborne disease infection:

- Accidental needle sticks: Puncture wounds from needles contaminated with diseased blood.
- Cuts from sharp instruments: Cuts from sharp instruments that have been in contact with infected blood.

- Direct contact with infected blood: Infected blood comes in contact with the eyes, nose, mouth, or skin.

Bloodborne diseases are sometimes passed from an infected mother to her infant. In the past, these diseases were transmitted to people through blood transfusions and organ donations from infected donors. New testing methods have made this mode of infection rare. Bloodborne diseases are **not** spread through casual contact, hugging, or kissing. Additionally, they cannot be spread by food or water, sharing utensils and dishes, coughing, or sneezing.

At-Risk Behaviors

Some behaviors put people at greater risk of contracting a bloodborne disease. Those behaviors include the following:

- Unprotected sex, including oral sex.
- Sharing needles to inject illegal drugs.

Each of these behaviors puts people in contact with blood, semen, or vaginal fluids, all of which can carry bloodborne pathogens. A notable exception is hepatitis C, which is rarely spread through sexual contact. Instead, HCV is transmitted by blood-to-blood contact, such as unsterilized injection equipment or infusion of inadequately screened blood and blood products.

Universal Precautions

As a health care worker, you should follow Standard Precautions in dealing with patients. Additionally, you should use **Universal Precautions** to prevent the transmission of bloodborne diseases. Universal Precautions are similar to Standard Precautions. You should avoid direct contact with blood, vaginal secretions, semen, pericardial fluid, amniotic fluid, peritoneal fluid, interstitial fluid, and pleural fluid. You do not need to take Universal Precautions for feces, nasal secretions, sputum, sweat, tears, urine, vomit, or saliva unless it is contaminated with blood.

Universal Precautions (you-neh-VER-sel pre-CAW-shens) A set of precautions that prevents the transmission of HIV, HBV, HCV, and other bloodborne pathogens when providing health care

CAUTION: You should always wear gloves when handling body fluids to prevent the spread of diseases, both bloodborne and not.

Universal Precautions require the use of the following protective equipment:

- Gloves
- Gowns
- Aprons
- Masks
- Protective eyewear
- Resuscitation equipment that prevents the spread of pathogens

Under Universal Precautions, you should also take steps to avoid injuries caused by contaminated scalpels, needles, and other sharp instruments. Surfaces and equipment that come in contact with infected blood should be sterilized using a bleach solution or as indicated by facility guidelines.

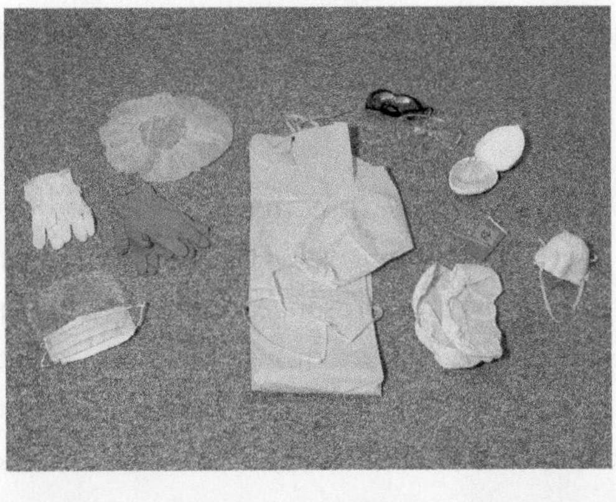

FIGURE 9.15

Protective clothing and gear includes gloves, masks, gowns, and goggles

Source: George Dodson/Pearson Education

TABLE 9.1 Standard Precautions: Examples of tasks and use of protective equipment

Task	Gloves	Gown	Mask	Protective Eyewear
Controlling spurting blood	Yes	Yes	Yes	Yes
Controlling minimal bleeding	Yes	No	No	No
Blood drawing	Yes	Yes	Yes	Yes
Oral or nasal suction	Yes	No	Yes	Yes
Handling/cleaning contaminated instruments	Yes	Yes	Yes	Yes
Measuring blood pressure	No	No	No	No

What to Do if You Are Exposed to Blood

If you are exposed to blood during work, you should:

- Wash accidental needle sticks and cuts with soap and water.
- If your nose, mouth, or skin is exposed, flush the affected area with water.
- If your eyes are exposed, flush with water, saline, or other sterile solutions as mandated by your facility.
- Always report the exposure to your manager. You will need to discuss the exposure with your facility's exposure management department to evaluate your risks and post-exposure treatment.

Post-exposure treatment depends on the type of exposure. Because health care workers are given the HBV vaccine, their risk of infection is low. Workers should be tested within a couple months of vaccination to make sure immunity is complete. Hepatitis B immune globulin and/or the HBV vaccine can be given after exposure to prevent infection. Treatment should start within twenty-four hours of exposure. Because post-exposure treatment is usually effective, routine follow-up is not recommended unless there are symptoms.

For HCV, no vaccine exists, nor does post-exposure medical treatment. This makes preventive measures important in the case of HCV. However, the incidence of HCV infection after exposure is relatively low when compared to HBV. A person who is exposed to HCV should be tested immediately after exposure and four-to-six months after exposure to see if he or she is infected.

As with HCV, no vaccine exists for HIV. The use of antiretroviral drugs after exposure has been shown to reduce the transmission of HIV. However, these drugs have serious side effects, so they are not used unless exposure is significant. Treatment should start as soon as possible. A person exposed to HIV should be tested for the virus as soon as possible after exposure. Testing should be repeated at six months and then again at one year.

Testing for Bloodborne Diseases

HBV and HCV infections have some external symptoms, such as jaundiced (yellowed) skin. However, HIV infection may not have external symptoms. A blood test can confirm the presence of any of these three diseases. A false positive is possible, so multiple tests are required to verify infection. As a health care worker, your facility likely has a routine blood testing procedure in place. You will need to undergo regular blood testing. If you are exposed to infected blood, you likely will need to be tested more often.

BUILD YOUR SKILLS *Safety Equipment*

Some health care institutions are providing new safety equipment designed to keep health professionals safe. Respirators filter air to keep health care workers safe from SARS, influenza, and other contagious diseases that are spread when infected patients cough or sneeze.

Needle safety devices and personal protective gear help to reduce the risk of being stuck by a needle. A needle stick doesn't just hurt; it can spread bloodborne pathogens, such as HIV, from infected patients. Needle safety devices either provide built-in needle shields or containers that separate the needle from the syringe right after blood is drawn. Puncture-resistant finger or arm guards also help to eliminate needle sticks.

Most facilities are now using needleless systems. Although it may be impossible to remove all use of needles from health care facilities, the use of needleless systems for intravenous fluid systems and covered needle systems for any necessary needle use has decreased the incidence of needle stick injuries. In most locations there is no longer any need to recap needles.

Why is it important to handle needles safely?

Ethical and Legal Issues

As a health care worker, your employer has certain obligations to keep you safe. The employer should provide protective equipment at all times. Your employer should also have practices in place that reduce your risk of exposure. You should also be vaccinated with the HBV vaccine. If you are exposed to a bloodborne disease, your employer should also offer management and treatment for the disease. Exposure to a bloodborne disease will be recorded in your confidential medical records whether you contract the disease or not. It may be reported to government agencies for disease tracking and research purposes. Regardless, your personal information will remain private.

People who have a bloodborne disease, including health care workers, have certain legal rights. A health care facility must maintain a patient's confidentiality. Participation in any treatment and testing must be voluntary. A facility should also offer adequate information, support, and referrals to help an infected individual and his or her family understand the disease and its treatment. Depending on state and federal laws, a health care facility must report bloodborne diseases and make an effort to warn other people who are at risk in a confidential manner.

GENERAL SAFETY AND INJURY AND ILLNESS PREVENTION

OSHA establishes guidelines for a safe work environment for all employers and their employees. The OSHA standards say that employees have *the right to know* what **hazards** are present in their environment. OSHA regulations require employers to train and offer immunizations to high-risk employees in the first ten days of a new job. A committed

hazards
(HA-zerds) Things that may cause harm to human, animal, or environmental health

partnership between the employer and employee is necessary to provide a safe environment for everyone.

OSHA Standards

This section explains the areas in which health care agencies and facilities must be in compliance; these include the:

- Ergonomic Program
- Injury and Illness Prevention Program
- Hazard Communication Program
- Exposure Control Plan

Ergonomic Program

Employers are changing the work environment to meet the expected OSHA ergonomic standards. You will spend a large portion of your day in the work environment. You should be comfortable, use good posture, and learn exercises to prevent getting stiff and sore. The safety officer where you work will help you adjust your environment to accomplish this. If you sit in a work station during the day, your chair, desk, and computer must be adjusted to fit your needs. If patients need to be lifted and moved in your workplace, there should be procedures and equipment in place to facilitate lifts and movements. This prevents physical problems caused by improper working conditions.

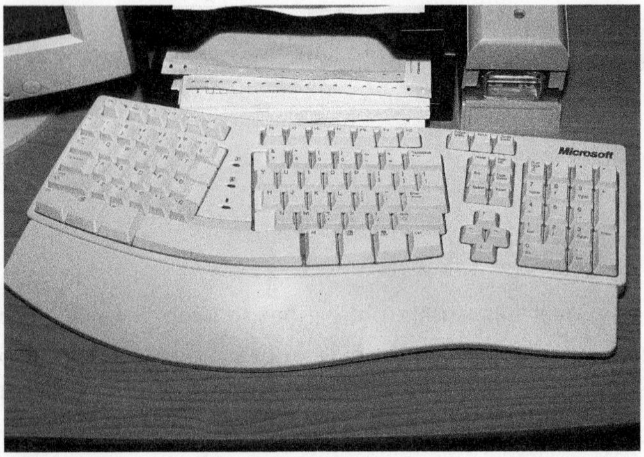

FIGURE 9.16

An ergonomically correct work station includes a well-adjusted desk, chair, and keyboard

Source: Michael Newman/PhotoEdit

You should get into the routine of stretching frequently during the day if you sit at a work station. Stretching and other simple exercises can reduce the risk of injury due to repetitive activities. The following exercises can reduce eyestrain, headaches, and tension in your back, neck, shoulders, and wrists:

1. ***Deep Breathing.*** Close your eyes. Inhale deeply and slowly through your nose. Exhale slowly through your mouth. Repeat at least four times.
2. ***Changing Focus.*** Look up from your computer screen and focus your eyes on a distant object. Look back at an object that is close and allow your eyes to focus on it. Repeat this exercise four times.
3. ***Arm and Hand Shake.*** Drop your arms and hands to your side and let them relax. Shake your relaxed hands for a few seconds. Then shake your hands and arms.
4. ***Finger Stretch.*** Grab the edge of your desk with your palms down and your thumb below the edge. Press down for a few seconds. Then press up for a few seconds. Turn your hands upside-down, so palms are facing up and your four fingers are below the edge. Repeat the exercise.
5. ***Ankle Stretch.*** Sit upright in your chair. Rotate both feet to the right, so that your ankles are stretched. Then rotate both feet to the left.

6. ***Body Stretch.*** Lock your hands behind your head. Lean back in your chair and arch your back.
7. ***Shoulder Shrug.*** Bring your shoulders up to your ears and try to press your shoulders and ears together. Hold for a few seconds. Let go of your shoulders and allow them to drop. Repeat four times.

APPLY IT STAYING FIT

Maintaining fitness is important when you are a health care professional. A fit body is strong and flexible and can help you to move patients and equipment without fatigue or injury. A fit mind can help you to handle the stresses of caring for people. Exercise can help you to maintain both a fit body and a fit mind. Lifting weights can help you to build strength in your arm, leg, and back muscles. Pilates, yoga, or dance can help you to strengthen muscles, improve balance, and focus your mind. Running or biking can help to increase your endurance. Any exercise can help you to work off stress.

After checking with your physician, choose some exercises that appeal to you. Make sure you exercise at least three times per week. Incorporate a variety of exercises into your weekly routine for different physical and mental benefits.

How can an exercise program help a health care worker to avoid injury on the job? Why should you check with your family doctor before beginning an exercise program?

Injury and Illness Prevention Program

The Injury and Illness Prevention Program (IIPP) **mandates** that every employer establish, implement, and maintain an effective IIPP. As a student or employee you are responsible for:

mandates (MAN-dates) Orders or commands

- Knowing who is responsible in the facility for the IIPP.
- Practicing policies and procedures that ensure safe and healthy work practices.
- Understanding the communication system used to keep you informed of hazards.
- Knowing what hazards are present and how to prevent injury from them.
- Knowing to whom to report an injury or illness during work hours and what documentation to complete.
- Knowing the location of the safety bulletin board (or communication book) in your facility. You are responsible for reading all items posted each month.

Your school or employer will test you for signs of tuberculosis (TB). Exposure to tuberculosis is determined by a TB skin test. If your TB test indicates exposure, you will need additional tests. You will also be offered hepatitis B vaccine. This vaccine protects you from getting hepatitis B while working in the health care environment.

Hazard Communication Program

The Hazard Communication Program mandates that employers inform employees of:

- Chemicals or hazards in the environment.
- Where chemicals or hazards are stored and used.
- How to interpret chemical labels and hazard signs.
- Methods and equipment for cleaning chemical spills.

- Personal protection equipment and its storage location.
- The hazard communication system.

As a student or employee, you are responsible for knowing:

- What chemicals or hazards are in your work area.
- Where the chemicals or hazards are stored or used.
- How to read and interpret container signs and labels.
- What to do when a chemical or **biohazard** spills.
- What personal protective equipment to wear when working with or around chemicals and biohazards.
- Your facility's system for informing you of hazards in the work area.

biohazard
(BIE-oh-ha-zerd) Biological materials or infectious agents that may cause harm to human, animal, or environmental health

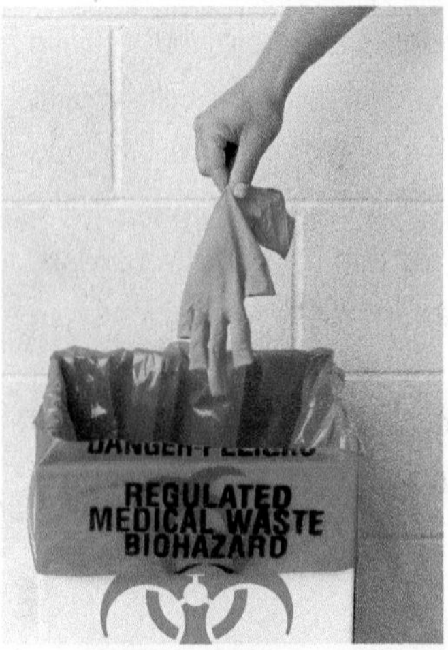

FIGURE 9.17

Following OSHA guidelines for the disposal of contaminated, biohazardous material

Source: George Dodson/Pearson Education

The way that harm is caused determines the following hazard category:

- *Chemical hazards* cause harm when a chemical is mixed with another chemical, causing a reaction. When a chemical reacts with another substance or because of temperature change, it creates a new chemical. For example, chlorine bleach mixed with ammonia creates a harmful (even deadly) gas called chloramines.
- *Health hazards* have the potential to harm a healthy body. For example, acid burns and destroys the skin.

Science Link Biohazardous Materials

Biohazardous materials are defined as biological materials or infectious agents that may cause harm to human, animal, or environmental health. Viruses that cause disease (such as the human immunodeficiency virus, or HIV) are biohazards. So are disease-causing bacteria (such as *E. coli*).

Plant toxins, allergens (such as pollen), and snake venom are biological agents that may cause disease, so they may be classified as biohazards. Certain types of recombinant DNA may also be classified as biohazards. This is DNA that has the potential to harm plants or animals if it escapes into the environment.

Viruses, bacteria, and other biohazardous material can be spread by blood or other body fluids.

Therefore, care must be taken to minimize patient and health care worker exposure to body fluids. Any equipment that is used on a patient must be sterilized before it is used on any other patient. Health care professionals must wear gloves, protective clothing, and (in some cases) masks when working with patients. Needles must be used carefully and discarded in a designated container after use. Any clothes or linens exposed to blood or other body fluids must be stored in properly labeled biohazard containers until they can be washed. Drawn blood must be transported carefully and stored in labeled safety cabinets or containers.

OSHA has developed procedures for the proper handling and disposal of biohazardous materials.

These procedures must be followed in every health care facility, for the safety of patients, visitors, and staff.

What is the difference between a biohazard and a chemical hazard?

Material Safety Data Sheets (MSDSs)

Product manufacturers prepare material safety data sheet (MSDS) forms to provide the information needed to handle chemicals safely. Employers must make the MSDSs available to employees. The Hazard Communication Program explains how the employer plans to keep people safe when chemicals are present. The communication system must explain:

- What hazards are present and where they are stored and used.
- What precautions to take when hazardous products are present. These precautions include:
  - Wearing appropriate personal protective equipment (PPE).
  - Ventilating rooms properly.
  - Keeping flammable products away from flames or other heat sources.
- How to use potentially hazardous products safely.
- Proper cleanup and disposal of hazardous products.
- First aid if exposure occurs.
- How to label containers with a chemical, by always including:
  - Product name.
  - Chemicals in the product.
  - Precautions for use of the product.

As a student or employee you are responsible for knowing where hazard communications are kept and how to access them. You find hazard information on manufacturer's literature. You may receive memorandums from your employer alerting you to new hazards in the environment. Most facilities keep hazard communications:

- In safety policy and procedure manuals.
- In material safety data sheet (MSDS) books.
- On the safety bulletin board.
- On product labels.
- On signs.

Exposure Control Program

An exposure control plan provides steps to reduce employee or student exposure to bloodborne pathogens. The plan includes the following:

- Determining the possibility of exposure under each position description.
- Developing a schedule and method for ensuring that the plan is enforced.
- Evaluating post-exposure.

Safe Work Practices

Safety is everyone's responsibility. Certain rules are important to all health care workers. To be a safe worker and to protect yourself, coworkers, visitors, and patients, learn the rules listed here.

- ***Walk! Never run in hallways.*** If you run, you may fall and injure yourself. You can collide with another person or object. You can injure someone else, or you might create panic.

MATERIAL SAFETY DATA SHEET

I Product Identification

COMPANY NAME: Calgon Vestal Laboratories
ADDRESS: 5035 Manchester Avenue
St. Louis, Missouri 63110
Nights: 314-802-2000
CHEMTREC: (800) 424-9300
PRODUCT NAME: Klenzyme
Product No.: 1103
SYNONYMS: Medical Apparatus and Instrument Presoak

II Hazardous Ingredients of Mixtures

Material	(CAS#)	% by Wt.	TLV	PEL
Subtilisins (Proteolytic enzymes)	(9014-01-1)	< 5	.06ppb	N/A
Sodium tetraborate, decahydrate	(1303-96-4)	< 5	5mg/m3	10mg/m3

III Physical Data

Vapor Pressure, mmHg: N/A
Evaporation Rate (ether = 1): N/A
Solubility in H_2O: Complete
Freezing Point F: N/A
Boiling Point F: > 212F
Specific Gravity H_2O = 1 @ 25C: 1.08
Vapor Density (Air = 1) 60–90 F: Undeterm.
% Volatile by wt: N/A
pH @ Undiluted Solution: N/A
pH as Distributed: 7.5–8.0
Appearance: Amber liquid
Odor: Typical, mild odor

IV Fire and Explosion

Flash Point F: N/A
Flammable Limits: N/A
Extinguishing Media: Not flammable. In event of fire, use water fog, CO_2, and dry chemical.
Special Fire Fighting Procedures: No special requirements given. As with any chemical fire, proper cautions should be taken, such as wearing a self-contained breathing apparatus.
Unusual Fire and Explosion Hazards: None known

V Reactivity Data

Stability-Conditions to avoid: Stable
Incompatibility: None known
Hazardous Decomposition Products: Propionaldehyde, CO, CO_2 in fire situations
Conditions Contributing to Hazardous Polymerization: Will not occur

VI Health Hazard Data

Effects of Overexposure (Medical Conditions Aggravated/Target Organ Effects)

A. *Acute* (Primary Route of Exposure)
Eyes & Skin: Upon contact, mildly irritating to eyes. Prolonged or repeated contact may irritate skin.
Inhalation: Spray mists or dusts from dried residues may result in respiratory irritation, coughing and/or difficulty in breathing.
Ingestion: May cause upset to gastrointestinal tract.

B. *Subchronic, Chronic, Other:* Subtilisins chronic exposure to dusts showed allergic sensitization with respiratory allergic reactions within minutes or delayed up to 24 hours.

VII Emergency and First Aid Procedures

Eyes: Immediately flush eyes with plenty of water for at least 15 minutes. See a physician.
Skin: Immediately wash with soap and plenty of water for at least 15 minutes while removing contaminated clothing. If irritation develops, seek medical aid.
Inhalation: Remove to fresh air. If not breathing, give artificial respiration. If breathing difficult, give oxygen if available. Seek medical aid and report all inhalation exposures to health and safety personnel.
Ingestion: Do not induce vomiting. Give water to dilute. Call a physician. Never give anything by mouth to an unconscious person.

VIII Spill or Leak Procedures

Spill Management: Contain spill and absorb material with an inert substance. Collect waste in suitable container.
Waste Disposal Methods: Dispose of in accordance with local, state, and federal regulations.

IX Protection Information/Control Measures

Respiratory: Not required under normal use
Eye: Safety glasses
Glove: Rubber
Other Clothing and Equipment: Clothes sufficient to avoid contact
Ventilation: Local exhaust

X Special Precautions

Precautions to be taken in Handling and Storing: Avoid exposure to high temperature or humidity. Wash hands thoroughly after use. Keep container closed when not in use.
Additional Information: Read and observe all labeled precautions.

Prepared by: R. C. Jente
Revision Date: 08/24/96
Seller makes no warranty, expressed or implied, concerning the use of this product other than indicated on the label. Buyer assumes all risks of use and/or handling of this material when such use and/or handling is contrary to label instructions.
While Seller believes that the information contained herein is accurate, such information is offered solely for its customers' consideration and verification under their specific use conditions. This information is not to be deemed a warranty or representation of any kind for which Seller assumes legal responsibility.

FIGURE 9.18

Example of a Material Safety Data Sheet form

- ***Walk on the right-hand side of the hall***, and not more than two **abreast**. It is important to leave hallways open so that there are no traffic jams. In an emergency, a traffic jam can cause a delay and mean the difference between life and death.
- ***Use handrails when using the stairs.*** This prevents falling and injuring yourself.
- ***Watch out for swinging doors.*** Be certain that someone is not on the other side of a swinging door. You might injure yourself or someone else.
- ***Don't play around.*** **Horseplay** is not tolerated. It is disturbing to others, may lead to accidents, causes confusion, and shows a lack of respect for patients and personnel.
- ***Always check labels.*** Never use anything from containers that are not labeled. Using the wrong contents can cause injury or death to a patient. Using the wrong contents may also damage or ruin equipment.
- ***Wipe up spills and place litter in containers.*** A wet floor can cause someone to slip and fall. If there is litter on the floor, someone may trip and be seriously injured.

abreast
(a-BREST) Side by side

horseplay
(HORS-play) Rowdy and childish behavior; acting inappropriately in a work environment

THE MORE YOU KNOW

Slips, Trips, and Falls

Slipping on wet surfaces, falling, and tripping over obstacles are among the most common injuries suffered by workers. The following are some OSHA recommendations to prevent these injuries from occurring:

- Clean only one half of a hallway or staircase at a time so that staff, visitors, and patients have a dry surface to walk on. Use warning signs to alert people to slippery floors.
- Clean all spills immediately and thoroughly.
- Keep floors dry and clean. This can be especially important in entry ways when people walk in out of the rain. Put down mats to help reduce slipping.
- Do not leave buckets, mops, or other supplies sitting in hallways when they are not in use.
- Use appropriate ladders or step stools to reach hard-to-reach places or to perform maintenance, such as when cleaning light fixtures.
- Use non-skid waxes in toilets and shower areas to reduce slipping.
- Immediately report damaged surfaces, poor or ineffective lighting in halls, stairways, or other areas, and other conditions that can lead to injury.
- Areas that are frequently wet or moist—such as an outside walkway with poor drainage—can become especially slippery due the growth of mold and fungi. Report such areas to your supervisor. Additionally, keep these areas clean. Use appropriate cleaners to reduce the growth of molds and fungi.
- Wear functional shoes with good grip.

Why are environmental services workers especially at risk for slipping, tripping, and falling?

- ***Dispose of sharps in designated containers.*** Used needles, broken glass, and other sharp objects should be deposited in specially marked safety containers to minimize injury.
- ***Follow instructions carefully.*** If you do not understand instructions or do not know how to do a task, always ask for instructions. If you do something incorrectly, you may cause a serious problem.
- ***Report any injury to yourself or others to your supervisor immediately.*** Reporting an injury ensures treatment for the injured without delay and correction of the potential hazard.
- ***Do not use electrical cords that are damaged.*** Frayed or damaged cords can cause shocks, burns, or fire.
- ***Report a shock you receive from electrical equipment to your supervisor.*** This prevents fire or a shock to someone else.
- ***Do not use malfunctioning equipment.*** It is dangerous and may cause serious injury to you or someone else.
- ***Make sure all medical supplies and equipment are secure.*** Sharp instruments, drugs, and chemicals may cause harm if taken by patients or other visitors to the health care facility. Keep these and other supplies in locked drawers or closets, if possible.
- ***Report unsafe conditions to your supervisor immediately.*** Safety is everyone's business. Be aware of your environment. Watch for unsafe conditions.
- ***Follow Standard Precaution guidelines.***

frayed
(FRAYD) Worn or tattered; such as electrical cords may be worn, causing wires to be exposed

shock
(SHOK) Convulsion of muscles and extreme stimulation of nerves when an electric current passes through the body

DISASTER PREPAREDNESS

Your facility is required to have a disaster plan. You are responsible for knowing the plan and responding when a disaster occurs.

Disaster Plan

To be prepared for any type of disaster you need to know the following:

- The floor plan of your facility.
- The nearest exit route.
- The location of alarms and fire extinguishers.
- How to use alarms and fire extinguishers.
- Your role as a health care worker when a disaster occurs.

The following are some basic rules to remember when a disaster strikes:

- Assess the situation; count to ten to calm yourself.
- Be sure that you are not in danger. (Placing yourself in danger only makes the situation worse.)
- Remove those who are in immediate danger if it is safe to do so.
- Notify others of the emergency according to facility policy.
- Use stairs, *not* the elevator.

Fire Causes and Prevention

Fire is often the result of a disaster. It is your responsibility to be alert to causes of fire and act to prevent fire when possible. There are three elements that must be present before a fire can start: oxygen, heat, and fuel. Most fires can be prevented if everyone is observant and careful.

observant
(ob-ZERV-ent) Quick to see and understand

The following are some ways you can help prevent fires:

- Restrict smoking to **designated** outdoor areas.
- Monitor garbage containers.
- Check electrical equipment for proper functioning and frayed electrical cord. If there is any problem, report it immediately.
- Take only the amount needed to complete the task when using flammable liquids. You would spill only the amount you poured, not the whole container. Keep flammable liquids in a container approved by the UL, a not-for-profit product safety testing and certification organization.

flammable
(FLA-meh-bul) Catches fire easily or burns quickly

There are four classes of fire extinguishers. Each type extinguishes a different type of fire.

- **Class A** extinguishers are the most common and put out fires in ordinary combustibles, such as wood, paper, cloth, and many plastics. These extinguishers contain pressurized water. Class A extinguishers have a green triangle marking of an "A" and depict a garbage can and wood pile burning.
- **Class B** extinguishers should be used on fires involving flammable liquids, such as grease, gasoline, and oil. These extinguishers contain carbon dioxide. Class B extinguishers have a red square marking of a "B" and depict a gasoline can with a burning puddle.
- **Class C** extinguishers should be used on energized electrical equipment or wiring where the electric non-conductivity of the extinguishing agent is important. These extinguishers contain potassium bicarbonate or potassium chloride. Class C extinguishers have a blue circle marking a "C" and depict an electric plug with burning outlet.
- **Class D** extinguishers are designed for use on combustible metals such as sodium, titanium, and magnesium. These extinguishers contain either sodium chloride or copper powder and are pressurized with nitrogen. Class D extinguishers have a yellow star marking of a "D." There is no picture designator for Class D extinguishers and they are not given a multi-purpose rating for use on other types of fires.
- In addition, there is a **Class ABC** extinguisher that can be used on wood, cloth, paper, flammable liquids, gasoline, grease and electrical equipment. A Class ABC fire extinguisher is designed to extinguish Class A, B, and C fires. It contains a graphite type chemical that is irritating to the skin.

Bioterrorism

Everyone must be aware of the dangers of chemical or biological disasters. Facilities have plans to provide for the safety of patients, physicians, staff, and visitors. These plans include *shelter-in* during a possible exposure.

Shelter-in is a nationally accepted term indicating the need to remain inside of the facility during a potential exposure to chemical and biological hazards. These plans include securing entrances and exits to the building and securing outside air sources. Your responsibility is to learn what your facility plan is and to follow the procedures that are in place.

FIGURE 9.19
How to operate a fire extinguisher

How to Operate a Fire Extinguisher

BACKGROUND: Health care facilities are required by law to establish safety boards and to inspect the facility regularly for any type of potential fire hazard. Equipment must be checked regularly and escape routes must be kept open.

Fire drills are performed at specific intervals to assure that the facility and its staff are equipped to handle any fire emergency. Nurses are educated and tested annually on their knowledge of the procedures for response to a fire and how to remove patients from danger. Fire extinguishers can be used for types A, B, or C fires.

A Trash, wood, or paper
B Liquids
C Electrical equipment
ABC Use on all fires

ALERT: Follow Standard Precautions.

PREPROCEDURE

1. First Response: **RACE**
   Rescue
   Alert appropriate facility officials
   Contain Fire
   Extinguish Fire

PROCEDURE

2. Locate fire extinguisher and check type.

NOTE: Every nurse should know the location of the closest fire extinguisher to his/her work station.

3. Hold fire extinguisher upright. Pull ring pin.
4. Stand back six to ten feet and direct flow towards base of the fire.
5. Squeeze lever, sweeping side to side.

POSTPROCEDURE

6. Replace or have extinguisher recharged after use.

APPLY IT EMERGENCY CODES

Specific emergency terms are common to all health care facilities, such as "no code" or "DNR." However, each facility has its own emergency terminology with which employees must be familiar. Many health care facilities combine the word *code* with other words or numbers to communicate particular kinds of emergencies when calling emergency medical teams to an area of the hospital (e.g., *code zero*, *code blue*, or *code 99*). Investigate the emergency codes that are used by a local hospital. List each code and its purpose.

BODY MECHANICS AND ERGONOMICS

Health care workers move, lift, and carry all types of equipment and supplies. They also help position or move patients. Moving patients can be particularly hazardous to your back, as the patient may struggle or twist during movement. Ergonomic practices suggest the use of specialized equipment for moving patients. Special equipment could include wheelchairs, walkers, canes, hydraulic lifts, or **gait belts**.

gait belt
(GATE belt) A safety device used to move a patient from one place to another; also used to help hold up a weak person while he or she walks

ambulate
(am-BUE-late) Walk

Of these items, the simplest and possibly most effective item for decreasing injuries to both the patient and the health care worker is the gait belt. Every facility should have gait belts available for use in all patient areas. Gait belts combined with good body mechanics allow the health care worker to safely lift, transfer, and **ambulate** the heavier and disabled patients with less personal strain or danger of injury.

When equipment is unavailable, ergonomic practices emphasize proper body mechanics during movement. When you use proper body mechanics, you save energy, prevent muscle strain, and increase your efficiency. Body mechanics is the coordination of body alignment, balance, and movement. When you use your body and your muscles properly, you are practicing good body mechanics. Good body mechanics require you to keep your body in a neutral, upright position. You should keep your back straight at all times. You should let your leg muscles do most of the work. You should never twist your body. You should never strain as you perform work.

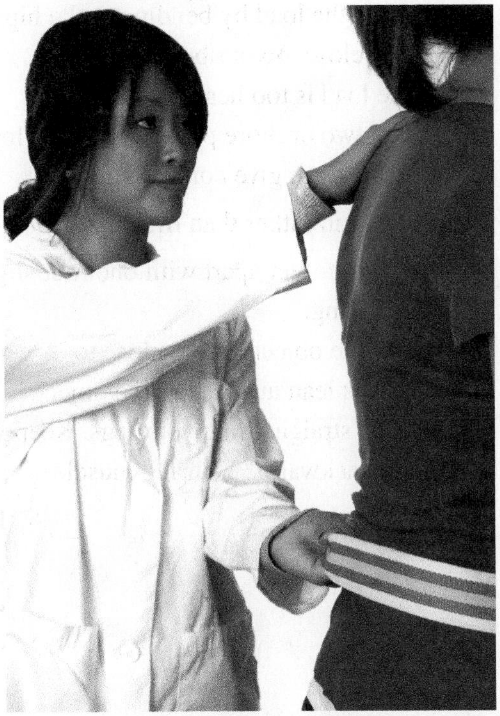

FIGURE 9.20

Ambulating a patient with a gait belt

Source: aceshot1/Shutterstock

It is essential to practice good body mechanics when you are lifting or moving patients to prevent strain and injury. You should also practice good body mechanics when you are performing simple tasks, such as checking blood pressure or entering data into a computer. Injuries from these simple tasks can develop over time if you use poor body mechanics. The following principles will help you to maintain good body mechanics.

load
(LODE) Weight of an object or person that is to be moved

gravity
(GRA-veh-tee) Natural force or pull toward the earth; in the body, the center of gravity is usually the center of the body

1. Stoop. Do not bend.
   - Stand close to the object. Create a base of support by placing your feet wide apart.
   - Place one foot slightly forward.
   - Bend at your hips and knees with your back straight, lower your body, and bring your hands down to the object.
   - Use the large muscles in your legs to return to a standing position.
2. Lift firmly and smoothly after you size up the load.
   - If you cannot easily pull the object to you (if the load is too heavy), *get help!*
   - Grasp the load firmly.
   - Lift by using the large muscles of your legs.
   - Keep the load close to your body.
   - Do not twist your body.
   - To change direction, shift your feet in the direction you want to go.
3. Always use the center of gravity when carrying a load.
   - Keep your back as straight as possible.
   - Keep the weight of the load close to the body and centered over your hips.

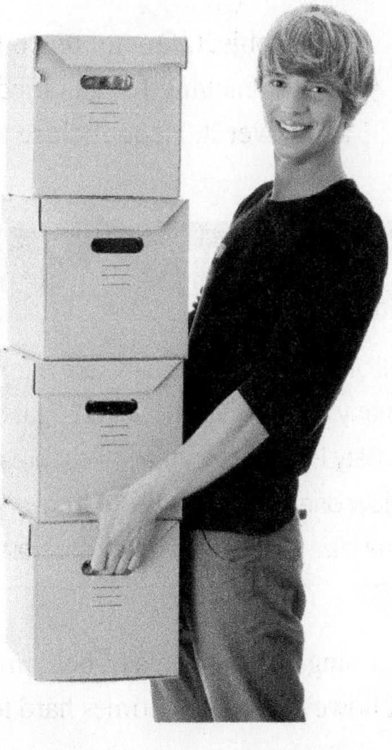

FIGURE 9.21

Using good body mechanics to carry a load

Source: Piotr Marcinski/Shutterstock

- Put down the load by bending at the hips and knees. Keep your back straight and the load close to your body.
  - If the load is too heavy, *get help!*
  - When two or more people carry the load, assign one person as the leader so that he or she can give commands.

4. Pulling: Pull rather than lift the load.
   - Place your feet apart with one foot slightly forward. Keep close to the object you are moving.
   - Grasp the object firmly, close to its center of gravity.
   - **Crouch**; lean away from the object.
   - Pull by straightening your legs. Keep your back straight.
   - Walk backwards. Your leg muscles should do all the work.

crouch
(KRAUCH) To stoop, using the large muscles of the legs to help maintain balance

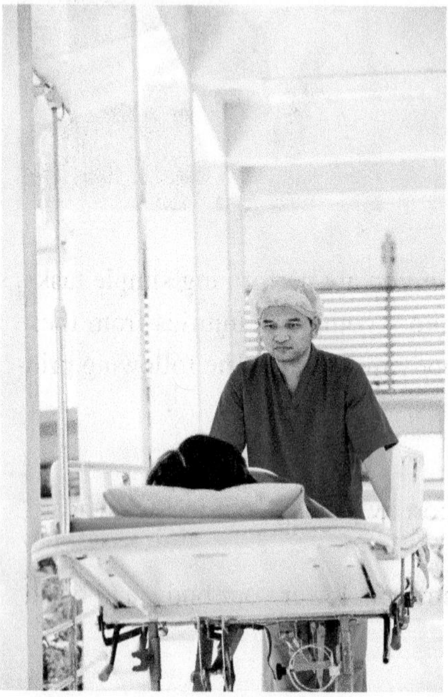

FIGURE 9.22
Pushing a cart by leaning forward with the chest and shoulders
Source: Apples Eyes Studio/Shutterstock

5. Pushing: Push rather than lift the load.
   - Stand close to the object to be moved.
   - Crouch down with your feet apart.
   - Bend your elbows and put your hands on the load at chest level.
   - Lean forward with your chest and shoulders near the object.
   - Keep your back straight.
   - Push with your legs.
6. Reaching: Carefully evaluate the distance.
   - Always use a stool or a ladder to reach objects that are too high.
   - Stand close to the object.
   - If you are standing on the floor, place your feet wide apart, one foot slightly forward.
   - Maintain good body **alignment**. Move close to the object. Do not reach to the point of straining.
   - When reaching for an object that is above your head, grip it with your palms up, and lower it. Keep it close to your body on the way down.

alignment
(a-LINE-ment) Keeping the body in proper position—in a straight line without twisting

APPLY IT CAREER-RELATED RISKS

Nearly all areas of health care are physically demanding. There are also risks associated with many types of health care occupations. With a partner, select a health career and research the safety issues within that career area. Use the Internet for your research, and, if possible, interview one or more person who works in the area you are researching. Share your findings with the class and compare and contrast the safety issues found for different career areas.

Using the principles of body mechanics can help you to avoid injury. As you are working, however, it is sometimes hard to determine whether your body is in the proper position.

One aspect of ergonomics is self-evaluation or evaluation by supervisors or coworkers. Evaluation can help you and your coworkers to correct bad habits and avoid injury. Evaluation can also help to identify problems in the workplace that may lead to poor body mechanics.

You can do the following to evaluate ergonomic practices:

1. ***Watch each other:*** Tell your coworkers if they are twisting their bodies or bending their backs when working with patients. Ask coworkers to watch your body mechanics as well.
2. ***Check equipment:*** Equipment that is faulty or hard to operate can cause you to strain muscles. Make sure brakes on wheelchairs are working, so that you do not hurt your back while moving a patient. Make sure other equipment is at the correct height (between the waist and the shoulders), so you do not have to bend to use it.
3. ***Discuss procedures:*** In some situations, good body mechanics alone may not be enough to prevent injury. Discuss whether you need to create lifting teams instead of having staff move patients by themselves. Also discuss how you can use equipment to help move patients.

To summarize, there are six important rules to remember when following the basic principles of body mechanics:

1. Keep your back straight.
2. Bend at the hips and knees.
3. Keep your feet approximately six to eight inches apart to provide a wide base of support.
4. Use the strongest muscles of your legs.
5. Do not twist your body.
6. Use the weight of your body to help push or pull.

When you learn to lift and move correctly, you protect yourself and others from injury.

REALITY CHECK

After reading about the prevalence and dangers of microorganisms and viruses in health care facilities, are you worried? You should be. This is serious business. People die from some of these infections. If you're going to work in a health care setting, you have to understand and follow infection control procedures. You have to understand the nature of microorganisms and viruses, how they affect the body, how they spread, and how to protect yourself and other people from infection. If you don't, you could contract a serious infection yourself or you could spread infections to other people. It will be up to you to follow Standard Precautions and avoid transmitting infectious disease.

If your job involves handling blood, body fluids contaminated with blood, semen, or vaginal secretions, extra steps must be taken to protect yourself and others from bloodborne diseases. This includes following Universal Precautions, using protective equipment properly, and avoiding risk factors. If you're going to work in surgery or in other areas that require sterile technique, following the principles of asepsis will be a crucial part of your job.

Safety in the health care workplace is essential, and goes well beyond preventing the spread of infections and disease. You must comply with OSHA standards and the policies and procedures your employer has in place to protect everyone in the environment. Failure to do so could cause serious harm. Make sure you are thoroughly familiar with safety precautions, workplace hazards, fire prevention and control, and disaster and bioterrorism policies and procedures. You may be called upon with little or no notice to rescue people or implement an emergency plan. This is no time to be searching for a policies and procedures manual. It's up to you remember this information and be able to apply it at a moment's notice.

Practicing good body mechanics and ergonomics will go a long way in protecting your own health and safety, especially if your job involves lifting and moving patients or other heavy objects. Learn everything you can about safety in the workplace, and comply with all of these safety precautions.

Key Points

- People are surrounded by microorganisms and viruses; they are in the air you breathe, on your skin, in your food, and on everything you touch.
- Some microorganisms and viruses are pathogens; other microorganisms are nonpathogens.
- Pathogens include some bacteria, some protists, some fungi, rickettsiae, and viruses.
- Since pathogens cause illness, it is important to understand how they are spread and how they can be controlled.
- Learning the signs and symptoms of infection will help you provide better patient care.
- Every health care worker must help prevent the spread of infection.
- Nosocomial infections are acquired while a patient is hospitalized and may extend their length of stay.
- Asepsis is the method used to destroy the environment that allows pathogens to live, breed, and spread.
- Major factors in the control of microorganisms are hand washing, disinfection, sterilization, and following Standard Precautions.
- Bloodborne diseases include HBV, HCV, and HIV.
- Although bloodborne diseases are rarely passed between a patient and caregiver, they still pose a significant risk.
- A caregiver must follow Standard Precautions and Universal Precautions. Universal Precautions reduce exposure to blood and blood-contaminated fluids, thus reducing exposure to bloodborne diseases.
- Health care facilities are obligated to provide protection and confidentiality to both its patients and its employees.
- Safety is the responsibility of all health care workers.
- Employers must inform employees of workplace risks and take steps to minimize those risks.

- Employees must follow rules and practice safe behavior to minimize risks of injury to themselves, coworkers, and patients.
- OSHA is very strict about enforcement of regulations that keep the work environment safe.
- Disaster preparedness is everyone's responsibility. Each person is responsible for responding to a disaster and being alert to potential hazards.
- Three elements are required to start a fire: oxygen, heat, and fuel.
- There are at least three ways to help prevent fires. These include checking for frayed electrical cords and malfunctioning equipment, careful handling of flammable liquids, and following proper oxygen procedures.
- Know the disaster plan for your facility.
- Move patients to safety if they are in danger. Know where to find the fire extinguishers and which exits to use. Do not use an elevator. Be calm and do not panic.

Section Review Questions

Answer each of the following questions. Indicate which page in the textbook led you to your answer.

1. Where are microorganisms and viruses found?
2. What conditions affect the growth of bacteria?
3. List five ways to prevent the spread of microorganisms and viruses.
4. List three ways by which bloodborne diseases are accidentally passed.
5. Explain why asepsis is important.
6. Describe the purpose of Universal Precautions.
7. List six pieces of personal protective equipment used in Universal Precautions.
8. Explain OSHA's role in workplace safety.
9. Identify what you are responsible for knowing and doing when a disaster occurs.
10. Discuss the importance of *ergonomics* and list six rules of correct body mechanics.

Learn By Doing

Complete Worksheets 1–5 in Section 9.2 of your *Student Activity Guide*.

CHAPTER 9 Review

Chapter Review Questions

Answer each of the following questions. Indicate which page in the textbook led you to your answer.

1. Describe the purpose of the USDA's MyPlate.
2. Explain the importance of water to the human body.
3. Identify the characteristics of three common eating disorders.
4. List four commonly abused substances; describe their negative impact on the human body.
5. Define *medical asepsis* and list five aseptic techniques.
6. List three examples of items that require sterilization.
7. List some of the Standard Precaution guidelines concerning the use of protective equipment.
8. List two behaviors that increase the risk of contracting bloodborne diseases.
9. Name places to find information about hazards in a facility.

Chapter Review Activities

1. Review the activities offered at a local senior center. How many of the activities focus on spiritual fitness? Speak with a local yoga, pilates, or tai chi instructor and ask for a demonstration at the senior center geared for that age group. What is the response of the participants?
2. Demonstrate appropriate hand washing techniques and explain how these procedures reduce the spread of infections and disease.
3. You have been assigned the task of identifying potential fire hazards in your facility. List the three elements required to start a fire, and identify four ways to prevent fires. Discuss the steps that your facility should take to protect workers, patients, and visitors from fire hazards.
4. Demonstrate the correct techniques for lifting and moving objects.

What If? Scenarios

What would you do in each of the following situations? Record your answer, explain it, and indicate which page in the textbook led you to your decision.

1. You no longer feel good about your self-image; you are overweight, rarely get any exercise, eat junk food most of the time, and smoke way too many cigarettes.
2. Your child spends almost three hours a day texting friends and using his computer, video games, and cell phone. He rarely leaves the house except to go to school.
3. There's a health fair at your school tomorrow that offers free health screenings.
4. A friend has been under a great deal of work-related stress; he's using alcohol and drugs to relieve his anxiety.
5. You have been asked to plan the menus for a two-day family reunion; your family expects nutritious meals.
6. Your best friend eats huge meals and then vomits; she has lost a lot of weight and seems to be depressed.
7. You accidentally cut your finger with a needle after treating a patient who has HCV.
8. You notice a coworker leaving the restroom without washing her hands; she doesn't cover her mouth and nose when she coughs or sneezes.
9. You notice there's an infestation of tiny flies living in the break room on your unit.
10. Your employer is encouraging you to take advantage of their free hepatitis B vaccine.
11. After sitting at your work station this week, you're experiencing eyestrain, headaches, and tension in your back, neck, shoulders, and wrists.

12. Your job includes lifting and moving patients, and you are concerned about possibly hurting your back.

13. You notice two electrical appliances with frayed cords sitting near a supply of flammable liquids in your department's store room.

Media Connection

Use the companion website for additional interactive learning activities.

Portfolio Connection

When you care for patients, it is important to know if they are eating a healthy diet. Food preferences and diet can be more of a source of distress and conflict for patients than the actual illness.

Choose an illness resulting from an eating disorder. Write a paragraph about the illness. Explain the symptoms, how the body is affected, and the treatment. Use the USDA's dietary guidelines to evaluate how the diet is nutritionally deficient.

Keep a copy of MyPlate in your portfolio. Write notes for yourself demonstrating how you would explain to patients the importance of a healthy and varied diet.

CHAPTER 10

Employment, Leadership, and Professional Development

Source: WavebreakmediaMicro/Fotolia LLC

SECTIONS

"My interest is in the future because I am going to spend the rest of my life there."

Charles F. Kettering, Inventor and engineer, 1876–1958

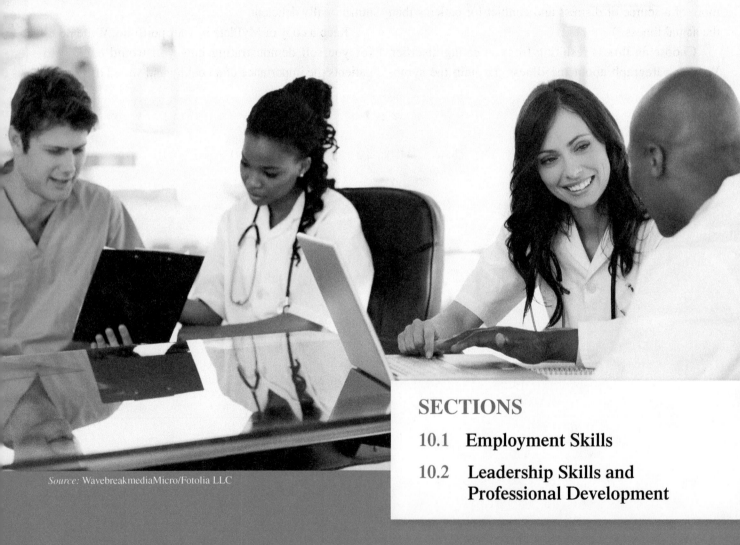

GETTING STARTED

Make a list of your **occupational preferences**. In what part of the country would you like to live and work after graduation? What type and size of health care facility would best meet your employment needs? How many hours per week do you want to work, and what shift and schedule would you prefer? How much compensation will you need? What **employment benefits** would you like to have? Are opportunities for additional training and career advancement important to you? What top three factors would be personally most important in accepting a job offer?

Employment Skills

SECTION 10.1

Background

Once you're ready to begin employment, effective job-seeking skills will help you find a job that matches your qualifications and your personal preferences. Job-seeking skills will help you identify labor trends and employment opportunities in the geographic area where you want to live and work. Once you've researched potential places to work, identified Employers of Choice in your town, and developed your professional **résumé** and **cover letter**, you'll be ready to start contacting employers.

occupational preferences (AH-cue-PAY-shen-al PRE-fer-en-sez) The types of work and work settings that you prefer

employment benefits (im-PLOY-ment BEH-ne-fits) Employer-paid insurance and retirement savings

résumé (RE-zeh-may) Document summarizing job qualifications

cover letter (kuh-VER le-TER) Letter introducing a job applicant to a potential employer

Objectives

After completing this section, you will be able to:

1. Define the key terms.
2. List three sources of information on job openings.
3. Describe four characteristics of a professional résumé.
4. Name five things you should do when filling out a job application form.
5. Explain why employers use pre-employment assessments.
6. Describe five ways to present a professional image during a job interview.
7. Discuss the difference between *traditional* and *behavioral* interview questions.
8. List three ways to convince interviewers that you are serious about wanting the job.
9. Describe what you should do if you don't get a job offer.
10. Discuss the role of compromising to eventually get the job you want.

FINDING THE RIGHT JOB FOR YOU

The job-seeking process starts with learning the skills you need to find a job that's a good match for you. These skills will help you narrow down the type of job to look for and the most productive ways to spend your time finding it.

Where are the best employment opportunities that match your qualifications and your occupational preferences? Your options will be somewhat governed by the health career that you choose. Depending on your occupation, you can consider hospitals, outpatient facilities, home care agencies, community health clinics, rehabilitation facilities, physician practices, mental health centers, public health organizations, school systems, diagnostic imaging centers, laboratories, urgent care clinics, and surgery centers as possible places of employment. You might be surprised by the variety of places that employ people with your education and skills.

You must answer many questions when identifying your occupational preferences. These include:

- Do you want to work close to where you live now or move to another location?
- Do you want to work in the same place throughout the year, work seasonal jobs in different parts of the country, or rotate among different companies as a temporary worker?
- Do you want a full-time or part-time job with employment benefits, or a supplemental job that provides flexibility in work schedules but no guaranteed work hours or employment benefits?
- Do you want a job where you can stay and grow with the organization over time, or just a place to launch your career?
- Do you want a small organization where you can become multiskilled and work in more than one area, or a large organization where you can become a specialist?
- Do you want a job that pays well but may require compromising on some of your other preferences, such as location, work schedule, or employment benefits?

Identifying your occupational preferences will help guide your job search; factors include:

- Geographic location (urban, rural, state, region, country)
- Type of employment setting (inpatient, outpatient, community-based, academic medical center)
- Size of the organization (small, large, statewide network, global organization)
- **Employment status** (full-time, part-time, supplemental)
- Work schedule/shift (days, evenings, nights, weekends, holidays, 10- or 12-hour shifts)
- Employment benefits (health, life, vision, and dental insurance; retirement and pension)
- Amount of compensation (pay) and paid time off for vacations and holidays
- Opportunities for advanced training, tuition assistance, and job promotions
- Length of employment prior to eligibility for the organization's retirement plan

employment status
(im-PLOY-ment STAY-tes) Hired to work full-time, part-time, or supplemental

Places to Find Employment Information

Once you've narrowed down the types of places you would like to work, investigate labor trends, job openings, salary ranges, employment benefits, and opportunities for career development. Labor trends forecast the supply and demand for different types of health care workers. Supply and demand changes over time and varies in different parts of the country.

When there is a shortage of nurses, for example:

- Demand increases.
- More nursing jobs are available to fill, with fewer nurses to fill them.
- Nurses have an easier time finding a job and may have several job offers from which to choose.
- Employers increase salaries and benefits to help recruit nurses.
- Employers offer a **hire-on bonus** as part of nurse recruitment.

hire-on bonus
(HIRE-on BOW-nes) Extra compensation for accepting a job offer

Conversely, when there is an oversupply of nurses:

- Demand decreases.
- More nurses are looking for jobs with fewer jobs to be filled.
- Nurses have a more difficult time finding a job, and there is more competition.
- Salaries and benefits remain steady.
- Hire-on bonuses for nurse recruitment temporarily disappear.

Nursing shortages are predicted to worsen as experienced nurses retire and leave the workforce. Yet not too long ago, nursing students just graduating from school had difficulty finding jobs in many parts of the country. The situation is similar in other professions, such as physical therapy, radiography, and respiratory therapy where supply and demand cycles have shifted over recent years.

Locate specific websites and other references to help you monitor the labor trends for the occupation you have chosen. By tracking the supply and demand for people in your field, you'll know the best times to apply for a job, and how difficult or easy it might be to find the kind of job for which you are looking.

FIGURE 10.1

Reviewing employment trends and searching for job opportunities

Source: Jace Tan/Shutterstock

THE MORE YOU KNOW

Health Care Employers of Choice

Identify which organizations are considered the Health Care Employers of Choice in your area. Employers of Choice:

- Actively support the growth, development, and job advancement of employees.
- Provide scholarships, tuition assistance, on-site continuing education, and advanced training for employees.
- Offer flexible work schedules for employees enrolled in school.
- Host an Employee Assistance Program (EAP) to help workers resolve personal issues and overcome barriers to job retention.
- Support a work environment that fosters continual improvement and lifelong learning.

If an employer has already helped you with a scholarship, part-time job, or another means of support while you are in school, show your loyalty. If the employer *took a chance* on you and invested in your education, then as a professional you have an obligation to re-pay that investment by working there for a sufficient period of time if the employer extends a job offer.

retention
(REE-ten-shen) The process of keeping

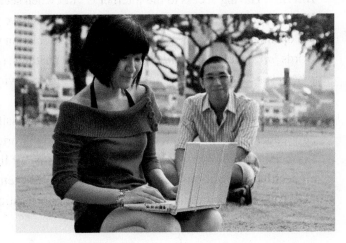

This is no time to take shortcuts on your homework. Make contacts with people who can help you investigate the best employment opportunities where you want to live and work. Landing your first professional job will launch your career and point it in the right direction. Making good decisions early in your career will increase your potential for a lifetime filled with satisfying and rewarding work.

retirement benefits (ri-TIRE-ment) Employer-funded pension contributions

Don't ignore the importance of **retirement benefits**. You probably won't think about retiring for many years, but your first professional job lays the foundation for your career and your life. If an employer is willing to invest in your retirement plan and perhaps even match the funds that you save yourself, you might be surprised how quickly those investments will grow over the years and provide a nice nest-egg when you're ready to retire.

Here are some places to find information about job openings:

- ***Internet.*** Having access to the Internet is vital when seeking jobs in health care. Most hospitals and many health care organizations have websites and may post their job openings online. Check out professional association websites and search the key words *job search* or *job link.* You can find job postings, career fairs, workshops for job-seekers, and tips on writing a résumé and interviewing. You can also post your résumé online for potential employers to view.
- ***Newspaper ads.*** Get into the habit of reading the classified advertisements in local newspapers and online news sites, and track job opportunities from week to week. Look under *Help Wanted.* There are different ways of listing jobs. Some papers list all health care positions under *Medical.* Others list them under a particular job title. Also become familiar with some of the abbreviations used by newspapers.

Common Abbreviations

appl.	applicant	immed.	immediately
asst.	assistant	incl.	included
cert.	certified	lic.	licensed
exp.	experience	suppl.	supplemental
FT	full time	PT	part time

- ***Employment settings.*** If you're looking for a position in a medical laboratory, apply directly to a laboratory. If you want to work in a hospital, go to the hospital's website or visit their **personnel department** or **human resources department**. Online sites and your telephone book offer an extensive list of possible employers.
- ***Health care workers.*** Speak with health care workers to get their opinions on the best places to work. They may have worked for numerous employers and can help you identify Employers of Choice in the area.
- ***Networking.*** By **networking**, you can help strengthen your interpersonal skills, identify job opportunities, and uncover the best places to work. Join a professional association, become a volunteer, or participate in community activities to widen your scope of collegial relationships.
- ***Friends and relatives.*** You may know someone who works in health care who can suggest a place to apply or introduce you to a possible employer.
- ***School counselors, placement coordinators, and librarians.*** Schools often have resource people who can help you track down job openings. They're a good resource for information on current employment trends and how to find job openings where you want to work.

personnel department (per-she-NEL di-PART-ment) People within an organization who recruit, select, and employ job applicants

human resources department (HYU-men REE-sors di-PART-ment) Current term for personnel department

networking (NET-werking) Interacting with a variety of people in different settings

- ***School bulletin boards.*** If you have a career center or a bulletin board where jobs are listed, be sure to check it daily.
- ***Occupational reference materials.*** Reference guides available online and in libraries list the locations, sizes, and other helpful details for health care organizations around the country.

Employment Agencies

employment agencies (im-PLOY-ment AY-jent-seez) Companies that connect job applicants with employers

Employment agencies help connect job applicants with employers who have jobs to fill. Some employment agencies specialize in health care jobs. Employers post their job openings with the agency, and then job-seekers review the postings to see which openings might be a good fit.

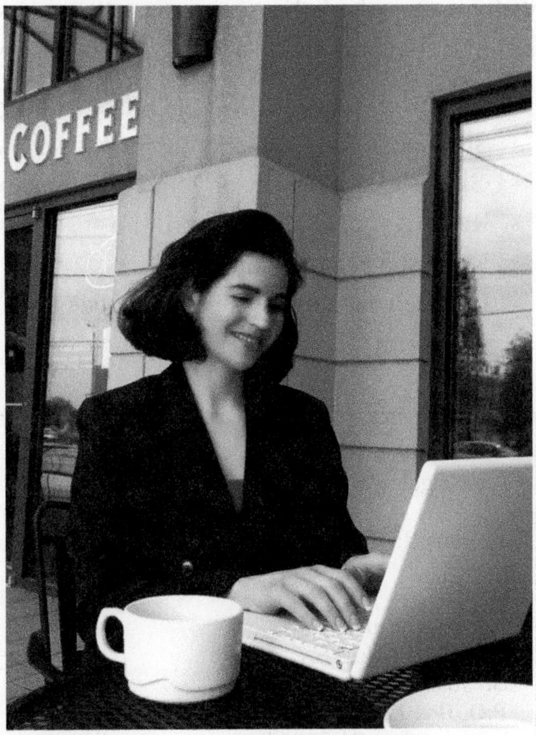

FIGURE 10.2

Job hunting via the Internet

Source: David Gilder/Shutterstock

- Public employment agencies are funded by tax dollars and don't charge a fee for their service. You can find public employment agencies online and in your telephone book under *Government Agencies*. Look for *Work One* or *One Stop* career centers sponsored by the U.S. Department of Labor's Employment and Training Administration.
- Private employment agencies charge for their services. Some charge the employer, while others charge the job-seeker. You can find information about private employment agencies online and in your telephone book. Depending on the health occupation you've chosen, you probably won't need the services of a private employment agency during the early stages of your career. Later on, if you seek an executive leadership position, you might find these services helpful and worth the expense.

Hundreds of websites such as *monster.com* now exist where you can find job openings, post your résumé, and apply for jobs online. Once you've set up your profile and posted your résumé, you can create alerts to e-mail you when new jobs have been posted. You can submit an application with the click of your mouse and keep track of the places where you've applied. Sites such as these can be especially helpful when looking for job opportunities beyond your region of the country.

APPLY IT ONLINE JOB SEEKING SITES

Conduct some online research to identify two websites that help job seekers. List the types of information provided on the sites and describe other kinds of resources that might be helpful. How do these sites benefit both job seekers and employers?

Cover Letters

Now that you know where to look for a job, you need to know how to contact the employer and present yourself in a professional manner. If you have a lead on a possible job, you may choose to call for information. Give your name, identify the job of interest, and ask how to apply.

You may be asked to submit a cover letter as part of your application materials. Even if a cover letter isn't required, providing one is still a good idea. Many employers now use online, electronic systems to manage the job application and selection process. Online job applications limit the amount of information, and the kinds of information, that you can submit. So your cover letter serves as your sales letter—a way to sell yourself to the employer in order to get an interview. Your cover letter should:

job application
(JOB a-pleh-KAY-shen) Form used to apply for a job; also known as an employment application

selection process
(se-LEK-shen PRAH-ses) Steps to determine which applicants are chosen

- Be neat and easy to read and reflect good grammar and correct spelling.
- State the job you're applying for and how you heard about the job opening.
- Give a brief overview of your education, experience, and qualifications.
- Refer to your résumé or portfolio.
- Request a personal interview.
- Provide your address, phone number, e-mail address, and the best way and times to reach you.

FIGURE 10.3
Sample cover letter

888 Whitegate Avenue
Los Angeles, CA 90820

January 25, 2014

Mr. E. B. Burns
Director of Nurses
St. Joseph's Hospital
P.O. Box 123
Los Angeles, CA 90880

Dear Mr. Burns:

I am responding to your advertisement in Nurses World on January 14, 2014. I am interested in applying for the position of nurse assistant. I graduated from Medical Technologies High School on December 15, 2010. I studied nursing assisting and am well qualified for this position. My course work included communication, CPR, and a core of courses that prepared me to be employed as a nursing assistant. I also worked in a hospital setting eight hours a week for sixteen weeks. My attendance is excellent, and I am very reliable. My goal is to use my skills as a nursing assistant and to be an exemplary employee.

My résumé is enclosed. Also included is a list of skills I have mastered. I know that I am well qualified for this position. I am looking forward to an opportunity to interview for this position. I will call on Monday, February 3, at 9:00 a.m. and hope to arrange an interview at that time.

If you require additional information, or want to contact me, please call me at (123) 456-7890 after 3:00 p.m.

Sincerely,

Mark Adams, CNA

BUILD YOUR SKILLS *Organizing Your Job Hunt*

Job hunting can lead to concerns about where you will live, how much money you will earn, and what direction your career will take. If these concerns cause you too much stress, they can affect your ability to present yourself well to prospective employers. Here are some tips to help organize your job hunt and manage your stress:

- Stay organized. Keep a good supply of résumés and cover letters on hand. Maintain a list of the places to which you have submitted job applications. Include details about the people who have interviewed you, including their names, job titles, and contact information. Keep track of follow-up phone calls and other communication.
- Plan ahead. Get clear directions to locate employers before the date of your interview. Visit the location in advance to identify the travel time.
- Use a schedule. Keep a clear and up-to-date schedule of all your appointments to avoid over-scheduling yourself. Have your schedule open in front of you when you make appointments for new and follow-up meetings and interviews.
- Join a job hunter's group. Groups offer good networking opportunities and emotional support.

Job hunting should be an exciting time. Managing the process so that you minimize stress can help you enjoy it and achieve success.

Résumés

In addition to your cover letter, potential employers need more details about you and your qualifications. This is accomplished by preparing a résumé. Even if a résumé isn't required, it's still a good idea to have one. Even if you lack significant postsecondary education or work experience, you still have important information to share with potential employers.

Résumés provide:

- A snapshot of your background, education, and work experience.
- A description of your experience that relates to the job for which you are applying.
- The qualifications you're presenting for consideration.
- Visible evidence of your written communication skills.

If you've never developed a résumé, you can find Microsoft Word templates on the Internet or references in your school library or local bookstore to give you some guidance and examples. You could also ask someone who writes or reviews résumés to assist you. Your résumé should be:

- Typed, professional in appearance, and concise.
- Available in multiple forms (print and electronic, such as a Word document).
- Easily faxed, scanned, sent as an e-mail attachment, or photocopied with good quality.
- Printed on plain white paper with no borders or graphics.
- Well organized and formatted, using bullets and underlining.

Organize the information and make sure your grammar and spelling are correct. The most current information should appear at the beginning of each section. Emphasize your educational background, skills, and abilities that match the qualifications for the job. If you are a young person with little or no job experience or postsecondary education:

- List your high school accomplishments and extracurricular activities, such as academic awards, sports, orchestra or choir, science fair entries, perfect attendance awards, or participation in school organizations.
- Mention leadership roles, computer skills, seminars, or training sessions you've attended, certificates you've earned, and distinctions you've received.
- Describe volunteer activities and community service.
- Include health care courses, clinical observations, and internship experience in health care facilities.

FIGURE 10.4

Sample résumé

800 E. Oak Street
Conway, AR 72032

Home: 501-666-8340
Cell: 501-620-9180

Mary Jane Rodgers

Career Plans	Complete 2-year Associate of Science Nursing Program Short-range: Nursing assistant Long-range: Complete a Bachelor of Science Program as a registered nurse
Experience	2010–present Henry's Hamburger Shop Conway, AR **Sales Clerk** • Food preparation • Counting inventory • Customer service • Operating a cash register and making change • Maintaining health standards 2008–2009 June Allison Conway, AR **Babysitter** • Meal preparation • Overnight care of two children, 8 and 10 years of age • Planning recreation
Family Responsibilities	• Prepare dinner 2–3 times a week • Weekly gardening • Perform minor household tasks
Education	Diploma candidate 2010 Hoover High School Conway, AR
Interests	Dancing, classical music, reading, skiing, member of Explorer Scouts Medical Post and Health Occupation Students of America
Skills and Strengths	Fluent in oral and written Spanish communication Proficient in Windows programs including Word, Excel, PowerPoint, and Outlook applications

Submitting supportive documents (such as copies of certificates, grade transcripts, or reference letters from a teacher or internship site supervisor) is usually permissible, but don't get carried away. Select one or two of the best items to submit with your résumé, and save the others for your interview in case you get a chance to present them in person.

APPLYING FOR JOBS

Once you have identified some potential job openings, it's time to the launch the job application process. This includes completing job applications, providing references, taking pre-employment assessments, and having your qualifications verified.

Job Applications

As with the résumé, the job application (also known as an employment application) conveys a lot of information about you, and it's an important part of the employment process. When employers receive a surplus of applications for a particular job opening, the application is typically the first item they use to screen applicants and narrow down the applicant pool. Employers screen job applications to:

screen
(SCREEN) To sift, filter, or separate

- Determine if your qualifications match those of the job.
- Evaluate how well you read and follow instructions.
- Assess your written communication skills, spelling, and grammar.
- Decide whether or not to proceed with an interview.

Many companies now require online applications. If you need to submit your application online, make sure you have the computer skills required to navigate the employer's website and enter your information electronically. If necessary, ask someone who is familiar with the process to help you.

RECENT DEVELOPMENTS

Online Applications on the Rise

If you're required to submit your job application online, you must have an e-mail account. Login on the job application website and set up your profile, username, and password. Employers can view this information, so make sure that your username and password are appropriate. Allow time to become familiar with how the computerized system works.

Keep your electronic résumé handy and expect to cut and paste sections from your résumé into your application. With many online systems, you can save a draft of your application and go back later to revise and complete it.

Pay attention to the knowledge, skills, abilities, and qualifications that are listed in the job posting, and identify some of the key words. Incorporate these key words in your application because computerized systems search for key words to find applicants who might be a good match.

If you aren't familiar with completing online job applications, expect to encounter some challenges until you've learned how to use the system. If you don't have basic computer skills, take some computer classes as soon as possible. If the organization where you want to work uses computers to manage job application process, they probably also rely on computerized systems for many other aspects of their business.

If the employer uses a paper application form, fill it out yourself and don't ask someone to do it for you. Type the information or make sure your writing is legible and neat.

Regardless of whether you complete your job application online or on paper, you should:

- Read the instructions and follow them.
- Use your best written communication skills and make sure all words are spelled correctly.
- List accurate dates for your education and work experience.
- List the *job number* if the employer uses a numbering system for job postings.
- Review the form to make sure you haven't left anything out.

If the application calls for a brief statement about why you're applying for the job, take some time to think about your answer before writing it. You might be surprised how much weight your answer carries in the selection process. Convince the reviewers that you're familiar with the job and their organization. Let them know that you believe you're a good match for the qualifications they're seeking. If space permits, describe briefly how hiring you would benefit the organization.

Your job application, cover letter, and résumé make that all-important first impression. Spend time making sure it's the impression you want to convey. These three documents will likely determine whether or not you get invited for an interview. Present your best qualities and don't undersell yourself. Stand on your own merits and avoid exaggerating your qualifications.

Be truthful—**never falsify your information**. Lying about your qualifications is dishonest, unethical, and unprofessional. If you misrepresent your qualifications and your lies are discovered, you will be disqualified as an applicant. If your dishonesty is discovered after you've started the job, you may be dismissed from the job.

Consider This *Dishonesty on Job Applications*

Research shows that 70% of applicants overstate their qualifications on job applications. More than one third lie about their experience and achievements and 12% fail to disclose criminal records. About a third of all job applicants admit to thinking about stealing from their employers.

What happens when these applicants become employees? About half of all new hires don't work out, often the result of dishonest behavior before and during employment. The result can be devastating to the companies that hire them. About 30% of all business failures in the U.S. are caused by employee theft. Employee theft is growing by 15% a year, and as much as 75% of internal theft is never detected. In addition to theft, work-related violent crimes affect about 2 million people every year.

If you've had a misdemeanor or a felony conviction, you must disclose it on your job application. Most employers conduct a criminal history background check as part of the employment process. A prior conviction may or may not eliminate you from consideration depending on the job you're applying for, the type of offense, how long ago it

APPLICATION FOR EMPLOYMENT

Mountain View Health Care Center is an equal opportunity employer and upholds the principles of equal opportunity employment. It is the policy of Mountain View Health Care Center to provide employment, compensation and other benefits related to employment based on qualifications and performance, without regard to race, color, religion, national origin, age, sex, veteran status or disability, or any other basis prohibited by federal or state law. As an equal opportunity employer, Mountain View Health Care Center intends to comply fully with all federal and state laws and the information requested on this application will not be used for any purpose prohibited by law. Disabled applicants may request any needed accommodation. This application is intended to allow you, the applicant, to provide Mountain View Health Care Center with the information and data so that your suitability and qualifications can be fairly determined for the position(s) for which you are applying. Please complete this application and answer all questions completely. Please print clearly in ink.

PLEASE PRINT CLEARLY—BE SURE TO SIGN THIS APPLICATION

Date

Name: Last First Middle

Social Security No.: Home Phone:

Address:

No. - Street

City State Zip

Have you been previously employed by Mountain View Health Care Center? ☐ Yes ☐ No
If "Yes", when? In what capacity?

How did you learn of the position for which you are applying:
☐ Newspaper/Print Advertisement ☐ Friend/Relative ☐ Employment Agency ☐ Job Service ☐ Radio/TV Advertisement

EMPLOYMENT DESIRED

Position(s) applied for
Shift Preferences: ☐ First Shift – Days ☐ Second Shift – Evenings ☐ Third Shift – Nights
☐ Full-time ☐ Part-time If "Part-time", number of shifts/hours desired:
Date available to start Salary requested

PERSONAL HISTORY

Are you a United States citizen or do you have an entry permit which allows you to lawfully work in the U.S.? ☐ Yes ☐ No
If applicable, Visa Type: Immigration No.:
Are you at least 18 years old? ☐ Yes ☐ No

Are you able to perform all of the duties required by the position for which you are applying, without endangering yourself or compromising the safety, health, or welfare of the Patients or other Staff Persons? ☐ Yes ☐ No
If "No," please explain:

EDUCATION

Name and Location Of School	Graduation Date	Course of Study/ Degree Issued
High School		
College		
Other		

LICENSURE/CERTIFICATION/REGISTRATION

Type of License/Certification	Registration Number

List any special skills or qualifications which you possess and feel are relevant to health care and the position for which you are applying.

FIGURE 10.5

Sample job application

EMPLOYMENT HISTORY

Please give accurate and complete information. Start with present or most recent employer.

May we contact and communicate with your present employer? ☐ Yes ☐ No

Employer Telephone No.

Address Employed from / to /

Name of Supervisor Hourly Pay: Start Last

Position and Responsibilities

Reason for Leaving

Employer Telephone No.

Address Employed from / to /

Name of Supervisor Hourly Pay: Start Last

Position and Responsibilities

Reason for Leaving

Employer Telephone No.

Address Employed from / to /

Name of Supervisor Hourly Pay: Start Last

Position and Responsibilities

Reason for Leaving

MILITARY SERVICE

Branch From To

What were your duties?

Did you receive any specialized training? ☐ Yes ☐ No

If "Yes", describe:

REFERENCES

Names of people whom we may contact for a reference.

Name Address Phone

Name Address Phone

Names of co-workers (no relatives) you have worked with and whom we may contact for a reference.

Name Address Phone

Name Address Phone

Please read the following statements completely and carefully before you initial and sign your name.

The Applicant HEREBY CERTIFIES that the answers given on this Application For Employment, including any statements or answers provided by the Applicant during interview, are true and correct. The Applicant fully authorizes Mountain View Health Care Center to contact any references, past and present employers, persons, schools, law enforcement agencies and any other sources of information which may be relevant to the Applicant and this Application For Employment. It is understood and agreed that any misrepresentation, false statement, or omission by the Applicant will be sufficient reason for rejection of the Application For Employment or for dismissal from employment at any time, without recourse or liability to Mountain View Health Care Center.

I have read, understand and agree to the above statement. (Please initial here). __________

SIGN HERE ________________________________ DATE ______________

FIGURE 10.5

(Continued)

occurred, and so forth. But if you fail to disclose the conviction and your employer discovers it later on, you could lose your job and do irreparable harm to your reputation.

Employers are increasingly searching the Internet to gather additional information on job applicants. They may run a credit report, visit social networking sites, and read blogs. Be very careful. Don't publish or share any personal information that you wouldn't want prospective employers to view or hear about.

credit report
(KRE-dit REE-port) A review of records to assess a person's financial status

blogs
(BLOGS) Similar to newspaper columns but published on the Internet instead of in print

Your job application form and résumé provide contact information that potential employers will use to set-up an interview. Make sure that the recorded message on your telephone reflects the image you want to convey to potential employers. Think twice about religious, political, or musical overtones in your recorded message. Refrain from having children record the message or answer your telephone when you're expecting a call from a potential employer. An inappropriate, unprofessional, or confusing message may be all it takes to screen out your application.

References

Most employers require references who can provide more information about job applicants. Choose your references carefully. Consider the following:

- One reference should be qualified to attest to your knowledge, competence, and potential for learning, such as a teacher.
- A second reference should be qualified to comment on your character, work ethic, and reliability, such as a previous employer or your internship site supervisor.

FIGURE 10.6

Lining up a reference for job applications

Source: ARENA Creative/Shutterstock

Consider the following when lining up references:

- Select people who are familiar with your skills, the quality of your work, and your ability to learn quickly.
- Ensure the credibility of your references; never use a spouse or relatives as a reference.
- Contact people ahead of time and ask for permission to list them as references.
- When asked, provide written permission for references to disclose information about your performance and qualifications.
- Identify the job you're applying for and when they might be contacted by the employer.
- Make sure you have accurate contact information for each reference, including their e-mail address.
- Choose references who have positive, insightful, and complimentary things to say about you.

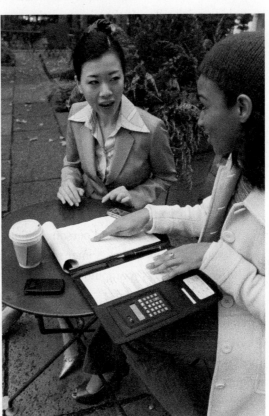

If you know someone who works for the organization to which you are applying, and if that person is familiar with you and the quality of your work, consider listing him or her as a reference. However, avoid *name dropping, pulling strings,* or *using connections* to try to enhance your chances of a job offer. Such attempts could have a negative effect and back-fire on you. Take the professional approach—stand on your own merits and get hired for the right reasons.

Because a frequent reason for terminating employees is poor attendance, employers are especially interested in the attendance record of job applicants. Employers are typically impressed by job applicants who can demonstrate effective time management skills and the ability to balance school, work, and a personal life with good results. When an employer contacts your references for feedback about your performance and reliability, expect your attendance to be one of the topics discussed.

Another topic that's frequently raised during reference checks is your people skills. Employers need to know if you can form positive relationships, function as a team player, treat people with respect, and display good customer service skills.

Choosing the right references and making sure they're well prepared to respond when contacted is critical. Employers often wait to check references until they're close to making a job offer. If there's more than one finalist for a job, the applicant with the best references will probably get the offer. Even if you're the only finalist, just one less-than-satisfactory reference is all it takes to lose the job at the last minute.

Pre-Employment Assessments

pre-employment assessments (pre-im-PLOY-ment a-SES-ments) Tests and other instruments used to measure knowledge, skills, and personality traits

Expect to take some written or computerized **pre-employment assessments** as part of the application and employment process. Employers need to know if your competencies and personal traits match the characteristics they're seeking. Some companies include an online assessment with their job applications. Other companies schedule half-day or full-day assessments to evaluate factors such as:

- Basic skills
- Work ethic, character, and personal values
- Personality traits and customer service skills
- Job-specific skills (computer skills, applied math, and so forth)

Pre-employment assessments are difficult to prepare for because they measure the accumulation of the knowledge, skills, and personal characteristics that you've developed over time. When taking pre-employment assessments, be well-rested and ready to concentrate. Make sure you understand the instructions before taking the assessment. Try to relax and just do your best. Answer all questions in an honest and consistent manner.

Some employers will share assessment results with applicants while others will not. When an employer is willing to share the results, ask for feedback on how well you performed to learn about your strong and weak points. If your scores indicate some weaknesses, work on strengthening those skills as you apply for other jobs. If you don't get an interview the first time you apply, enhance your qualifications and reapply later. Some employers require a waiting period of a few months before accepting another job application from the same person.

Verifying Qualifications

Most health care jobs today require a minimum of a high school diploma or a GED. While a few jobs exist for people without a high school diploma or a GED, opportunities for advancement will be limited until workers return to school and complete their secondary education. Most health care jobs now require successful completion of a postsecondary education or college degree program as well as a professional license, certification, or registration.

Depending on the type of job for which you are applying, you may need to submit supporting documentation such as an **official transcript** from each of the schools you've attended; copies of diplomas, certificates of completion, or college degrees; and verification of active status of professional licenses, certifications, registrations, or other credentials required for the job.

official transcript (ah-FIH-shel TRAN-script) Grade report that is printed, sealed, and mailed directly to the recipient to prevent tampering by the applicant

JOB INTERVIEWS

Once you've submitted your job application, résumé, references, and supportive documentation, completed your pre-employment assessments, and survived the screening process, it's time for your job interview.

Preparing for an Interview

Making a good impression during an interview pulls together just about everything discussed in this textbook. The objective is to present yourself as a competent, motivated, and caring professional who is well-qualified and prepared for the job. Interviewers will be looking for information about your academic achievements, occupational experiences, interpersonal skills, and personal qualities to help decide if you are a good fit for the organization and the position. Don't just show up for an interview. Do your homework first.

Research the Organization

Learn as much as you can about the job and the organization ahead of time so you can talk intelligently about the opportunity for which you are applying. If you're applying for a job in an outpatient clinic, find out more about the kinds of patients it sees, the on-site services it provides, the kinds of workers it employs, the hours it is open, and so forth. If it's obvious during the interview that you aren't familiar with the organization, the interviewers will wonder if you're really serious about wanting the job or not. If you take time to research the organization first, interviewers will be impressed with your interest and may give you some extra consideration in the selection process. To research the organization you should:

- Review their website, newspaper employment ads, and brochures.
- Read articles about the organization online and in local newspapers and magazines.
- Find out if they have won any recent awards or been featured in special reports.
- Speak with people who are familiar with the organization, such as employees, patients, and vendors.
- Spend some time on-site before your interview to observe the environment.

Even if you've already answered a question on the application form about why you're applying for the job, expect to be asked this question again during the interview. Familiarity with the organization and the job will help convince interviewers that you're a good match for the opening. Someone may ask, "What did you do to investigate this job and our organization to make sure this is a good match for you?" If you've done your homework, you'll have several examples to share with interviewers.

Anticipating Interview Questions

Interviewers use traditional and behavioral questioning techniques:

traditional questions (treh-DIH-shen-al KWES-chens) Ask how you *would* behave in certain situations

behavioral questions (bi-HAY-vyer-al KWES-chens) Ask how you *did* behave in certain situations

Traditional questions ask how you *would* behave in certain situations.

Behavioral questions ask how you *did* behave in certain situations.

Many interviewers believe that past performance is the best predictor of future performance and that's why they use behavioral questions. Behavioral questions are more probing and call for more thought and specific answers. Here are some examples to illustrate the difference:

- ***Traditional:*** "What weakness might prevent you from being successful in this job?"
  Behavioral: "Describe a weakness that you had in the past and explain what you did to overcome it."
- ***Traditional:*** "How would you handle stress in this job?"
  Behavioral: "Describe a previous stressful situation and how you handled it."
- ***Traditional:*** "What are your goals for the next five years?"
  Behavioral: "What were your goals when you started school and how successful have you been in accomplishing them?"

Once you've answered a behavioral question, expect more detailed follow-up questions such as these:

- Why did you try that approach?
- What did you do or say that led to that outcome?
- How would you do things differently the next time?
- What did you learn from the experience?

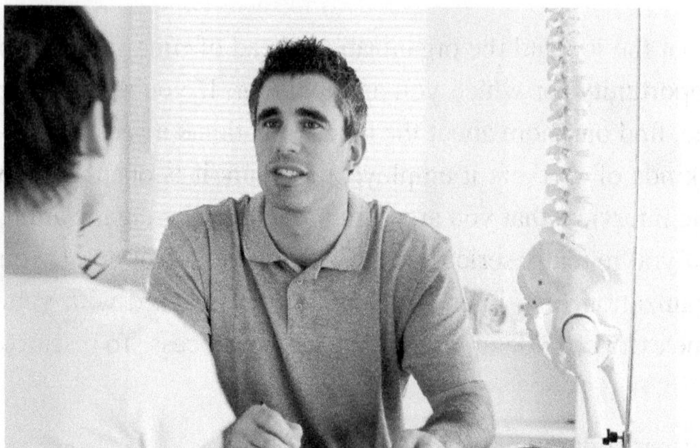

FIGURE 10.7

Meeting for an interview

Source: wavebreakmedia/Shutterstock

Prepare for both traditional and behavioral questions since you won't know until you get there which approach the interviewers will use. It could be a combination of both types of questions.

Refresh your memory about challenges that you've faced, projects you've worked on, and goals you've achieved. Have some personal stories in mind in case you're asked for examples. Knowing as much as you can about the job description and the skills that your interviewer seeks will help you anticipate the types of questions that might be asked.

Practice at home or at school with someone firing questions at you in a mock interview setting. Be prepared to answer questions such as:

- Why are you interested in this job?
- Have you had a job that didn't turn out as expected? What did you do about it?
- What specifically have you done to investigate this job?
- How can you be sure this job is right for you?

- Have you ever been fired from a job? If so, why were you fired, and how did you react?
- Have you experienced conflict with a former supervisor? If so, how did you resolve it?
- What do you think it would take to be successful in this job?
- What have you done to prepare for this job?
- Did you need to learn something new in your previous job? If so, how did you do that?
- What strengths would you bring to this job and this organization?
- How did you support the reputation of the organization where you used to work?
- What appeals to you about working for this organization?
- Why should we select you over other applicants?
- Have you ever applied for a job and didn't get it? If so, what did you do?

The more questions you can anticipate in advance, the better prepared you will be. Expect some *what if?* questions, such as:

- What would you do if you had to be late for work one morning?
- What would you do if you observed a coworker stealing from the organization?
- What will you do if you're not selected for this job?

Interviewing is a two-way process. At some point during the session, the interviewer will probably ask, "What questions do you have for me?" You'll need to be well prepared for this because your response will carry some weight in the selection process. Here are some examples of questions that you might ask:

- Is this job full-time, part-time job, or supplemental?
- What would my work schedule be?
- Does this job include employment benefits? If so, where could I get more information about the benefits?
- Once I'm on the job, what additional training or duties should I expect?
- Do you offer tuition assistance for employees who want to get more education or training or work on college degrees?
- How soon would I become **vested** in the retirement plan?

vested
(VES-ted) Fully enrolled in, and eligible for, benefits

When it comes to asking questions about how much the job pays, keep reading.

Participating in an Interview

The big day has finally arrived. Do the following immediately prior to your interview:

- Review this chapter again to make sure the information is fresh on your mind.
- Get plenty of sleep and eat a good breakfast or lunch before your appointment.
- Make sure you know exactly where to go, how to get there, and where to park.
- Plan to arrive at least fifteen minutes early.
- If you get delayed, call the contact person to let them know why you can't be there on time, apologize for any inconvenience, and ask if you need to reschedule.

Allow plenty of time for the interview itself. Other applicants may be scheduled for interviews during the same time period as you, so interviewers could be running late, and you might be kept waiting.

It should go without saying but must be mentioned—don't bring children with you to your interview. Having children present is disruptive and an indication that you lack reliable childcare. If your childcare plans fall through, it's better to reschedule your interview than to arrive with a child.

Once you've arrived at the right time and place, it's important to make a positive and professional first impression. Your appearance *will speak louder than words.* Interviewers could be your age or younger, but it's more likely they'll be older than you and perhaps about the same age as your parents. What type of clothing and personal image would they consider professional and appropriate for an interview? This is no time to think about styles and fashion trends or to wear something outrageous in order to be remembered or to *stand out in the crowd.* You definitely want to make a lasting impression, but it should be based on your qualifications and friendly personality, not your unconventional appearance. Interviewers are going to *size you up* by assessing how well their patients, customers, business associates, and coworkers might react to you and your appearance if you were to get the job. So it's important to look your very best.

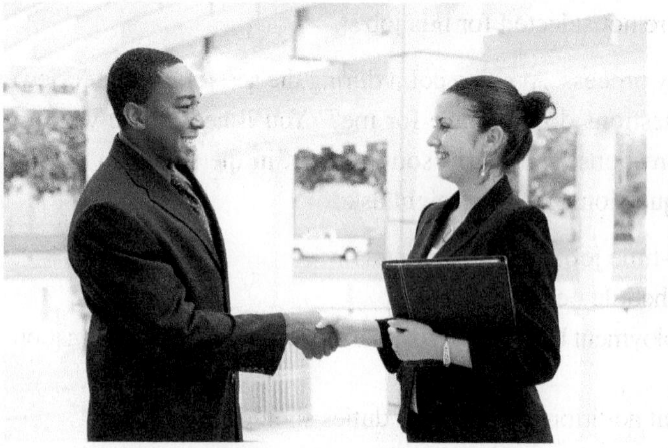

FIGURE 10.8
Presenting a professional image
Source: Stephen Coburn/Shutterstock

Revisit earlier portions of this textbook to refresh your memory about appropriate clothing and how to present a professional image. The importance of wearing appropriate clothing cannot be stressed too much. Men should wear a suit or sport coat with a tie. Women should wear a business suit or professional-looking skirt, blouse, and jacket. Proper shoes and accessories are important. Avoid low necklines, ripped or baggy pants, or evening wear. *Dress for success* even if you have to borrow clothes.

Bring several copies of your résumé with you. Bring a list of references that includes contact information and e-mail addresses. Also bring a notepad and a pen. On the notepad, list some personal accomplishments and stories to recall in case you are asked. Jot down examples of how you've handled stress in the past and a situation where you've had to learn something new, in case you are asked. Have some questions ready to ask the interviewer when the opportunity arises. If you dropped out of school or have gaps in your employment history, be prepared to explain why.

Here are some documents to have ready:

- Your career portfolio.
- Thank you notes from coworkers, patients, or physicians.
- Awards or **citations** that you've received.
- Grade reports and transcripts for courses or educational programs completed.
- Copies of professional certificates and other evidence of your performance and professional growth.

citations
(sie-TAY-shens) Honorable mention for receiving an outcome or result

Bring copies of the most relevant items to your interview, but don't overwhelm the interviewer with papers. Select just a few items that relate most closely to the job you're applying for and have them ready in case you need them.

SMILE! Smiling is one of the easiest ways to make a good first impression. As soon as you are called into the room, thank the person for the interview. Don't sit down until shown a seat and until the person conducting the interview has been seated. Offer a firm handshake. Never hug the interviewer! Try to remember the names of the people to whom you are introduced. Apply your best interpersonal communication skills and personality traits. Remember the importance of customer service in health care. All health care employers seek job applicants with pleasant personalities who can relate well to other people. Practice your best people skills during the interview. It's okay to be nervous. In fact, interviewers might wonder what's wrong with you if you aren't nervous. But try to maintain your composure and self-confidence.

During your interview:

- Describe the skills and abilities you would bring to the job.
- Convince interviewers that you would make a positive contribution to their organization and serve as an effective member of their team.
- Remember why you chose a career in health care; let your enthusiasm and commitment to helping people show.
- Be sincere; don't just make up answers that you think interviewers want to hear.
- Share some brief personal stories as examples of how you've overcome challenges and achieved your goals in the past.
- Be yourself; don't pretend to be someone you *think* would be more appealing to the interviewers.
- Trust the interviewers to recognize a good match when they see one; you want to be a good match for the job, and you want the job to be a good match for you.
- Be honest; if you're asked why you left school or terminated employment, tell the truth.
- Be prepared to answer questions about your attendance, transportation, and the back-up plans you will have in place in case things don't go as expected.

Here are some more things to think about:

- Sit up straight, don't chew gum or bite your fingernails, and try to relax.
- Pay attention to your body language and the non-verbal messages you are sending.
- Convey a positive attitude; don't express anger about a former teacher, job, or supervisor.
- Don't *carry baggage* from your past into what could become a new situation and fresh start.
- Display self-confidence and a genuine interest in what is being discussed.
- Don't ramble; stay on track and focus on the message you want to convey.
- Don't let your guard down; everything that you say and do will be taken into account.

Even if you decide early in the interview that you aren't interested in the job, continue to *put your best foot forward*. A few years from now you may want to apply there again. The person who interviews you at one organization may know the people who do the hiring at other organizations. Never pass up an opportunity to make a good impression.

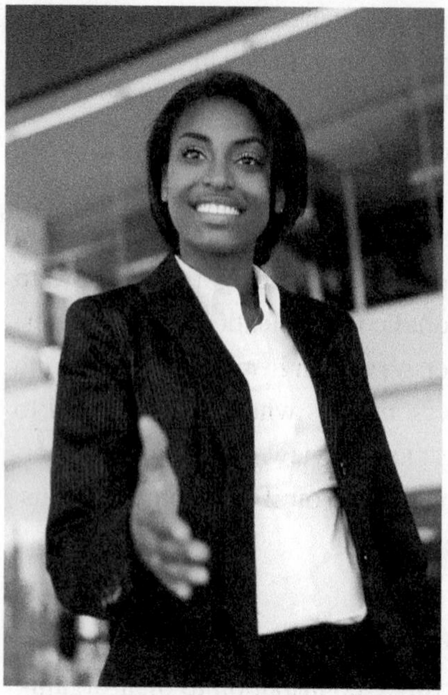

FIGURE 10.9
Making a good first impression
Source: Stephen Coburn/Shutterstock

Some interview sessions are quite formal, while others are more conversational and informal. If you're invited to lunch or dinner, and it feels like a social setting, you are still being sized-up as a potential employee. Don't be surprised if you're interviewed by more than one person, perhaps at the same time. Having one person fire questions at you can be intimidating enough without having two or three people doing the same thing during the same session. Sometimes employers have no choice but to have multiple people interview an applicant at the same time. Occasionally, it's done intentionally to see how well an applicant performs under pressure.

Answer questions thoughtfully. Concentrate on each question and think before you answer. Don't just blurt out the first thought that pops into your head, but don't ponder too long either. Employers need to know if you can think and respond quickly. Let your interviewer know that you're always eager to learn new things. If you present yourself as someone who resists change, you'll likely lose points in the selection process.

Some interviewers ask intimidating, strange, or confusing questions just to see how applicants perform under stress. Don't let these kinds of questions shake your confidence. Interviewers are not supposed to raise the following topics during an interview:

- Age, race, ethnicity, religious or political beliefs.
- Marital status, number and age of children, and pregnancies.
- Lifestyle preferences (heterosexual, homosexual, bisexual, transsexual).

discriminate
(dis-KRI-meh-nate) To treat a person or group unfairly on the basis of prejudice

Unfortunately, some interviewers do ask inappropriate questions and then use the information to **discriminate** against job applicants during the selection process. Therefore, it's important to be prepared for these kinds of questions and have responses in mind.

For example, an interviewer might ask a young female applicant: When do you plan to start a family? How many children do you plan to have? Or, how old are your children and who takes care of them while you're at work? With questions such as these, interviewers are concerned about the applicant's ability to manage parenthood and a full-time job at the same time. Which of the following responses would be most appropriate?

- You aren't supposed to ask questions like that so I'm not going to answer.
- I know that balancing my personal and professional lives will be a challenge. But I've been working part-time and taking care of my elderly grandmother for the past two years while enrolled in school full-time. So I know I have the skills and the support I need to manage a job and my family successfully.

It should be obvious which of these two responses would be best received by the person asking the questions.

Language Arts Link — Equal Employment Opportunities

Dating back to the early 1960s, women and minorities had significantly fewer opportunities for employment than they have today. Federal and state laws, Supreme Court decisions, and presidential orders have led employers to hire people who, just a few years ago, would not have been considered for employment. *Equal opportunity employment* is now an integral part of the workplace in most companies, but improvements still need to be made.

Title VII of the Civil Rights Act of 1964, as amended in 1972, states that it is illegal for an employer to discriminate in hiring, firing, promoting, or compensating people based on their race, color, sex, religion, or national origin. The Age Discrimination in Employment Act of 1967, as amended in 1978 and 1986, prohibits age discrimination. The Rehabilitation Act of 1973 and the Americans with Disabilities Act of 1990 prohibit discrimination against workers who are qualified for a job, but have physical or mental disabilities.

Research one of these laws or another law (such the Child Labor law) that prohibits unfair and inappropriate employment practices. Prepare an oral report to present to your classmates and teacher to share what you have learned. Include a statement that describes the purpose of your report. Create an outline that organizes the material to be covered in a logical sequence. Ask another person to review your outline and offer some feedback before giving your presentation. Use printed materials or other visual aids to help explain your topic.

What led to the law that you chose? Who had to fight for it, and why was the law passed? What benefits have resulted from the law? How might this law change in the future?

Remember that interviewing is a two-way process. When the interviewer says, "What questions do you have for me?" consider asking:

- "What characteristics are you looking for in an ideal applicant?" (Gather some important information and create an opportunity to describe how your qualifications match what the interviewer is seeking.)
- "What is the potential for growth and advancement within your organization?" (This question conveys that you are ambitious and seeking an organization with which you can grow.)

Jot down the responses along with any other information that you don't want to forget. Interviewers will notice that you are organized, pay attention to details, and record important information. Avoid asking for information that's already available in printed materials or on the organization's website. Interviewers will wonder why you aren't better prepared.

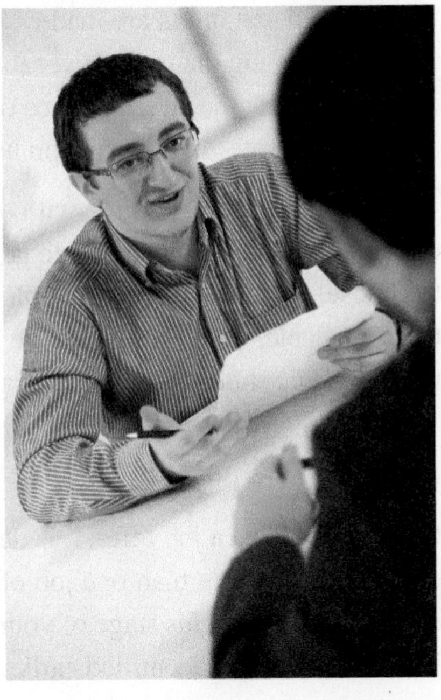

FIGURE 10.10

Asking questions during a job interview

Source: EmiliaUngur/Shutterstock

Not everyone agrees on whether or not to ask questions about pay and benefits during the first interview. Although pay and benefits are important, it's best to focus on the primary responsibilities of the job and the qualifications being sought by the employer first. If you know there's going to be a second follow-up interview, wait for that appointment to ask about pay and benefits. Or, let the interviewer take the lead in bringing up the discussion during your first interview.

Give some thought ahead of time to what your pay and benefit requirements would be in case you're asked those questions during your first interview. Saying, "I don't know" or, "I haven't really thought about it" indicates you haven't done your homework. Before your interview, investigate customary pay ranges for the job you are seeking by using occupational references, speaking with a counselor or placement advisor at school, or asking a human resources consultant or manager where you would be working. Keep in mind that pay rates are based on the geographic location of the health care facility.

How much pay do you need? It is okay to say, "The salary is negotiable," but have an acceptable range in mind in case you get pinned down or a job offer is extended. If you've done your homework, you've already identified what is most important in selecting the best offer. Instead of focusing on starting pay and benefits, new graduates should be more concerned about the job itself, support for continuing education, and opportunities to gain new skills and valuable work experience.

After the Interview

Regardless of whether you still want the job or not, you should follow-up the interview with a letter thanking the employer for the opportunity to interview. This demonstrates courtesy and good manners, and it also puts your name and communication skills in front of the decision-makers one more time. Since the majority of job applicants fail to follow-up, delivering a hand-written thank you letter or sending a thank-you e-mail message within 24 hours after your interview will make a good impression. Your thank you correspondence also provides an opportunity to restate how excited you are about joining the organization. You can also follow-up on something that was discussed or forgotten during the interview.

If you want the job, do the following:

- Contact the interviewer and ask if there is anything else you can do to verify your qualifications or answer any remaining questions.
- Try to wait patiently. It can take several weeks before employment decisions are finalized and offers are made.
- Avoid calling the interviewer to ask if a decision has been made yet. You don't want to become an annoyance or appear desperate. Most organizations will notify all applicants when a position has been filled.

Expect some competition with other job applicants. When employers face shortages of qualified workers, it's easier to get a job, and you may have several offers from which to choose. But when there's a surplus of qualified job applicants for the number of positions available, competition can be fierce. If you've mastered everything so far in this textbook, you should be in good shape to land the job you desire.

CONSIDERING JOB OFFERS

Once you receive a job offer, it is decision-making time. You may even have the luxury of considering more than one job offer at the same time. To help ensure that this is the right job for you at this stage of your career, compare the offer with the list of important job factors that you identified earlier in this chapter.

888 Whitegate Avenue
Los Angeles, CA 90820

February 10, 2014

Mr. E. B. Burns
Director of Nurses
St. Joseph's Hospital
P.O. Box 123
Los Angeles, CA 90880

Dear Mr. Burns:

Thank you for interviewing me yesterday afternoon. The position interests me very much, and I know that I will do a good job for you. I hope that you will give me an opportunity to work for the nursing department at St. Joseph's.

Sincerely,

Mark Adams, CNA

FIGURE 10.11
Sample thank you letter

How well does the job match what you're looking for? Confer with your parents, teacher, advisor, or role model to help you analyze the situation and make the right decision. If this is your first health care job, you might not get everything for which you are hoping. Identify your top priorities and consider making some compromises if the job might move you closer to what you're looking for in the future.

Math Link Comparing the Value of Job Offers

Math comes in handy when calculating the value of different job offers. You make the best job choice when you take all of the benefits of a job into consideration. Some jobs pay less, but have excellent benefits. Other jobs pay a high salary, but provide only minimum benefits.

Calculate the full value of three different job offers by determining the dollar value of the salary, health insurance, paid vacation time, stock or retirement benefits, and life insurance benefits. Compare your findings and evaluate which job is best for you. If you need some additional data, go online or use library resources to find the information you need.

Job #1 offers the following: Starting salary—$35,000, comprehensive health insurance plan valued at $750 per month, 2 weeks paid vacation, no retirement, no stock or life insurance.

Job #2 offers the following: Starting salary—$32,000, comprehensive health insurance plan valued at $200 per month, 3 weeks paid vacation, employer retirement plan valued at $150 per month.

Job #3 offers the following: Starting salary—$27,000, no health insurance, 2 weeks paid vacation, 20 shares of company stock valued at $500 each and vested (employee earns it) after 1 year on the job.

Which of these jobs provides the most value? Why? Show your work to prove your point.

Once you've accepted a job offer, the offer will likely be contingent based on passing a pre-employment physical exam and a drug screen. Employers can ill afford to hire people with substance abuse problems. This is one example where making a poor first impression usually won't result in a getting a second chance. Some employers now also screen for nicotine and refuse to hire people who smoke.

If you don't get selected for the job, at least you will know that you did your best, and you will have learned something of value in the process. If you believe you are well qualified, don't give up; employers value **perseverance**. Ask for feedback on how to enhance your qualifications, follow the advice, and then reapply. It's not unusual for applicants to be turned down the first time and then hired later on. If you reapply and are turned down a second time, work with an adviser or mentor to revisit your goals and identify ways to increase your qualifications.

perseverance (per-she-VIR-ence) To remain constant to a purpose

If you're seeking employment in a large or specialized facility or in a town where the competition for jobs is fierce, consider applying for a job in a smaller facility or in another town first and then making a move later on. Gaining work experience with a good reference someplace else may be the key to securing the job you really want. Graduating from school and landing your first job isn't the end of your journey, it's really just the beginning.

REALITY CHECK

When filling out job applications, developing a résumé, and participating in interviews it's absolutely essential to be honest with everything that you say and do. There are plenty of examples of people who lied about their identities, education, work experiences, credentials, or criminal histories and got caught. Some of these people got caught prior to receiving a job offer. Others were already on-the-job before the employer discovered their dishonesty. In some cases, it might take an employer several months to realize that an employee had falsified information on his or her job application.

If you lie about your identity or qualifications or fail to disclose personal information that would have disqualified you from employment, it really doesn't matter how long you're on the job before someone finds out. You can be fired at any time for fraud and dishonesty. In most health care organizations, once you've been fired under conditions such as these, you won't get a second chance. You'll never be eligible for rehire.

It's small world. More than likely, your supervisor networks with leaders from other organizations in your area. Once you've developed a reputation for dishonesty and fraud, word spreads. This is especially true in small towns and in geographic areas with a limited number of health care employers. All it takes is one dishonest act to make a negative, and sometimes permanent, impact on a person's future employment opportunities.

Key Points

- Identify your occupational preferences and labor trends where you want to work.
- Look for the best job opportunities that match your qualifications and interests.
- Include a cover letter with your résumé and job application.
- Make sure your résumé is accurate and conveys a professional image.

- Be honest and accurate in describing your qualifications.
- Disclose any misdemeanors or felonies on job applications.
- When applying online, allow time to learn how to navigate the computerized system.
- Expect a criminal history background check and drug screen as part of the employment process.
- Identify appropriate references and ask if they would be willing to serve.
- Expect employers to ask questions about your attendance record.
- Expect to take some pre-employment assessments as part of the job application process.
- Prepare for a job interview by having answers ready for the questions you expect to be asked.
- Present a professional image during your interview, including appearance and behavior.
- When considering job offers, you might have to make some compromises to eventually secure the job you want.
- Landing your first professional job is just the beginning of your journey.

Section Review Questions

Answer each of the following questions. Indicate which page in the textbook led you to your answer.

1. List three sources of information on job openings.
2. Describe four characteristics of a professional résumé.
3. What are five things that you should do when filling out a job application?
4. Why do employers use pre-employment assessments?
5. Describe five ways to present a professional image during a job interview.
6. Give two examples to illustrate the difference between *traditional* and *behavioral* interview questions.
7. What are three ways to convince interviewers that you are serious about wanting the job?

Learn By Doing

Complete Worksheets 1–5 in Section 10.1 of your *Student Activity Guide.*

Leadership Skills and Professional Development

SECTION 10.2

Background

Creating and maintaining an environment that fosters excellence is an important aspect of providing quality patient care. Every health care facility needs effective leaders who can inspire others to fulfill the mission, vision, and values of the organization.

Becoming a health care leader requires time, patience, and a commitment to learning new skills.

Health care professionals must be lifelong learners. A well thought-out career plan with realistic goals can help workers develop their **potential** and achieve success through professional development activities.

potential
(peh-TEN-shel) Existing as a possibility

Objectives

After completing this section, you will be able to:

1. Define the key terms.
2. Explain why effective leadership is crucial in health care.
3. Describe four characteristics of effective leaders.
4. Identify three ways to develop leadership skills.
5. List two benefits of participating in a health care professional association.
6. Describe the goals and role of HOSA.
7. Explain why health care workers must be lifelong learners.
8. Describe five resources for professional development.
9. Discuss the benefits of having a career plan.
10. Explain how succession planning creates opportunities for job advancement.

BECOMING A PROFESSIONAL LEADER

Once you've graduated from high school, completed your postsecondary health care education, and launched your health career, you'll need to start thinking about professional development and the importance of lifelong learning. It's never too early to plan ahead. Regardless of which profession you choose or where you decide to work, developing some leadership skills is a great way to start working towards career advancement.

Like most other kinds of businesses, health care organizations need people with effective leadership skills. Working in a leadership role can be stressful, but the rewards often outweigh the negatives. Successful leaders have the ability to articulate a vision, outline a plan of action, and direct individuals and groups toward achieving common goals. Effective leadership is crucial in health care where the pace of change is rapid, the challenges are difficult, and the stakes are high. Health care is a complex life and death business. Its leaders must be capable, strong, dedicated, compassionate, empathetic, and sensitive to the needs of others. Leadership is providing the guidance, encouragement, and support that people need to achieve success.

While the **perks** associated with leadership jobs might look attractive, there are good reasons why people in leadership positions often report stress and burnout. Effective leadership requires the following:

perks
(PERKS) Benefits that come with status

- Hard work and long hours to complete your own work while facilitating the work of other people; many leaders don't get paid overtime like hourly employees do.
- Maintaining your technical and patient care skills while developing your leadership skills.
- Communication skills to resolve conflicts among adults who really ought to behave better.

- Managing stress while meeting impossible deadlines and attempting to do more, with less, and get better outcomes.
- Being careful about everything you say and do.
- Mastering new software, tracking emerging trends, and keeping up with industry developments.

RECENT DEVELOPMENTS

The High Demand for Effective Health Care Leaders

As in other U.S. industries, people with effective leadership skills are in high demand in health care. Because of health care reform and the rapid pace of change, leaders are playing an increasingly important role in understanding and communicating the dynamics of change and determining how health care organizations must respond in order to remain viable. Today's leaders must be willing to take calculated risks and change the way they have conducted business in the past. Leaders must revisit their corporate missions and values and realign their goals and operations to meet current and emerging needs. They must increase productivity, patient satisfaction, patient safety, quality of care, and the volume of patients served while reducing costs and adjusting to new methods of delivering services and securing reimbursement. Leaders must educate their employees about the forces of change and engage all stakeholders in the transition. They must demonstrate effective operational and analytical skills to gain a higher market share among competitors and strengthen their organization's financial bottom line and their reputation for quality and service.

Unless you've been in a leadership position yourself, it's hard to imagine the stress involved in keeping so many different things in balance. It's easy to be critical of leaders who do things that you don't agree with or who don't respond as quickly as you would like. The next time you encounter leaders in your school or organization, think about what it must be like to walk in their shoes, and consider giving them a break. Leaders are just like the rest of us, human beings trying to do their very best each and every day. No one is perfect and sometimes our leaders fall short.

Aside from the drawbacks of leadership roles, leaders do enjoy lots of benefits, including:

- Receiving higher pay than employees who work at lower levels of the organization.
- Being exempt in many cases from **clocking in and out**, and having more flexibility in their work schedules.
- Receiving more paid time off and working fewer weekends and holidays.
- Having nice offices or cubicles, helpful assistants, and clerical support.
- Getting to attend workshops and going on employer-paid business trips.

clocking in and out (CLOK-ing in and AUT) Using a time clock or electronic system to record hours worked

But many of the people who experience high levels of job satisfaction in leadership roles will tell you it's not the pay or the benefits that make them look forward to coming to work each day. Leaders have the opportunity to:

- Articulate a vision, layout a plan, and stimulate a collaborative effort.
- Help the organization fulfill its mission and reach new heights.

FIGURE 10.12

Articulating a vision to stimulate collaborative effort

Source: Dmitriy Shironosov/ Shutterstock

- Encourage people to learn, grow, and achieve their goals.
- Make improvements to benefit employees, the organization, and the patients.

Employees who work in an environment geared for excellence are more likely to take pride in their work, perform at high levels, and continually seek ways to improve patient care and customer service. Leaders should do the following:

- Facilitate excellence among individuals and the group as a whole.
- Provide the resources and tools that employees need to do their work.
- Act as advocates for individuals and the group within the organization.
- Monitor the performance and outcomes of individuals and the group.
- Adapt their leadership styles to meet the needs of the group at any given time.

In addition, effective leaders should:

- Respect the rights, dignity, opinions, and abilities of others.
- Display self-confidence and a willingness to take a stand.
- Practice good listening skills and respect the opinions of people who disagree with them.
- Value diversity and emphasize the benefits of individual differences.
- Communicate effectively and state instructions and ideas clearly.
- Be willing to work as hard as everyone else works.
- Complete tasks on time and according to expectations.
- Display optimism and a can-do attitude.
- Remain open-minded and willing to change and compromise.
- Praise others and give credit where credit is due.

Effective leaders don't expect subordinates to do something they aren't willing to do themselves. They openly support the organization's mission, vision, and values and encourage other people to do the same. They discuss matters privately when they disagree with an employer's policy or action.

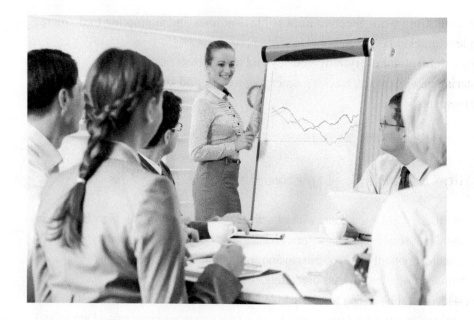

Consider This *Leadership Styles and Teamwork*

Three effective leaders might display three different leadership styles. Each leadership style has a different effect on teamwork.

A *democratic* leader will make the final decisions, but invite other members of the team to contribute to the decision-making process. This usually increases job satisfaction because members of the team feel appreciated and respected. In addition, this leadership style can help to develop skills of team members. A democratic style of leadership may lead to better outcomes because everyone's suggestions have been taken into consideration.

Conversely, an *autocratic* leader exercises absolute power over the team. Members have little opportunity to offer suggestions, and often resent being treated in this manner. Sometimes this style of leadership may be acceptable when supervising routine functions performed by lower-skilled employees. But most of the time, autocratic leadership results in low morale, high turnover, and absenteeism.

A leader might take a *laissez-faire* approach. This French phrase means *leave it be* and is used to describe a leader who leaves team members alone to do their work. This loose style of leadership works best with an experienced staff that routinely gets good results. Workers who need direct supervision and more support may feel abandoned by a *laissez-faire* leader. This can lead to a lack of respect for their leader and less than desirable outcomes.

When applying leadership skills, successful team leaders must:

- Organize and coordinate the team's activities.
- Encourage input and feedback from team members.
- Motivate all team members to work toward established goals.
- Assist in solving problems.
- Monitor the progress of the team.
- Provide reports and feedback to all team members on the effectiveness of the team.

morale
(meh-RAL) The mental or emotional spirit of a person or a group

Developing Leadership Skills

It's not unusual for a health care worker to get promoted into a leadership role before acquiring basic leadership skills. If this happens to you, you'll need to ramp up quickly. But if you have the luxury of time to prepare before moving into a leadership position, many options are available to gain some leadership skills. For example, you can:

- Sign up for leadership classes, read some books, and review online resources.
- Work alongside an experienced and skilled leader and observe his or her behavior.
- Function as part of a team, and observe other people's leadership skills as you develop your own.
- Volunteer to serve on committees at school, work, church, and so forth.
- Participate in athletics, school clubs, and community organizations.
- Help organize special events and projects with family and friends.

FIGURE 10.13

Participating in a community organization to gain leadership skills

Source: Pojoslaw/Shutterstock

All of these activities will provide valuable experience in working with other people and collaborating to achieve desired outcomes. However, don't overlook the importance of being an effective follower. When you collaborate with other people, you will fluctuate between leading and following based on the needs of the group at any particular time.

Becoming an experienced leader in your profession will take some time and patience. Here are a few places to start:

- Become well-skilled and experienced in your health care discipline.
- Develop your critical thinking skills and learn to make thoughtful decisions.
- Strengthen your verbal and written communication skills, and your negotiating and conflict resolution skills.
- Learn about other cultures and develop respect and appreciation for people who are different from you.

If you have the opportunity, job shadow a health care leader to see what a typical day involves. Ask what types of skills are important and how he or she learned them. If you're interested in pursuing a leadership role, take some assessments to identify your strengths and weaknesses, enroll in classes to overcome skill gaps, line up a mentor who can give you some advice, and become active in a professional association.

FIGURE 10.14

Taking classes to prepare for a leadership role

Source: wavebreakmedia/Shutterstock

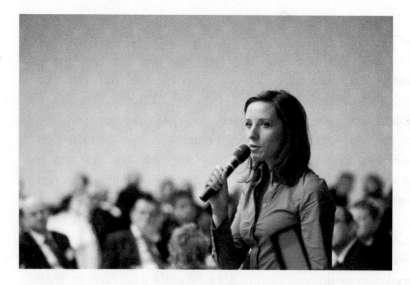

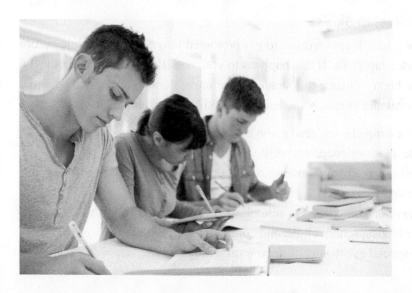

Community Service Leadership and Professional Development

Volunteer in a community service organization to help develop and practice your leadership skills. Once you have become active, offer to assist the organization in reviewing and updating its mission, vision, and values. What is the primary purpose of the organization? Who does it serve? Has its role in community changed in the recent past? If so, how and why has its role changed? Offer to help members develop short- and long-term SMART goals to fulfill their organization's mission and purpose. How can volunteering in community service organizations provide additional opportunities for professional development?

Participating in Professional Associations

Becoming active in a professional association, such as HOSA or SkillsUSA, is one of the best ways to develop and practice leadership skills. Membership in a student organization or a health care professional association provides the opportunity to gain knowledge and practical experience in working with a wide variety of people.

APPLY IT HEALTH CARE PROFESSIONAL AND TRADE ASSOCIATIONS

Identify a health care occupation of interest to you. Conduct some research to find out if there is a professional or trade association for workers in this discipline. If so, what is the purpose of the association? Who is eligible to join and what are the requirements for membership? Are members charged a fee to belong? What resources, activities, and benefits does the association provide for its members? Does the association offer, or require, continuing education for membership? If so, describe the educational offerings and/or requirements.

Health care has numerous professional associations to help workers remain current with emerging trends, new medical procedures, and advancements in technology. Most of these organizations are discipline-specific, such as nursing, radiography, or medical assisting, and have local, state, and national chapters working together on common goals. Belonging to a health care professional association provides:

- Opportunities to develop leadership skills through elected offices and committee work.
- Updates on new medical procedures and technological advances.
- Information on salary ranges, employment trends, and job postings.
- Updates on current **legislative issues**.
- Interaction with other health care professionals.
- Pooled funding to support improvements in the occupation or profession.
- Influence as a united group to encourage positive change.

legislative issues
(LEH-jes-lay-tiv IH-shews)
Topics involving local, state, and national law-making

You can find professional associations by checking Internet sites, reading professional journals, attending continuing education sessions, asking fellow colleagues, and reading reference materials about the profession. Consider participating in professional Internet organizations such as LinkedIn to connect with other people who share common interests and goals.

BUILD YOUR SKILLS *Becoming a Member of HOSA*

HOSA (formerly Health Occupations Students of America) is the student organization for health occupation students at the secondary, postsecondary, and college level. HOSA's primary goals are to:

- Promote career opportunities in the health care industry.
- Enhance and promote the delivery of quality health care to all people.
- Encourage all health occupations students and instructors to be actively involved in current health care issues.

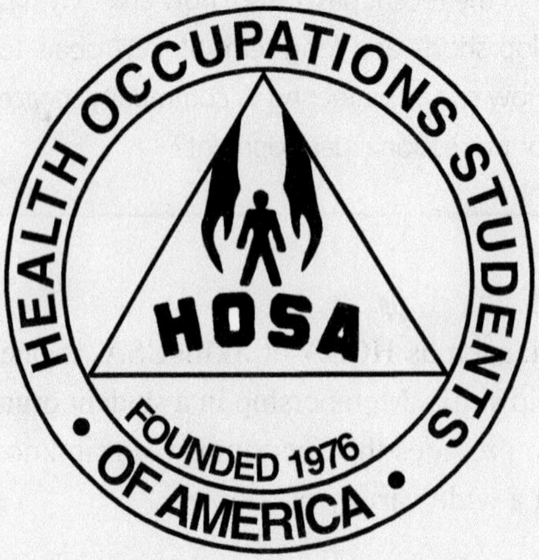

FIGURE 10.15
Emblem of HOSA, reprinted with permission of HOSA

HOSA provides many opportunities for students to learn and achieve. One such opportunity is the skills competitions. Competitions are at three levels—local, state, and national—with students advancing on to the next levels by winning the previous ones. HOSA offers more than forty-six different events divided into categories based on the curriculum. Competitive event categories include:

Category I. Health Science Events, such as:

- Dental spelling
- Dental terminology
- Medical spelling
- Medical terminology
- Medical math

Category II. Health Professions Events, such as:

- Administrative assistant
- Biotechnology
- Clinical nursing
- Nursing specialty
- Dental assisting
- Home health aid

Category III. Emergency Preparedness Events, such as:

- CPR/First Aid
- Emergency Medical Technician
- First aid/rescue breathing
- Community Emergency Response Team (CERT)

Category IV. Leadership Events, such as:

- Extemporaneous writing
- Medical photography

extemporaneous
(ek-stem-peh-RAY-nee-us)
Spoken without preparation or notes

- Extemporaneous health poster
- Extemporaneous writing
- Job seeking skills
- Prepared speaking
- Interviewing skills

Category V. Teamwork Events, such as:

- Community awareness
- Creative problem solving
- HOSA Bowl participation
- Forensic medicine
- Medical reading

Category VI. Recognition, such as:

- Outstanding HOSA chapter
- National recognition program

Competition requirements include the following:

- Student must be an active HOSA member.
- Student must be identified as either a secondary student (currently enrolled in a high school) or a postsecondary student (graduate from high school or over eighteen years of age).

Students attending HOSA functions follow a strict code of conduct and official HOSA uniform and competitive event dress codes. Experiencing the challenges, structure, and competition in HOSA teaches students how to reach for and achieve their highest potential. In addition, HOSA also offers many scholarship and leadership opportunities at the local, state, and national levels. (Health Occupations Students of America)

CAREER DEVELOPMENT

Lifelong learning is a critical component of professional growth and development because all health care professionals must continue to learn at every stage of their health career. Health care workers have many opportunities for **professional development** through involvement in professional associations, employer- and college-based educational programs and courses, and working with mentors and role models. Developing short- and long-term goals as part of a well-constructed career plan helps people identify next steps and stay on track. Health care professionals should always be on the lookout for new opportunities and anticipate revising their career plan periodically.

professional development (pre-FESH-nel di-VEH-lep-ment) Education for people who have begun their careers and need to continue growing

Reasons to Grow as a Professional

Why must health care professionals be lifelong learners?

- ***Ethical behavior demands it.*** If you expect to provide the best, most up-to-date service to your patients, you need to learn the latest developments in your field.

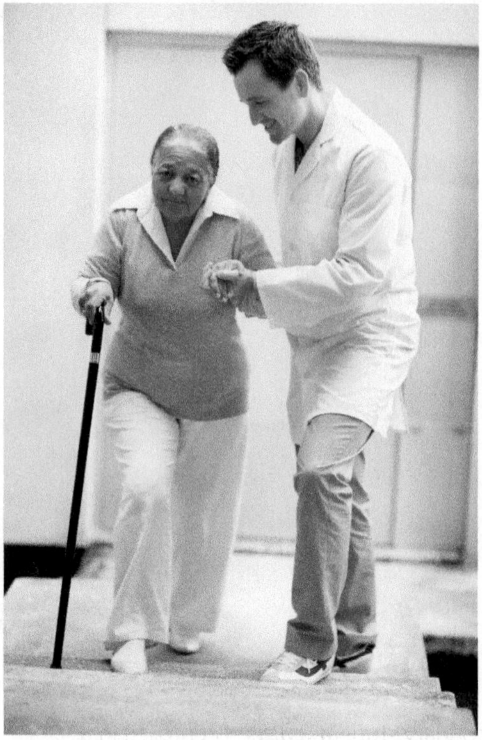

FIGURE 10.16
Caring for an elderly patient
Source: Yuri Arcurs/Shutterstock

Providing outdated, substandard care would be unethical and dangerous. In fact, many licensed professionals, such as doctors, nurses, and EMTs, must participate in a specific number of hours of continuing education each year to maintain their license.

- ***Technology changes.*** Medical technology changes rapidly. Diagnostic equipment that was unavailable a generation ago is part of routine medical care today. Computers and software programs are more important than ever before. Advancements in technology enable professionals to provide new services and better care to patients, but only when professionals learn to use the technology safely and effectively.
- ***Patient needs change.*** The population you serve as a health care professional is dynamic. As the elderly population increases, you'll need to learn more about geriatrics and the health care needs of seniors. If you work in direct patient care and a new disease or pathogen emerges, you'll need to learn as much as you can about this recent development and how to treat your patients while protecting yourself.
- ***Responsibilities increase.*** To advance in your career, you'll need more knowledge and skills to manage your new responsibilities. For example, you might need to learn how to read budget reports, interview job applicants, or increase productivity.
- ***Job descriptions change.*** Nothing is static when it comes to job duties in health care.

dynamic
(dy-NA-mik) In motion, energetic and vigorous

static
(STA-tik) Stationary and motionless

Language Arts Link — Continuing Education for Health Care Professionals

Identify a health care occupation of interest to you, and research the continuing education (CE) expectations for people working in that discipline. Who establishes CE expectations for this occupation? Is CE required, or recommended? If CE is required, how much CE must a worker obtain and over what period of time? (For example, the requirement might be 24 clock hours of CE over a two-year period.) What types of education are considered *continuing education*? Where can workers obtain CE? How are CE activities reported, and who keeps track of CE hours? What resources are available to support continuing education?

Create a poster to report your information. Make sure work is accurate and your grammar and spelling are correct. Exchange your poster with a classmate and ask for feedback on ways to make it more interesting and insightful. Revise your poster based on the feedback you receive, and share it with your classmates and teacher.

Why does this health care occupation require or recommend continuing education? What might happen if workers in this field fail to continue their education?

Employers constantly reorganize departments, redesign work, and reassign staff. As the organization changes, so do job titles, job descriptions, and job duties. When jobs become obsolete, they are replaced by new jobs. Two jobs might be merged into one, with employees becoming cross-trained to work in both areas. To maintain your current job and to prepare for advancement, expect to always be involved in professional development activities.

Resources for Professional Development

Where can you get professional development? Many resources are available for the professional development of people working in health care; these include:

- ***Associations.*** Many professional associations provide meetings, courses, workshops, journals, online modules, and other opportunities for professional development.
- ***Employer training courses.*** Many employers offer training courses to develop their employees. Employer programs include classes to improve customer service, communication skills, computer literacy, and competence in using new equipment and software. Employers may offer **tuition assistance** for employees who wish to return to school and work on advanced degrees and professional certifications. In some cases a **work commitment** may be required to repay the investment the organization has made in the employee's education.
- ***Colleges and universities.*** Many colleges and universities offer classes that can help you learn more about your profession. A variety of courses are now offered online for the convenience of working professionals.
- ***Journals.*** Professional journals help alert people to the latest developments in their fields. Journals also provide opportunities for health care professionals to write articles and become published authors.

tuition assistance
(too-WIH-shen eh-SIS-tens) Paying for a portion of college tuition fees

work commitment
(WERK keh-MIT-ment) A written agreement to work for an employer for a specified period of time

FIGURE 10.17

Classroom for employer-sponsored training

Source: CandyBox Images/Folotia LLC

APPLY IT PREPARING FOR HOSA COMPETITION

Ask your teacher for guidance and directions on how to prepare for the HOSA skills competition. Should you want to compete in the Nursing Assistant skills competition, for example, you will have to demonstrate skills such as handwashing, making an occupied/unoccupied bed, or transferring a patient. If you choose to compete in a teamwork event such as Parliamentary Procedure, you will have to demonstrate your leadership skills and your understanding of parliamentary procedure by conducting a simulated business meeting.

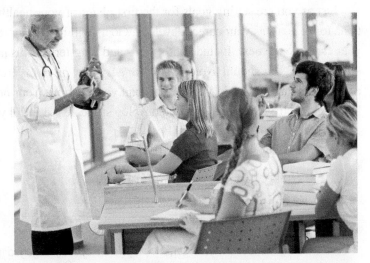

YOUR CAREER PLAN

A career plan is a strategy for your growth and development as a health care professional. Developing a plan requires forethought about the current status of your career, where you wish to be in a few years, what steps you need to take to achieve your goals, and how you will overcome any obstacles along the way.

Some health care organizations encourage or require their employees to have a career plan. The plan might be developed by the employee, with input from his or her supervisor to make sure the individual's goals align with the organization's business goals. The plan outlines the knowledge and skills the employee expects to acquire during the coming year with specific learning and performance goals identified. When it's time for the employee's annual performance evaluation, his or her performance will be rated at least in part by how well he or she achieved the goals that were set.

reactionary (re-AK-sheh-nair-ee) Responding to a stimulus or influence

It's still a good idea to have a career plan even if your employer doesn't require one. You need to have a pretty good idea about where you are headed and how you're going to get there. Otherwise you'll be in a **reactionary** mode instead of planning ahead. Many health occupations have career ladders for workers to climb, moving from entry-level jobs to higher skilled jobs and potentially into more specialized jobs requiring additional education and credentials. In some occupations you can also *move laterally* instead of *up the ladder,* broadening your knowledge and skills. Identify the career ladders available in your occupation and think about what direction you might like to head in the future. It's your career, so take charge of it.

Just as you are setting goals for the first phase of your health career, you should continue to set goals as your career develops. Goals will help you progress from one phase of your career to the next. Include both short- and long-term goals in your career plan. When setting goals, you should avoid *taking the easy way out.* You probably have the ability to accomplish much more in your career than you imagine. Your network of supporters can help you identify your strengths and develop strategies to fulfill your potential.

THE MORE YOU KNOW

Taking Advantage of Retirements

succession planning (sek-SHE-shen PLA-ning) A proactive approach to identifying and preparing employees to fill positions when other workers retire

An increasing number of health care employers are actively engaged in **succession planning**. Succession planning is a proactive approach to identifying and preparing employees to fill positions as other workers retire. As the health care workforce ages and more employees retire, employers will need a steady supply of well qualified people to step in and take their places. Retirements create opportunities for advancement. So it's important for you to plan ahead and be ready when these opportunities arise. Including your supervisor in career planning can help pave the way for your next career move.

Changing Careers

As time passes and you revisit your career plan, you might find that you are growing in a different direction than you expected. For example, you might discover that you really enjoy training people in a new skill and decide to make teaching the focus of your career. Or perhaps you like participating in a research project and decide to pursue research as a career track. Working in direct patient care for a prolonged period of time can be emotionally and physically exhausting for some people, so switching careers to focus on education or research might be the answer.

People change careers for lots of other reasons, too. Some people get tired and simply need a change. Jobs may become outdated and replaced with other kinds of duties. Switching careers might open new opportunities for advancement. Sometimes people discover health occupations they didn't know existed and decide to make a change. If you decide you would like to change careers, use the same process to investigate your new career that you used to find your first one.

Balancing Priorities and Career Advancement

As you set goals and proceed with your career plan, keep your priorities in mind and strike a good balance between your personal and professional lives. Take things one step at a time and try to avoid overloading yourself. Enjoy your life and spend quality time with family and friends.

It's not unusual for health care workers to wonder if the time they're spending at work and on career advancement activities is negatively affecting their families. They may be setting a good example for their children through hard work, self-discipline, sacrifice, and perseverance. However, balancing the goals of a dynamic career with the demands of a busy personal life is a challenge for many health care professionals.

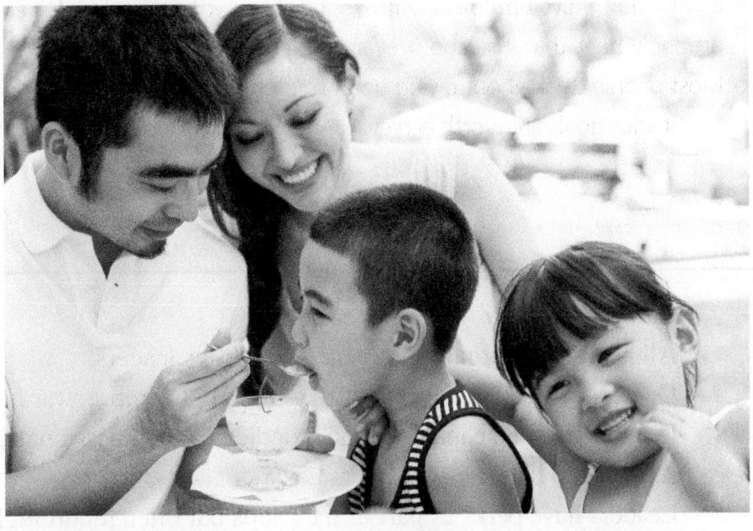

FIGURE 10.18

Setting aside time for family fun

Source: ZINQ Stock/Shutterstock

Achieving your goals and reaping the benefits of a successful health career may require some adjustments. Don't be surprised if your goals change over time and don't become discouraged if attaining a goal takes longer than you had anticipated. Adjustments and delays are part of the process as you learn more about yourself, what you want out of your career, and what's going to work best for you and your family. The important thing is to have a career plan with realistic goals and be headed down the road to where you eventually want to be.

Expecting the Unexpected

Even if you are well on your way to achieving your goals, keep your eyes open for new opportunities when you least expect them. If options arise to train in a different discipline, move from an inpatient to outpatient setting, transfer to a new clinic or hospital within the network, or advance into a leadership role, seize the opportunity and let it work to your advantage. Many of the skills you develop in one job can serve as transferable skills for another job. You never know what might be out there, just waiting for you around the next corner. It's all part of lifelong learning and the health career journey.

Expect to take some risks along the way. Risk taking *does not* mean being foolish or haphazard in making decisions. But it *does* mean taking some cautious steps that force you to stretch a little bit. If you don't try, you'll never know what you could have achieved.

REALITY CHECK

One way to think about career planning and professional development is to view yourself as the *Leader of Your Career*. As you now know, leaders articulate a vision, outline a plan of action, and direct individuals and groups toward achieving common goals. As the Leader of Your Career, you should envision your future, set realistic goals, and assemble a network of classmates, teachers, mentors, role models, family members, and friends to help provide encouragement and support on your way to success.

Don't expect things to work out exactly as planned. When the going gets rough (and it will), don't give up. Speak with your network of supporters for encouragement. You'll probably hear that just about everyone else has experienced set-backs in their careers. Most people think about giving up at one point or another in their professional lives.

If your goals are worth achieving, they're worth fighting for. So hang in there.

Key Points

- All health care organizations need effective leaders.
- Developing leadership skills is a good way to work towards career advancement.
- Leaders must be capable, strong, dedicated, compassionate, empathetic, and sensitive to the needs of others.
- Leaders have perks as part of their jobs but often report high stress and burnout.
- Leaders create an environment based on excellence, and they seek to fulfill the organization's mission, vision, and values.
- Many opportunities are available to develop your leadership skills and engage in professional development.
- Job shadowing a health care leader to see what a typical day involves can help you learn more about the roles and responsibilities of leaders.
- Lifelong learning and professional development are crucial for health care professionals.

- Health care workers can participate in professional development activities through professional associations, employer- and college-based educational programs and courses, and working with mentors and role models.
- Workers should develop a career plan with short- and long-term goals and expect their plans to change over time.
- Avoid taking *the easy way out;* focus on developing your full potential.
- Avoid overloading yourself and take time to enjoy family and friends.
- Watch for unexpected opportunities and take advantage of them.
- When the going gets rough, hang in there.

Section Review Questions

Answer each of the following questions. Indicate which page in the textbook led you to your answer.

1. Discuss four characteristics of effective leaders.
2. Identify three ways to develop leadership skills.
3. List two benefits of joining a health care professional association.
4. Describe five resources for professional development.
5. Discuss the goals and role of HOSA.
6. List the benefits of having a career plan.
7. Explain the role that *succession planning* plays in creating opportunities for job advancement.

Learn By Doing

Complete Worksheets 1–5 in Section 10.2 of your *Student Activity Guide*.

CHAPTER 10 Review

Chapter Review Questions

Answer each of the following questions. Indicate which page in the textbook led you to your answer.

1. Why should you take extra care in filling out a job application?
2. What might happen if you falsify information on a job application or résumé?
3. Why do interviewers ask behavioral interview questions?
4. What should you do if you don't get the job offer you want?
5. What role does compromise play in eventually getting the job you want?
6. Explain why health care workers must be lifelong learners.
7. List three reasons why health care workers must grow as professionals.
8. Why should health care workers take careful risks in career planning?

Chapter Review Activities

1. Locate newspaper ads and online listings of job openings in the area of the country where you want to work. How much information do these ads provide? Make a list of other resources you can use to find out more information about these job opportunities.
2. Identify two health care professions, one which is projected to grow in terms of the demand for workers and one that is projected to remain stagnant or decline in the demand for workers. List the factors involved in each of these trends. Describe how these factors and labor trends impact employment opportunities in the two professions.
3. Interview your mentor or role model. Ask if his or her career goals changed over time. If so, why did his or her career goals change? When and how did the goals change? What happened as a result? Does your mentor or role model wish he or she had done something differently with respect to career planning? If so, what and why?
4. Speak with your teacher or a supervisor or manager. In what types of professional development activities does this person participate? Is professional development required or just recommended and encouraged?

What If? Scenarios

What would you do in each of the following situations? Record your answer, explain it, and indicate which page in the textbook led you to your decision.

1. You have just graduated from school, moved to a new town, and need to find a good job. But you don't know anyone in town, and you aren't familiar with area health care employers.
2. Your career seems to be stagnant and going nowhere. You're beginning to wonder if it's time for a change.
3. You have a job interview at 8:00 a.m. Saturday morning. Your friends are having a party Friday night that starts at 9:00 p.m., and they want you to join them.
4. The job for which you would like to apply requires five years of previous work experience. You have three years of work experience in a large hospital that, to you, seems comparable to five years in a smaller hospital. A small change on your résumé would make you appear eligible for the job even though it wouldn't be totally accurate.
5. Last semester, your grades dropped because you had to spend a lot of time caring for an injured

family member. The educational program to which you have applied requires a high school transcript as part of the application process. You have a copy of your transcript, and it would be easy to scan the document, change your grades, and submit the revised version. After all, your grades would have been better if not for helping with a family emergency.

6. After deciding to apply for a clinic job, you find out that your mother knows the clinic's director. Just a few months ago, she helped the director refinance his home mortgage. Your mother has offered to speak with the clinic's director on your behalf.
7. You've applied for the same job twice and have yet to receive a job offer.
8. The organization where you work is opening a new hospital in a nearby town. Your manager is encouraging you to apply for one of the supervisor positions. The job opening sounds good, but you're afraid that you don't have the leadership skills needed to be successful.

Media Connection

Use the companion website for additional interactive learning activities.

Portfolio Connection

It's time to make sure that your career portfolio includes several important documents. Insert copies of your résumé, cover letters, thank you letters, and reference letters in your portfolio. Include detailed information about your references and how to contact them. Keep all of your correspondence with potential employers handy and well organized. Also insert copies of your career plan, including your short- and long-term SMART goals. Include any documents or details that relate to your career plan so you can find them later when you need them.

Hiring decisions can take several months, and you may be interacting with several employers at the same time. Keep an updated list of the job applications and cover letters that you submit, the interviews that you undergo, and the correspondence that you send and receive. If an employer who interviewed you six weeks ago contacts you for a second interview, you'll need to refresh your memory about your interactions with this organization before you return for another interview. Make sure you have the interviewer's name and job title in your records, plus details about the other people you met during your first interview. Review the notes you took during your first interview and spend more time preparing for your follow-up interview. This is where having a well-organized portfolio will be worth the time you've invested.

Make extra copies of portfolio materials that you might want to share with interviewers when you get the chance. These items could include grade transcripts, perfect attendance certificates, job performance reviews, special awards and recognitions, thank you letters from community service activities, and so forth. Always give interviewers *copies* of your documents, not the *originals*. Keep your originals in a secure place where you can easily access them when more copies are needed.

Your career portfolio is a *living* and *evolving* collection of documents and records. This means that your portfolio must be kept current and complete, especially as things change during your career. Add a copy of your evaluation after you undergo a job performance review. Insert letters you receive from patients, physicians, and coworkers. Keep copies of certificates of completion, continuing education records, and professional certifications, licenses, and college degrees that you earn. As your goals change, keep your career plan and your short- and long-term SMART goals up-to-date in your portfolio.

Maintaining your portfolio will help you develop effective organizational skills. You'll have quick and easy access to career-related documents as you need them. Years from now, your portfolio will reveal the history of your career—the courageous steps you took and the daunting challenges you overcame on your road to success. It all starts here, with a binder of documents and information about YOU.

Closing Thoughts

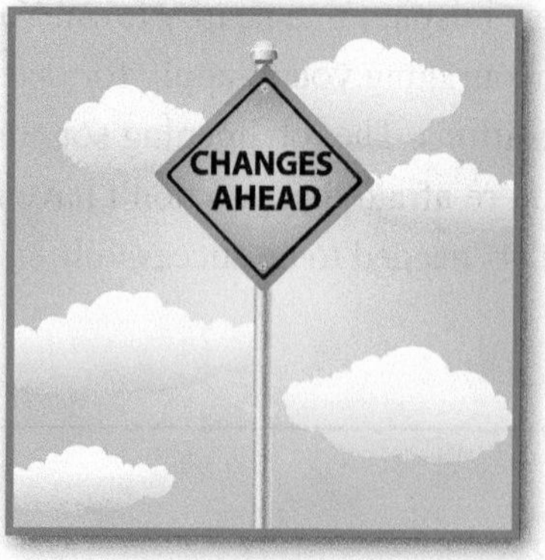

Source: mamanamsai/Shutterstock

There's time left for one last Reality Check and some closing thoughts.

You'll soon be joining an industry that's on the brink of change. As the demand for health care services grows, so will the expense and the difficulty of paying for it. Obesity will soon reach crisis level; caring for aging baby boomers will require even more resources; cancer and other life-threatening diseases will challenge researchers well into the future; and emerging medical technologies will raise additional moral, ethical, and legal issues. With so many demands on the U.S. health care system, it's clear that major change is on the horizon.

Speaking of major changes, your life is about to undergo change as well. You're thinking about your future and making some important decisions. You're taking on more responsibility, and soon you'll be *out on your own*. Before long, you'll be entering the job market as a health care professional.

Change can be a good thing, especially if you anticipate change and are well prepared for it. That's what this book is all about—your future and how to prepare for it.

The future can be exciting and scary at the same time. Remember this quote?

> *Life is unsafe at any speed, and therein lies much of its fascination.*
> (Journalist Edgar Ansel Mowrer, 1892–1977)

Let's take a quick look at some of the things you've learned, how they fit together, and where to go from here.

THINGS TO DO

1. Choose your occupation and your career carefully. Do lots of research; be aware of labor trends and projections; and consider your personal values, interests, motivations, personality traits, knowledge, skills, and abilities in finding the perfect career match for you.
2. Have a plan and expect it to change. Know where you're headed and how you're going to get there. Expect things to change, but stay on the right track and take advantage of unexpected opportunities when they arise. Keep your SMART goals up-to-date and share them with people who can help you succeed.

3. Set yourself up for success. Use good judgment and make thoughtful decisions. Build your resources and your network of supporters. When you need some help, don't hesitate to ask for it. Don't let other people discourage you or prevent you from reaching your goals. If your goals are worth achieving, they're worth fighting for, so hang in there. Keep an optimistic attitude and surround yourself with people who have a positive influence on your life.
4. Keep your priorities straight. Your job and your career should be high on your list, as well as your health and wellness and your commitment to spending quality time with family and friends. Reliability, dependability, accountability, and trustworthiness are the keys to earning self-respect and the respect of others.
5. Never stop learning. If you expect to excel in health care, you must always be a student. Continually sharpen your skills, maintain your competence, and participate in continuing education every chance that you get. Remember that knowledge is the key to just about everything.
6. Develop your leadership skills. No matter where life takes you, your ability to articulate a vision and make it a reality through collaboration with others will serve you well.

THINGS TO THINK ABOUT AND REMEMBER

1. Who you are as a person makes a difference. If you want to be seen by others as a professional, you must earn and maintain that honor every day that you come to work. Demonstrating a strong work ethic, meeting legal and ethical responsibilities, and displaying character traits that reflect compassion and respect for others are the keys to a professional reputation. Represent your employer with dignity, pride, and loyalty. Always *do the right thing* because *it's the right thing to do.*
2. It's all about the patient. When you work in health care, it's not about you or your job title or your schedule for the day. It's always about the patient. How your patients feel about their health care experiences can have a significant impact on the success of your organization. *High tech* drives advancement in health care and medicine, but it can never replace the importance of *high touch.*
3. Care about quality and safety. Health care is an extremely complex industry with life and death literally hanging in the balance. It's easy for things to *fall through the cracks* and cause problems. Pay attention to details and find ways to improve quality of care. Help create and maintain an environment where patients, coworkers, and others feel safe and *in good hands.*

Source: Nejron Photo/Shutterstock

4. Keep up with current events. This is your career, so be aware of what's going on in the health care industry, in your profession, and in your place of employment. Get involved and help shape the future.
5. Make positive ripples with everything you say and do. Stop and think before you act. Be present in the moment, and act with intention and self-awareness. Consider the impact that your attitude, appearance, and behavior have on other people. Respect other people's opinions and values, and do your best to improve the lives of those around you.

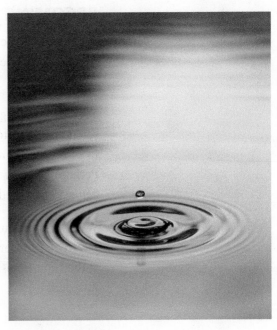

NEXT STEPS

1. Complete your education. If you decide to focus on just one goal right now, make it "to graduate." You'll need a strong academic foundation upon which to build your career and your future. It all starts with earning good grades and completing your education.
2. Develop your skills. Focus on your soft skills as well as your hard skills. Improve your ability to communicate, resolve conflict, and solve problems through critical thinking. Hone your computer skills and your ability to manage your time, personal finances, and stress. Learn to appreciate and accept people who are different from you. Embrace diversity and find ways to make it work for you and for the people around you.
3. Accept responsibility. Adopt the attitude, "the buck stops here." Make your own decisions with the support of your family and friends, and then accept the consequences. Admit when you've made a mistake and learn from it. This is your life, so seize control of it. Take some calculated risks to stretch a bit and develop your full potential. When the going gets rough, hang in there.

BECOMING THE CEO OF YOUR LIFE

Whether you decide to care for patients directly or serve in a support role behind-the-scenes, you'll be part of a nationwide workforce that strives to improve the lives of others.

Today's amazing health care system was built by those who came before you—the scientists, inventors, physicians, nurses, and others who devoted their work and their lives to improving medical science and the health and wellness of those they serve. Perhaps one day *you* will be among those who change the course of medicine for the better, recognized for your efforts in the history books of the future.

When you graduate from school, you'll become the *Chief Executive Officer of Your Life*. You can start preparing now by making the right decisions, for the right reasons, at the right times. The time you spend now planning for your future will be time well invested.

IT'S REALLY UP TO YOU

If you have researched health care occupations and are sure that a health career is a good match for you . . .

If you have given careful thought to your future and have the support of your family and other key people in your life . . .

If you have the courage and the motivation it takes to tackle and overcome tough challenges . . .

And if you're serious about serving the needs of others and making a difference in their lives as well as your own . . .

then go for it!

Become a health care professional and make a difference.

WHERE WILL YOU FIT IN?

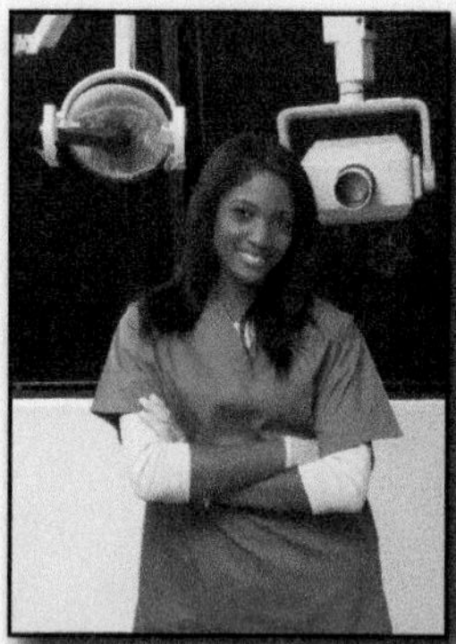

Source: OLJ Studio/Shutterstock

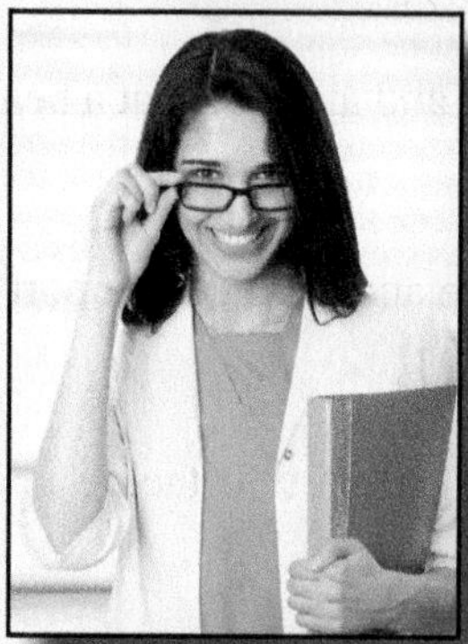

Source: Konstantin Chagin/Shutterstock

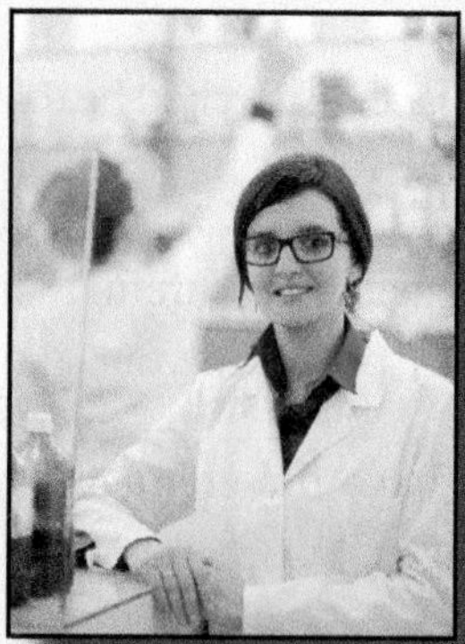

Source: shock/Shutterstock

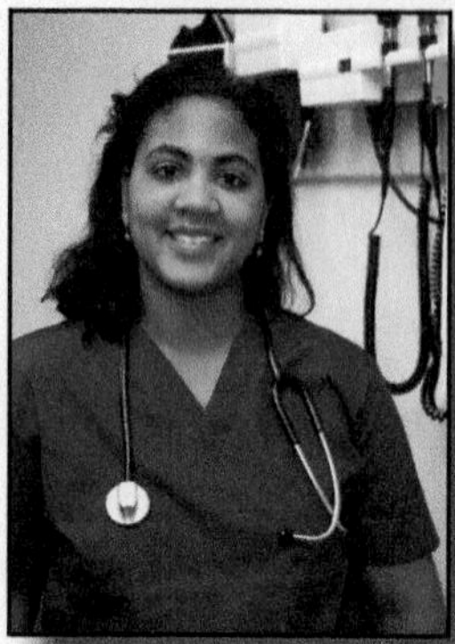

Source: Rob Marmion/Shutterstock

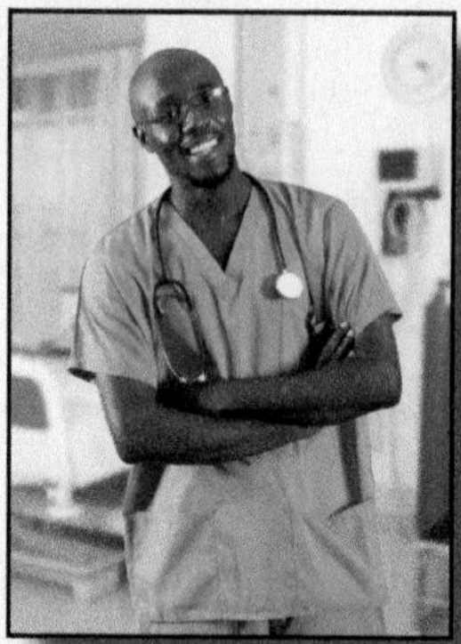

Source: michaeljung/Shutterstock

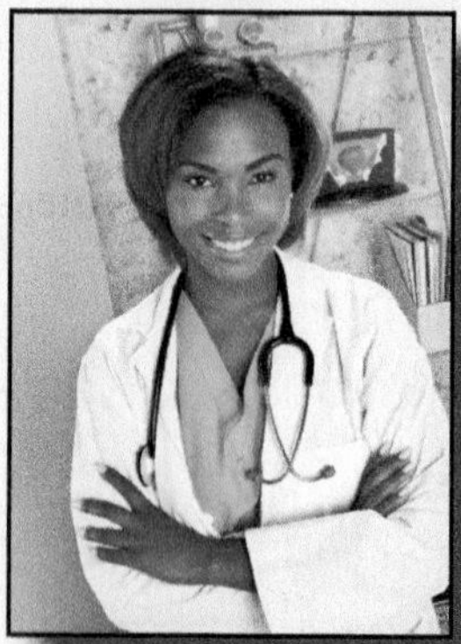

Source: REDAV/Shutterstock

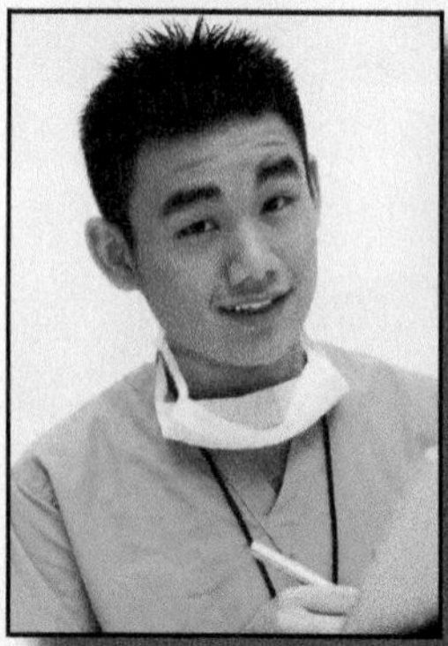

Source: Blend Images/Shutterstock

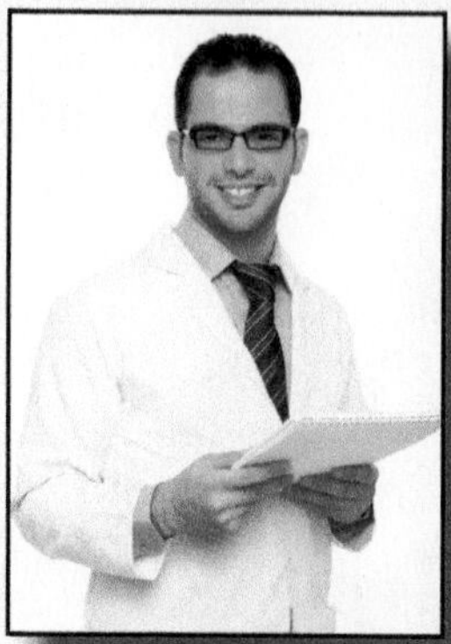

Source: Ebtikar/Shutterstock

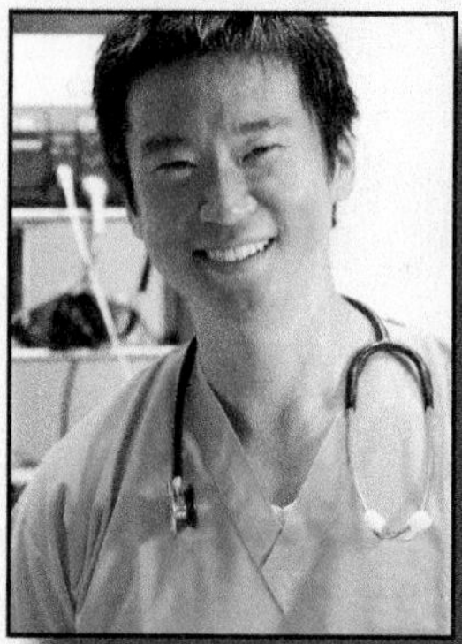

Source: James Peragine/Shutterstock

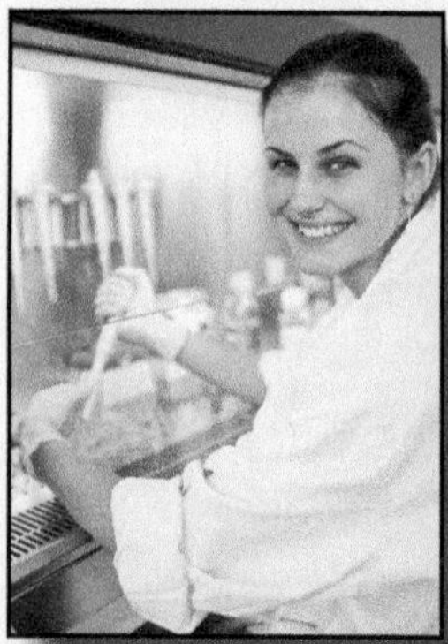

Source: lightpoet/Shutterstock

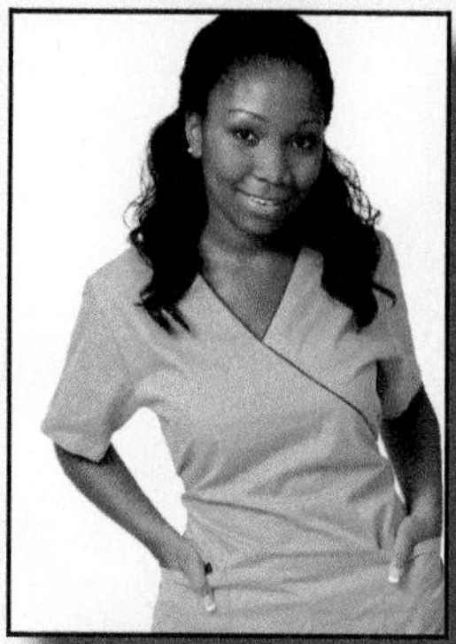

Source: Aspen Photo/Shutterstock

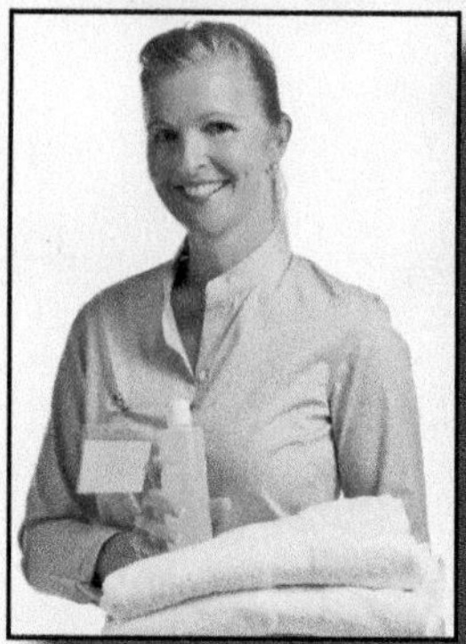

Source: AVAVA/Shutterstock

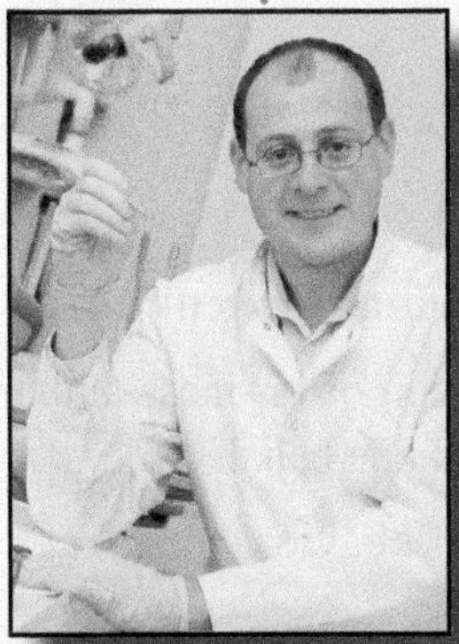

Source: Dmitry Kalinovsky/ Shutterstock

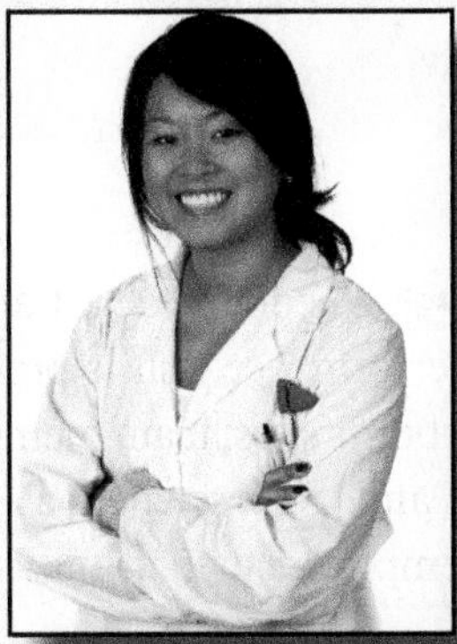

Source: aceshot1/Shutterstock

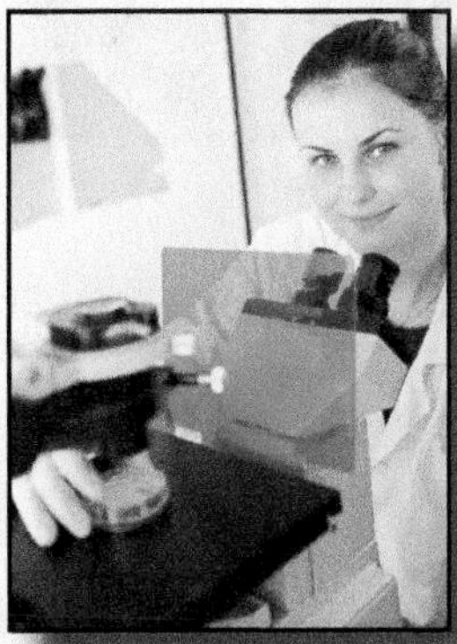

Source: lightpoet/Shutterstock

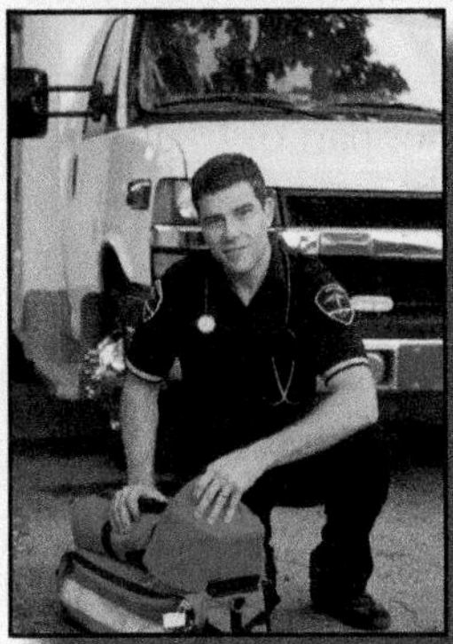

Source: Tyler Olson/Shutterstock

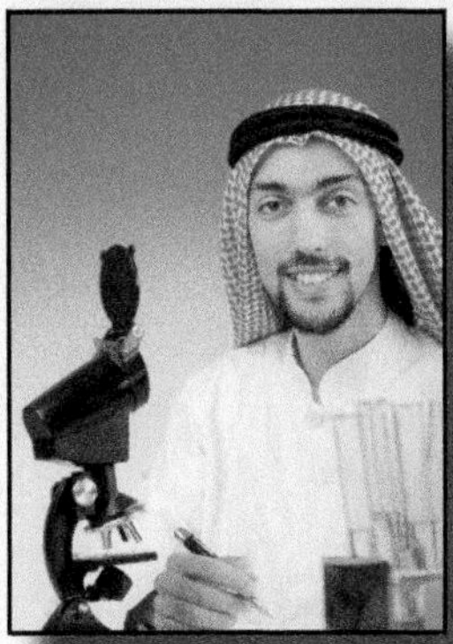

Source: Elnur/Shutterstock

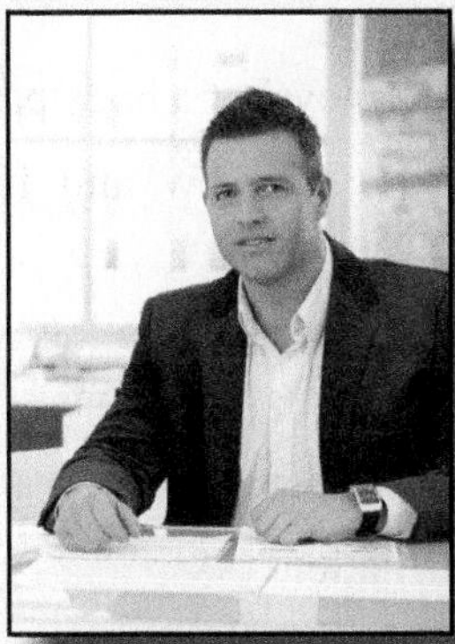

Source: StockLite/Shutterstock

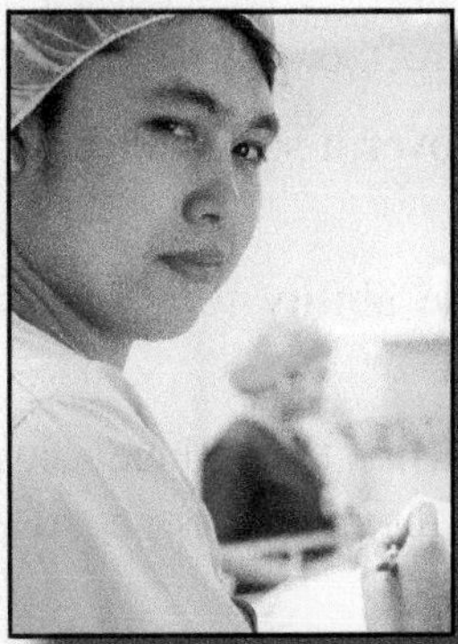

Source: pedalist/Shutterstock

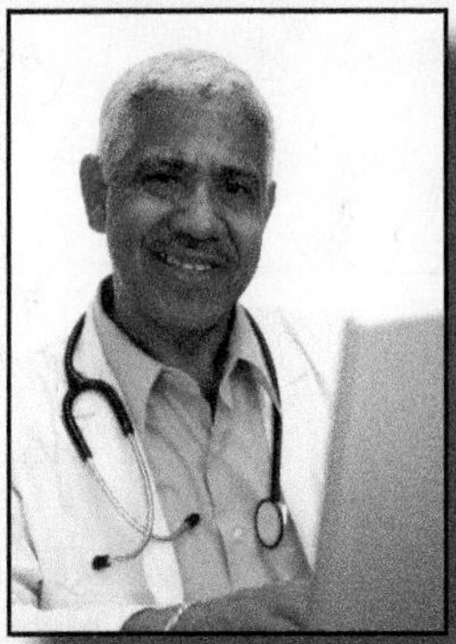

Source: Rob Marmion/ Shutterstock

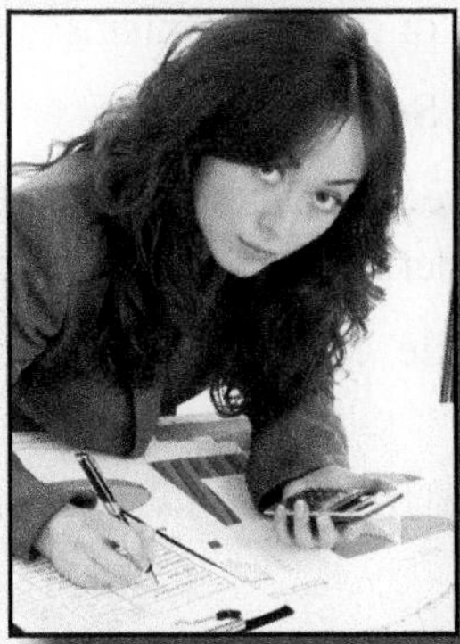

Source: Zadorozhnyi Viktor/ Shutterstock

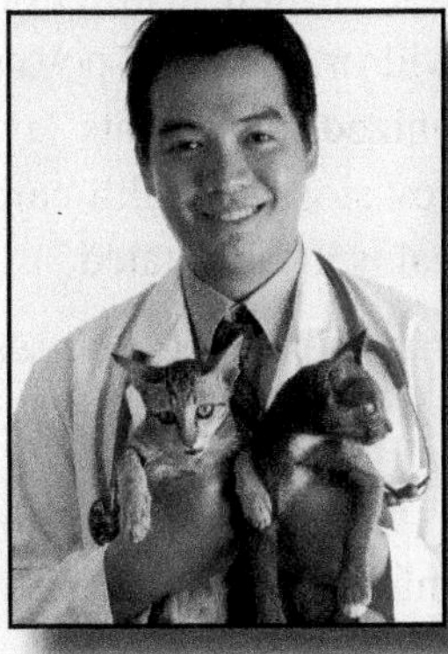

Source: william casey/ Shutterstock

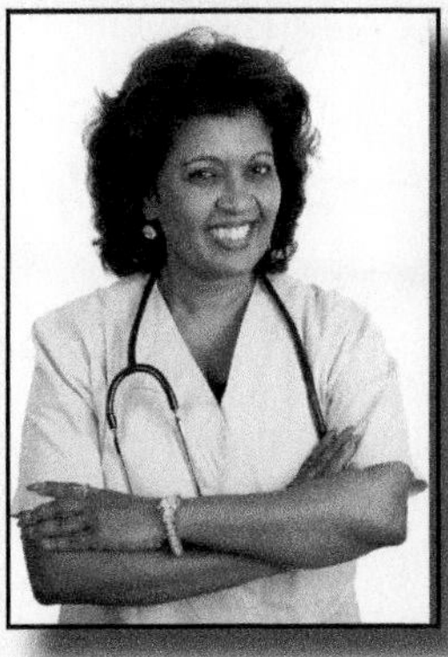

Source: Lisa F. Young/ Shutterstock

GLOSSARY

360-degree feedback Feedback about an employee's job performance that is provided by peers, subordinates, team members, customers, and others who have worked with the employee who is undergoing evaluation

abreast Side by side

absorption To take up liquid or other matter

accountability Willing to accept responsibility and the consequences of one's actions

accountable care organizations Networks where hospitals and doctors work together and share accountability to manage all of the health care needs of a large group of Medicare patients for an extended period of time

accreditation Certified as having met set standards

accurate Exact, correct, or precise

acute Severe, but over a short period of time

adaptive skills The ability to adjust to change

addiction A compulsion to continue using a substance even though it has negative consequences

ad hoc For a specific purpose

advance directive A written instruction such as a living will or a durable power of attorney recognized under state law relating to the provision of health care when the individual is incapacitated

advanced placement High school courses that qualify for college credit

adverse To oppose

adverse effects Unfavorable or harmful outcomes

advocates People or groups that speak or write in support of something or someone

aerobic Requiring oxygen

agent A person or business authorized to act on another's behalf

aggressive Behavior aimed at causing harm or pain

alignment Keeping the body in proper position—in a straight line without twisting

alternative medicine Using healing arts which are not part of traditional medical practice in the United States

ambulate Walk

ambulatory Able to walk

amenities Pleasant and attractive features or benefits

amino acids Compounds found in living cells that contain carbon, oxygen, hydrogen, and nitrogen and join together to form proteins

amputation Removal of a body part

anaerobic Able to grow and function without oxygen

anatomy The science of dealing with the structure of animals and plants

anesthesia Loss of feeling or sensation

annoyance Irritation

anonymous Not named or identified

antiseptic Substance that slows or stops the growth of microorganisms

appropriate Suitable, correct

apps Software applications for smartphones and computerized hand-held devices

asepsis Sterile condition, free from all germs

aseptic Free from the living germs of disease

aseptic technique Method used to make the environment, the worker, and the patient as germ-free as possible

assertive Bold, confident, self-assured

assessments Tools or processes to gather information

atrophy To shrink and become weak

attachment A file linked to an e-mail message

attitude A manner of acting, feeling, or thinking that shows one's disposition or opinion

audiology The study of hearing disorders

autoclaves Sterilizers that use steam under pressure to kill all forms of bacteria on objects that pathogens live on and can transfer infection

bacteria A disease-causing microorganism

bactericidal Kills bacteria

bacteriostatic Slows or stops the growth of bacteria

barriers Things that obstruct or impede

basic skills Fundamental aptitudes in reading, language, and math

baseline data Gathering information before a change begins to better understand the current situation

behavioral questions Ask how job applicants behaved in the past

benchmark A standard by which something can be measured or compared

benefits Payments and assistance based on an agreement

best practice A method or technique that has consistently shown superior results through research and experience as compared with other methods and techniques

bias Favoring one way over another, based in having had some experience

bingeing Eating or drinking excessively

bioethics Ethical decisions that are related to life issues

biohazard Biological materials or infectious agents that may cause harm to human, animal, or environmental health

blind carbon copy An e-mail feature that allows a person to send an e-mail to multiple people without them seeing the other receivers' e-mail addresses

blogs Similar to newspaper columns but published on the Internet instead of in print

bloodborne Carried in the blood

body The main part of a letter or other written document

body language Nonverbal messages communicated by posture, hand gestures, facial expressions, and so on.

body mass index (BMI) Measure of body fat based on height and weight for adult men and women

boilerplate language Standard language used repeatedly without change

bulk A greater amount

calorie Unit of measure of the fuel value of food

capabilities Potential abilities

carbohydrates Groups of organic compounds that include sugars, starches, celluloses, and gums that provide major sources of energy

carbon copy An e-mail feature that allows a person to send a copy of an e-mail to another person

career ladder A vertical sequence of job positions to move up in rank and pay

career lattice Related job positions offering both vertical and lateral movement

career plan Strategy for a person's professional growth and development

caregivers Health care workers who provide direct, hands-on patient care

cellulose The primary component of plant cell walls which provides the fiber and bulk necessary for optimal functioning of the digestive tract

central processing unit The part of a computer that interprets and carries out instructions; also known as the CPU

certifications Credentials from a state agency or a professional association awarding permission to use a special professional title; must meet pre-established competency standards

chain of infection A chain of events, all interconnected, is required for an infection to spread

character A person's moral behavior and qualities

chart To write observations or records of patient care

cheating Deceiving by trickery

chief complaint The primary reason why a patient seeks medical care

chiropractic The method of adjusting the segments of the spinal column

cholesterol A type of lipid or fat found in the body; produced by the liver or eaten in food

chronic Occurs frequently over a long period of time

citations Honorable mention for receiving an outcome or result

civility Politeness, consideration

civil law The body of law governing certain relationships between people, such as marriage, contracts, and torts

clergy People who perform religious functions

clerical Of or pertaining to keeping records, filing, typing, or other general office tasks

clinical internship A real-life learning experience obtained through working on-site in a health care facility or other setting while enrolled as a student

clinical trials Research to evaluate the effectiveness and safety of a medical procedure, device, or drug

cliques Small, exclusive circles of people

clocking in and out Using a time clock or electronic system to record hours worked

clone A group of cells that is genetically identical to the unit from which it was derived

closing The ending portion of letter

code of ethics Principles of conduct for decision making and behavior

cognitive Based on facts and logical conclusions

coherent Capable of understanding

cohesiveness State of being well integrated or unified

co-insurance A percentage the subscriber is required to pay of every medical bill

colleagues Fellow workers in the same profession

coma Deep sleep, unconscious state for a period of time

communicable Capable of being passed directly or indirectly from one person or thing to another

comparative data Information gathered from multiple sources that is analyzed to identify similarities and differences

compensation Payment

competence Possessing necessary knowledge and skills

complementary medicine Combining alternative medical approaches with traditional medical practices

compliance Acting in accordance with laws and with a company's rules, policies, and procedures

compromise A settlement of disagreement between parties by each party agreeing to give up something that it wants

concise Expressed in few words

conduct Standard of behavior

confidential Limited to persons authorized to use information or documents

confidentiality Maintaining the privacy of certain matters

conflict A contradiction, fight, or disagreement

conflict of interest An inappropriate relationship between personal interests and official responsibilities

conflict resolution Overcoming disagreements between two or more people

confrontation To face boldly, defiantly, or antagonistically

congenital Existing at, or before, birth

conscience Moral judgment that prohibits or opposes the violation of a previously recognized ethical principle

consensus Reaching a decision that all members agree to support

consent Approve, agree

constant Fixed, unchanging

constructive criticism Offering positive input on another person's weaknesses with the goal of their improvement

consumers People who purchase or use a product or service

contaminated Soiled, unclean, not suitable for use

contingency plans Backup plans in case the original plans don't work

continuing education Additional instruction for adults who have completed their formal education

continuity Continuous, connected and coordinated

continuous quality improvement (CQI) The regular use of methods and tools to identify, prevent, and reduce the impact of process failures

contract A legally binding exchange of promises or an agreement between parties that the law will enforce

convalescence The gradual recovery of health and strength after illness

convents Establishments of nuns

cooperation Acting or working together for a common purpose

co-payment A set amount the subscriber pays for each medical service

corporate mission Special duties, functions, or purposes of a company

corporate values Beliefs held in high esteem by a company

corrective action Steps taken to overcome a job performance problem

cosmetic Something done for the sake of appearance

courtesy Polite behavior, gestures, and remarks

cover page The first page of a fax or a written report

cover letter Letter introducing a job applicant to a potential employer

credentials Letters or certificates given to a person to show that he/she has the right to exercise a certain authority

credible Worthy of belief or trust

credit report A review of records to assess a person's financial status

criminal history background check A review of legal records to search for misdemeanors and felonies

criminal law The body of law that defines criminal offenses, deals with the apprehension, charging, and trial of suspected persons, and fixes penalties applicable to convicted offenders

critical thinking Using reasoning and evidence to make decisions about what to do or believe without being biased by emotions

crouch To stoop, using the large muscles of the legs to help maintain balance

cultural competence The ability to interact effectively with people from different cultures

cultures Groups of people who share the same values, norms, and behaviors

custodial Marked by watching and protecting rather than seeking to cure

data mining Sifting through large amounts of data to find significant information

debilitating Causing weakness or impairment

decompose To decay, to break down

deductible An amount the subscriber must pay before the insurance begins to pay

defamatory Statement that causes injury to another person's reputation

defense mechanisms Mental devices that help people cope with various situations

defensive medicine Medical practices aimed at avoiding lawsuits rather than benefitting the patient

deficiency A disease caused by lack of a nutrient

delegate To give another person responsibility for doing a specific task

deviation Departure from a standard or norm

diagnostic Deciding the nature of a disease or condition

dialect A variety of language that is distinct to a culture

dictate Record patient information for medical records

digestion The process of making food absorbable by dissolving it and breaking it down into simpler chemical compounds that occur in the living body chiefly through the action of enzymes secreted into the alimentary canal

dignity The degree of worth, merit, or honor

diligent Careful in one's work

dilemma A difficult situation or problem that requires making a choice

directive Something that serves to guide or impel towards an action or goal

disability Something a person is unable to do well due to a physical or mental impairment

discharging The act of releasing or allowing to leave

discipline A branch of knowledge or learning (nursing, medical assisting, surgical technology, and so on)

discretion Being careful about what one says and does

discriminate To treat a person or group unfairly on the basis of prejudice

disinfection Process of freeing from microorganisms by physical or chemical means

dismissal Involuntary termination from a job

disparities Lack of similarity or equality (health disparities: unfair and misdiagnosis and treatment)

dispense To distribute or pass out

dissection Act or process of dividing, taking apart

diversity Differences, dissimilarities, variations

divulge To make known

documentation A record of something

domain name The Internet address for a web page

dose The quantity of a medicine or a drug that is administered at one time

dress code Standards for attire and appearance

drug screen Lab test to detect illegal substances in a job applicant

durable power of attorney A type of advance medical directive in which legal documents provide the power of attorney, or the authorization to act on someone else's behalf in a legal or business matter, to another person in the case of an incapacitating medical condition

dynamic In motion, energetic and vigorous

education Acquiring knowledge and information

electronic health records Medical records kept via computer; also known as EHRs

eligibility The quality or state of being qualified

elimination Process of expelling or removing, especially waste products from the human body

emancipated Legally considered an adult

embryos Living human beings during the first eight weeks of development in the uterus

emoticons Use of punctuation marks and letters in an e-mail message to convey the sender's emotions

empathy Understanding and relating to another person's emotions or situation

employers of choice Companies where people like to work

employment agencies Companies that connect job applicants with employers

employment benefits Employer-paid insurance and retirement savings

employment status Hired to work full-time, part-time, or supplemental

empowered To give authority, to enable or permit

endowments Gifts of property or money given to a group or an organization

engaged Involved

engagement Securing the attention of a person

enterotoxin Poisonous substance that is produced in, or originates in, the contents of the intestine

entry-level A starting position for someone with little or no experience

environmental sanitation Methods used to keep the environment clean and to promote health

epidemics Diseases affecting many people at the same time

ergonomic An object or practice designed to reduce injury

error Something done incorrectly through ignorance or carelessness

essential Necessary

ethics A system of moral principles

etiquette Acceptable standards of behavior in a polite society

euthanize To painlessly end the life, or permit the death, of a hopelessly sick or injured animal or individual for reasons of mercy

excreted When waste matter is discharged from the blood, tissues, or organs

executive summary A brief overview listing the major points of a business document

exempt To be free or released from some liability or requirement to which others are subject

exorcise To force out evil spirits

expertise High degree of skill or knowledge

expressed consent Giving approval verbally or in writing

expressed contracts Contracts in which terms are written out in the document

extemporaneous Spoken without preparation or notes

extract Identify and take out or emphasize

extrinsic Motivated by external influences

extroverts People who focus on the outer world

facilitator A person responsible for leading or coordinating a group or discussion

facilities Places designed or built to serve a special function; such as a hospital, clinic, or doctor's office

facsimile or fax machine A device that sends and receives printed pages or images as electronic signals over telephone lines

false hope Looking forward to something that probably won't happen

fats Groups of organic compounds that, together with carbohydrates and proteins, constitute the primary structural material of living cells; also known as lipids

feces Solid waste that is evacuated from the body through the anus; also known as stools

felony A major offense with extensive jail time as a penalty

first responders The first people to appear and take action in emergency situations

flammable Catches fire easily or burns quickly

flash drive A small memory device used to store and transport files among computers; also known as a thumb drive or jump drive

font Style of type

formal Structured, in accordance with accepted forms and regulations

fraud Intentional deceit through false information or misrepresentation

frayed Worn or tattered; such as electrical cords may be worn, causing wires to be exposed

front-line workers Employees who have the most frequent contact with a company's customers

full-time Working approximately 40 hours per week

gait belt A safety device used to move a patient from one place to another; also used to help hold up a weak person while he or she walks

gatekeepers People who monitor the actions of other people and who control access to something

GED General Educational Development test; a high school equivalency credential

generalized Affecting all of the body

genes A portion of DNA that contains instructions for a trait

genetics Traits passed from parent to child through heredity

geriatric Specializing in health care for elderly patients

goals Aim, objects, or ends that one strives to attain

golden rule Treat other people the way you want to be treated

GPA Grade point average; a measure of a student's academic achievement in school

grammar System of word structures and arrangements

gravity Natural force or pull toward the earth; in the body, the center of gravity is usually the center of the body

groomed Clean and neat

gross domestic product (GDP) The total market value of all goods and services produced in one year

gross misconduct Unacceptable behavior of a serious nature, often leading to job dismissal

group norms Expectations or guidelines for group behavior

H-CAPS/HCAHPS Hospital Consumer Assessment of Healthcare Providers and Systems; survey to collect data about the patient's perception of his or her hospital experience

harass To behave in an offensively annoying or manipulative way

hard skills The ability to perform the technical, hands-on duties of a job

hazards Things that may cause harm to human, animal, or environmental health

healing environments Physical spaces designed to reduce stress, ensure safety, and uplift the spirits of patients, visitors, and staff

health care exchanges Open marketplaces where buyers and sellers of health insurance come together to help consumers compare and shop for coverage

health risk assessments Questionnaires that identify which health issues a person needs to focus on based on his or her medical history and lifestyle

HEDIS Health Plan Employer Data and Information System, an organization that provides quality care guidelines

hemoglobin Complex chemical in the blood; carries oxygen and carbon dioxide

heredity Passed from parent to child

hierarchy A group of people or units arranged by rank

HIPAA Health Insurance Portability and Accountability Act of 1996; national standards to protect the privacy of a patient's personal health information

hire-on bonus Extra compensation for accepting a job offer

HITECH Act Health Information Technology for Economic and Clinical Health Act of 2009; national standards to protect the confidentiality of electronically transmitted patient health information

holistic Pertaining to the whole; considering all factors

homeostasis Constant balance within the body; balance is maintained by the heartbeat, blood-making mechanisms, electrolytes, and hormone secretions

horseplay Rowdy and childish behavior; acting inappropriately in a work environment

HOSA The student organization for health occupation students at the secondary, postsecondary, adult, and college level

host The organism from which a microorganism takes nourishment; the microorganism gives nothing in return and causes disease or illness

hostile workplace An uncomfortable or unsafe work environment

hotline Direct and immediate telephone assistance

human resources department Current term for personnel department

hygiene Body cleanliness

hypertension Elevation of the blood pressure

hypothesis An explanation for an observation that is based on scientific research and can be tested

immunizations Substances given to make disease organisms harmless to the patient; may be given orally or by injection, such as for tetanus and polio

impaired A reduced ability to function properly

impartial Not favoring one side or opinion over another

impatience Restlessness

impending About to happen

implied consent Giving approval through an action

implied contracts Contracts in which some terms are not specifically stated, but are understood by the parties based on the nature of the transaction

incapacitated Permanently or temporarily impaired due to a mental and/or physical condition

inclusive A tendency to include everyone

inconsistent Not satisfied by the same set of values

indifferent Showing no interest or concern

infant mortality rate The number of infants that die during the first year of life

inferior Lower or less than

infirmity Unsound or unhealthy state of being

initiative Taking the first step or move

inoculation To introduce an antibody or antigen to prevent a disease

input To enter data into a computer for processing

institutional accreditation A quality assurance process to ensure that a school meets high quality standards

insubordination Refusal to complete an assigned task

integrity Of sound moral principle

intellectual stimulation Causing deep thought

intentional Something done on purpose

interdependence The need to rely on one another

interdisciplinary Involving two or more disciplines

interests Things that draw the attention of a person

Internet The worldwide computer network with information on many subjects

Internet search engines Programs that search documents for keywords and produce lists where the keywords were found

internship A real-life learning experience obtained by working on-site in a health care facility while enrolled as a student

interpersonal relationships Connections between or among people

interpersonal skills The ability to interact with other people

intervention The act of interfering to change an outcome

intranet A private computer network with limited access

intravenously Directly into a vein

intrinsic Motivated by internal influences

introverts People who focus on their inner world

intuitive Based on instinct and feeling

invasive Entering the body

invincible Incapable of being overcome

isolated Separated, lack of contact with others

job application An online or paper form used to apply for a job; also known as an employment application

job description A document that describes a worker's job duties

job outlook The demand of a career in a certain field

job shadowing Observing workers to see what their jobs are like

journal A written record of a person's thoughts and experiences

judgment Comparison of options to decide which is best

judgmental Having or expressing a critical point of view

justice Fairness; applying good rules equally to all people

labeling Describing a person with a word that limits them

labor projections Estimates of the number of positions needed in the future based on labor trends

labor trends Forces that impact employers, workers, and those seeking work

lactation The body's process of producing milk to feed newborn babies

law A rule of conduct or procedure recognized by a community as binding or enforceable by authority

learning style The method in which a student learns best

legal disability A person has a disability for legal purposes if he or she has a physical or mental impairment which has a substantial and long-term adverse effect on his or her ability to carry out normal day-to-day activities

legible Hand-writing that can be read and accurately interpreted by another person

legislation A law or body of laws

legislative issues Topics involving local, state, and national law-making

letterhead Professional stationery imprinted with business contact information

liable Legally responsible

licenses Credentials from a state agency awarding legal permission to practice; must meet pre-established qualifications

life expectancy The number of years of life remaining at any given age

living will A will in which the signer requests not to be kept alive by medical life-support systems in the event of a terminal illness

load Weight of an object or person that is to be moved

localized Affecting one area of the body

logo Graphic image that represents a company or organization

long-term goals Aims that will take a relatively long time to achieve

malnutrition Poor nutrition caused by an insufficient or poorly balanced diet or by a medical condition

malpractice Negligence, failure to meet the standard of care or conduct prescribed by a profession

managed care A health care system where primary care doctors act as gatekeepers to manage each patient's care in a cost-effective manner

mandates Orders or commands

manners Standards of behavior based on thoughtfulness and consideration of other people

maternal Relating to the mother or from the mother

mature Having reached adult development

Medicaid A government program that provides health care for low-income people and families and for people with certain disabilities

medical homes Organizations that deliver primary care through a comprehensive team approach that ensures quality outcomes

Medicare A government program that provides health care primarily for people 65 and older

memorandum A short note written to help a person remember something, or to remind a person to do something; also known as a memo

mental illness Health condition that changes a person's thoughts, emotions, and behavior and affects that person's ability to undertake daily functions

mentor A wise, loyal adviser

metabolism Collection of chemical reactions that takes place in the body's cells to convert the fuel in food into energy

metabolize To break down substances in cells to obtain energy

metrics A set of measurements that quantify results

microbiology The branch of biology dealing with the structure, function, uses, and modes of existence of microscopic organisms

microorganisms Organisms so small that they can only be seen through a microscope

midwives Non-physician women who deliver babies

minerals Inorganic elements that occur in nature; essential to every cell

minor Under the legal age of full responsibility

misdemeanor A minor offense with a fine and/or short jail sentence as a penalty

misrepresentations Untruths, lies

mission statement A summary describing aims, values, and an overall plan

mistake To understand, interpret, or estimate incorrectly

mobility The ability to move from place to place without restriction

monasteries Homes for men following religious standards

moral convictions Strong and absolute beliefs about what is right or wrong

morale The mental or emotional spirit of a person or a group

morals Capability of differentiating between right and wrong

mortality rate The ratio of deaths in an area to the population of that area, over a one-year period

motivations Forces that move you to set goals and achieve them

multiskilled Cross-trained to perform more than one function, often in more than one discipline

negligence Failure to perform in a reasonably prudent manner

networking Interacting with a variety of people in different settings

noninvasive Not involving penetration of the skin

nonpathogenic Not disease-causing

nosocomial infection An infection acquired while in a health care setting, such as a hospital

notarized Certified as to the validity of a signature

novice Someone new in a field or activity, a beginner

nutrients Chemical compounds found in food

obese Weighing more than 20% over a person's ideal weight

objective What is real or actual; not affected by feelings

obligation Moral responsibility

observant Quick to see and understand

observations Something that is noted

obstacles Things that stand in the way or oppose progress

obstetrics The branch of medical science concerned with childbirth

occupation A person's job to earn a living

occupational preferences The types of work and work settings that an individual prefers

occupational therapy Helps to give people skills for everyday activities in order to lead satisfying lives

office politics Clique-like relationships among groups of coworkers that involve scheming and plotting

official transcript Grade report that is printed, sealed, and mailed directly to the recipient to prevent tampering by the applicant

ombudsman A social worker, nurse, or trained volunteer who ensures that patients/residents are properly cared for and respected

optimists People who look on the bright side of things

organizational chart Illustration showing the components of a company and how they fit together

parasites Organisms obtaining nourishment from other organisms they are living in or on

pathogenic Disease-causing

perseverance To remain constant to a purpose

preferences Giving priority or advantage to some things over other things

prestigious Admired and respected, of high esteem

proactive Anticipating and acting in advance

project To show or reflect

proteins Complex compounds found in plant and animal tissue, essential for heat, energy, and growth

protist An organism belonging to the kingdom that includes protozoans, bacteria, and single-celled algae and fungi

purging Causing oneself to vomit

orthopedics The medical specialty concerned with correcting problems with the skeletal system

outcome data Information gathered after a change has occurred to examine the impact or results

outpatient A place to receive medical care without being admitted to a hospital; or a person who receives medical care someplace other than a hospital

output To produce information; turn out

over-the-counter drugs Medications and supplements that don't require a prescription

paralysis Loss of sensation and muscle function

part-time Working approximately 20 hours a week

passive Accepting or allowing an action without response

passive-aggressive Appearing passive, but aggressive in behavior

password A secret series of numbers and letters that identifies the person who should have access to a computer, file, or program

pasteurization To heat food for a period of time to destroy certain microorganisms

pathogens Microorganisms or viruses that can cause disease

payers Someone that covers the expense for goods received or services rendered

PDR *Physician's Desk Reference;* contains information on medical diseases, conditions, and drugs

peers People at the same rank

penmanship Handwriting

people skills Personality characteristics that enhance your ability to interact effectively with other people; also known as soft skills

performance evaluation Measurement of success in executing job duties

perioperative Three phases of surgery, from the time a decision is made to have surgery, through the operation itself, and until the patient has recovered

perks Benefits that come with status

perspective The manner in which a person views something

personal digital assistant A small, mobile, hand-held computerized device; also known as a PDA

personal financial management The ability to make sound decisions about personal finances

personal image The total impression created by a person

personal management skills The ability to manage time, finances, stress, and change

personal skills The ability to manage aspects of your life outside of work

personal values Things of great worth and importance

personality Distinctive individual qualities of a person, relating to patterns of behavior and attitudes

personnel department People within an organization who recruit, select, and employ job applicants

perspective The manner in which a person views something

pessimists People who look on the dark side of things

phlebotomy The practice of opening a vein by incision or puncture to remove blood

physiology The branch of biology dealing with the functions and activities of living organisms and their parts

podiatry The diagnosis and treatment of foot disorders

polite Courteous, having good manners

portfolio Collection of materials that demonstrate knowledge, skills, and abilities

postsecondary After high school

posture The position of the body or parts of the body

potential Existing as a possibility

predators Organisms or beings that destroy

pre-employment assessments Tests and other instruments used to measure knowledge, skills, and personality traits

prejudge To decide or make a decision before having the facts (prejudice)

premium The periodic payment to Medicare, an insurance company, or a health care plan for health care or prescription drug coverage

prenatal Occurring before birth

prerequisites Required or necessary as a prior condition

preventive Actions taken to avoid a medical condition

primary care Basic medical care that a patient receives upon first contact with the health care system, before being referred to specialists

primitive Ancient or prehistoric

principal First, or among the first, in importance or rank

priorities Having precedence in time, order, and importance

probationary period A testing or trial period to meet requirements

problem solving Using a systematic process to solve problems

process Set of actions or steps that must be accomplished correctly and in the proper order

procrastinate To postpone or delay taking action

productivity The power to reach goals and get results

profane Improper and contemptible

professional associations Organizations composed of people from the same occupation

professional development Education for people who have begun their careers and need to continue growing

professionals People with experience and skills who are engaged in a specific occupation for pay or as a means of livelihood (see Section 1.1 for the definition of "health care professionals" as presented in this text)

program A planned set of courses and activities to prepare students for a particular career

programmatic accreditation A quality assurance process to ensure that an educational program meets high quality standards

prohibit To not allow

projections Estimates of the number of positions needed in the future

proofread Reviewing a document for errors

prosthetics Artificial parts made for the body, such as teeth, feet, legs, arms, hands, eyes, or breasts

protocol Policies and procedures

providers Doctors, health care workers, and health care organizations that offer health care services

proxy decision maker The advocate for a patient who isn't competent to make decisions about his or her own medical care

prudent Careful or cautious

psychiatry The practice or science of diagnosing and treating mental disorders

psychology The science of the mind or mental states and processes

punctual Arriving on time

quackery The practice of pretending to cure disease

quarantine Isolating a person or animal to prevent the spread of disease

rational Based on reason, logical

rationed A fixed portion or amount

reactionary Responding to a stimulus or influence

reactive Responding to something that has happened

readmission A quick return to the hospital after discharge

reasoning Forming conclusions based on coherent and logical thinking

recipient A person or thing that receives

recognition Receiving credit for achievement

recreational therapy Uses play, recreation, and leisure activities to improve physical, cognitive, social, and emotional functioning; the primary goal is to develop lifetime leisure skills

refer To send to

reference A person who can provide information about a job applicant

registration A list of individuals on an official record who meet the qualifications for an occupation

regulate To control or adjust

rehabilitation Process that helps people who have been disabled by sickness or injury to recover as many of their original abilities for activities of daily living as possible

reimbursement To pay back or compensate for money spent

reliable Can be counted upon; trustworthy

remarkable Unusual, uncommon, and extraordinary

remedial Correcting a deficiency

replicate To reproduce or make an exact copy

reportable incident Any event that can have an adverse effect on the health, safety, or welfare of people in the facility

reputation A person's character, values, and behavior as viewed by others

resistance The ability of the body to protect itself from disease

respect Feeling or showing honor or esteem

respiration The inhaling and exhaling of air, or breathing

responsibility A sense of duty binding someone to a course of action

résumé Document summarizing job qualifications

retention The process of keeping

retirement benefits Employer-funded pension contributions

rickettsiae Parasitic microorganisms that live on another living organism and cause disease

rigors Things that are hard or severe

role A position, responsibility, or duty

role model A person whom someone aspires to be like

root cause The factor that, when fixed, will solve a problem and prevent it from happening again

rotation Movement from one place to another

salmonella A rod-shaped bacterium found in the intestine that can cause food poisoning, gastroenteritis, and typhoid fever

salutation Greeting

samples room A place where health care facilities keep samples of drugs and medical supplies

saprophytes Organisms that live on dead organic matter

scope of practice Boundaries that determine what a worker may and may not do as part of his or her job

screen To sift, filter, or separate

screenings Tests or examinations that are done to find a disease or condition before symptoms appear

secondary High school

selection process Steps to determine which applicants are chosen

self-awareness Understanding where you are, what you're doing, and why you're doing it

self-discovery The process of learning about one's self

self-esteem Belief in oneself, self-respect

self-image The mental picture that a person has of himself or herself

self-worth Importance and value in oneself

sentinel event An unexpected occurrence involving death or serious physical or psychological injury, or the risk thereof

sexual harassment Unwelcome, sexually-oriented advances or comments

shock Convulsion of muscles and extreme stimulation of nerves when an electric current passes through the body

short-term goals Aims that will take a relatively short time to achieve

Six Sigma A strategy that uses data and statistical analysis to measure and improve an organization's operational performance

skills Capabilities that can be acquired and developed through a learning, practice, and repetition

slang The informal language of a particular group

SMART goals Goals that are specific, measurable, attainable, relevant, and time bound

smartphones Mobile telephones that have advanced computing and connectivity features

social networking sites Internet places for people to publish and share personal information

social services Activities and resources to support well-being for individuals and families

socioeconomic status Social status in a community based on income, education, occupation, and so forth

soft skills Personality characteristics that enhance your ability to interact effectively with other people; also known as people skills

specialists People devoted to a particular occupation or branch of study

specialties Fields of study or professional work, such as pediatrics, orthopedics, obstetrics

spell check Software that verifies the correct spelling of words

spirochetes Slender, coil-shaped organisms

staffing level The number of people with certain qualifications who are assigned to work at a given time

stagnant Without motion; dull, sluggish

stakeholders People with a keen interest in a project or organization; may be end-users of a product or service

standard of care The type of care that would be reasonably expected under similar situations

Standard Precautions Guidelines designed to reduce the risk of transmission of microorganisms from recognized and unrecognized sources of infection in the hospital

standards Accepted basis of comparison in measuring quality or value

static Stationary and motionless

stereotypes Beliefs that are mainly false about a group of people

sterilized Made free from all living organisms

stethoscope An instrument used to hear sound in the body, such as heartbeat, lung sounds and bowel sounds

stimulate To cause an activity or heightened action

stress management The ability to deal with stress and overcome stressful situations

subjective Affected by a state of mind or feelings

subject line A statement describing the subject of a letter

subordinates People at a lower rank

succession planning A proactive approach to identifying and preparing employees to fill positions when other workers retire

superstitious Trusting in magic or chance

supplemental Flexible work schedule with no guaranteed hours or benefits

surgical Repairing or removing a body part by cutting

surrogate Substitute

susceptible Capable of being affected or infected; the body can be attacked by microorganisms and become ill

sympathy Feeling sorrow or pity for another person

symptoms A sign or indication of something

synergy People working together in a cooperative action

system A coordinated body of methods or plans of procedure

systematic A methodical procedure or plan

systems perspective Stepping back to view an entire process to see how each component connects with the others

taboos Banned from social custom

tasks Pieces of work, or functions to be performed, as part of a job

telemedicine The use of telecommunications technology to provide patient care in remote areas where patients and caregivers cannot meet in person

telerobotics Robots controlled from a distance using wireless connections; used in conducting remote surgery

texting Sending real-time, short text messages between cell phones or other handheld devices; also known as text messaging

therapeutic Treating or curing a disease or condition

thesaurus Reference source for locating alternate words with similar meanings

time management The ability to organize and allocate one's time to increase productivity

tomography Radiographic technique that produces a scan showing detailed cross-sections of tissue

torts Under civil law, wrongs committed by one person against another

toxicity A disease caused by too much of a nutrient

toxins Poisonous substances

traditional Customary beliefs passed from generation to generation

traditional questions Ask how job applicants would behave in the future

training Building skills

traits Characteristics or qualities related to one's personality

transferable skills Skills acquired in one job that are applicable in another job

transmitting Causing to go from one person to another person

transparency Open, clear, and capable of being seen

trends General direction or movement

trust To place confidence in the honesty, integrity, and reliability of another person

trustworthiness Ability to have confidence in the honesty, integrity, and reliability of another person

tuition assistance Paying for a portion of college tuition fees

tweets Text-based messages of up to 140 characters

unbiased Free from prejudice and favoritism

unethical A violation of standards of conduct and moral judgment

Universal Precautions A set of precautions that prevents the transmission of HIV, HBV, HCV, and other bloodborne pathogens when providing health care

up-code Modifying the classification of a procedure to increase financial reimbursement

urology The study of the urine and urinary organs in health and disease

username A unique identifier composed of letters and numbers used as a means of initial identification to gain access to a computer system or Internet service provider

vaccine A weakened bacteria or virus given to a person to build immunity against a disease

values Important elements in a person's life

vendors People who work for companies with which your company does business

vested Fully enrolled in, and eligible for, benefits

viruses Genetic material that is surrounded by a protective coat and that can only reproduce inside a host cell; can only be seen under a microscope

vision A mental image to imagine what the future could be

vision statement A vivid and idealized picture of the future

vitality The ability of an organism to go on living

vitamins Groups of substances necessary for normal functioning and maintenance of health

web browser A software application that allows users to locate and access Internet web pages

website A group of pages on the Internet developed by a person or organization about a topic

whistle blower A person who exposes the illegal or unethical practices of another person or of a company

work commitment A written agreement to work for an employer for a specified period of time

work ethic Attitudes and behaviors that support good work performance

workplace bullies Employees who intimidate and belittle their coworkers

work values Global aspects of work that are important to a person's satisfaction

INDEX

J